W9-CFA-350

OCULAR TUMORS IN ANIMALS AND HUMANS

OCULAR TUMORS IN ANIMALS AND HUMANS

Edited by

Robert L. Peiffer, Jr., and Kenneth B. Simons

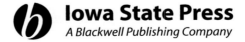
Iowa State Press
A Blackwell Publishing Company

About the Editors

Robert L. Peiffer, Jr., DVM, PhD, DAVCO is Professor of Comparative Ophthalmology in the Departments of Ophthalmology and Pathology, University of North Carolina, School of Medicine. He has won international awards for his ophthalmological research and holds memberships in the American Veterinary Medical Association, American Association of Ophthalmic Pathologists, and the International Society of Ophthalmic Pathology.

Kenneth B. Simons, MD, is Professor of Ophthalmology and Pathology, and Senior Associate Dean for Academic Affairs at the Medical College of Wisconsin. He received his BS degree from the University of Massachusetts and his MD degree from Boston University. He completed his ophthalmology residency training at the University of North Carolina and pursued additional fellowship training in ophthalmic pathology at the Jules Stein Eye Institute, University of California, Los Angeles.

Iowa State Press
2121 State Avenue, Ames, Iowa 50014

Orders: 1-800-862-6657
Office: 1-515-292-0140
Fax: 1-515-292-3348
Web site: www.iowastatepress.com

∞ Printed on acid-free paper in the United States of America

First edition, 2002

Library of Congress Cataloging-in-Publication Data

Ocular tumors in animals and humans / [edited by] Robert L. Peiffer, Jr., Kenneth B. Simons.—1st ed.
   p. ; cm.
Includes bibliographical references and index.
   ISBN 0-8138-2388-9 (alk. paper)
   1. Eye—Tumors—Pathophysiology. 2. Veterinary ophthalmology. 3. Tumors in animals.
   [DNLM: 1. Eye Neoplasms. 2. Eye Neoplasms—veterinary. WW 149 O214 2001]
   I. Peiffer, Jr., Robert L. II. Simons, Kenneth B.
RC280.E9 O29 2001
616.99′284—dc21   2001006198

The last digit is the print number: 9 8 7 6 5 4 3 2 1

DEDICATION

To Kathleen, to Wendy, to the children

CONTENTS

CONTRIBUTORS

CONTRIBUTORS: *ANIMAL*

Daniel M. Albert, MD, MS [*Chapter 10*]
Frederick A. Davis, Professor and Chair, and
    Lorenz E. Zimmerman, Professor
Department of Ophthalmology and Visual Sciences
University of Wisconsin Medical School
Madison, WI 53292

Nedim C. Buyukmihci, VMD, DACVO [*Chapter 9*]
Professor of Ophthalmology
Department of Surgical and Radiological
    Sciences
School of Veterinary Medicine
University of California
Davis, CA 95616

William C. Carlton, DVM, PhD, DSc (Hon)
    [*Chapters 5 and 12*]
Leslie Morton Hutchings Distinguished
    Professor Emeritus of Veterinary Pathology
Department of Veterinary Pathobiology
School of Veterinary Medicine
Purdue University
West Lafayette, IN 47907

Bernard Clerc, MD [*Chapter 6*]
Department of Ophthalmology
d'Alfort Veterinary School
94704 Maisons Alfort
France

Richard R. Dubielzig, DVM, DACVP
    [*Chapters 8 and 11*]
Professor of Pathology
School of Veterinary Medicine
University of Wisconsin
Madison, WI 53706

Jeffrey I. Everitt, DVM, DACVP, DACLAM
    [*Chapter 14*]
Senior Scientist
CIIT Centers for Health Research
Research Triangle Park, NC 27709-2137

Craig A. Fischer, DVM, DACVO [*Chapter 5*]
Animal Eye Clinics of Florida
Clearwater, FL 34622

Gia Klauss, DVM [*Chapter 10*]
School of Veterinary Medicine
University of Wisconsin
Madison, WI 53706

Denise M. Lindley, DVM, MS, DACVO
    [*Chapter 5*]
Animal Eye Consultants
Crestwood, IL 60445-1824

John R.B. Mould, BA, BVSc, DVOphthal,
    MRCVS [*Chapter 7*]
Lecturer in Veterinary Ophthalmology
Glasgow University Medical School
Glasgow G61 1QH, Scotland

Robert L. Peiffer, Jr., DVM, PhD, DACVO
    [*Chapters 1 and 6*]
Professor of Ophthalmology and Pathology
School of Medicine
University of North Carolina
Chapel Hill, NC 27599

Claudio Peruccio, DECVO [*Chapter 7*]
Department of Animal Pathology
Faculty of Veterinary Medicine
University of Turin
1005 Grugliasco, Italy

Simon M. Petersen-Jones, DVetMed, PhD, DVOphthal, DECVO, MRCVS [*Chapter 7*]
Assistant Professor, Comparative Ophthalmology
Department of Small Animal Clinical Sciences
Michigan State University
D-20-8 Veterinary Medical Center
East Lansing, MI 48824-1314

Alessandra Ratto, DVM [*Chapter 7*]
Laboratory of Comparative Oncology
National Institute for Cancer Research
16132 Genoa, Italy

Ron C. Riis, DVM, DACVO [*Chapters 2 and 6*]
New York State College of Veterinary Medicine
Cornell University
Ithaca, NY 14853

John A. Shadduck, DVM, PhD [*Chapter 14*]
President, Shadduck Consulting LLC
2916 Shore Road
Fort Collins, CO 80524

Herbert E. Whiteley, DVM, PhD [*Chapter 14*]
Office of the Dean
College of Veterinary Medicine
University of Illinois
Urbana, IL 61801

Brian P. Wilcock, DVM, PhD [*Chapter 3*]
Professor of Pathology
Ontario Veterinary College
University of Guelph
Guelph, Ontario N1G 2W1, Canada

CONTRIBUTORS: *HUMAN*

Daniel M. Albert, MD, MS [*Chapter 10*]
Frederick A. Davis, Professor and Chair, and Lorenz E. Zimmerman, Professor
Department of Ophthalmology and Visual Sciences
University of Wisconsin Medical School
Madison, WI 53292

Jonathan D. Boniuk, MD [*Chapter 3*]
Riverdale, NY 10413

Thomas W. Bouldin, MD [*Chapter 9*]
Professor of Pathology and Laboratory Medicine
Department of Pathology and Ophthalmology
School of Medicine
University of North Carolina
Chapel Hill, NC 27514

Harry Brown, OD, MD [*Chapter 4*]
Professor of Pathology and Ophthalmology
Harry and Bernice Jones Eye Institute
University of Arkansas for Medical Sciences
Little Rock, AR 72205

Karen E. Chancellor, MD [*Chapter 9*]
Associate Chief Medical Examiner
North Carolina Office of the Chief Medical Examiner
and
Clinical Assistant Professor
Department of Pathology
School of Medicine
University of North Carolina
Chapel Hill, NC 27614

Robin L. Grendahl, MD [*Chapter 11*]
Anchorage, AK 99508

Hans E. Grossniklaus, MD [*Chapter 12*]
Professor of Ophthalmology and Pathology
Emory University School of Medicine
Emory Eye Center BT 428
Atlanta, GA 30322

J. William Harbour, MD [*Chapter 7*]
Assistant Professor of Ophthalmology, Molecular Oncology, and Cell Biology
Washington University School of Medicine
St. Louis, MO 63110

Amy K. Hutchinson, MD [*Chapter 12*]
Assistant Professor of Ophthalmology
Medical University of South Carolina
Charleston, SC 29425

Marilyn C. Kincaid, BA, MD [*Chapter 13*]
Clinical Professor of Ophthalmology and Pathology
Departments of Ophthalmology and Pathology
St. Louis University School of Medicine
St. Louis, MO 63013

Jacques Lasudry, MD [*Chapter 10*]
1200 Brussels, Belgium

Guy G. Massry, MD [*Chapter 13*]
Sinskey Eye Institute
Santa Monica, CA 90404

James C. Orcutt, MD, PhD [*Chapter 11*]
Professor of Ophthalmology
Department of Ophthalmology
University of Washington
VA Medical Center
Seattle, WA 98108

Robert L. Peiffer, Jr., DVM, PhD, DACVO
    [*Chapter 6*]
Professor of Ophthalmology and Pathology
School of Medicine
University of North Carolina
Chapel Hill, NC 27599

Pearl S. Rosenbaum, MD [*Chapter 3*]
Department of Ophthalmology and Pathology
Montefiore Medical Center
University Hospital of Albert Einstein College
    of Medicine
Bronx, NY 10467

Joseph W. Sassani, MD [*Chapter 7*]
Professor of Ophthalmology and Pathology
Milton S. Hershey Medical Center
Penn State University
Hershey, PA 17033

Kenneth B. Simons, MD [*Chapters 1, 2, and 11*]
Professor of Ophthalmology and Pathology
Senior Associate Dean for Academic Affairs
Medical College of Wisconsin
Milwaukee, WI 53226

Nasreen A. Syed, MD [*Chapter 11*]
Director of Ophthalmic Pathology
Scheie Eye Institute
and
Assistant Professor of Ophthalmology
Departments of Ophthalmology and Pathology
University of Pennsylvania
Philadelphia, PA 19104

Holly Van Hecke, BM, MM, MD [*Chapter 5*]
Eye Physicians of Watertown
Watertown, WI 53098

Connie M. Vitali, MD [*Chapter 2*]
Clinical Assistant Professor of Pathology
University of Illinois
College of Medicine
Rockford, IL 61103

FOREWORD

The subspecialty of ocular oncology has attracted the interest of a number of specialists in ophthalmology and veterinary medicine in recent years. A few ophthalmology departments have individuals who specialize almost exclusively in ophthalmic oncology. This centralization of a unique subspecialty has greatly improved methods of diagnosis and management of patients with tumors of the eyelids, conjunctiva, intraocular structures, and orbit.

There are several recent textbooks that cover well the subject of ocular tumors in humans. Bob Peiffer and Ken Simons, who have extensive experience in the pathology of tumors in all species, have conceptualized and completed an authoritative textbook on the unusual and fascinating subject of tumors in animals as well as humans. The concept of combining animal and human ocular oncology into one text represents an unusual approach. In addition to their own exhaustive contributions to this magnificent treatise, Bob Peiffer and Ken Simons have solicited the contributions of a number of other well-known experts in veterinary medicine, clinical ophthalmology, and ophthalmic pathology.

The result is *Ocular Tumors in Animals and Humans*, a comprehensive work that includes clinical and histopathologic characteristics of virtually all important ophthalmic tumors and pseudotumors in a wide variety of species. The book is well organized, being divided into anatomic sites in the ocular region, which are further divided into lesions that arise from specific ocular and adnexal tissues. The clinical illustrations and photomicrographs are bountiful and excellent. Each chapter has a thorough bibliography that includes almost all pertinent references.

All ophthalmologists and veterinary medicine specialists who have an interest in tumors in and around the eye will find it a useful source of reference and fascinating reading. *Ocular Tumors in Animals and Humans* is a highly informative book that will be a standard reference source for many years.

Jerry A. Shields, MD
Director, Ocular Oncology Service
Wills Eye Hospital
and Professor of Ophthalmology
Thomas Jefferson University
Philadelphia, PA, USA

PREFACE

As I struggled to create an introduction that would provide the reader with insight into the purpose and scope of this text, as well as to justify its creation, it occurred to me that perhaps the most meaningful background that I could provide would be to relate this text to the events of my career and my evolution as a comparative ophthalmic pathologist.

I was attracted to ophthalmology as a specialty for four reasons. First, it encompassed both medical and surgical aspects of disease management. Second, there was an alluring mystique surrounding the specialty associated with the uniqueness and sensitivity of the eye as well as the sophistication of the instrumentation that ophthalmologists utilized. Thirdly, seeds of interest had been planted and nurtured by Dr. Don Carter at Iowa State University, where I interned, and Drs. Andy Lavignette and Bill Carlton at Purdue University, during the first year of a surgical residency. Dr. Carlton provided me with my introduction to ophthalmic pathology when he allowed me to attend the course that he offered to his graduate students. Lastly, I was fortunate to be awarded an NIH postdoctoral fellowship in comparative ophthalmology at the University of Minnesota, my alma mater. These events unraveled by happenstance and circumstance as much as decision making on my part.

As there was no structured program in place to train a veterinary ophthalmologist, I was compelled to design my own and was fortunate enough to come into contact with Dr. John Harris, Chairman of the Department of Ophthalmology in the School of Medicine at the University of Minnesota. He was broad-minded enough to offer all of the resources that were available through his nationally recognized department to his own residents to this young veterinarian. I suspect that his motivations were based on a combination of generosity of spirit as well as curiosity.

These were busy times as I recollect trying to acquire the skills necessary to be a competent clinical veterinary ophthalmologist and do justice to my thesis research, which involved inherited glaucoma in beagles (no doubt the passage of time has somewhat romanticized these early years). These events were superimposed, of course, on the social and political context of the seventies, and I suspect that I am not alone in my generation in looking upon the somewhat Bohemian experiences as a graduate student as perhaps the most interesting years of my life.

The story of this book really begins as I began to prepare and organize material from my clinical cases to submit to the American College of Veterinary Ophthalmologists, a requisite to achieve the highly esteemed membership in this organization. Although the pathology department in the College of Veterinary Medicine was nationally recognized for its excellence, there was no individual who had developed an interest in ophthalmic pathology and no technicians who were experienced in the preparation of ophthalmic tissues. Slides that came back from enucleated globes portrayed the organ in every possible geometric configuration but spherical, and tissue relationships (indeed, if some tissues could be identified at all) were significantly distorted. Because of the prominent pigmentation found in the canine uvea, "melanoma" was a frequent diagnosis, even though clinical observations supported alternative diagnoses. I had just begun to participate in the weekly pathology rounds at the medical school, where Drs. Charlotte Hill and Hugh Monahan had developed an outstanding program for both service and resident education. I asked Charlotte if she would be kind enough to allow me to process my animal globes through her laboratory, and her agreement to do so was a key event in the evolution of this text.

Virginia Havener was the ophthalmic histotechnologist in Charlotte's lab, and Virginia took me under her wing to teach me both the basics and subtleties of how one gets from a tissue in a bottle to a diagnosis that will contribute to optimal patient management. My experiences led to an increasing fascination, even infatuation, for ophthalmic pathology and I suspect that I spent more time in the ocular pathology laboratory, located in the bowels of the hospital at the University of Minnesota at that time, than anywhere else during my postdoctoral period.

Charlotte was kind enough to invite me to attend and present a case report at the Georgiana Dvork Theobold Midwestern Society of Ophthalmic Pathology, and I remember the trek across the plains to attend my first meeting in Omaha, hosted by Drs. Jerry Christiansen and Harold Gifford. My associations with the ocular pathologists that I have come into contact with through this organization over the years have served as a stimulus for personal growth; Dr. Harry Brown is one of these individuals who has contributed to this text. Dr. Jerry Shields, who has been a pioneer of human ophthalmic oncology, provided both inspiration and insight during these periodic contacts. Space does not allow acknowledgment of all of the valued colleagues that the Theobald and later the Hogan Societies introduced me to.

As my experience with tissues from my patients, as well as with the human tissues that came through the laboratory at the University of Minnesota, grew, I was struck by both similarities and differences in the way that the eye responded to disease when one began to cross species lines. I was particularly interested in the comparative aspects of ocular neoplasia, and frustrated by the lack of information regarding ocular tumors in animals. Our knowledge at that time consisted predominantly of case reports and small series; there was a tendency for investigators to assume that animal ocular tumors were inherently identical to human tumors, both in terms of morphology and biologic behavior. This early work by such individuals as Leon Saunders and Charles

Barron was the foundation of our current understanding. Closer scrutiny revealed interesting similarities but striking differences.

In 1978, Dr. David Eifrig, who I had met and interacted with as a post doc while he was on the faculty as a retinologist at the University of Minnesota, invited me to Chapel Hill to oversee the ocular pathology laboratories and the resident ophthalmic pathology training in his fledgling department at the University of North Carolina (UNC). I had recently accepted my first academic position in the College of Veterinary Medicine at the University of Florida in Gainesville, but the challenge and opportunity of this offer made the decision to move not extremely difficult. David packed me off for a summer at the Armed Forces Institute of Pathology, where my exposure to their materials, other young ocular pathologists in training, and the teaching of Drs. Zimmerman, McLean, and Hidayat provided me with both additional substance and the courage to beat the path I had chosen. Dr. Marilyn Kincaid was one of the young pathologists with whom I crossed paths just north of Washington.

At UNC, I was fortunate to inherit Mrs. Doris Brown, a wonderful and delightful lady as well as an ocular histotechnologist *par excellence* whose role in the development of the program was invaluable. In addition to providing diagnostic services and training the residents, we developed a comparative ophthalmic pathology laboratory and, bolstered by the support of submissions of practicing veterinary ophthalmologists throughout the country and indeed the world, were able to develop an archive of animal ocular tissues that has been utilized to train young veterinary ocular pathologists and ophthalmologists as well as for retrospective research that hopefully has strengthened the foundations of our understanding of animal ocular oncology. I have been privileged along the way to work with valued human pathologist colleagues, initially Dr. Stanley Lipper and currently Dr. Tom Bouldin.

In this light, I would be sorely remiss not to mention my veterinary pathologist friend and colleague, Dr. Brian Wilcock. While at the University of Guelph, Brian's interest in ocular pathology paralleled my own, and our collaborations have enhanced the numbers and validity of our observations.

Ophthalmic pathology has changed over my years of involvement; what was once a department-supported ophthalmic pathology laboratory has, because of fiscal realities, become incorporated into the Department of Pathology. In the early years, there were few pathologists with inclinations toward the eye, and ocular pathology was largely within the realm of clinical ophthalmologists who had received additional training in ocular pathology; now pathologists are claiming this turf, and the trends are to train individuals who are formally exposed to both pathology and ophthalmology. However, the importance of providing students, be they in veterinary or human medicine, or pre- or postdoctoral degree programs, with training in the pathology of the eye has remained constant and will, I hope, continue to be so. I do not try to train my students to become ophthalmic pathologists; rather, I try to provide them with an appreciation of disease at a cellular and subcellular level. Occasionally, you will come across a student who heeds the siren's song: Dr. Ken Simons is such an individual. We were scheduled to have brunch with Ken, a resident in our program, on a lovely summer Sunday morning in 1982, but we had to cancel abruptly because of the birth of our first child. Ken went on to do an ocular pathology fellowship under Dr. Bob Foos at UCLA and then to the Medical College of Wisconsin, where I suspect unfortunately his duties as an administrator limit the time that he spends at his microscope. Ken is responsible not only for parts of the text that he himself has written but for organizing and overseeing the contributions of the human sections of this text.

This then is an encapsulated sequence of the events and cast of characters that have led to this book. As our knowledge of ocular tumors and animals has expanded (although still lacking), the similarities and differences become evermore compelling. There are obvious advantages of enhanced understanding of ocular tumors in terms of patient management for both M.D. ophthalmologists and veterinary ophthalmologists; the need for this understanding increases as our clinical diagnostics and treatment modalities become increasingly sophisticated and technology evolves. Similarities and differences across species lines are not only intellectually fascinating but practical in the sense of model systems and investigations into the validity of interspecies applications. My personal experiences have shown to me the excitement that can be generated and the progress that can be made when you bring together individuals and ideas from seemingly diverse arenas of the biologic sciences. From this perspective, we hope that this text will be of value to all those with an interest in ocular tumors.

Robert L. Peiffer, Jr.
Chapel Hill, NC
May 2001

ACKNOWLEDGMENTS

The editors would like to acknowledge all those whose endeavors have made this text possible. To our contributing authors—we are indebted for the quality of their work and their patience over several years of preparation. To our colleagues—we recognize that without the submission of tissues the pathologist is lost indeed. For our families who have shown tolerance as we try to achieve balance between our personal and professional lives—we are blessed.

The vision of Iowa State University Press in undertaking the production of the first truly comparative ophthalmology text has been inspirational and the competency and professionalism of their staff has made the effort enjoyable.

OCULAR TUMORS IN ANIMALS AND HUMANS

ORBITAL TUMORS

Robert L. Peiffer, Jr., and Kenneth B. Simons

ANIMALS

Historical Perspectives. Definitive knowledge of orbital tumors in animals is somewhat limited for a variety of reasons related to low incidence and the limitations of clinical diagnosis and management. Refinement and application of contemporary diagnostic techniques—notably ultrasound and imaging by computer-assisted tomography and magnetic resonance imaging, as well as enhanced practitioner awareness—have recently contributed to early diagnosis and more effective management.

Terminology. In general, although the anatomy of the bony orbital rim and walls will vary among species, orbital anatomy and contents are quite consistent, the notable exception being the harderian gland found in lagomorphs and rodents. Proliferative diseases may arise from the bony walls; the connective tissue that lines the orbit, muscles, globe, and other structures; the orbital fat; the extraocular muscles; the vessels and nerves that course through this space; the lacrimal gland; the gland of the third eyelid; or the zygomatic salivary gland. Tumors of the optic nerve and secondary orbital tumors are discussed in separate chapters.

Noninfectious inflammatory disease is uncommon in animals as compared with humans; dysthyroid ophthalmopathy has been described in a monkey as an isolated example.[1] Young dogs—notably golden retrievers—are subject to an immune-mediated extraocular myositis. Craniomandibular osteopathy and eosinophilic myositis can indirectly involve the orbit.[2,3] Immune-mediated posterior scleritis may mimic orbital proliferative processes. Otherwise, such conditions as orbital pseudotumor and the granulomatous proliferative diseases encountered in humans have not been well documented in animals; case reports of a pseudotumor in a bush baby (a prosimian),[4] eosinophilic orbital cellulitis in a cat,[5] and bilateral fibrosing pseudotumor in a cat[6] are found in the literature. Infectious inflammatory disease[7–11]—orbital cellulitis or abscessation—may occur as an extension of processes involving the molars, the adjacent sinuses, or the periorbital glands, and foreign bodies may occasionally be encountered. Clinical and histopathologic distinction from neoplasms is usually not difficult.

Cystic orbital disease is infrequent and most frequently includes zygomatic salivary gland mucoceles or lacrimal cysts.[12,13] A case of hydrops, apparently from lacrimal and/or conjunctival secretions, following alleged enucleation has been described,[14] and air can gain access to the orbit either from the adjacent sinuses[15] or via the nasolacrimal system after enucleation.[16] Vascular malformations can result in a pulsating exophthalmos.[17,18]

Incidence and Epidemiology. Orbital tumors are in general uncommon; in a study of cats from Auburn University, of 16,655 admitted over a 16-year period, 530 (3.1%) had a diagnosis of neoplasia; of these, 21 involved the orbit and only 3 of these were primary.[19]

Although statistical data are limited, incidence in dogs is likely somewhat higher. From 1968 to 1979 at the University of Pennsylvania, 25 cases of canine orbital tumors were diagnosed; one was an inflammatory pseudotumor and the remainder were neoplastic processes, of which 3 were benign and 21 malignant. Of the malignant neoplasms, 56% were primary and, of the secondary tumors, the most commonly encountered was four cases of nasal carcinomas with extension to the orbit. There was no breed or sex predisposition; ages ranged from 1.5 to 15 years, with a mean of 8.5 years.[20]

Twenty-three cases were retrieved from the 1975–89 files at Cornell, ranging from 2 to 14 years, with a mean of 8 years. No breed or laterality predisposition was noted, with 15 females represented. Seventeen tumors were classified as primary, and 21 of the 23 were malignancies.[21] Diversity characterizes the nature of these orbital tumors. In the Pennsylvania series, mesenchymal tumors were slightly more commonly encountered than epithelial tumors; extension of nasal or sinus carcinomas was most commonly encountered, with three multilobular osteochondromas and two each of fibrosarcomas and anaplastic sarcomas, with all other diagnoses represented solitarily. The Cornell series included six osteosarcomas, four mast cell sarcomas, four reticulum cell sarcomas, and two fibrosarcomas. Lymphosarcoma is a relatively common secondary orbital neoplasm, involving three of the 21 cases in the aforementioned feline series; in cats, extension of oral, nasal, and adnexal squamous carcinoma is likewise encountered.[22]

Clinical Signs. Usually, space-occupying orbital lesions are present as exophthalmos with resistance to retropulsion; rarely, sclerosing neoplasms and inflammatory processes can result in enophthalmos.[23] Depending on location and extent, the globe may be deviated, the third eyelid protruded, ocular motility impaired, and, if the optic nerve is compressed or stretched, an afferent pupillary defect and/or visual impairment may be present with or without optic disc changes upon ophthalmoscopy. Anterior extension may be present as orbital rim or subconjunctival masses.

Tumors in the posterior orbit are likely to result in exophthalmos without deviation; tumors elsewhere result in deviation away from the mass. As might be expected, benign tumors are slow growing; malignant tumors may grow quite rapidly, can be associated with signs related to involvement of the adjacent sinuses, and may be visible extending into the oral cavity just posterior to the last upper molar. In contrast to inflammatory disease, orbital neoplasms are generally painless.

Diagnostic workup should include skull radiographs, ultrasound, and computer-assisted tomography or magnetic resonance imaging to define location and extent of involvement.[24–37] Biopsy is generally required to establish definitive diagnosis and may take the form of tissue sampling of oral or anterior orbital and subconjunctival masses; fine-needle aspiration biopsy of deeper orbital tumors; or exploratory orbitotomy.

Gross Light-Microscopic and Histochemical Features. Described primary orbital neoplasms and their histologic features are described in Table 1.1; the multitude of primary and secondary neoplasms that might be encountered makes inclusive discussion impossible, and readers are directed to more general references in this regard.

Immunohistochemistry and Ultrastructure. Because of the diversity of types of orbital neoplasms, a comprehensive discussion of this topic would involve a lengthy discussion of immunohistochemistry and ultrastructural morphology of both solid and lymphoid tumors, topics elegantly presented by others to whom readers are referred,[38,39] and only essential general principles that are discussed below.

This is not at all to distract from the usefulness of these techniques to a pathologist's quest of a definitive diagnosis of an orbital tumor. Not uncommonly, the neoplasms will have few distinguishing light-microscopic characteristics and are thus labeled *undifferentiated*. Determining cell of origin, whether a primary or metastatic lesion, and probable site of origin of a metastatic lesion are important factors in management and can be enhanced by these ancillary techniques.

Immunohistochemistry can be performed on formalin-fixed paraffin-embedded tissues; fresh (less than 2 weeks) 10% formaldehyde will ensure optimal reactivity. Immunohistochemical detection of the presence or absence of intermediate filaments (cytokeratin, actin, vimentin, desmin, and glial fibrillary acidic protein, hematopoietic markers, S-100 protein, and HMB-45, among others) can be useful in clarifying diagnostic confusion that may accompany small round cell neoplasms; spindle cell carcinomas, melanomas, and sarcomas; epithelial neoplasms; and pleomorphic neoplasms. Histiocytic tumors

Table 1.1—Reported orbital tumors in animals

Neoplasm	Species	Gross	Histologic Features	Immunohistochemical Features
Osteoma	Dog/cat[31]	Firm, white	Bone production (Fig 1.1, a-e)	
Osteosarcoma	Dog/cat	Firm, white	Spindles or trabeculae of osteoid bone and cartilage; fibular stroma; pleomorphic spindle mesenchymal cells (Fig. 1.2)	
Parosteal osteoma/ Osteosarcoma	Dog/cat[32,33]	Granular, friable, gritty	Island and cords of chonroid tissues with calcified ossified centers surrounded by a zone of plump spindle cells (Fig. 1.3)	
Chondrosarcoma	Dog	Translucent, grayish white	Cartilage with a fibrillary matrix and undifferentiated mesenchymal cells (Fig. 1.4)	
Hemangiosarcoma	Dog/cat	Red	Pleomorphic vascular endothelial cells with small vascular channels (Fig. 1.5)	
Rhabdomyosarcoma	Dog	Nodular gray-pink +/- hemorrhage, necrosis	Pleomorphic mesenchymal cells with variable ribbon or strap-like cells and multinucleated giant cells. The mesenchymal cells are positive with Masion's trichrome. Cross striations enhanced by Heidehan's iron, hematoxylin, or phosphotungstic acid hematoxylin	Actin and myosin fibers
Neurofibrosarcoma	Dog		Whorls of spindle cells about nerves	
Lacrimal gland adenoma/ adenocarcinoma	Dog	Pink, lobulated (Fig. 1.6)	Cords and sheets of epithelial cells (Fig. 1.7)	
Zygomatic salivary gland adenoma/ adenocarcinoma	Dog[34,35]	Pink, lobulated	Columnar epithelial cells in ductal formations or sheets of cells with a loose stroma	
Third eyelid gland adenocarcinoma	Dog[36]	Sheets of epithelial cells	Columnar epithelial cells in ductal formations or sheets of cells with a loose stroma	
Harderian gland adenoma	Mice	Pink, lobulated	Papillary epithelial proliferations +/- cysts; cells have foamy cytoplasm and basally located nuclei (Fig. 1.8)	
Granular cell myoblastoma	Dog[37]	Firm	Large polyhedral cells with granular cytoplasm; granules have features of lysosomes	
Fibrosarcoma	Dog	Firm, white to gray	Undifferentiated spindle cells in herring-bone patterns (Fig. 1.9 a-e)	

5

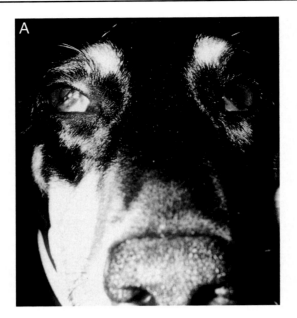

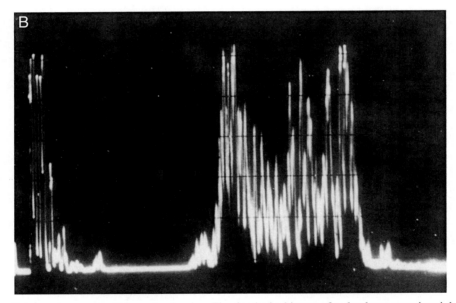

FIG. 1.1—Osteoma in a young Doberman pinscher. The dog had a history of a slowly progressive right exoph-thalmos with prominent protrusion of the third eyelid (**A**). A lateral to medial A scan defined a mass with high reflective spikes (**B**). (continued)

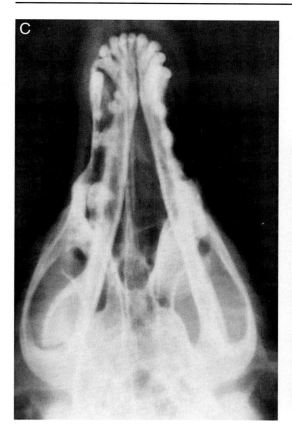

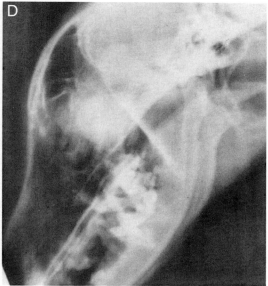

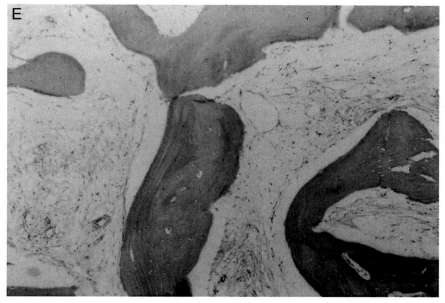

FIG. 1.1 (continued)—Radiographs showed a circumscribed bony lesion of the medial orbital wall **(C and D),** which was excised via lateral orbitotomy. The tumor was composed of sheets of cancellous bone within a connective tissue matrix **(E).** Hematoxylin-eosin, ×100.

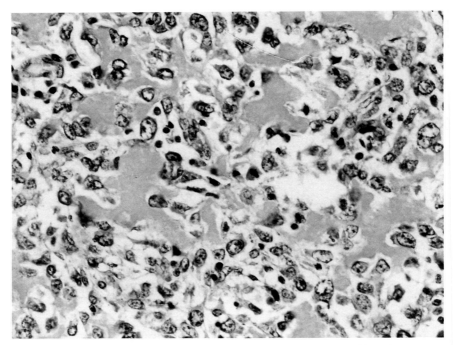

FIG. 1.2—Orbital osteosarcoma composed of spicules of osteoid produced by undifferentiated mesenchymal cells. Hematoxylin-eosin, ×300. (Courtesy of Dr. W. Carlton.)

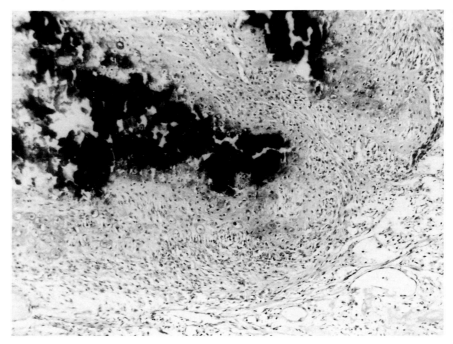

FIG. 1.3—Paraosteal osteoma. Foci of chondroid tissue with mineralized centers are found surrounded by spindle mesenchymal cells. Hematoxylin-eosin, ×88. (Courtesy of Dr. W. Carlton.)

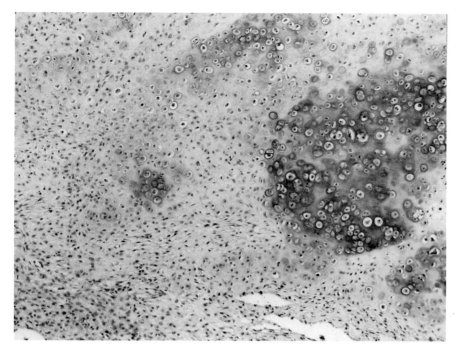

FIG. 1.4—Orbital chondrosarcoma. Islands of hyaline cartilage are surrounded by undifferentiated mesenchymal cells. Hematoxylin-eosin, ×88. (Courtesy of Dr. W. Carlton.)

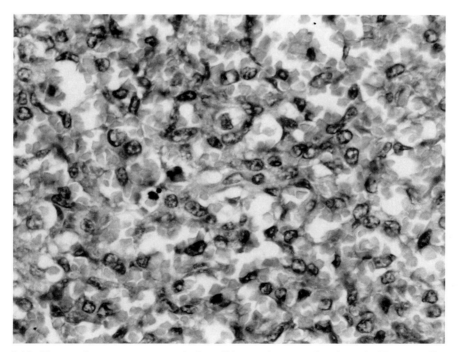

FIG. 1.5—Orbital hemangiosarcoma composed of small incomplete vascular channels. Hematoxylin-eosin, ×350. (Courtesy of Dr. W. Carlton.)

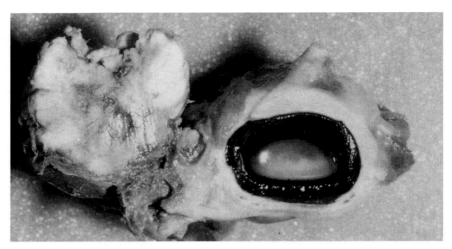

FIG. 1.6—Lacrimal gland adenocarcinoma from a Labrador retriever following exenteration.

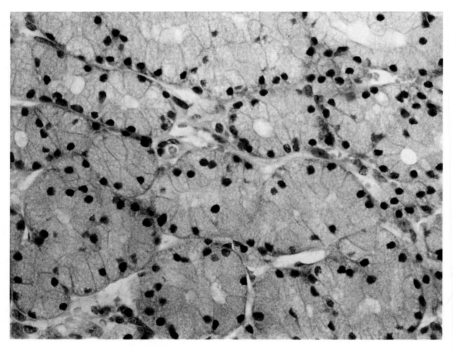

FIG. 1.7—Lacrimal gland adenoma composed of lobules of acini of tall columnar epithelial cells with fine granular cytoplasm and small round dense basally located nuclei. Hematoxylin-eosin, ×350. (Courtesy of Dr. W. Carlton.)

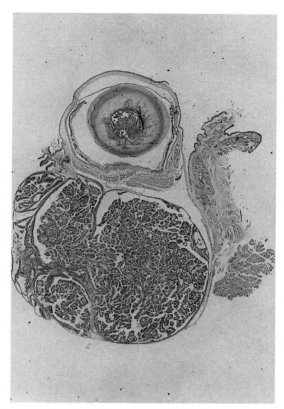

FIG. 1.8—Harderian gland adenoma in a rat with prominent papillary formations. Hematoxylin-eosin, ×35. (Courtesy of Dr. W. Carlton.)

have characteristic antigen phenotypes, and factor VIII positivity characterizes neoplasms of vascular origin. Interpretation of results should be somewhat circumspect as technical variables can affect expression, and species differences in regard to both antigen presentation and antibody sensitivity may exist.

Management and Prognosis. Management decisions and prognosis are determined by the extent and nature of the tumor as determined by imaging, biopsy, and/or surgical exploration. Lateral orbitotomy[40] provides optimal exposure for circumscribed lesions; an anterior approach is generally preferred for exenteration if a diffuse process is present. Inflammatory disease may benefit from medical treatment. Benign neoplasms of both soft tissue and bone can be excised successfully, frequently with preservation of eye and vision. Unfortunately, these tumors are in the minority. The anatomic relationships of the orbit make total excision of invasive malignancy difficult at best, and extension to and through adjacent soft tissues and bone is the rule rather than the exception. Surgeon and oncologist should combine their efforts in these cases, as well as those where orbital tumors are secondary. Exenteration and radiation therapy may prolong life and provide an occasional cure, but, in general, a guarded prognosis, at best, is indicated.

HUMANS

Orbital tumors in humans represent a diverse group of disease entities. Although occasional

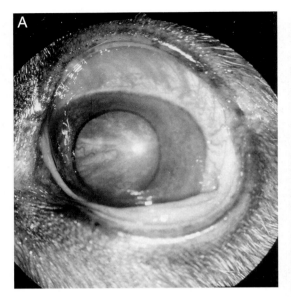

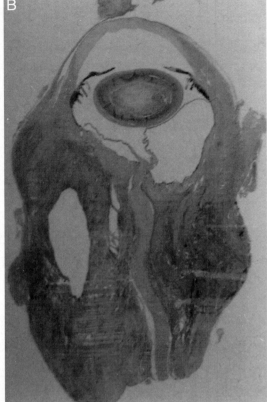

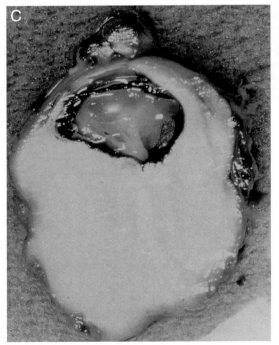

FIG. 1.9—Orbital fibrosarcoma in an elderly golden retriever. Clinically, there was exophthalmos, intense episcleral injection, and a retinal detachment (**A**). The tumor filled the orbit, compressing the sclera and surrounding the optic nerve (**B and C**). **C,** ×2; (continued)

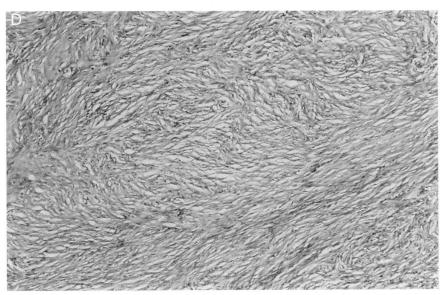

FIG. 1.9 (continued)—Spindle cells in a herring-bone pattern characterized the histopathology **(D)**. Hematoxylin-eosin; **D,** ×100.

sclerosing processes can result in enophthalmos, the common clinical presentation of these diseases is usually that of exophthalmos, the character of which depends on the nature and location of the particular lesion. Over the past several decades, ultrasound, computerized axial tomography, and magnetic resonance imaging have joined plain radiographs and biopsy as invaluable tools in the diagnosis and management of these diseases.[41]

Immunohistochemistry and electron microscopy have evolved into valuable tools for pathologists,[42,43] and imaging-guided fine-needle aspiration biopsy has provided a simple alternative to more radical procedures.[44] As with animal orbital tumors, the topic is vast, and here we address only cardinal aspects.

A discussion of lymphoid tumors of the orbit, orbital tumors arising from the optic nerve, and neoplasms that involve the orbit by extension or metastasis from distant sites are presented in other chapters. Here we review orbital inflammatory processes and present orbital tumors in two broad categories: those that tend to affect children and those that tend to affect adults.

Orbital Inflammatory Syndromes. Occurring most frequently in the young, orbital cellulitis is the result of an extension of a bacterial sinusitis through the orbital walls; *Staphylococcus aureus, Streptococcus,* and occasionally anaerobes are commonly cultured. *Hemophilus influenzae* may cause orbital cellulitis by hematogenous spread without associated sinusitis. The inflammatory response is suppurative, and septic cavernous sinus thrombosis may be a catastrophic complication if effective antimicrobial therapy is not initiated.[45,46]

Chronic nongranulomatous orbital inflammation is most commonly associated with either dysthyroid ophthalmopathy, or Grave's disease, and orbital pseudotumor. Approximately 10% of patients with Grave's disease develop infiltrative orbital myopathy, usually bilateral with edema and resultant proptosis, extraocular motility imbalances with resulting diplopia, and optic nerve compression. Computer-assisted tomography and ultrasound show increased thickness of the extraocular muscles (Figure 1.10), preferentially the inferior and medial rectus, with sparing of the tendonous insertion. Histopathologically,

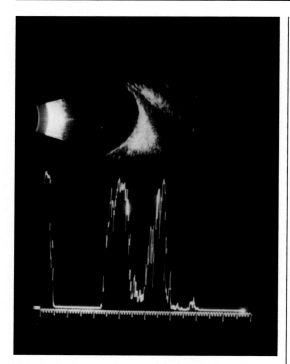

FIG. 1.10—B-scan ultrasound **(top)** showing left medial rectus enlargement within the belly of the muscle. A scan **(bottom)** demonstrates low reflectivity in the posterior aspect of the muscle. (Photos courtesy of Michael F. Lewandowski, RDMS.)

the involved muscles are characterized by a predominantly lymphocytic-plasmacytic infiltration, with mast cells and histiocytes in small numbers, fibrosis, and increased amounts of extracellular mucopolysaccharides, probably produced by the endomysial fibroblasts.[47,48] Therapeutic options include high doses of systemic corticosteroids and, if the optic nerve is compressed, localized radiotherapy or decompressive orbital surgery.

Orbital pseudotumor has no recognizable cause, occurs both in children and adults, and may be unilateral, bilateral, or alternating. Onset is much more rapid than that which occurs with Grave's disease or orbital lymphomatous tumors, and, in contrast to the former, involves the muscle tendons, orbital fat, and lacrimal gland. On histopathologic examination, a mononuclear inflammatory cell infiltrate, frequently in combi-

nation with eosinophils and a variably present circulating eosinophilia is seen. Involvement of the periosteum of the cavernous sinus may produce painful external ophthalmoplegia (Tolosa-Hunt syndrome). Uncommonly, extensive orbital sclerosis may occur. The disease is usually steroid responsive, with radiotherapy used in resistant cases.

A mononuclear dacryoadenitis may occur as an isolated finding or in association with Sjögren's syndrome. Granulomatous vasculidites, including Wegner's granulomatosis and giant cell cranial arteritis, may involve the orbital vessels; polyarteritis nodosa and thrombophlebitis may also affect the orbital vessels with nongranulomatous infiltrates. Sarcoidosis can affect the lacrimal gland, extraocular muscles, the optic nerve, or involve the orbit by extension from an involved sinus. Erdheim-Chester disease may have orbital infiltration with Touton giant cells and lipid-laden macrophages as part of systemic involvement.

Orbital inflammation of infectious etiology includes orbital phycomycosis, which occurs as a necrotizing vasculitis in debilitated patients; aspergillosis; and tubercular involvement of the lacrimal gland.

Parasitic involvement of orbital tissues may be encountered with trichinosis, which may lodge in the extraocular vessels, or by the development of *Ecchinococcus* or *Taenia saginata* cysts.[49] Sinus mucoceles may extend through the thin orbital bones to present as cystic orbital lesions

Orbital Neoplasms. In contrast to animals, the majority of expanding orbital neoplasms are benign, with a predominance of lymphoproliferative conditions, followed by vascular lesions. Developmental disorders predominate in children.

Orbital Tumors of Children. Congenital malformations of the orbit and its structures may cause proptosis; of these, meningoceles, encephaloceles, or ectopic brain tissue are the most common. Microphthalmos with cyst formation (Figure 1.11) may also present as a space-occupying orbital lesion, as may ectopic lacrimal gland.

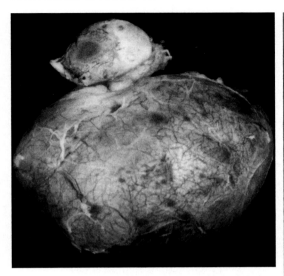

FIG. 1.11—Gross photograph showing microphthalmos with large cyst. Note the "neck" extending from the globe into the cyst.

The two most important congenital orbital tumors are teratomas and dermoid cysts. Teratomas arise from aberrant germ cells and, related to their tendency to affect midline structures, may involve the orbit. Although these congenital tumors are benign, they can become quite massive, with resultant dramatic proptosis. Histologically, elements of all three of the embryonic germ layers are present. The lesions are frequently cystic and are usually well circumscribed, if not encapsulated. Local excision with preservation of a functional globe may be possible in some cases.[50]

Orbital dermoid cysts are choristomas that arise as a result of sequestration of surface epidermis during embryogenesis, frequently between the suture lines of the orbital bones. This is the most common orbital tumor of childhood and is usually located superotemporal, although superonasal and deep orbital lesions have been documented. Radiographs frequently will reveal a bony defect due to expansion of the cyst. The lesions are encapsulated and with careful dissection can be totally removed. Histologically, the cyst wall is lined by keratinized stratified squamous epithelium with associated adnexal structures; the cyst lumen is filled with keratin and with sebaceous and sudoriferous material, as well as hair shafts. This is a slowly expansive lesion that may not become symptomatic until later in life; spontaneous or traumatic rupture of the cyst releases the contents that stimulate a lipogranulomatous inflammatory response.

VASCULAR TUMORS. Vascular tumors of childhood include capillary hemangiomas, lymphangiomas, and arteriovenous formations associated with Wyburn-Mason syndrome. Capillary hemangiomas (Figure 1.12) are predominantly lesions of the lid and anterior orbit[51] and are addressed in the chapter on lid tumors. Lymphangiomas (Figure 1.13), although classified as choristomas, are diagnosed usually in early childhood from age 2–3 onward, though later onset has been documented. They may be fairly localized lesions, or extensively infiltrate the orbital tissues, in which case their diffuse nature makes total removal quite difficult; in these cases, debulking is frequently beneficial. Histopathologically, lymphangiomas are composed of a monolayer of endothelial cells around a lumen containing proteinaceous fluid. Lymphoid follicles may be identified between the channels and may account for the worsening of the associated proptosis during upper respiratory infections.[52] Hemorrhage into the delicate channels may result in acute exacerbation and the formation of a so-called chocolate cyst.[53]

RHABDOMYOSARCOMA. Rhabdomyosarcomas are the most common mesenchymal primary orbital tumor of childhood; awareness of them and early diagnosis are vital because chemotherapy and radiotherapy can result in cures in up to 80% of the cases of this aggressive malignancy. Although the disease has been described from close to birth to well into the second decade, it generally affects children from 4 to 10 years of age, with a median of about 7 years, and a slight male predisposition. There is predilection for the superior orbit, and it is generally accepted that these tumors do not arise from the extraocular muscles but from ectopic rests of primitive skeletal muscle. Clinically, rapid growth and

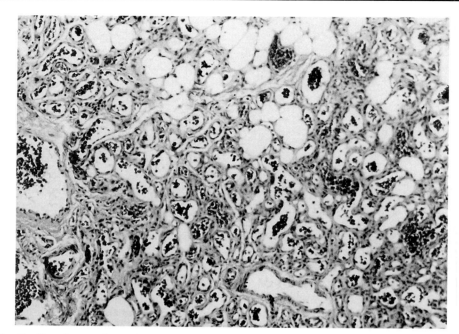

FIG. 1.12—Capillary hemangioma showing small, delicate, thin-walled channels filled with erythrocytes. Hematoxylin-eosin, ×40.

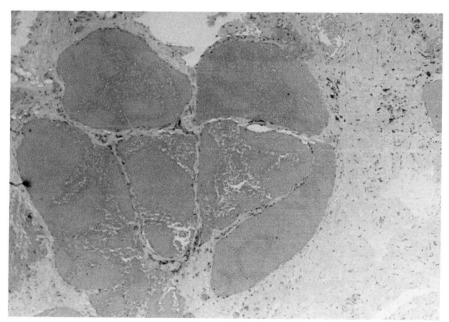

FIG. 1.13—Lymphangioma demonstrating a monolayer of endothelial cells around a lumen of proteinaceous fluid. Hematoxylin-eosin, ×25.

progression of proptosis is the hallmark of the disease. Anterior lesions may present as conjunctival masses. Extension into the periorbital sinuses may be present in up to 40%–50% of cases.[54]

Four histopathologic types have been described, of which the embryonic type accounts for almost 80%; biopsy of embryonic rhabdomyosarcoma will show undifferentiated spindle cells with hyperchromatic nucleoli. The cells will be arranged in fascicles, occasionally alternating with myxoid zones. The cytoplasm is bipolar and frequently will show eosinophilia due to the presence of cytoplasmic muscle filaments that are seen by light microscopy in about 50% of cases. Electron microscopy will demonstrate the thick (150 mm) myosin and thinner actin filaments, often demonstrating sarcomeric organization. Immunohistochemistry is often valuable with consistent positivity for desmin and 2-sarcomeric actin whereas antibodies to myoglobin, vimentin, and enolase are less reliable.[55]

In the alveolar form of rhabdomyosarcoma, more rounded rhabdomyoblasts with intensely eosinophilic cytoplasm align along connective tissue septae containing blood vessels, providing an overall pattern somewhat suggestive of the alveoli of the lungs. This lesion has the tendency to involve the inferior orbit and is considered the most aggressive form of rhabdomyosarcoma, frequently producing regional metastases. Botryoid rhabdomyosarcoma is a variant of the embryonal type that presents as a subconjunctival lesion, producing grapelike excrescences of tissue.

In a differentiated rhabdomyosarcoma, which tends to occur in somewhat older individuals, the neoplastic cells are remarkable for their large straplike appearance, which closely resemble degenerating mature striated muscle.

NEUROFIBROMAS. Orbital neurofibromas in the first decade of life are almost invariably associated with neurofibromatosis; those neurofibromas and schwannomas that occur in individuals from age 20 on tend to be isolated. These neoplasms are difficult to manage because of the infiltrating nature of the tumor and its intimate association with adjacent tissues, and debulking is frequently the only surgical option. Histologically, there are diffuse infiltrating nerve twiglets, which have a somewhat organoid appearance in that each unit is surrounded by perineurium that encloses axons, Schwann cells, and endoneural fibroblasts, and that mimic disorganized peripheral nerves.[56]

FIBRO-OSSEOUS AND CARTILAGINOUS TUMORS. Fibrous dysplasia and ossifying fibroma represent two fibro-osseous lesions that may involve the orbit. The former is relatively benign, but may affect vision as a result of encroachment on the optic canal,[57] whereas the latter is more aggressive and circumscribed, frequently involving the orbital roof.[58] Histologically, fibrous dysplasia (Figure 1.14) consists of immature woven bone set in a fibrous stroma with absence of osteoblasts rimming the trabeculae; ossifying fibroma is composed of more mature lamellar bone, in which there are lamellar lines and osteoblasts rimming the trabeculae; the stroma is active and highly vascularized.

Osteogenic sarcoma and chondrosarcoma are aggressive malignancies that may arise spontaneously from the orbital bones and paranasal sinuses in children; patients that have had radiation therapy to treat retinoblastoma are at risk. Stromal cells will be hyperchromatic and mitotically active, and are more disorganized than in the preceding two conditions.

HISTIOCYTIC DISORDERS. Proliferative histiocytic disorders may occur in children. Juvenile xanthogranuloma rarely involves the orbit compared to iris and eyelids. Eosinophilic granuloma is a localized lesion with a tendency to develop along the superotemporal orbital rim with lysis of adjacent bone; curettage and low doses of radiotherapy can be curative. Letterer-Siwe disease, Hand-Schüller-Christian disease, and sinus histiocytosis with massive lymphadenopathy may involve the orbit as a component of systemic disease.

ORBITAL TUMORS OF ADULTS

VASCULAR TUMORS. Cavernous hemangioma (Figure 1.15) is the most common adult vascular tumor, usually affecting individuals after the third decade, with a predisposition for females. Proliferation is usually intraconal, and a slowly progressive painless proptosis may affect vision by optic nerve compression or induced hyperopia, with resultant

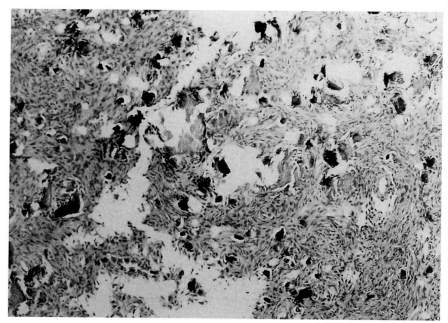

FIG. 1.14—Fragments of immature woven bone within a fibrous stroma typical of fibrous dysplasia. Hematoxylin-eosin, ×33.

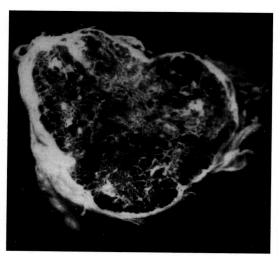

FIG. 1.15—Gross photograph of cavernous hemangioma showing encapsulated tumor with large blood-filled spaces.

retinal striae as the globe is compressed. Histopathologically, the lesions consist of encapsulated large vascular spaces with thick fibrous septae (Figure 1.16); there are no large feeding or drainage vessels, and careful en bloc excision is curative.[59]

Hemangiopericytomas (Figure 1.17) are uncommon encapsulated hypervascular and hypercellular lesions that tend to occur in middle-aged individuals with male predisposition. At surgery, it has a distinctive blue appearance. Microscopically (Figure 1.18), the tumor is composed of plump pericytes surrounding a rich capillary network; reticular staining demonstrates individual cells surrounded by this fiber. Factor VIII positivity may be useful in diagnosis. Malignant potential of this tumor is demonstrated by its tendency to recur when incompletely excised, and late metastases may occur.[60,61]

Other vascular tumors, including arteriovenous malformations and fistulas, orbital varix, venous angioma, vascular leiomyoma, papillary endothelial hypoplasia, angiosarcoma, and angiolymphoid hyperplasia with eosinophilia (Kimura's disease) are uncommon, but may present with signs of space-occupying orbital lesions.

FIBROBLASTIC AND OTHER MESENCHYMAL TUMORS. Fibrous histiocytomas are the most common primary orbital mesenchymal tumor of adults, occurring at a mean age of 43 years and

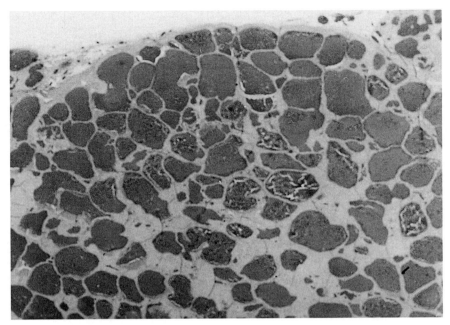

FIG. 1.16—Photomicrograph showing large vascular spaces with intervening dense fibrous septae of typical cavernous hemangioma. Hematoxylin-eosin, ×5.

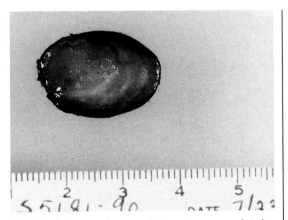

FIG. 1.17—Gross photograph showing encapsulated appearance of hemangiopericytoma.

with a slight predilection for the superior orbit. Although the majority of the lesions are benign, a small percentage have malignant histologic features and, if incompletely removed, may be recurrent and locally invasive; metastasis is quite uncommon, however. Histologically, the lesions are circumscribed and partially encapsulated. The tumor is composed of two populations of cells—

fibroblasts and histiocytes—with the former predominant. The latter may contain lipid and be multinucleated. The cells typically array in a storiform or spiral pattern (Figure 1.19).[62]

There are also less common orbital mesenchymal tumors, which include fibromas and fibrosarcoma, leiomyoma, and leiomyosarcoma;[63] lipoma and liposarcoma; nodular fasciitis; and myxomas.

NEURAL TUMORS. Neural tumors are uncommon in adults, but neurofibromas and schwannomas (neurilemomas) have been described. Histologically, neurofibromas are circumscribed lesions consisting of wavy bundles of Schwann cells surrounding axons. Neurilemomas are characterized by a proliferation of Schwann cells without axons and display cellular areas of palisading nucleoli (Antoni A pattern) or areas of myxoid change (Antoni B pattern).

LACRIMAL GLAND TUMORS. Lacrimal gland tumors are common causes of superior temporal space-occupying orbital lesions in adults. Of lacrimal gland tumors, approximately half are inflammatory or lymphoid lesions (sarcoidosis

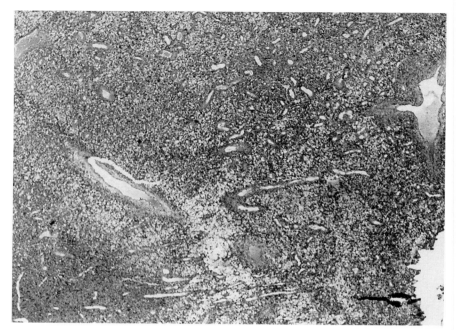

FIG. 1.18—Photomicrograph of hemangiopericytoma showing rich capillary network surrounded by pericytes. Hematoxylin-eosin, ×10.

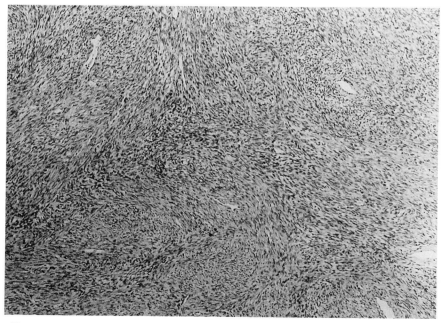

FIG. 1.19—Characteristic storiform or matted appearance of a benign fibrous histiocytoma. Hematoxylin-eosin, ×10.

has a distinct predisposition for the lacrimal gland), and the other half are epithelial parenchymal neoplasms. These neoplasms tend to arise from the posterior pole of the gland. In general, lacrimal gland tumors are quite similar to their salivary gland counterparts.[64,65]

Benign mixed tumor (pleomorphic adenoma) usually presents in the third and fourth decades as a slowly progressive painless lesion, with a male predisposition. Radiographically, there may be corticated attenuation of the lacrimal fossa due to pressure exerted by the mass; imaging will demonstrate a well-defined lesion. Microscopically, the lesion is encapsulated and is characterized by bilayered ductules and a myxoid stroma, which may show chondroid change or osteoid deposition. In long-standing cases or following incomplete excision, transformation to a malignant mixed tumor may occur; en bloc excision via lateral orbitotomy is the treatment of choice, and incisional biopsy is contraindicated.

Adenoid cystic carcinoma affects a similar age group as benign mixed tumor, but patients typically present with a more rapidly progressive clinical history, pain, and motility disturbance; in addition, there is a female predisposition. Radiographic studies may disclose irregular erosion of the contiguous orbital rim and lacrimal fossa. Histologically, the lesion is unencapsulated, with a tendency for perineural involvement and extension. Microscopically, the tumor is composed of rather bland-appearing basaloid cells arranged in ducts and nests, the "lumens" within these nests creating a cribiform or "Swiss cheese" pattern. Hyaline basement membrane-like material may surround the nests and cords of cells. Adenoid cystic carcinomas are aggressive invasive malignancies. After confirmation by incisional biopsy, radical excision of involved tissue is the treatment of choice. Long-term survival is poor, with a 10% 20-year survival rate.

Squamous cell carcinoma, undifferentiated carcinoma, mucoepidermoid carcinoma, and adenocarcinoma may all arise de novo in the lacrimal gland. Oncocytomas occur as an uncommon benign neoplasm.

OTHER ORBITAL TUMORS OF ADULTS. Sinus mucoceles may expand through the thin orbital bone to involve the orbit. Orbital amyloid deposition may occur, usually as a localized process.

REFERENCES

1. Peiffer RL, Grimson BS, McCartney WN, Johnson PJ, Wilkerson B. Dystroid orbital disease in *Macaca* fascicularis. *J Med Primatol* 10:219, 1981.
2. Whitney JC. Eosinophilic myositis in a dog. *Vet Rec* 67:1140, 1955.
3. Glauberg A, Beaumont PR. Sudden blindness as the presenting sign of eosinophilic myositis: a case report. *J Am Anim Hosp Assoc* 15:609, 1979.
4. Haines P, Moncure C. Pseudotumor of the orbit in a prosimian primate (lesser bushbaby: *Galago senegalenses*). *J Med Primatol* 2:369, 1973.
5. Dziezyc J, Barton CL. Exophthalmia in a cat caused by an eosinophilic infiltrate. *Prog Vet Comp Ophthalmol* 2:91, 1992.
6. Miller SA, Van der Woerdt A, Bartick TE. Retrobulbar pseudotumor of the orbit in a cat. *J Am Vet Med Assoc* 216:356, 2000.
7. Koch SA. Medical orbital abscess in a collie dog. *J Am Vet Med Assoc* 156:1905, 1970.
8. Peiffer RL, Janke BH. Orbital cellulitis, sinusitis, and pneumonitis caused by *Penicillium* sp. in a cat. *J Am Vet Med Assoc* 176:449, 1980.
9. Roberts SR, Thompson TJ. *Pneumonyssus caninum* and orbital cellulitis in the dog. *J Am Vet Med Assoc* 155:731, 1969.
10. Rebhun WC, Edwards NJ. Cryptococcosis involving the orbit of a dog. *Vet Med Small Anim Clin* 72:1447, 1977.
11. Wilkinson GT, Sutton RH, Gromo LR. *Aspergillus* spp. infection associated with orbital cellulitis and sinusitis in a cat. *J Small Anim Pract* 23:127, 1982.
12. Martin CL. Orbital mucocele in a dog. *VM SAC* 66:36, 1971.
13. Schmidt GM, Betts CW. Zygomatic salivary mucoceles in the dog. *J Am Vet Med Assoc* 171:940, 1978.
14. Munger RL. Orbital hydrops secondary to alleged enucleation. *Can Pract* 7:70, 1980.
15. Bryan GM. Subconjunctival emphysema in a cat. *VM SAC* 72:1087, 1973.
16. Bedford PAL. Orbital pneumatosis as an unusual complication of enucleation. *J Small Anim Pract* 20:551, 1979.
17. Rubin LF, Patterson DF. Arteriovenous fistula of the orbit in a dog. *Cornell Vet* 55:471, 1965.
18. Komar G, Schuster A. A rare ophthalmological picture of disease (exophthalmos pusans) in a dog. *Berl Munch Tiertartzl Wochenschr* 80:359, 1967.
19. Gilger BC, McLaughlin SA, Whitley RD, Wright J. Orbital neoplasms in cats: 21 cases (1974–1990). *J Am Vet Med Assoc* 201:1083, 1992.

20. Gross S, Aguirre G, Harvey C. Tumors involving the orbit of the dog. *Proc Am Coll Vet Ophthalmol* 10:229, 1979.

21. Kern TJ. Orbital neoplasia in 23 dogs. *J Am Vet Med Assoc* 186:489, 1985.

22. Peiffer RL, Spencer C, Dopp SA. Nasal squamous cell carcinoma with periocular extension and metastasis in a cat. *Feline Pract* 8:43, 1978.

23. Pentlarge VW, Powell-Johnson G, Martin CL. Orbital neoplasia with enophthalmos in a cat. *J Am Vet Med Assoc* 195:1249, 1989.

24. Ackerman N, Munger RJ. Intraconal contrast orbitography in the dog. *Am J Vet Res* 40:911, 1979.

25. Dziezyc J, Hager DA, Millichamp NJ. Two-dimensional real-time ocular ultrasonography in the diagnosis of ocular lesions in dogs. *J Am Vet Med Assoc* 23:501, 1987.

26. Morgan RV. Ultrasonography of retrobulbar diseases of the dog and cat. *J Am Anim Hosp Assoc* 25:393, 1989.

27. Stuhr CM, Scagliotti RH. Retrobulbar ultrasound in mesaticephalic and doli-chocephalic dog using a temporal approach. *Vet Comp Ophthalmol* 662:91. 1996.

28. LeCouteur RA, Fike JR, Scagliotti RH, Cann CE. Computed tomography of orbital tumors in the dog. *J Am Vet Med Assoc* 180:910, 1982.

29. Calia CM, Krischner SE, Baer KE, Stefanacci JD. The use of computed tomography scan for the evaluation of orbital disease in cats and dogs. *Vet Comp Ophthalmol* 4:24, 1994.

30. Grahn BH, Stewart WA, Towner RA. Magnetic resonance imaging of the canine and feline eye, orbit and optic nerves and its clinical application. *Can Vet J* 34:418, 1993.

31. Knecht CD, Green JA. Osteoma of the zygomatic arch in a cat. *J Am Vet Med Assoc* 171:1077, 1977.

32. Pletcher JM, Koch SA, Stedham MA. Orbital chondroma rodens in a dog. *J Am Vet Med Assoc* 175:187, 1979.

33. Cottrill NB, Carter JD, Pechman RD. Bilateral orbital parosteal osteoma in a cat. *J Am Anim Hosp Assoc* 23:405, 1987.

34. Buykmichi N, Robin LF, Harvey CE. Exophthalmus secondary zygomatic adenocarcinoma in a dog. *J Am Vet Med Assoc* 167:162, 1975.

35. Ratto A, Peiffer RL, Peruccio C, Rossi L. Zygomatic salivary gland adenocarcinoma in a dog. *Prog Vet Comp Ophthalmol* 1:59, 1991.

36. Wilcock BP, Peiffer RL. Adenocarcinoma of the gland of the third eyelid in seven dogs. *Am Vet Med Assoc* 193:1549, 1988.

37. Holscher MA. Granular cell myoblastoma (schwannoma) in the orbit and cerebrum of two dogs. *Canine Pract* 10:35, 1983.

38. Wick MR. Immunohistochemistry in the diagnosis of solid malignant tumors. In: Jenette JC, ed. *Immunohistology in Diagnostic Pathology.* Boca Raton, FL: CRC, 1989:161.

39. Chadially F. *Ultrastructural Pathology of the Cell and Matrix.* London: Butterworths, 1988.

40. Slatter DH. Lateral orbitotomy by zygomatic arch resection in the dog. *J Am Vet Med Assoc* 175:1179, 1979.

41. Shields JA, Shields, CL, Davison LA. Recent advances in the diagnosis of orbital tumors. *Trans Pa Acad Ophthalmol* 38:473, 1986.

42. Reifler DM, Kinis SR, Kenderdell JS, Dekker JR, Fisher LJ. Immunocytologic methods in the diagnosis of orbital tumors. *Henry Ford Hosp Med J* 33:171, 1985.

43. Orcutt JC, Reeh MJ, Gown AM, Lindquist TD. Diagnosis of orbit and periorbital tumors: use of monoclonal antibodies to cytoplasmic antigens (intermediate filaments). *Ophthalmic Plast Reconstr Surg* 3:159, 1987.

44. Czerniak B, Woyke S, Daniel B, Krzysztolik Z, Koss LG. Diagnosis of orbital tumors by aspiration biopsy guided by computerized tomography. *Cancer* 54:2385, 1984.

45. Macy JI, Mandelbaum SH, Minckler DA. Orbital cellulitis. *Ophthalmology* 87:1309, 1980.

46. Weiss A, Friendly D, Eglin K, et al. Bacterial periorbital and orbital cellulitis in childhood. *Ophthalmology* 90:195, 1983.

47. Trokel SL, Jakobiec FA. Correlation of CT scanning and pathologic features of ophthalmic Graves' disease. *Ophthalmology* 88:553, 1981.

48. Hufnagel TJ, Hickey WF, Cobbs WH, et al. Immunohistochemical and ultrastructural studies on the exenterated orbital tissues of a patient with Graves' disease. *Ophthalmology* 91:1411, 1984.

49. Kennerdell JS, Dresner SC. The nonspecific orbital inflammatory syndromes. *Surv Ophthalmol* 29:93, 1984.

50. Chang DA, Dallow RL, Walton DS. Congenital orbital teratoma: report of a case with visual preservation. *J Pediatr Ophthalmol Strabismus* 17:88, 1980.

51. Bergstrom K, Enoksson P, Gamstrorp I, Naeser P. Haemangioendothelioma of the orbit. *Ophthalmologica* 177:115, 1978.

52. Harris GJ, Sakol PJ, Bonovolonta G, De Concili-iis C. An analysis of thirty cases of orbital lymphangioma: pathophysiologic consideration and management recommendations. *Ophthalmology* 97:1583, 1990.

53. Reese AB, Howard GM. Unusual manifestations of ocular lymphangioma and lymphangiectasis. *Surv Ophthalmol* 18:226, 1973.

54. Jones IS, Reese AB, Krout J. Orbital rhabdomyosarcoma: an analysis of 62 cases. *Trans Am Ophthalmol Soc* 63:223, 1965.

55. Sun XL, Zheng BH, Li B, Li LQ, Soejima K, Kanda M. Orbital rhabdomyosarcoma: immunohistochemical studies of seven cases. *Chin Med J [Engl]* 103:485, 1990.

56. Moore JG. Neonatal neurofibromatosis. *Br J Ophthalmol* 46:682, 1962.

57. Liakos GM, Walker CB, Carruth JS. Ocular complications in craniofacial fibrous dysplasia. *Br J Ophthalmol* 63:611, 1979.

58. Fu YS, Pezin KH. Non-epithelial tumors of the nasal cavity, paranasal sinuses, and nasopharynx: a clinicopathological study: II. Osseous and bibro-osseous lesions including osteoma, fibrous dysplasia, ossifying fibroma, osteoblastoma, giant cell tumor and osteosarcoma. *Cancer* 33:1289, 1974.

59. Garner A. Cavernous haemangioma of the orbit: a consideration of its origin and development. *Orbit* 7:149, 1988.

60. Croxatto JO, Font RL. Hemangiopericytoma of the orbit: a clinicopathologic study of 30 cases. *Hum Pathol* 13:210, 1982.

61. Jakobiec FA, Howard GM, Jones IS, Wolff M. Hemangiopericytoma of the orbit. *Am J Ophthalmol* 78:816, 1974.

62. Jakobiec FA, Howard GM, Jones IS, Tannenbaum M. Fibrous histiocytomata of the orbit. *Am J Ophthalmol* 77:333, 1974.

63. Jakobiec FA, Howard GM, Rosen M, Wolff M. Leiomyoma and leiomyosarcoma of the orbit. *Am J Ophthalmol* 80:1028, 1975.

64. Shields CL, Shields JA, Eagle RC, Rathmell JP. Clinicopathologic review of 142 cases of lacrimal gland lesions. *Ophthalmology* 96:431, 1989.

65. Font RL, Gamel JW. Epithelial tumors of the lacrimal gland: an analysis of 265 cases. In: Jakobiec FA, ed. *Ocular and Adnexal Tumors*. Birmingham, AL: Aesculapius, 1978:787.

2 EYELID TUMORS

Ronald C. Riis, Connie M. Vitali, and Kenneth B. Simons

ANIMALS

Eyelid neoplasms occur infrequently in cats, cows, dogs, and horses. The differential diagnosis of an eyelid neoplasm in cats and cows would be rather limited, squamous cell carcinoma being the only common lid tumor. The dog eyelid neoplasms have included adenoma of the sebaceous glands,[1–3] papilloma,[1,3,4] melanoma,[1,4,5] histiocytoma,[2,5] mastocytoma,[5] basal cell carcinoma,[5] squamous cell carcinoma,[3,6,7] adenocarcinoma,[5] fibroma, lipoma,[5] and others (these are listed in order of prevalence). A nonneoplastic eyelid tumor of dogs composed of lymphocytic and histiocytic cells is discussed under the histiocytomas.[8–10] The horse eyelid tumors include squamous cell carcinoma, sarcoids, *Habronema*, melanoma, histiocytoma, mastocytoma, pericytoma, and lymphocytoma in relative incidence. Horse lid neoplasms rarely reported include adenocarcinoma,[11] adenoma,[12] angiosarcoma,[13] basal cell carcinoma,[12] hemangiosarcoma,[14,15] and schwannoma[15,16] (Figure 2.1).

A survey of 202 dog eyelid tumors found that, histopathologically, 82.1% were either sebaceous gland tumors (44%), melanomas (20.8%), or papillomas (17.3%). Benign tumors (73.3%) were more prevalent than malignant (26.7%), and epithelial tumors outnumbered tumors of mesenchymal origin 134 to 23. Malignant cutaneous neoplasms of dogs were less prevalent on eyelids than in other regions of skin. The occurrence of more tumors on the upper eyelid (40.2%) than on the lower eyelid (30.2%) was not considered significant, and no sex predilection was found. Eyelid tumors in dogs appear to be primary, which are generally benign and, when malignant, do not metastasize and infrequently recur.[5]

Sebaceous Gland Neoplasms. Meibomian adenomas and adenocarcinomas are the most frequent eyelid tumors in dogs of middle to advanced age, comprising 44% of canine eyelid tumors.[5,17,18]

Sebaceous adenomas have a multilobular arrangement with large vacuolated cells in the center and smaller reserve cells at the periphery of each lobule (Figures 2.2–2.7). Sebaceous adenocarcinomas generally resemble benign adenomas grossly and microscopically in structure and cell arrangement, but adenocarcinomas have a greater percentage of proliferative reserve cells and fewer large foam cells. Proliferation of reserve cells is prominent in sebaceous adenocarcinomas accompanied by hyperchromatism and mitotic activity. Hemorrhage from hypervascularization and pigmentation from proliferative melanocytes are often a characteristic.[5] Meibomian tumors are managed by excision, cryoablation, or a combination thereof.[18] Lid tumor recurrence rates between dogs treated with cryosurgery and those treated surgically were not significantly different (15.1% and 10.5%, respectively). The mean recurrence time after cryosurgery was 7.4 months [±1.9 standard equivalent measure (SEM)], and 28.3 months (±7.2 SEM) after surgical excision. The long-term side effects were similar using either treatment, but the overall cosmetic appearance was better with cryosurgery.[19]

Squamous Cell Carcinoma. The lids of all animals are prone to solar dermatitis or keratosis especially if the skin is nonpigmented. The preneoplastic lesion may appear as an erythematous, scaly area, or slightly raised with a brown crusty

Ocular Adnexal Tumors in Animals

Graph 1   Data obtained from March 1, 1964
to November 30, 1994

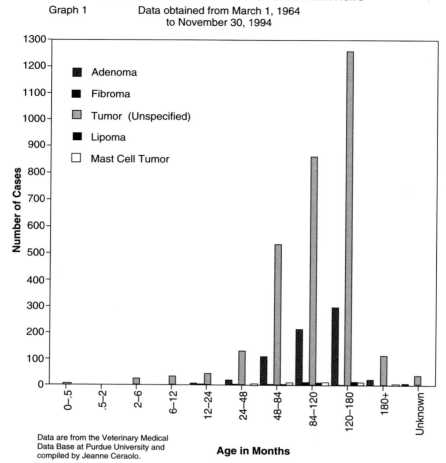

Data are from the Veterinary Medical
Data Base at Purdue University and
compiled by Jeanne Ceraolo.

Age in Months

FIG. 2.1—Ocular adnexal tumors in animals. Data obtained from 1 March 1964 to 30 November 1994. **A:** Adenoma, fibroma, unspecified tumor, lipoma, and mast cell tumor. (continued)

surface (Figure 2.8). The next stage is an ulcer covered by a fibrinopurulent exudate. As the tumor infiltrates, the underlying tissue responds, making a firm intradermal and subcutaneous mass.[20,21] In animals, particularly white cats with blue eyes, the preneoplastic and early neoplastic changes are effectively treated with cryotherapy.[22] Squamous cell carcinoma of the cat eyelid appears to be predominantly malignant (Figures 2.9 and 2.10). White-faced cattle and horses with lid squamous cell carcinomas seem to be neglected until they progress to later stages of the neoplasia with extensive tissue destruction and ulceration.[23–26]

HORSES. The most common neoplasia of the horse eye is squamous cell carcinoma. Risk factors for this neoplasm include age (middle to older horses; average, 9.4 years), breed (appaloosa and draft), coat color (white and gray), and geographic latitude. Actinic radiation has a definite effect.[27] Tumors of the eyelid have a poorer prognosis than those arising on the limbus, and the more extensive the tumor, the poorer is the prognosis.[27] Tumor recurrence after treatment reduces survival time (Figure 2.11).[28]

The treatment of squamous cell carcinoma of the lids of horses ranges from complete surgical excision, radiation [radioactive gold 198, iridium

Ocular Adnexal Tumors in Animals

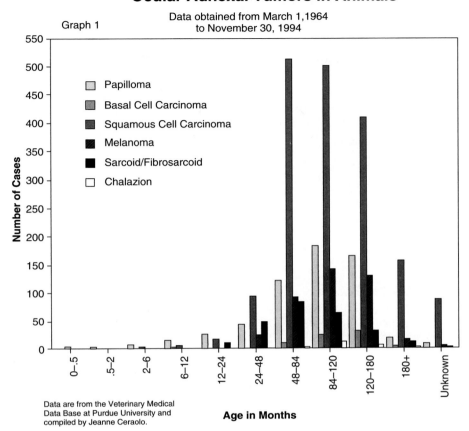

Graph 1

Data obtained from March 1,1964
to November 30, 1994

Legend:
- Papilloma
- Basal Cell Carcinoma
- Squamous Cell Carcinoma
- Melanoma
- Sarcoid/Fibrosarcoid
- Chalazion

Y-axis: Number of Cases (0 to 550)

X-axis: Age in Months — 0–.5, .5–2, 2–6, 6–12, 12–24, 24–48, 48–84, 84–120, 120–180, 180+, Unknown

Data are from the Veterinary Medical
Data Base at Purdue University and
compiled by Jeanne Ceraolo.

FIG. 2.1 (continued)—**B:** Papilloma, basal cell carcinoma, squamous cell carcinoma, melanoma, sarcoid/fibrosarcoid, and chalazion. (Data are from the Veterinary Data Base at Purdue University and compiled by Jeanne Ceraolo.)

192, or cesium 157 implants, or topical beta (strontium 90)], to hypothermia, hyperthermia, immunotherapy [bacillus Calmette-Guérin (BCG)], and carbon dioxide laser or YAG-laser therapy. The horse with squamous cell carcinoma has a guarded prognosis because it is predisposed to further tumor development within 2 years of the initial tumor diagnosis, even if the initial site was completely eradicated.[29,30]

CATTLE. Squamous cell carcinomas in cattle occur principally in older purebred or crossbred white-faced cattle. Hereford cattle have an inheritable tendency to develop this neoplasia. Occasionally, Simmental and Holstein Friesian cattle develop lid squamous cell carcinomas but rarely do other breeds. It has not been reported in black Aberdeen Angus cattle.

Sixty-six percent of the squamous cell tumors originate at the lateral limbus, followed in incidence by the medial limbus, lower eyelid, nictitans, and the medial canthal area. Hereford herds in semi-arid regions with abundant sunlight, especially at higher altitudes, have an incidence of ocular squamous cell tumors as high as 40%, with up to 10% of these being carcinomas. Since cattle with eye tumors are usually marketed rather than treated, nearly 80% of the eye tumors of cattle at slaughter have squamous cell carcinomas.[31] Meat inspectors identify metastatic

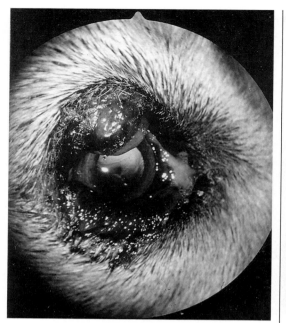

FIG. 2.2—Dog upper-lid sebaceous adenoma. This is the most common lid tumor in dogs. Incisional curettage and cryosurgery is an ideal therapy.

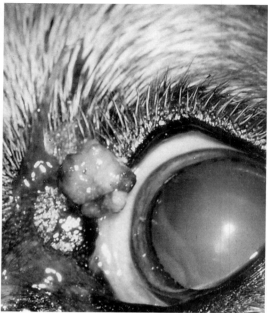

FIG. 2.3—Dog upper-lid sebaceous adenoma that is predominantly external and small can be removed by lid wedge resection and marginal repair.

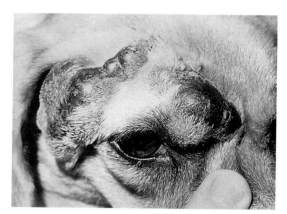

FIG. 2.4—Dog lids and lateral face with extensive sebaceous adenomas.

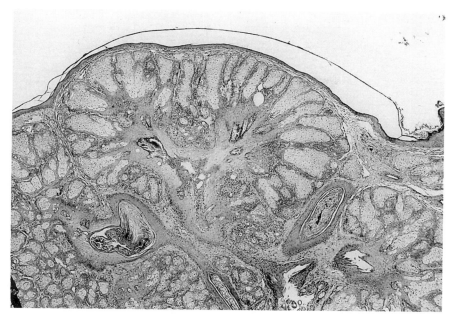

FIG. 2.5—Dog lid sebaceous adenoma. Lobules showing sebaceous hyperplasia and ductal occlusion. Hematoxylin-eosin, ×35.

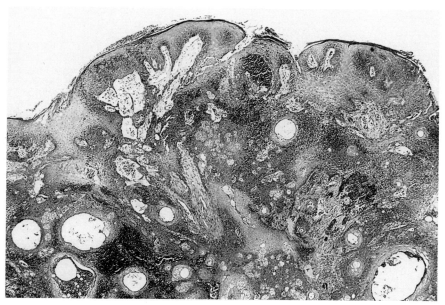

FIG. 2.6—Dog lid sebaceous adenoma with basal cell components (darker cells). Hematoxylin-eosin, ×35.

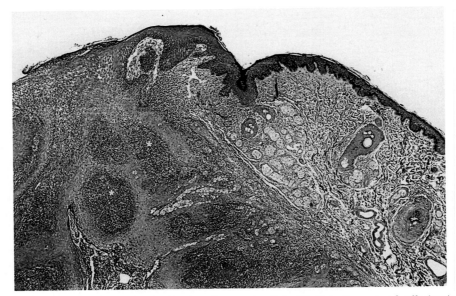

FIG. 2.7—Dog sebaceous adenoma infiltrating into the margin of the lid. Note the nests of cells (star). Hematoxylin-eosin, ×35.

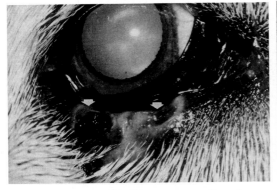

FIG. 2.8—Dog lower lid with squamous cell carcinoma historically present for 8 months. Surface serum or hemorrhage scabs recurrently slough, leaving a raw eroded lid margin. Hyperthermia alternating with hypothermia treatments destroyed the neoplasm and eventually the lid healed fairly cosmetically. Arrows identify two erosive sites.

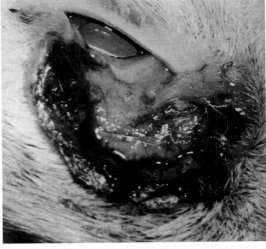

FIG. 2.9—Cat lower eyelid with squamous cell carcinoma. Severe erosion of the lid challenged a surgical excision even after the neoplasm was decreased in size by cryotherapy.

lesions in the ipsilateral parotid, lateral retropharyngeal lymph nodes, lungs, and parenchyma. Of all the cattle with ocular squamous cell carcinomas at slaughter, about 54% have metastatic lesions (Figure 2.12).

In a study comparing surgical excision to hyperthermia as the only treatment of similar ocular squamous cell carcinomas in cattle, the overall effectiveness of surgery was 46%, whereas it was 92% for hyperthermia.[31]

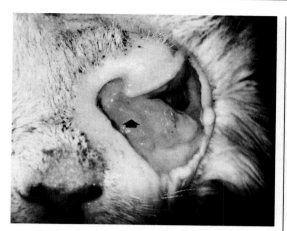

FIG. 2.10—Cat lids with squamous cell carcinoma after 2 weeks of cobalt radiation therapy. The neoplasm was arrested. The eye developed a cataractous lens secondary to radiation despite protective shielding. Adipose tissue is labeled with an arrow.

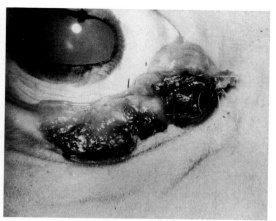

FIG. 2.11—Horse lower lid with squamous cell carcinoma. The neoplasm was surgically debulked and injected with a purified bacillus Calmette-Guérin cell wall preparation. Immunotherapy routes are successful, but the injections stimulate inflammation that temporarily disfigures the lids as much as the neoplasm.

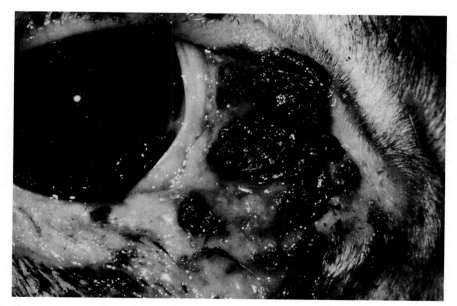

FIG. 2.12—Cow squamous cell carcinoma of the medial canthal area. These neoplasms have a distinct odor that in part is likely related to the necrosis and sepsis of the neoplasm.

Squamous cell carcinoma of the eye arises from the limbus, nictitans, or eyelid in cattle, horses, cats, and dogs, respectively. Ocular squamous cell carcinoma in cattle is the most economically significant neoplasm in domestic animals. It is relatively rare in dogs. Squamous cell tumors of cattle account for a tremendous economic loss. Much research and many classic studies have been devoted to "cancer eye" in cattle.[32,33]

Squamous cell carcinomas have a variable histologic appearance, and these features help in grading the neoplastic characteristics (Broder's classification):

Grade I squamous cell carcinomas are well-differentiated tumors composed of tumor cells with abundant eosinophilic cytoplasm, intercellular bridges, and concentric laminated masses of keratin with the classic *keratin pearls*. Mitotic activity is minimal, as is nuclear pleomorphism. Tumor cell invasion into the subcutis is accompanied by proliferations of fibrous connective tissue.

Grade II and III squamous cell carcinomas are moderately differentiated, composed of tumor cells with less eosinophilic cytoplasm, more nuclei pleomorphism, and hyperchromatism. Mitotic activity and bizarre morphology are prominent. Fewer keratin pearls are found as well as intercellular bridges. Invasion is more prominent with smaller tumor islands than with the well-differentiated tumors.

Grade IV squamous cell carcinomas show little squamous differentiation. The cell cytoplasm appears amphophilic with nuclei that are extremely pleomorphic and hyperchromatic. There are many mitotic cells. These tumors show deep or severe infiltration.

Metastasis is more likely to occur with poorly differentiated tumors of grades III and IV. Metastases are uncommon and usually are via lymphatics to regional lymph nodes and lungs. Squamous cell carcinoma of the eyelids may recur at the site of local excision mainly because wide resection is difficult.

Combination therapy for lid squamous cell carcinomas is advised. This includes debulking and the use of either thermotherapy, cryotherapy, immunotherapy (BCG injection), or radiation therapy alone or in conjunction with radiation sensitizers. Photodynamic therapy of squamous cell carcinoma in a cat has been described using chloroaluminum sulfonated phthalocyanine (CASPc) activated in the tumor by an argon laser emitting 675-nm light energy.[23] Chemotherapy with cisplatin has been used to treat squamous cell carcinoma in a dog at dosages of 40–60 mg/m^2 of body surface at 21-day intervals.[24] Chemotherapy of squamous cell carcinoma with bleomycin, benzaldehyde, thioproline, and acral retinoids has been ineffective.[25]

In a retrospective study, papilloma virus structural antigens were demonstrated in five of nine dog cutaneous squamous cell carcinomas, suggesting that papilloma viruses have an etiologic role in squamous cell tumors. Squamous cell carcinomas have occurred at the injection sites of live canine oral papillomavirus vaccine in some dogs.[25] Squamous cell carcinoma is fairly common in the lid and conjunctiva of horses and cows, but is rare in dogs. Solar radiation has been suggested in the pathogenesis of squamous cell carcinoma, hemangiomas, and hemangiosarcomas in dogs,[26] cats, cows, and horses (Figures 2.13–2.16).

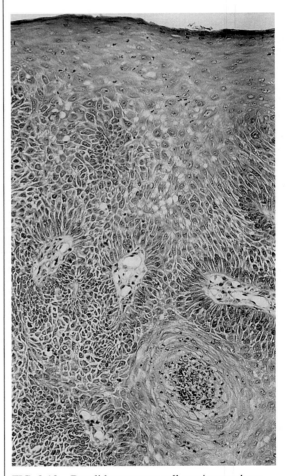

FIG. 2.13—Dog lid squamous cell carcinoma showing hyperplastic projections away from the surface epithelium. The surface appears as an acanthomatous plaque. The cellular differentiation is moderate. Hematoxylin-eosin, ×140.

Papilloma. Papillomas involving the lids have been reported in dogs, cows, horses, and sheep. In all cases, papillomas look similar, with a rough surface that is lobulated, elevated, and papillary. Microscopically, the lesion is made up of hyperplastic squamous epithelial fronds containing cores of vascularized connective tissue. Papillomas involve only the superficial epithelial layers (Figures 2.17–2.19).

Clinically, papilloma and squamous cell carcinoma can both look papillary and lobulated with a cauliflower-like appearance. Squamous cell carcinomas of long standing invade locally, causing deeper tissue destruction and infiltration. Squamous cell carcinomas grow more slowly than papillomas.[34] Management of papillomas has been good by excision alone in older animals, but excision should be followed by cryotherapy in younger animals.

Papillomatous lesions are common on the face of horses younger than 24 months of age. These tumors have a warty character occurring in clusters of 2–10 cm in diameter. Papillomatosis is the infectious variety caused by the papilloma virus. Vaccination protection against the virus is recommended for foals 2–3 months of age, especially if there is an environmental history of the disease. Papilloma viruses have been demonstrated in

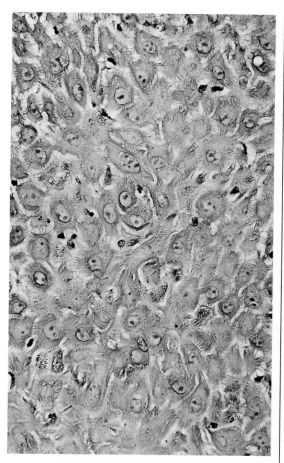

FIG. 2.14—Cow lid squamous cell carcinoma. This lid neoplasm was well differentiated and characterized by intercellular bridges, abundant cytoplasm, homogeneous nuclear patterns, and very few mitotic cells. Hematoxylin-eosin, ×40.

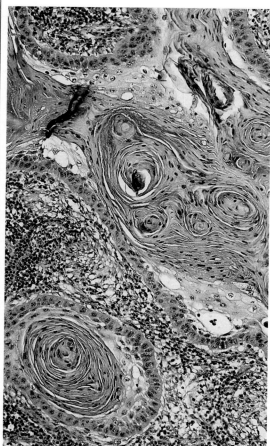

FIG. 2.15—Cow squamous cell carcinoma invasive into the lids and nictitans. This neoplasm was well differentiated with typical keratin pearls. Hematoxylin-eosin, ×140.

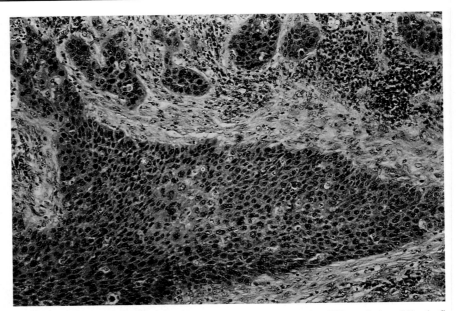

FIG. 2.16—Horse lid with squamous cell carcinoma with moderate cellular differentiation. Mitotic figures are evident (circle), and a more pleomorphic population of cells (*) is present in the center of the photograph. Surrounding inflammation is a common finding. Hematoxylin-eosin, ×140.

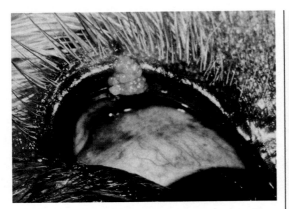

FIG. 2.17—Dog lid tumors are common in the middle to older age groups. This pedunculated marginal lid tumor was classified as a fibropapilloma histopathologically.

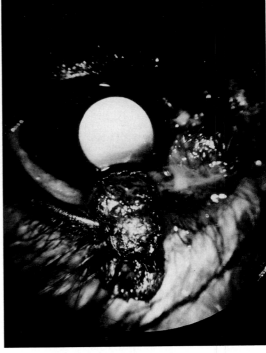

FIG. 2.18—Dog lid papilloma. These neoplasms were debulked and the bases treated with cryosurgery. The results were considered satisfactory.

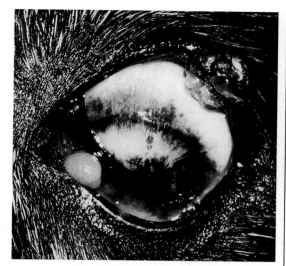

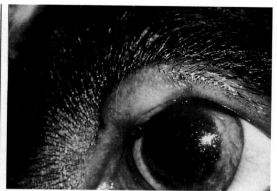

FIG. 2.20—Dog upper-lid histiocytoma. These neoplasms are characterized by rapid growth in young dogs.

FIG. 2.19—Dog lids with two neoplasms: a sebaceous adenoma on the upper lid and a fibropapilloma on the bottom lid. The eye is a phthisical cataractous globe.

plaques and cutaneous horns around cow eyes,[35] as well as in hyperkeratotic lesions of sheep,[36] rabbits,[37] and mice lids.[38]

Histiocytic Tumors. Nodular lesions of the lid, nictitans, and globe may be seen singularly or concurrently. Terms such as nodular granulomatous episclerokeratitis, fibrous histiocytoma, proliferative keratoconjunctivitis, pseudotumor, collie granuloma, and ocular nodular fasciitis have been used to describe apparently similar lesions. The cellular makeup of these lesions includes lymphocytes, plasma cells, monocytes, fibrocytes, and histiocytes. The predominant cell type varies, and the primary cell origin is undetermined, although the larger cell types are consistent with histiocytes. Occasionally, multinucleated cells are noted. The morphology of these lesions no doubt accounts for the many names given to this tumor. Although this lesion has been seen in many breeds of dogs and even cats and horses, it is most frequently diagnosed in the collie type breed. The nodular lesions of the lid are thought to be immune-mediated reactive granulomas of unknown etiology.[39] Excision, cryoablation, intralesional corticosteroids, and topical or systemic immunomodulators, including interferon, alone or in combination are therapeutic options.

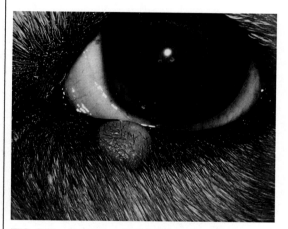

FIG. 2.21—Dog lower-lid histiocytoma. Although these tumors spontaneously regress, they will regress even more quickly if treated with cryosurgery.

Solitary histiocytomas are classically benign and minimally invasive. Histiocytomas involve both the dermis and the subcutis. They are usually found in 2- to 3-year-old dogs, appearing as either papillary or pedunculated dome-shaped lesions. Histiocytomas may have a central ulcerated zone.[34] The author's (R.C.R.) experience with management of histiocytomas has been good with cryosurgery. If the lid tumor is concurrent with other tumors, chemotherapy management with azathioprine as the drug of choice is suggested. Occasionally, corticosteroids are used as an adjunctive treatment (Figures 2.20–2.24).

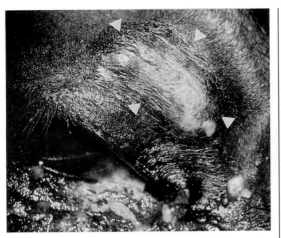

FIG. 2.22—Horse upper lid with a histiocytoma with enough bulk to cause ptosis. The triangles outline the borders of the tumor.

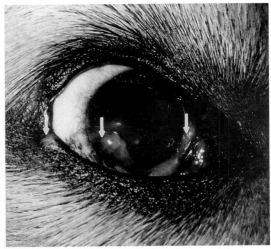

FIG. 2.23—Dog lid, limbus, and nictitans with tumors best responsive to azathioprine and/or cryosurgery. These tumors have been histologically called *fibrous histiocytomas* or *nodular granulomatous episcleroker-atitis* among many other descriptive names.

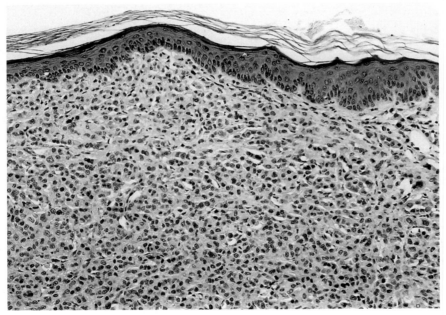

FIG. 2.24—Dog lid fibrous histiocytoma with a mixed population of cell types: mononuclear cells (lymphocytes, plasma cells, monocytes, and histiocytes), fibroblasts or fibrocytes, and occasionally giant cells. Hematoxylin-eosin, ×140.

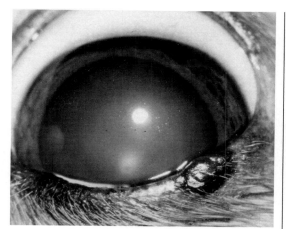

FIG. 2.25—Dog lid melanoma that had slowly expanded into adjacent tissue over 2 years of observation. Full-thickness lid resection was curative.

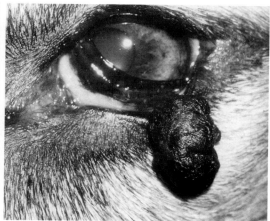

FIG. 2.26—Dog lid with a marginal pedunculated melanoma growing mainly onto the external surface. Lid function was impaired as the neoplasm grew slowly over several years.

Melanomas. Neuroepithelial cells of the neural crest are probably the origin of dermoepidermal melanocytes. Melanomas of the eyelid of dogs accounted for approximately 20% in one study;[5] 8% of those melanomas were classified as malignant. Malignancy of skin melanomas is determined by invasiveness of the dermis and epithelium, inflammatory infiltrates, and atypical cells.[40]

Melanomas of the lids of animals are usually pigmented and have a history of a nodule enlarging until it develops into either an external pedunculated mass or an infiltrative internal mass (Figures 2.25–2.27). Local recurrence is frequent following conservative excision; however, the prognosis for animals with malignant melanomas is fair if the margins are free of neoplastic cells. If the melanoma has mature, smaller cells surrounded by connective tissue fibrils as the cells progress from epidermal to the deeper dermal tissue, the melanoma is less malignant (Figures 2.28 and 2.29). Malignant melanoma cells tend to be larger and pleomorphic, containing large nuclei and prominent nucleoli. Mitotic activity may be difficult to judge without bleaching the histosection. Ulceration and inflammation are components of many neoplastic melanomas.

Malignant melanomas of the lid of young animals are rare. The case shown in Figures 2.30

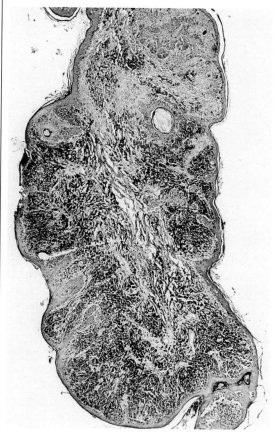

FIG. 2.27—Gross histopathology of the preceding figure. Hematoxylin-eosin, ×35.

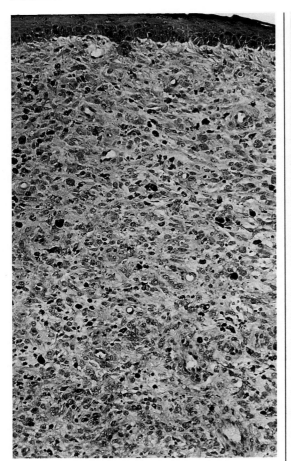

FIG. 2.28—Dog lid marginal melanoma with growth over a 6-month period. Cell types were generally similar with some cells heavily pigmented. Hematoxylin-eosin, ×140.

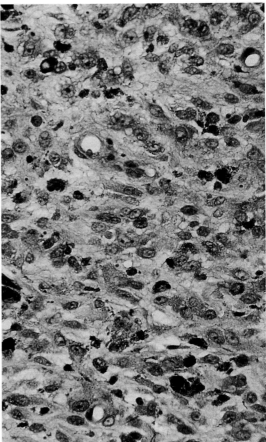

FIG. 2.29—Dog lid melanoma from the preceding figure at a higher magnification. The larger cell types predominate, and their abundant cytoplasm gives this neoplasm an open appearance. Hematoxylin-eosin, ×350.

and 2.31 is in an 8-week-old Labrador puppy with extensive lid-orbital involvement. Metastasis to the regional lymph node and thoracic nodes was found. Occasionally, poorly pigmented melanomas act aggressively to locally invade and metastasize (Figures 2.32–2.34).

Generally, horses are infrequently affected by lid melanomas, except the gray and white-coated breeds (Arabian, Lippizan, Percheron, and pinto) have an increased risk for cutaneous melanomas (Figure 2.35). Historically, melanomas of the skin are localized, slow-growing,

and pigmented neoplasms that do not metastasize. Surgical excisional therapy and/or cryotherapy has been successful management of lid horse melanomas.[41]

Basal Cell Carcinoma. Basal cell carcinomas of the lids of animals are quite uncommon and may be multilobulated and variably pigmented. The surface may show ulceration.[42] Basal cell carcinomas have also been called basal cell epitheliomas, basalomas, and "rodent ulcers." They are minimally aggressive neoplasms in

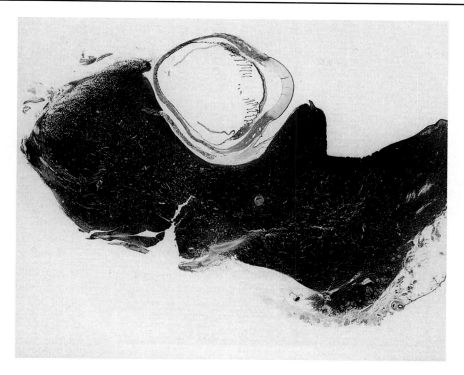

FIG. 2.30—A 9-week-old pup presented with swollen lids and orbital involvement. This gross histopathology preparation shows the extent of growth. It is rare to see congenital melanomas. ×2.4. (From David Covitz, DVM.)

dogs and cats, arising from the basal cells of the epidermis, hair follicles, sebaceous glands, and sweat glands. Basal cell tumors occur in dogs and cats at an average age of 7 and 9 years, respectively. Microscopically, the basal cell carcinoma involves only the superficial dermal tissue, but with potential to progress locally with projections away from the primary lesions. Full-thickness eyelid sections are recommended in their excisional treatment.

Sarcoid. The most common lid tumor in horses, donkeys, and mules younger than 7 years of age is the sarcoid. There is no predilection for horses of any particular gender or coat color,[43,44] although thoroughbreds may be genetically at highest risk. Sarcoids are fibroblastic tumors that are considered benign, but may be disfiguring and aggressive in their growth characteristics.

Sarcoids basically are of three types: (1) verrucous or wartlike, characterized by a dry, cauliflower, hairless lesion of usually less than 6 cm in diameter; (2) fibroblastic granulomatous tissue as large or greater than 20 cm in diameter; and (3) a mixture of types 1 and 2. The histologic diagnosis of a sarcoid may be fibroma, dermatofibroma, or fibrogranuloma. The cause of equine sarcoid remains uncertain, but bovine papilloma virus[45] (BPV 1 and 2) and a C-type retrovirus[46] have been implicated. Genetics, immunity, and infection probably all play a role in the sarcoid etiology.

Sarcoids that are small and localized can be treated with either hyperthermia or hypothermia. Larger sarcoids respond to immunotherapy using a purified commercial-killed BCG product[47] and cryosurgery.[43,48] A series of three intralesional BCG injections are given every 2 weeks. Debulking of

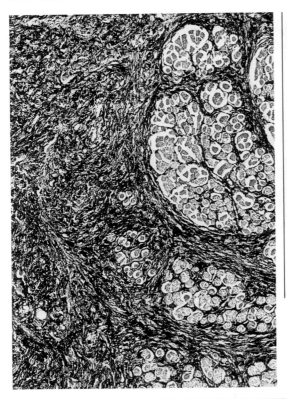

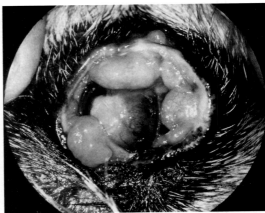

FIG. 2.32—Dog lid neoplasms that were thought to be papillomas, but rapid regrowth from previous excisions indicated an aggressive tumor. Metastasis to the orbit and lymphatics followed. Melanoma was ultimately diagnosed.

FIG. 2.31—A 9-week-old puppy melanoma of the lid and orbit in the same case as preceding figure. Note the infiltrating malignant melanoma cell patterns into the orbicularis muscle. Metastasis to the lymph nodes of the neck and thorax were also found.

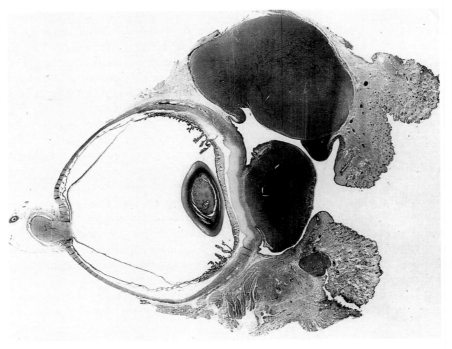

FIG. 2.33—Gross histopathology of the preceding eye neoplasm, with extension to the cornea shown. Hematoxylin-eosin, ×3.

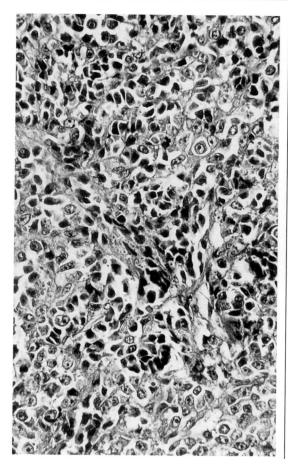

FIG. 2.34—Dog lid melanoma of the preceding two figures showing the cellular morphology. Note the variable melanin content throughout. Hematoxylin-eosin, ×350.

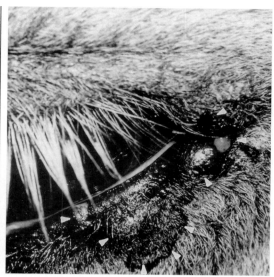

FIG. 2.35—Horse lower-lid melanoma with multifocal tumors causing minimal lid dysfunction. Several cryosurgical treatments arrested the growth, and a 3-year follow-up found no new growth.

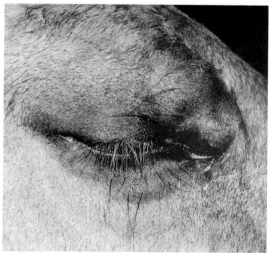

FIG. 2.36—Horse with an upper-lid swelling biopsied and diagnosed as a sarcoid. These tumors are considered the most common skin neoplasm in horses.

the lesion is recommended before the BCG injections (Figures 2.36–2.41).

Habronemiasis. Horse lid tumors occurring in the spring or summer may be due to granulomas caused by the parasite larvae of *Habronema.* These tumors are usually larger than 2 cm in diameter, hemorrhagic, and sometimes draining an exudate (Figure 2.42). Cytologic evaluation of the exudate shows predominantly eosinophils and mast cells. If the tumor displays a yellowish concentration on the conjunctival side of the lid or within the lid, surgical excision is recommended. The material removed histologically is necrotic inflammatory tissue. Systemic ivermectin treatment is effective.[49,50]

Chalazion. Chalazion (internal hordeolum) of the meibomian glands manifests as either solitary

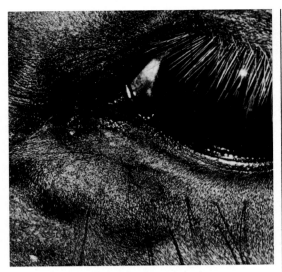

FIG. 2.37—Horse lid neoplasm diagnosed as a dermatofibroma. This neoplasm was treated as a sarcoid with immunotherapy (bacillus Calmette-Guérin).

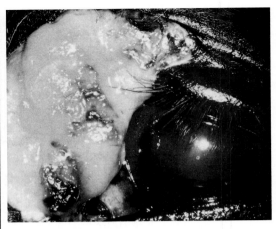

FIG. 2.39—Horse lid medial canthal sarcoid that is the verrucous type of sarcoid tumor with surface crusting and necrosis-associated inflammation. After surgical debulking and multiple immunotherapy (bacillus Calmette-Guérin) treatments, the results were satisfactory.

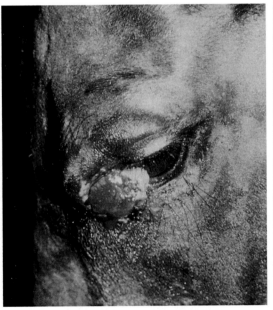

FIG. 2.38—Horse with a medial canthal sarcoid. The pedunculated nature of the neoplasm facilitated excision. Tissue at the base was treated by cryotherapy with satisfactory results. (From M. Neaderland, DVM.)

or multiple lesions of the glands, with resultant inflammation involving the conjunctival surface of the eyelids (Figure 2.43). This is seen more frequently in middle-aged dogs as chronic painless inflammation. Solitary abscess *stye* or multiple abscesses on the eyelid margins are external hordeolums or *styes* that involve the follicular glands of the cilia (Figure 2.44). These occur more frequently acutely in young animals, causing a painful squint, and are usually caused by *Staphylococcus* organisms (Figures 2.45 and 2.46). Chalazion may be associated with meibomian gland neoplasia when glandular obstruction causes glandular contents to be released interstitially, resulting in a granulomatous foreign-body response. Use of topical antibiotics and hot compresses is the usual treatment, but surgical excision may be required. Stubborn cases are aided by the use of parental as well as topical antibiotics (Figures 2.47 and 2.48).[51]

Eyelid Cysts. Cysts of the lid and conjunctiva may be congenital, inflammatory, traumatic, or secondary to a foreign body and rarely from a primary or secondary neoplasm. Surgical excision to remove the cyst and small fistulous tracts carefully is recommended. Recurrence of the cyst might increase the suspicion of neoplasia. The histologic findings in cystic cases included dif-

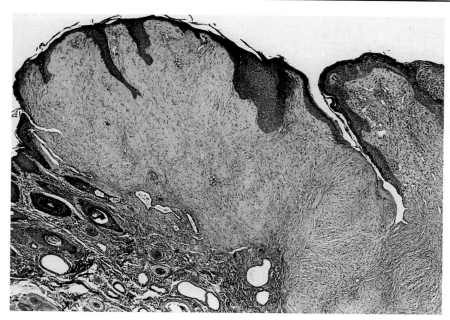

FIG. 2.40—Horse lid sarcoid with a low-magnification view of the tumor growth. The tumor infiltrates the dermis and destroys the adnexal structures. The overlying epithelium extends rete ridges into the tumor, a characteristic feature of sarcoids. Hematoxylin-eosin, ×35.

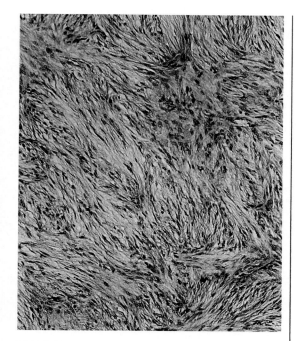

FIG. 2.41—Horse lid fibrosarcoma histopathology. This tumor responded to several treatments of bacillus Calmette-Guérin cell wall injections. Note the pattern of spiral cells forming intersecting fascicles characteristic of sarcoid.

fuse inflammation of the cyst wall and glandular tissues, or the cyst wall contained glandular acini. Flattened cuboidal epithelium and dilated intralobular ducts characterize secretion stasis. Adenocarcinomas have been the predominate neoplasm invading the orbit and lids. These neoplasms are usually from zygomatic salivary glands (Figures 2.49–2.51).[52–56]

Mast Cell Tumors. Mast cell tumors of the lid and conjunctiva have been reported.[57] Ocular mast cell tumors of the lid, nictitans, globe, and orbit have been described.[58–60] Mast cell tumors in dogs, usually noted in their advanced years, have common skin sites on the trunk and extremities. When found, the tumors can be easily diagnosed by cytology because of the cell's basophilic granular cytoplasm. Histopathology of the tumor is necessary to classify the tumors into Patnaik's grading system of mastocytomas.[61] The clinical staging of mast cell tumors should include regional lymph node aspirates, buffy-coat smears, bone marrow aspirates, and abdominal radiographs.

Metastasis of mast cell tumors is to regional lymphoid tissues or skin. Paraneoplastic syndromes

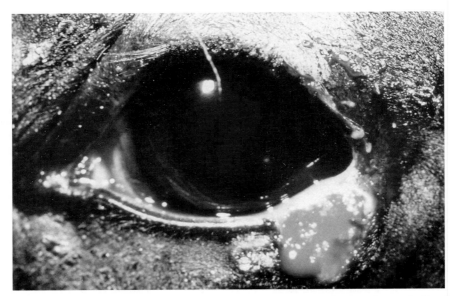

FIG. 2.42—Horse lid inflammation from the parasitic larva *Habronema.* The lid must be surgically cleaned of the caseous material, which is inspissated cellular debris and larvae. Medicate the wound with topical antibiotic-corticosteroid ointment. (From W.C. Rebhun, DVM.)

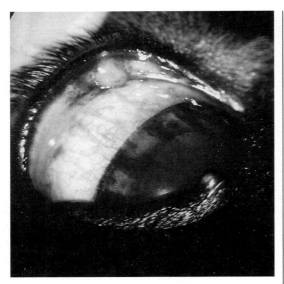

FIG. 2.43—Dog lid chalazion or inflammation of the meibomian gland. An incision on the conjunctival surface perpendicular to the margin over the swelling allows for curettage and relieves the congested inflammation. Topical antibiotics are recommended.

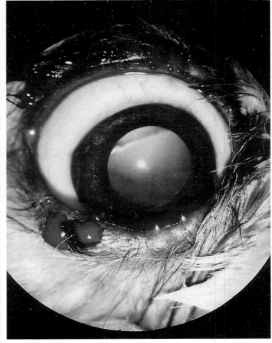

FIG. 2.44—Dog blepharitis with hemorrhagic exudative fistulas across the lid margins.

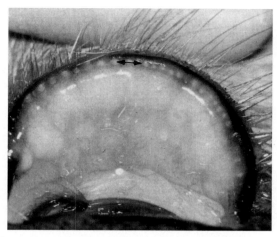

FIG. 2.45—Dog (puppy) lids swollen with painful inflammation from a *Staphylococcus* infection. The cytology from the expressed meibomian glands produced a diagnostic picture of septic inflammation that was confirmed by culture. The arrow points to the inflamed gland openings across the lid margin.

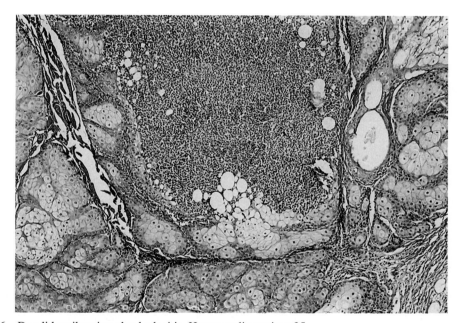

FIG. 2.46—Dog lid meibomian gland adenitis. Hematoxylin-eosin, ×35.

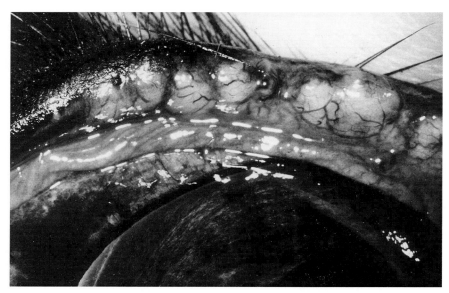

FIG. 2.47—Horse eyelid with conjunctival lesions on all four lids appearing much like chalazion. The lid swellings were well tolerated by the horse and presented over several years without change.

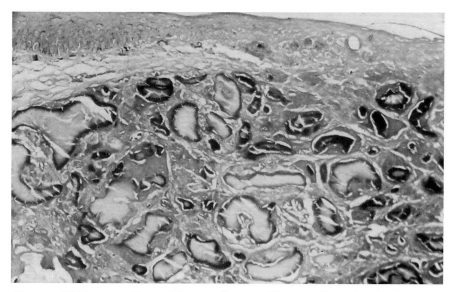

FIG. 2.48—Horse eyelid biopsy specimen of the preceding case. Hematoxylin-eosin-stained samples identified concretions of material that generated no inflammatory response. Congo red and crystal violet stained the material positively. Immunospecific stain for amyloid A was positive. Polarized light showed areas of intense polarization. This chalazion-like lesion was lid amyloidosis.

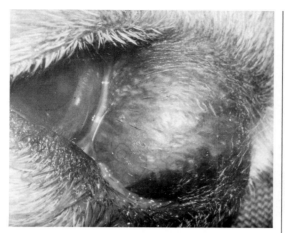

FIG. 2.49—Dog lid with medial canthal swelling caused by a cystic tumor from the accessory lacrimal tissue of the nictitans or the zygomatic salivary gland.

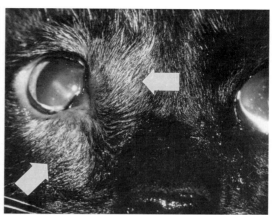

FIG. 2.51—Cat medial canthal tumor causing a firm infiltration into the upper and lower lids was diagnosed as an adenocarcinoma of the nictitans most probably arising from the accessory lacrimal gland.

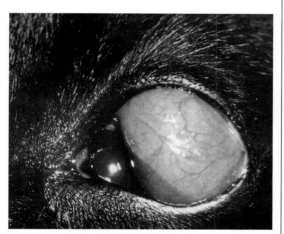

FIG. 2.50—Dog upper lid with cystic conjunctival distention from the primary lacrimal gland.

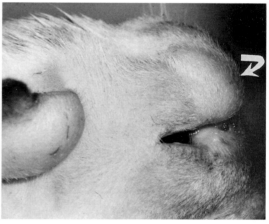

FIG. 2.52—Cat with mastocytoma of the lids and ears. This lateral view shows the swelling of the lids (arrows) that severely compromised the lid function.

secondary to the mast cell degranulation can cause functional impairment with lid mast cell tumors.

The prognosis of a mastocytoma case is based on degree of mast cell differentiation, mitotic activity of the cells, and the extent of infiltration of the tumor into adjacent tissue.[62] Biologic behavior of mast cell tumors is somewhat unpredictable, however. Tumors can remain quiescent or slow growing for years and then suddenly become highly aggressive. Mast cell tumors have been referred to as "the syphilitic lesion of the dog" because of their variable manifestations (Figures 2.52–2.56).[63]

Keratoacanthoma. Keratoacanthomas of the animal eyelid have been reported in cattle and dogs. These lesions are umbilicated, with a keratin or parakeratin-filled crypt that is lined by a layer of stratified squamous epithelium that exhibits pseudoepitheliomatous hyperplasia.

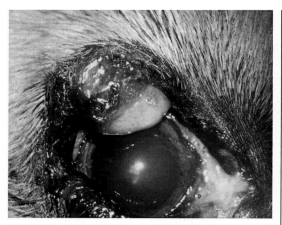

FIG. 2.53—Dog lid with a mast cell tumor growing from the margin and conjunctival surface.

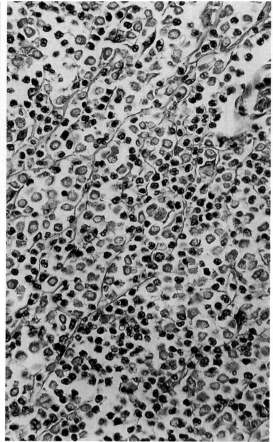

FIG. 2.54—Dog lid mastocytoma histopathology section. Note the large, dark cells: cytoplasmic granules account for these characteristics. ×350.

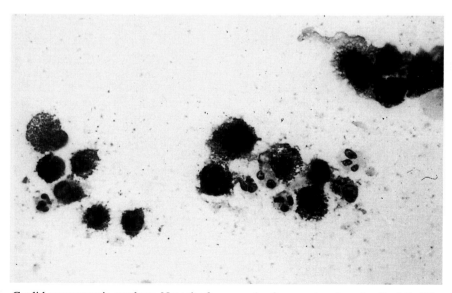

FIG. 2.55—Cat lid mastocytosis cytology. Note the free granules from ruptured mast cells. All of the vital stains will accentuate the mast cell granules to aid the diagnosis. Wright's stain, ×1000.

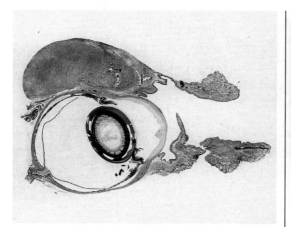

FIG. 2.56—Dog lid mastocytoma extending into the orbit but not penetrating the globe.

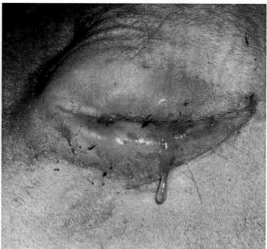

FIG. 2.57—Horse lid swollen and exuding serum. The diagnosis was a pericytoma fibroma.

These lesions are usually 0.5–2.0 cm in diameter. Keratoacanthomas seem to appear suddenly, but do not change in size after 2–3 months, allowing differentiation between the biologic behavior of squamous cell carcinoma and keratoacanthoma. Another differentiating feature is the total regression of a keratoacanthoma that occurs after several months.[64] Benign keratoacanthomas occur more often on the lower eyelid of cattle, where they appear as hyperkeratotic growths coated with lacrimal secretions and debris.[31]

Lymphomatous Lesions. Lymphomas of the lids are almost always an ocular manifestation of systemic malignant lymphoma, with multiple sites throughout the body. These tumors are usually predominantly lymphocytic, with plasma cells and histiocytes also present in significant numbers. Most isolated lymphoid lid tumors have normal blood morphology reports, but some leukemic animals have abnormal morphology of lymphoreticular components within the bone marrow. Some dogs, especially German shepherds, present with isolated lid swellings that are benign lymphoid infiltrations responsive to local corticosteroid treatment. Ocular manifestations of systemic leukemia often infiltrate cow lids and orbit. Lymphosarcoma of the horse eyelid has been rarely reported to be the cause of lid swelling (Figures 2.57 and 2.58).[65,66]

Xanthomatosis. Multiple eyelid or subcutaneous tumors containing lipid occur in cats.

Tumors range from 3 to 8 mm in diameter; they are soft, glistening, and brownish white on section. Cats with xanthomas may have increased serum lipid levels, or those whose serum levels are normal may have intracellular defects in fat metabolism.[67] Regardless of their circulating lipid levels, the tumors are not treated unless they interfere with lid function (Figure 2.59).

HUMANS

As in animals, tumors of the human eyelid are basically those tumors found in skin. Because of certain environmental and anatomic factors, however, the frequency of certain tumors differs from skin elsewhere. For example, the eyelid skin is commonly exposed to sunlight, so those lesions related to solar damage more frequently involve the lid as opposed to the torso. Another example is the relative frequency of sebaceous tumors; because of the large number of sebaceous glands found in the eyelid, tumors of sebaceous origin have a higher incidence on the eyelid than elsewhere on the skin.

A brief review of normal eyelid histology will enable one to predict which skin lesions are likely to occur in the eyelid. The eyelid is composed of six basic layers: the skin, subcutis, orbicularis muscle, septum and tarsus, smooth muscle of Müller, and palpebral conjunctiva. The skin is composed of keratinized stratified

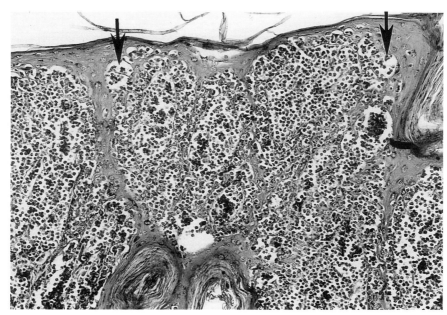

FIG. 2.58—Cow lid with lymphocytic infiltrates from periocular lymphocytic leukemia. Tumors with epitheliotrophic character (arrow) show infiltrative lymphocytes into the epithelium (epidermal necrosis) or so-called Pautrier's microabscesses. Hematoxylin-eosin, ×140.

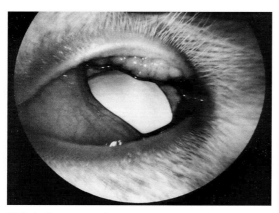

FIG. 2.59—Cat eyelid conjunctival swellings that would appear and disappear with a blink. The swellings are lipid accumulation referred to as *xanthomas.*

squamous epithelium overlying dermis. Within the epidermis are melanocytes and the normal complement of maturing squamous cells. Hair follicles and their associated sweat and sebaceous glands extend from the dermis to the skin surface.

The two groups of sebaceous glands in the eyelid are the glands of Zeis and the meibomian glands. Deep in the connective tissue, anterior to the tarsus, the roots of the eyelashes form pilosebaceous units that are called the glands of Zeis. Posterior to the eyelashes, within the tarsus, are sebaceous glands known as meibomian glands. These do not have an associated hair follicle.

Eyelashes originate at the lid margin. The apocrine sweat glands associated with the cilia are the glands of Moll. Eccrine sweat glands are found throughout the skin of the lids. Accessory lacrimal glands are found in the substantia propria of the conjunctiva. These are called Krause's glands and Wolfring's glands.

Among the mesenchymal elements comprising the lid are muscle (smooth and striated), adipose tissue, nerve, lymphatics, and vessels.

By far, epithelial lesions comprise the majority of eyelid tumors: those derived from the epidermis and skin appendages, and those derived from sebaceous and sweat glands. Other tumor types include mesenchymal lesions, vascular tumors, and melanocytic neoplasms.

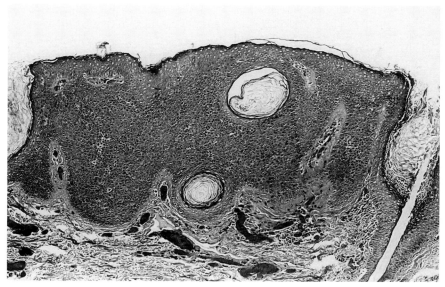

FIG. 2.60—Although there are several histologic patterns of seborrheic keratosis, the typical pattern is that of flat, thickened epidermis composed of benign basaloid cells with cystic collections of keratin called *horn cysts.*

Benign Epithelial Tumors

SEBORRHEIC KERATOSIS. Seborrheic keratosis is the most common benign neoplasm of the eyelid.[68] Usually found in middle-aged and older individuals, it is a spontaneously arising, occasionally pigmented, elevated, variably verrucous, granular to velvety growth[69] that characteristically appears to have been "pasted on." The cause of usual seborrheic keratosis has yet to be elucidated. However, these lesions have gained ominous fame in a rare paraneoplastic syndrome, Leser-Trélat, in which multiple new seborrheic keratoses or those of increasing size are associated with malignancy, most commonly of the gastrointestinal tract.[70] This manifestation has been postulated to be linked to overproduction of α-transforming growth factor by the primary tumor.[71]

Histologically, lesions are exophytic and usually well demarcated from the adjacent epidermis. They are composed of small, benign, basaloid cells containing variable melanin. Keratin production is often exuberant, producing keratin-filled cysts known as *horn cysts* or, when originating from down growth of surface keratin, as *pseudo-horn cysts* (Figure 2.60). Histologic subtypes include hyperkeratotic, adenoidal, and acanthotic variants. Again, melanin content is variable, resulting in a differential clinical diagnosis of melanoma or nevus. When inflamed, seborrheic keratoses undergo squamous differentiation resulting in whorls of squamous cells called *squamous eddies,* with enlarged nuclei and scattered mitoses, raising the histologic differential diagnosis of squamous cell carcinoma (Figure 2.61).[69,72]

Occasionally, similar histologic features may be seen to involve the epithelium of hair follicles and are termed inverted follicular keratoses. Although some authors place follicular keratoses within the spectrum of seborrheic keratoses, others separate the two entities.[73] The natural course of seborrheic keratoses is indolent, and malignant degeneration into basal or squamous cell carcinoma is rare.[69] Curettage, excision, and carbon dioxide laser vaporization are curative.

SQUAMOUS PAPILLOMA. Squamous papilloma is a nonspecific term that describes lesions of the eyelid that contain benign hyperplastic squamous epithelium. Seen in middle-aged or elderly patients, papillomas may be sessile or pedunculated. Typically, they are firm with a nodular or convoluted surface showing variable pigmentation.[74] Clinically, they may be mistaken for verrucae nevi (because they may be pigmented), seborrheic keratoses, and actinic keratoses.

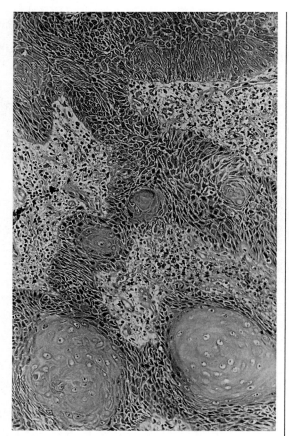

FIG. 2.61—Histologic features of an irritated seborrheic keratosis include whorls of benign squamous cells and proliferating basaloid cells.

Histologically, they are composed of hyperplastic, hyperkeratotic benign squamous epithelium overlying a fibrovascular stroma (Figure 2.62).

Their natural clinical course is indolent with slow growth. Therapy is by excision or laser ablation.

KERATOACANTHOMA. Keratoacanthomas are tumors found on sun exposed skin, usually in middle-aged to elderly individuals. Clinically, it can mimic squamous cell carcinoma, but follows an indolent course and, if left untreated, may spontaneously regress. Males are affected more than females by the lesion, which grows from a small papule to a 1- to 2.5-cm keratotic mass with a characteristic central crater within weeks to months.

Histologically, providing that sections are taken to include the crater, the architecture is distinctive. The symmetric cup-shaped lesion is well demarcated from the adjacent uninvolved epidermis. The crater, bounded by a well-defined lip of benign squamous epithelium, contains laminated keratin. The epithelium lining the crater is hyperplastic and, cytologically, the squamous cells contain abundant glycogen, resulting in a glassy cytoplasm (Figure 2.63). Should the section unfortunately be taken from the edge of the lesion, the architecture may be obscured, and the crater may be absent. In this case, the proliferating, endophytic squamous cells appear irregular and asymmetric, mimicking squamous cell carcinoma. In fact, occasionally, the differentiation of keratoacanthoma from squamous cell carcinoma cannot be made with absolute certainty; however, definite stromal invasion by single cells, vascular invasion, and lymphatic invasion require a diagnosis of carcinoma. If the tumor involves the lower reticular dermis, a feature rarely seen in keratoacanthoma, the diagnosis of carcinoma must be seriously considered.[69]

The natural course is toward complete regression, but aggressive behavior has been reported in some patients, particularly those who are immunocompromised. Therapy is variable, and biopsy may be required to provide a definitive diagnosis. In such cases, excisional biopsy, rather than a shave or incisional biopsy, is recommended, as the lesion's architecture is critical in establishing a diagnosis.

CORNU CUTANEUM. Also known as a cutaneous horn, this is a cone-shaped, hyperkeratotic mass that may overlie another lesion such as solar keratosis, squamous cell carcinoma, or even sebaceous carcinoma.[75]

Malignant and Premalignant Epithelial Lesions

SOLAR ELASTOSIS AND KERATOSIS. Exposure to sunlight has a dramatic effect on aging skin, with microscopic changes seen by age 30. The changes begin with hyperplasia of the elastic fibers and degeneration of the collagen in the upper dermis (Figure 2.64). When the collagen

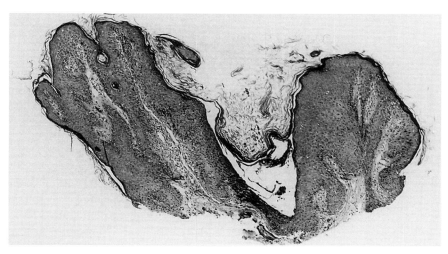

FIG. 2.62—Note the folded, papillomatous, hyperplastic epithelium of this squamous papilloma. The supporting stroma is fibrovascular.

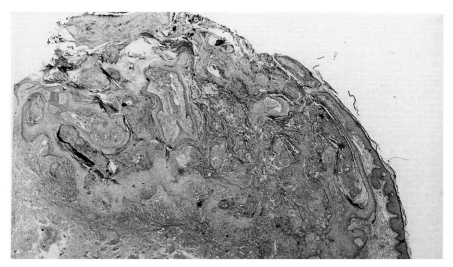

FIG. 2.63—This section of a keratoacanthoma nicely demonstrates the low-power architecture of a central crater surrounded by an epithelial lip. The high-power photograph shows the cytology of the squamous cells, particularly the glassy cytoplasm. As these may be mitotically active and have worrisome cytologic features, attention to the architecture of the lesion is critical in differentiating a keratoacanthoma from a squamous cell carcinoma.

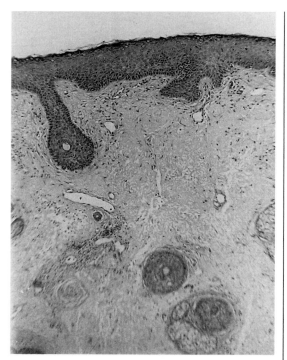

FIG. 2.64—One of the first histologic signs of sun damage to the skin is solar elastosis, a degenerative process of elastic fibers in the dermis. Note the amorphous areas in the upper dermis. Also observe that the overlying epidermis shows no dysplastic changes.

degenerates, it is replaced by amorphous basophilic material. Although these changes have been called senile elastosis, the more appropriate terminology is solar or actinic elastosis, implicating exposure to sunlight as the cause.

As sun damage continues, potentially premalignant epidermal lesions develop in which the keratinocytes become progressively dysplastic. These actinic or solar keratoses may progress to squamous cell carcinoma; however, it is important to recognize that such progression is not inevitable.

Clinically, solar keratoses are found on sun-exposed areas of light-skinned individuals. They usually measure less than 1 cm in diameter[69] and have a rough, scaly surface. Lesions may be pigmented or erythematous. Occasionally, mounds of keratin give the appearance of a cutaneous horn.

Histologically, actinic keratoses usually show degeneration of the collagen in the upper dermis

and, by definition, always show varying degrees of epidermal dysplasia. The changes begin in the basal layer and may progress to involve all layers of the epidermis (carcinoma in situ). The keratinocytes show cytoatypia with enlarged, hyperchromatic nuclei and an increased nuclear-to-cytoplasmic ratio. Some cells may acquire dense orange cytoplasm indicating inappropriate keratin formation or dyskeratosis. As the epithelium becomes dysplastic, orderly maturation is perturbed. Depending on the degree of dysplasia, mitoses, normally found in the basal layer only, may be found throughout the epidermis. Some may even be atypical (Figure 2.65). Associated hyperkeratosis and parakeratosis may be present, and a chronic inflammatory infiltrate is usually found in the upper dermis.

Recognizing that not all actinic keratoses progress to carcinoma, therapy is based on symptoms, size, and location of the lesion. Surgical excision or cryotherapy, with follow-up, are recommended.

SQUAMOUS CELL CARCINOMA IN SITU. Characteristically, epidermal dysplasia begins at the basal layer and progresses upward. The term squamous cell carcinoma in situ or Bowen's disease indicates that all layers of epidermis are dysplastic; however, the dermis has not been invaded by tumor.

Clinically, the lesions present as erythematous, keratotic plagues that are usually larger than actinic keratoses.[76] In long-standing lesions, horny plugs tend to develop.[77] In a study of 22 cases, duration of symptoms prior to referral ranged from a few weeks to 10 years.[77]

Histologically, full-thickness dysplasia may involve both the surface epithelium and that surrounding skin appendages (Figure 2.66). Although some lesions may be hyperkeratotic and papillary, others may be nonkeratotic and flat.

Surgical excision is the treatment of choice.[77]

SQUAMOUS CELL CARCINOMA. Invasive squamous cell carcinoma may arise de novo or in the setting of a precancerous dermatosis such as solar keratosis or Bowen's disease. It is also seen following carcinogenic insults like ionizing irradiation and in genetic disorders like xeroderma pigmentosum, an autosomal recessive disorder of

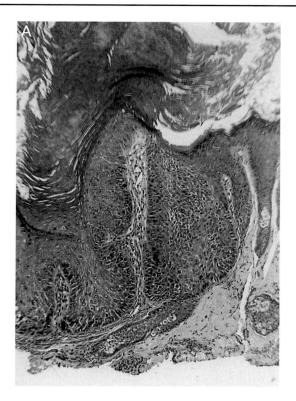

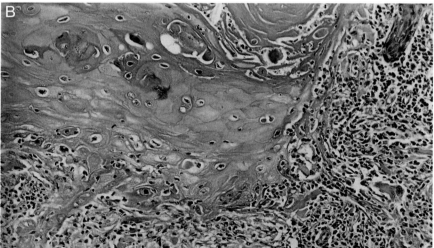

FIG. 2.65—In this actinic keratosis, solar degeneration is also observed **(A).** Additionally, however, one observes dysplastic changes in the lower epidermis **(B).**

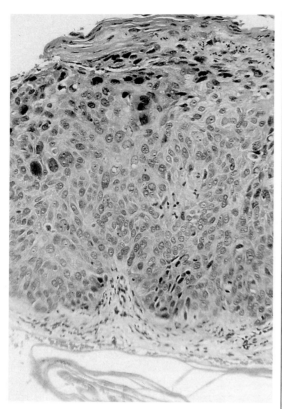

FIG. 2.66—The full-thickness epidermal dysplasia seen in this photograph represents squamous cell carcinoma in situ. Note the large, atypical cells extending to the surface. Also observe the lack of invasion through the basement membrane.

ultraviolet-light-damaged DNA.[78] Another recently implicated villain in the development of eyelid squamous cell carcinoma is human papilloma virus (HPV), whose genome has been detected within the lesions by the sensitive polymerase chain reaction technique.[79]

Whether arising de novo or in a preexisting lesion, squamous cell carcinoma, by definition, is a malignant proliferation of epidermal cells retaining characteristics of the suprabasal epidermis.[69] An invasive squamous cell carcinoma is one that has disrupted the basement membrane and has invaded the dermis or deeper.

Squamous cell carcinoma is the second most frequent eyelid malignancy,[80] with an incidence relative to all malignant lid tumors of between 2.4% and 30.2%.[81] With a tendency for lower-lid and lid-margin involvement, squamous cell carcinoma presents frequently as an irregular lesion with rolled edges and central ulceration.[82] Bleeding, due to ulceration, may be reported. Occasionally, the growth may be nodular or cystic. Squamous cell carcinoma may also underlie a cutaneous horn.[80] Because of these nonspecific characteristics, the clinical diagnosis may be difficult to establish. In one study of 31 squamous cell carcinomas, preoperative clinical diagnoses were correct in only four cases. Frequent misdiagnoses were basal cell carcinoma and senile keratosis.[82]

Histologically, the picture is that of an invasive epithelial malignancy that may sometimes be seen arising from an intraepithelial lesion (carcinoma in situ). The overall architecture is asymmetric, with surface ulceration common. The tumor invades the dermis in nests and sheets. Characteristically, malignant cells have rather distinct cytoplasmic borders; a moderate amount of eosinophilic, sometimes keratinized cytoplasm; large, pleomorphic, hyperchromatic nuclei; and prominent nucleoli. Intercellular bridges may identify the squamous nature of the cells. Keratin formation is variable, ranging from absent to present in individual cells to abundant pearls (Figure 2.67). The infiltrated dermis may exhibit a desmoplastic response to tumor, a feature that may help distinguish carcinoma from benign lesions that mimic cancer. Usually, a chronic inflammatory infiltrate is present within the dermis, and, in ulcerated or infected lesions, an acute inflammatory infiltrate and suppuration may be seen as well. The degree of differentiation of this lesion is judged by how well tumor cells resemble their cell of origin. Well-differentiated tumors may produce abundant keratin and easily identified intercellular bridges whereas poorly differentiated tumors may show no keratin formation, and intracellular bridges may not be detected by light microscopy. In the latter, immunohistochemical stains for cytokeratins or electron microscopy may allow classification of the tumor.

Squamous cell carcinoma may be locally aggressive. It also may invade vascular and lymphatic channels, spreading to regional lymph nodes or producing distant metastases. Regional lymph node metastases have been reported to range from 1.3% to 21.4%.[76] The lymphatic drainage for most of the upper lid and the lateral canthus is to the parotid nodes. The drainage for most of the lower lid and the medial canthus is to the submaxillary nodes.[81] Finally, perineural invasion is a mode of spread that allows invasion of the orbit, periorbital tissue, and cranium.

After biopsy-proven diagnosis and staging, the preferred mode of treatment is resection, with frozen-section monitoring of margins. Alternative or adjuvant therapy such as irradiation, cryotherapy, or chemotherapy may be required in nonsurgical patients or in advanced disease.[76]

BASAL CELL CARCINOMA. Representing about 90% of all malignant eyelid tumors,[83] basal cell carcinoma is the most common malignant tumor of the eyelid, frequently occurring on the lower lid. Most occur in older patients; however, these lesions are also seen in patients 20–40 years old.[84] Like squamous cell carcinoma, the major etiologic association appears to be exposure to sunlight.[80]

Clinically, these lesions present as small, pearly, firm nodules with fine telangiectatic blood vessels on the surface. As they grow, central umbilication or erosion may develop, resulting in a "rodent ulcer" with rolled edges. Lesions may also be pigmented, raising the clinical differential diagnosis of a melanocytic lesion. Perhaps the most worrisome variant, however, is the highly invasive, morphea-form basal cell carcinoma that manifests as a pale, indurated plaque. Accounting for about 15% of basal cell carcinomas,[83] these differ clinically and histologically from typical basal cell carcinoma and are known to be particularly difficult to resect completely, as strands of tumor commonly infiltrate well beyond the grossly apparent lesion.[85]

Histologically, basal cell carcinomas arise from the basal layer of epidermis and infiltrate the dermis in cords and nests. The tumor cells are fairly uniform, small basophilic cells with high nuclear-to-cytoplasmic ratios. Mitoses are variable. Peripheral palisading of tumor cells and retraction artifact surrounding nests are characteristic of this tumor (Figure 2.68). In the morphea-form basal cell carcinoma, cords of tumor diffusely invade the dermis into deeper tissues, including muscle, resulting in a brisk desmoplastic stromal reaction (Figure 2.68F).

Usually, any damage done by basal cell carcinoma is local. Metastases are rare; however, spinal metastases and meningeal carcinomatosis from basal cell carcinoma of the lid have been reported.[86] Intraocular invasion has been reported as well.[87]

Recommended therapy for a biopsy-proven lesion is complete excision, with frozen-section analysis of the margins, particularly in cases of large lesions, recurrent lesions, or morphea-form types.[88–90] The Mohs' technique or chemosurgery is another treatment option, with the clinically apparent tumor excised and the surrounding tissue sampled and analyzed by frozen section. For nonsurgical patients, radiation therapy may be therapeutic,[80] and cisplatinum chemotherapy, while not curative, may result in partial tumor regression.[91]

Adnexal Tumors. Tumors of the skin appendages are first categorized by their similarity to mature appendages with respect to pilar, eccrine, apocrine, or sebaceous differentiation. They are further classified by their degree of differentiation, from lesions that distinctly resemble the appendage of origin to those whose origin is difficult to determine. Most skin appendage tumors are benign; however, malignant degeneration has been reported. Particularly in the eyelid where sebaceous glands are concentrated, one must be aware of sebaceous carcinoma.

TUMORS WITH PILAR DIFFERENTIATION

TRICHOFOLLICULOMA. Trichofolliculoma is a tumor of pilar differentiation that closely resembles the hair follicle. The small lesion characteristically contains a central pore from which immature white hairs protrude (Winer's dilated pore).[92] Lack of the wisps of fine hair has led to clinical misdiagnosis.[93]

Histologically, a cystic space representing the primary hair follicle is present within the dermis.

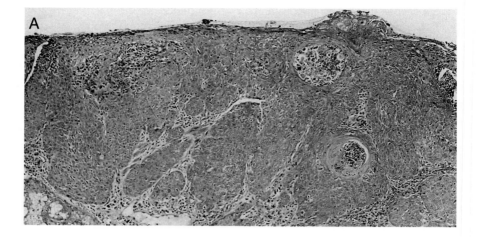

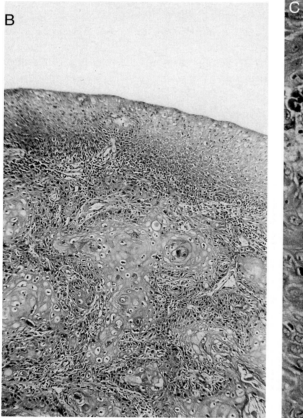

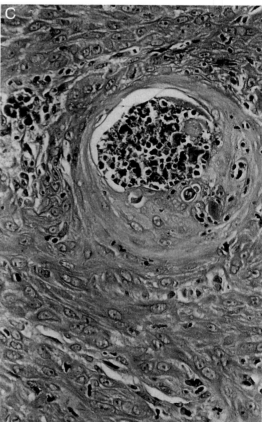

FIG. 2.67—In contrast to the lack of invasion in squamous cell carcinoma in situ, this invasive squamous cell carcinoma clearly demonstrates nests of tumor cells beyond the basement membrane (**A**). The squamous differentiation of the tumor is recognized by the nesting architecture. Additionally, the individual cell keratinization and intercellular bridges seen confirm the nature of the malignant cells (**B and C**). (continued)

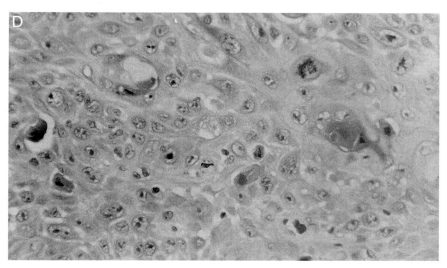

FIG. 2.67 (continued)—Note the nuclear pleomorphism and the atypical mitoses **(D).**

It is lined by squamous epithelium and contains keratin and fragments of hair shaft (Figure 2.69). Occasionally, when orientation and sectioning are optimal, one observes the cyst communicating with the epidermis. Radiating from the cyst wall are secondary follicles that may contain hair papillae. These secondary follicles have outer and inner root sheaths and may contain small groups of sebaceous glands within their walls. Complete excision is recommended.

TRICHOLEMMOMAS. Tricholemmoma is a benign tumor arising from the outer sheath of the hair follicle. Clinically, the lesion is small, nodular, and usually solitary. Sometimes, it has an irregular surface.[94] In one review of 31 cases, patient age ranged from 22 to 88 years.[95]

Histologically, the tumor is well defined and variably verrucous, with acanthotic lobules of epithelium extending into the dermis. The peripheral cells may palisade, resembling basal cell carcinoma. Occasionally, the lobules surround a hair follicle. Pathologically, the differential diagnosis may include verruca vulgaris because of the hyperkeratosis, basal cell carcinoma, and squamous cell carcinoma. In fact, misdiagnosis as squamous cell carcinoma has been well documented. Positive periodic acid-Schiff (PAS) staining not resistant to diastase confirms the presence of glycogen in the epithelium and may aid in the diagnosis.[96]

Of special note is the importance of multiple tricholemmomas seen in Cowden's disease, an autosomal dominant genodermatosis in which mucocutaneous lesions are related to carcinomas of the breast and thyroid. Although complete excision to prevent recurrence is the preferred treatment, the required margin of resection is narrower than for a malignant tumor.[97]

TRICHOEPITHELIOMA. Trichoepithelioma is a tumor of hair matrix cells that unsuccessfully attempt to form hair shafts, resulting in horn cysts. It is less differentiated than the trichofolliculoma, although they are similar in that they both represent all elements of the pilosebaceous apparatus.[69] Clinically, the lesions are often multiple, are more common in the young, and present as asymptomatic, flesh-colored nodules.[94]

Histologically, the basaloid cells form nests and cords within a fibrotic, occasionally desmoplastic stroma. The characteristic horn cysts show abrupt keratinization in the nests of basaloid cells. Because of the desmoplasia, this

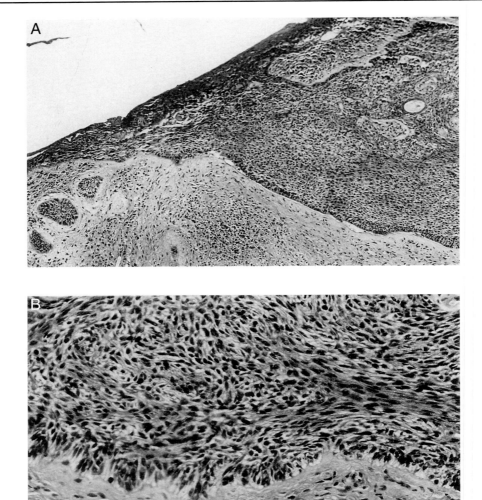

FIG. 2.68—Photographs of basal cell carcinomas. **A:** A low-power view of a tumor that is continuous with the overlying epidermis. **B:** On high power, the basaloid cells at the lesion's edge show prominent palisading of their nuclei. (continued)

abrupt keratinization is an important finding to differentiate trichoepithelioma from the morphea-form variant of basal cell carcinoma.

PILOMATRIXOMA. Pilomatrixoma, also known as benign calcified epithelioma of Malherbe, is a benign neoplasm of skin appendages with both hair matrix and cortex differentiation.[69] First described in 1880 by Malherbe and Chenantais,[98] the lesion was thought to be of sebaceous gland origin. Subsequently, special studies that included electron microscopy revealed the tumor's association with hair cells.[99]

Clinically, the tumor has a predilection for the head and neck and, when involving the eyelid, the most common site is the upper lid, followed

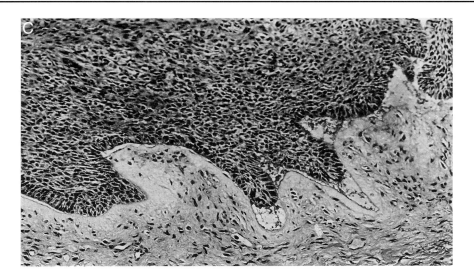

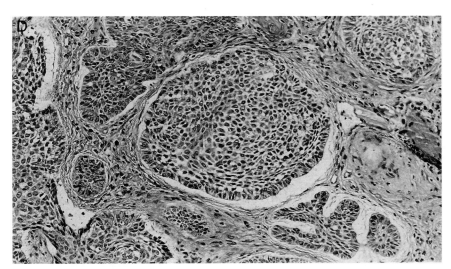

FIG. 2.68 (continued)—**C and D:** Characteristic retraction artifact. Note the separation of the tumor cells from the surrounding dermis. In addition to the nesting pattern seen in **A–D,** basal cell carcinoma may show other microscopic patterns, such as a cordlike arrangement of cells **(E).** (continued)

by the brow.[100] In a case report and review, Perez and Nicholson described six clinical features: onset in childhood or young adulthood, average size of 1 cm or less, firm to cystic consistency, moderate growth rate, pink to red-purple hue with subepithelial patches of yellow, and intact overlying skin with telangiectatic vessels.[101] Involvement of older age groups, however, has been reported. In one study of 67 cases, the age range was 2–78 years.[100]

Microscopically, a low-power profile reveals ill-defined eosinophilic material within a fibrous stroma. The eosinophilic material is composed of cell remnants that are devoid of nuclei, known as ghost or shadow cells. Basaloid cells occupy the periphery of young lesions, and one may

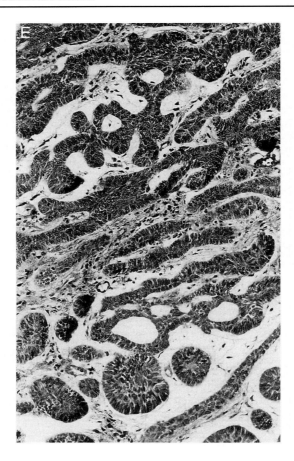

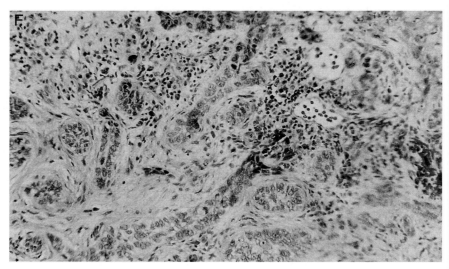

FIG. 2.68 (continued)—One particularly important clinical and histologic variant is the morphea-form basal cell carcinoma, a tumor that is difficult to resect and has a high recurrence rate. **F:** The small, infiltrative nests and cords of this variant amid a sclerotic stroma.

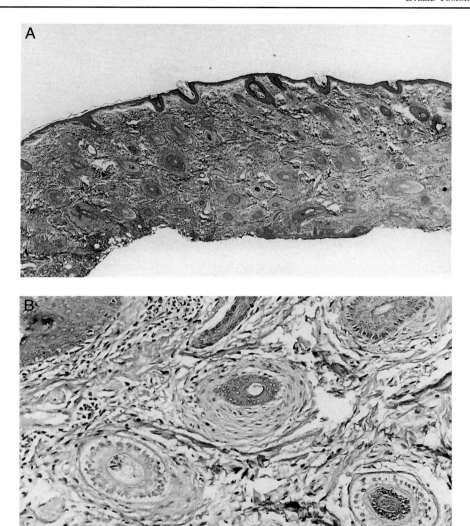

FIG. 2.69—An attempt at hair-shaft formation is seen in the low-power view of this trichofolliculoma **(A).** On higher power, one observes small round nests of epithelial cells within the dermis. Among the clues to the differentiation of this tumor is the actual hair shaft present in the center of some of these nests **(B).**

observe a transition from these cells to ghost cells. Keratinization is frequently observed, and a granulomatous response is common. As the lesions age, dystrophic calcification may be seen and, in older lesions, ossification may be observed (Figure 2.70).

Therapy is by excision, although curettage has been reported.[102]

TUMORS WITH ECCRINE OR APOCRINE DIFFERENTIATION. Eccrine tumors outnumber apocrine tumors, but, in many instances, the precise origin cannot be distinguished. The eccrine tumors involving the eyelid are the syringoma and the chondroid syringoma, the spiradenoma, and the eccrine acrospiroma. As mentioned, apocrine tumors are less common,

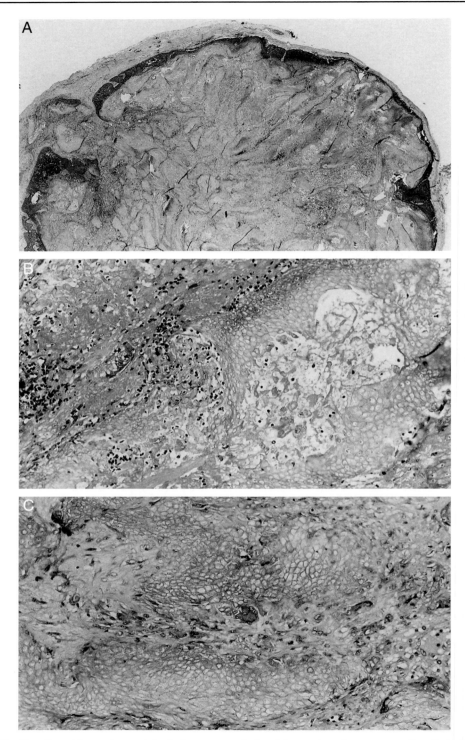

FIG. 2.70—The pilomatrixoma is a nodular lesion composed of mainly anucleated squamous cells called *ghost cells.* Peripheral basal cells are seen in the low-power micrograph (**A**), and ghost cells are recognized on the high-power views (**B and C**). A granulomatous response to the tumor is common. Note the multinucleated giant cell in **C.**

and these include the syringocystadenoma papilliferum and the hidradenoma papilliferum. The rare oncocytoma is thought to be of apocrine origin. Hidrocystomas may be of either eccrine or apocrine origin. Sweat gland carcinoma is extremely rare and may be of either eccrine or apocrine origin.

BENIGN ECCRINE TUMORS. Evidence that a tumor is of eccrine origin includes a tumor within the dermis that communicates with the epidermis and is composed of ducts lined by two cell layers. The two best-differentiated eccrine tumors are the syringoma and the eccrine hidrocystoma. An example of a less differentiated eccrine tumor occurring in the eyelid is the eccrine acrospiroma.

The syringoma is an adenoma of eccrine differentiation. Monoclonal antibody studies indicate a ductal origin of the tumor.[103] Syringoma is a common tumor of the sweat glands of the lid, occurring in over half the cases reviewed by Ni and colleagues from 1959 to 1980.[104] Lesions may be numerous, usually occur on the lower lid, and primarily affect women during puberty or later.[105] Familial cases have been reported.[103] Syringomas are small yellow to light brown papules 1–3 mm in diameter. Growing slowly, they persist asymptomatically.[94] Histologically, tadpole-shaped ducts lined by two rows of usually flat epithelial cells are imbedded in a fibrous stroma. Some ducts near the surface are dilated and contain keratin; however, solid strands of basophilic epithelial cells may also be seen (Figure 2.71). In some cases, the stroma may be fibrotic, raising both the clinical and histologic differential diagnosis of fibrosing or morpheaform basal cell carcinoma.[106]

Chondroid syringomas are similar to pleomorphic adenomas of the lacrimal and salivary glands. First described in 1859 by Bilroth,[107] they are uncommonly reported to involve the eyelid. Of the 55 sweat gland tumors reviewed by Ni and coworkers, six were chondroid syringomas.[104] Clinically, they are firm, intradermal or subcutaneous, sometimes polypoid lesions. Histologically, they consist of tubules lined by two cell layers within a mucoid stroma that may show chondroid differentiation. Interestingly, many tumors show both eccrine and

apocrine features. Malignant degeneration may occur, and complete excision is the recommended therapy.

The eccrine acrospiroma, also known as clear cell hidradenoma, is a benign rare lesion of the eyelid.[108] The lesions present as nodules that rarely may be ulcerated. Histologically, lesions are well delineated, nodular, and solid or cystic. Cells range from round to oval, with bland nuclei. Mitoses may be observed. Complete surgical excision is the treatment of choice.

Eccrine spiradenoma is another benign neoplasm rarely reported to involve the eyelid.[109] Clinically, spiradenomas are solitary, circumscribed nodules that are often painful. Histologically, lesions are composed of two cell populations: large, pale cells surrounded by small, round cells. Primitive tubular structures surrounded by eosinophilic dense basement membrane material are seen. Conservative excision is curative.

BENIGN APOCRINE TUMORS. Due to their secretory activity, apocrine cells show characteristic secretory features, particularly apical snouting or decapitation secretion. The cells have abundant, eosinophilic, granular cytoplasm with small cytoplasmic detachments along their luminal borders. These histologic features help to distinguish apocrine from eccrine cells.

Almost always found on the perineal area, hidradenoma papilliferum is another adnexal tumor infrequently reported to involve the eyelid.[110] Clinically, the tumor is slow growing and nodular. Histologically, dermal cysts are filled by elongated papillary structures with fibrovascular cores. These papillae are lined by cuboidal or columnar cells exhibiting apocrine characteristics, particularly apical secretory snouts. Excision is curative.

In contrast to hidradenoma papilliferum, syringocystadenoma papilliferum is multinodular or verrucous.[111] In addition, its usual location differs from hidradenoma papilliferum, being found mainly on the scalp or face. Microscopically, however, these two lesions share several features. Apocrine cells with apical snouts line papillary structures. In syringocystadenoma papilliferum, however, the papillae are blunt, and the surface of the lesion is

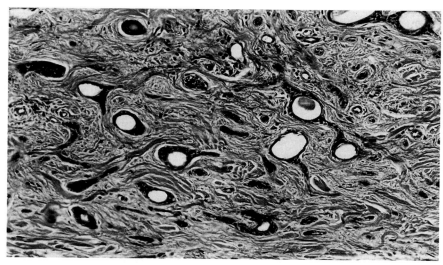

FIG. 2.71—Small, cystic structures lined by two layers of epithelial cells are arranged haphazardly in the dermis. The tadpole shape of these structures is characteristic of syringoma. Because the dermis may be variably sclerotic, morphea-form basal cell carcinoma may be in the differential diagnosis. However, the abrupt keratinization seen in the center of one of the cysts here is a good clue to the diagnosis of syringoma.

papillary. A dense lymphoplasmacytic infiltrate, not seen in hidradenoma papilliferum, is often present.

Hidrocystomas may have either apocrine or eccrine features.[112,113] Clinically, they are dome-shaped, translucent papules, probably representing a nonneoplastic process, perhaps an obstructed secretory duct. Microscopically, cystic spaces are lined by cells exhibiting apocrine or eccrine characteristics, although these may be difficult to discern. They may occasionally be multiple[112] and have been reported in association with ectodermal dysplasia.[114]

Oncocytomas are uncommon tumors arising from duct epithelium. There have been case reports of such tumors involving the eyelid.[115,116] In one report,[115] a 72-year-old man presented with a slowly enlarging, nontender, bluish, partially cystic mass on the left medial upper eyelid. Biopsy revealed a cystic and papillary tumor composed of cells characteristic of oncocytoma. These uniform cells had abundant granular, eosinophilic cytoplasm, and numerous cytoplasmic mitochondria, confirmed by electron microscopy, supported the diagnosis. Inter-

estingly, an adjacent apocrine gland remnant suggested an apocrine origin in this particular case.

CARCINOMA OF SWEAT GLAND ORIGIN. Carcinoma of sweat gland origin may involve eccrine or apocrine sweat glands;[104] however, eccrine carcinomas predominate. Some take the form of mucinous carcinoma,[117–120] and others retain syringomatous features.[121,122]

Although rare, mucinous carcinomas are found primarily on the head, most often the eyelids.[117,123] A review of the literature found an age range of 8–84 years, with primary mucinous eccrine carcinoma arising in the head and neck region in about 75% of patients.[120] Typically, these slowly enlarging lesions are pink, flesh-colored, or blue nodules, plaques, or lobulated masses.[123]

Microscopically, the primarily dermal tumors are composed of mucin pools that contain malignant cells sometimes forming small ductal structures. Mucin-poor forms have also been described[124] in which the mucin is demonstrated in individual cells and mucin pools are lacking.

Although most tumors are localized to the dermis, some invade the subcutis. Histochemical staining has shown the mucin to be a nonsulfated mucosubstance containing sialic acid.[117]

Although metastatic disease is uncommon, local recurrence is a problem. In one study of 20 patients with mucinous adenocarcinoma, eight developed recurrent disease, with one developing metastatic disease and one dying of disease. A review of the literature found the recurrence rate with mucinous carcinomas of the eyelid to be 34%.[120] Although uncommon, both regional and distant metastases have been reported.[117] As mucinous sweat gland carcinoma has been reported to be resistant to both chemotherapy and radiation,[120] complete excision with clear surgical margins is desired.

Another type of sweat gland carcinoma that has been described is the signet-ring type carcinoma, characterized by individual tumor cells invading a sclerotic stroma.[125] Although only a few cases have been reported in the literature, this cancer appears to affect elderly men who present with slowly progressing, diffusely thickened lids. The main differential diagnosis is metastatic carcinoma. The apocrine versus eccrine origin is debated.

Malignant syringoma involving the eyelid has also been described.[126] Clinically, features suggesting malignancy are large size and a solitary lesion. Although only minimal cellular atypia may be present, characteristics that favor malignancy include subcutaneous, muscular, and perineural invasion. Most tumors are indolent, and prognosis may be related to the degree of anaplasia. Complete excision is the therapy of choice.

Malignant tumors of Moll's glands have rarely been described. The evidence of apocrine origin includes a two-cell-layer glandular structure with the inner cells retaining secretory appearance and the outer, spindle cells representing myoepithelium.[121] Decapitation secretion has been reported. In the few cases reported, highly aggressive behavior has been documented.

TUMORS WITH SEBACEOUS DIFFERENTIATION

BENIGN SEBACEOUS NEOPLASMS. Sebaceous adenoma and sebaceous epithelioma are benign neoplasms with a curious association with visceral malignancy, particularly colon carcinoma. Arising from the meibomian glands or the glands of Zeis, they usually present as yellowish subepithelial nodules. Their color is due to their lipid content.

Histologically, a fibrotic stroma surrounding nests of cells and the basaloid nature of the cells enable one to distinguish these neoplasms from simple sebaceous hyperplasia. On the opposite end of the spectrum, one of the most helpful clues to the benignity of this lesion is the overall architecture. Unlike their malignant counterparts, sebaceous adenomas and epitheliomas are well-circumscribed nodules that lack pagetoid spread and an invasive or destructive pattern. The distinction between adenoma and epithelioma is based mainly on cell maturation manifested by the degree of lipid content in the tumor. Tumor cells of the adenoma contain prominent lipid, whereas epithelioma have few lipidized cells. In either case, complete excision of the adenoma or epithelioma is curative.

Of interest is the association of sebaceous neoplasms with visceral malignancy, known as Muir-Torre syndrome. In one retrospective study of 59 patients with sebaceous lesions,[127] 25 (42%) were found to have a visceral malignancy, and some had multiple malignancies (urogenital, hematologic, breast). Most (72%) had a family history of cancer. The association was found to be much higher with sebaceous adenoma and epithelioma than with sebaceous hyperplasia. Although multiple sebaceous lesions have been classically reported in Muir-Torre syndrome, investigators have also identified similar associations with single lesions.[127,128] It has therefore been recommended that patients presenting with sebaceous adenomas or epitheliomas be evaluated for an undiagnosed visceral malignancy.[128,129]

MALIGNANT SEBACEOUS NEOPLASMS. Sebaceous gland carcinoma, a tumor arising from meibomian glands and the glands of Zeis, is particularly interesting in the pathology of the human eyelid for several reasons. Relative to other anatomic sites, the concentration of sebaceous glands (meibomian and Zeis) is high, and the incidence of sebaceous carcinoma is also increased over other sites, comprising 1%–5½% percent of eyelid cancers.[105] In addition, sebaceous carcinomas frequently masquerade as benign inflammatory conditions like the chalazion, earning the dubious distinction of the masquerade syndrome.[130]

Usually affecting patients between decades 5 and 9, this tumor is encountered more often in women than in men,[131] and occurs most commonly on the upper lid.[132,133] Although sebaceous carcinoma occurs worldwide, a much higher percentage has been reported in the Far East, where a study of a group of patients from Shanghai found a 33% incidence of sebaceous carcinoma among malignant lid tumors.[133] An association with radiation exposure has been recognized in some cases.[131,134,135]

Not to be underemphasized is the difficulty of establishing the clinical diagnosis, as this cancer easily mimics inflammatory processes and benign neoplasms as well as other malignancies. Furthermore, appropriately including sebaceous carcinoma in the clinical differential diagnosis is crucial to specimen handling and to establishing the diagnosis. Resembling a chalazion, one common presentation is as a painless slow-growing mass that persists even after curettage.[136] The conjunctiva may be involved, showing erythema and roughening, resulting in a misdiagnosis of blepharoconjunctivitis.[133] Even a case of superior limbic keratoconjunctivitis has been reported to be a masquerading sebaceous carcinoma on biopsy.[137] Basal cell carcinoma and squamous cell carcinoma are among the malignant foils.[132,136] Symptoms range from little discomfort in the slow-growing, small tumors to occasional proptosis and severe pain secondary to nerve involvement in rapidly progressing lesions. Some patients report a sensation of a foreign body present in the eye.[133]

The suspicion of sebaceous carcinoma should alert the surgeon to provide the pathologist with fresh tissue for appropriate specimen handling. The histologic workup will include a lipid stain performed on fresh-frozen tissue to identify the lipid nature of the neoplastic cells. Because lipid is lost during specimen fixation and processing, submission of fresh tissue for frozen-section consultation is mandatory. The demon-

stration of lipid within tumor cells is invaluable in making the diagnosis of sebaceous carcinoma, as it is negative in both basal cell and squamous carcinomas.[138]

Histologically, depending on the degree of differentiation, the tumor may retain the lobular architecture of meibomian or Zeis glands. Cells are large and vesicular with prominent nucleoli. Containing abundant lipid, the cells sometimes have frothy cytoplasm that stains orange by oil red O lipid stain. The overall architecture is that of an invasive neoplasm and, cytologically, cells show distinctly atypical features (Figure 2.72).

A most interesting histologic feature of sebaceous carcinoma is the tendency of tumor cells to show intraepithelial or pagetoid spread.[139] The recognition of this phenomenon is important and may help avoid misdiagnosis.[140] It is unknown whether these changes are due to a field effect of the carcinogen on the epithelium or due to intraepithelial migration of malignant cells.[131] Interestingly, this intraepithelial spread is associated with a poorer prognosis, and DNA ploidy studies have shown that tumors with pagetoid spread have aneuploid DNA content and exhibit more anaplasia.[141]

The histologic differential diagnosis mainly includes basal cell and squamous cell carcinoma. Unlike basal cell carcinoma, sebaceous carcinoma does not exhibit peripheral palisading of cells. One of the most difficult differential diagnoses is squamous cell carcinoma, particularly when one considers intraepithelial conjunctival spread of sebaceous carcinoma. This may be so extensive that it mimics an intraepithelial squamous lesion. Squamous cell carcinoma, however, should not contain lipid, and therefore a lipid stain is crucial. To differentiate from adenocarcinoma of the glands of Moll, mucopolysaccharide staining should be negative in a sebaceous lesion and positive in an adenocarcinoma of the glands of Moll. The benign lesions in the clinical differential diagnosis are usually excluded by the malignant histology.

Factors that lean toward a poorer prognosis are long duration of symptoms, vascular or lymphatic infiltration, orbital extension, poor histologic differentiation, multicentric origin, and upper-lid location.[142] Recurrence has been reported in 9%–36% of sebaceous carcinomas, orbital inva-

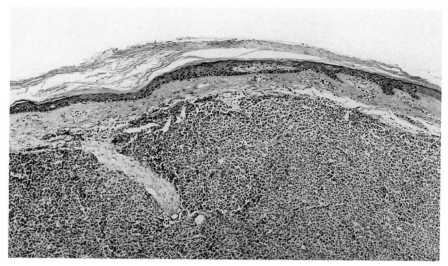

FIG. 2.72—Sebaceous carcinoma.

sion in 6%–17% of cases, and regional lymph node involvement in 17%–28% of cases.[131] Metastases to the parotid lymph nodes have also been reported.[143] Intracranial extension is well documented.[144,145] The mortality rate is reported to be 6%–30% in one review[131] and 30%–83% in another.[142] According to one study of 40 sebaceous carcinoma cases, the mortality rate has improved from 24% in patients treated before 1970 to zero cases in patients treated after 1970.[132] This has been attributed to more astute recognition of disease and aggressive surgical therapy.

Complete surgical excision with generous margins is the preferred therapy. Although some surgeons have tried therapy with the Mohs' technique,[142] recurrence has been reported[146] and, therefore, wide local excision has been advocated.[138] For tumors that have invaded the orbit, exenteration is required. Adjuvant radiation therapy may be necessary.[131,142]

Merkel Cell Carcinoma. Merkel cells are specialized dendritic cells with neuroendocrine features, and Merkel cell carcinoma is a rare eyelid tumor. The average age at the time of diagnosis is 66–73 years.[147] Approximately 10% of all Merkel cell carcinomas involve the eyelid or periocular region.[147] The upper lid is more frequently involved than the lower lid.

Clinically, the tumor presents as a subepithelial, painless, bulging nodule with a characteristic pink to red to violet hue. Occasionally, ulceration has been reported. Reports of presentation as recurrent chalazion[148] and as basal cell carcinoma[149] are noted.

Microscopically, Merkel cell carcinomas are dermal lesions, frequently penetrating fat or muscle. These tumors are composed of small, basophilic cells with scant cytoplasm. Cells are arranged in a nesting, organoid, or trabecular pattern (Figure 2.73). Their cytologic and architectural features suggest a neuroendocrine tumor; however, malignant lymphoma should be included in the differential diagnosis. In these cases, immunoperoxidase stains for differentiating antigens are indicated. These may include leukocyte common antigen to exclude lymphoma. Grimelius stain, a silver stain that detects argyrophilic granules, may also be helpful in identifying the neuroendocrine characteristics of tumor. Other immunohistochemical stains that have been reported to be positive in Merkel cell carcinoma include neuron-specific enolase, epithelial membrane antigen, and metenkephalin.[150] Electron microscopy is most useful and may demonstrate the neuroendocrine granules characteristic of this tumor. These are cytoplasmic dense-core granules averaging from

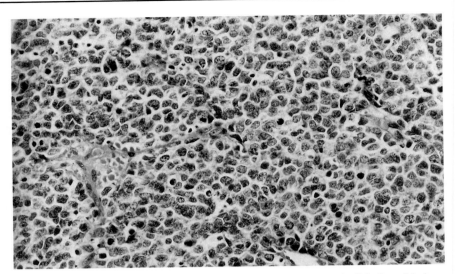

FIG. 2.73—This Merkel cell carcinoma produced a smooth bulging nodule on the lid of an elderly man. Histologically, it is characterized by expansion of the dermis by fairly uniform cells with round to oval nuclei and stippled chromatin. The differential diagnosis included lymphoma, which was excluded by negative immunoperoxidase stains for leukocyte common antigen and B- and T-cell antigens. Positive neuroendocrine antigens and electron microscopy supported the diagnosis of Merkel cell carcinoma. Extensive workup for a primary small cell carcinoma, particularly from the lung, was negative.

80 to 150 nm in diameter. Paranuclear aggregates of intermediate filaments are also present.

Once the neuroendocrine nature of the tumor is confirmed, one faces another diagnostic dilemma. Perhaps the most difficult differential diagnosis is metastatic small cell carcinoma, most commonly of lung origin, and metastatic carcinoid tumor. Both demonstrate immunoperoxidase staining and electron-microscopic characteristics similar to those of Merkel cell carcinoma. Therefore, it is imperative that a thorough search for a primary small cell carcinoma be completed prior to establishing the diagnosis of Merkel cell carcinoma.

The high tendency for recurrence and metastases prompts aggressive treatment with wide local excision, possible radiation therapy, and perhaps chemotherapy. As these tumors are radiation sensitive, irradiation may be an option in nonsurgical candidates and perhaps in patients with lymph node metastases.[149]

Vascular Tumors. Vascular lesions of the eyelid are uncommon and may be divided into those that are neoplastic and those that are reactive or inflammatory. Benign neoplastic vascular lesions that have been reported to involve the eyelid include capillary hemangioma, cavernous hemangioma, lymphangioma, and glomus tumor. Malignant neoplasms include Kaposi's sarcoma and angiosarcoma.

INFLAMMATORY VASCULAR LESIONS. Reactive vascular lesions may clinically simulate a neoplasm. One such vascular lesion is the pyogenic granuloma, an exaggerated form of granulation tissue. This frequently ulcerated nodule has a classic epidermal collarette, histologically. The stroma is edematous, inflamed, and highly vascular. Mitoses may be seen (Figure 2.74). A rare intravenous variant of the lesion has been reported in the eyelid.[151]

NEOPLASTIC VASCULAR LESIONS. Capillary hemangioma is the most common periocular vascular tumor in infants and children, usually presenting before 2 months of age. Although spontaneous involution may occur, visual complications,

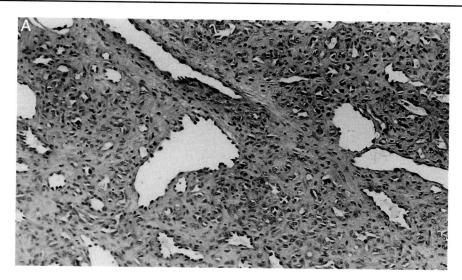

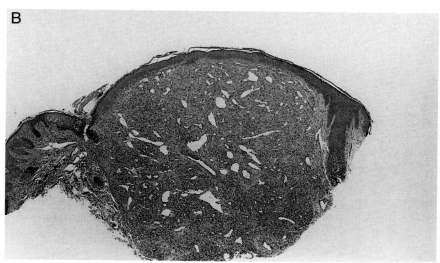

FIG. 2.74—Low-power study of a pyogenic granuloma shows the characteristic architecture of a well-circumscribed nodule surrounded by an epithelial collarette. The features are invaluable in establishing the diagnosis **(A).** High power shows vascular channels of various sizes set in an inflammatory background **(B).**

particularly amblyopia and strabismus, may result from tumor presence during development.[152] A soft red mass is present on physical examination. Histologically, lesions are composed of lobules of capillaries with proliferating endothelial cells. Management may be by corticosteroids, careful surgical dissection,[153] or laser photocoagulation.[154]

Cavernous hemangiomas, which occur later in life, are bluish, deep lesions composed of large vascular channels with thick walls (Figure 2.75). Surgical intervention may be indicated.

Lymphangiomas of the eyelid comprise only a small group of such tumors involving the eye as a whole.[155–157] They may be congenital or acquired and may present cosmetic problems. Generally, lymphangiomas of the orbit have been classified as superficial, deep, or combined. Lesions involving the lid only are classified as superficial,[157]

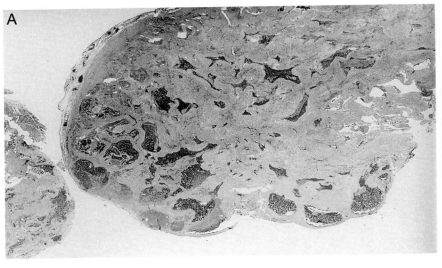

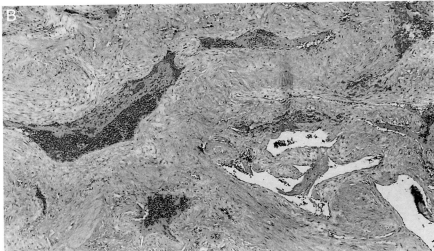

FIG. 2.75—This hemangioma is well circumscribed and composed of thick-walled vascular structures of various sizes (**A**). On a high-power profile, note that the endothelial cells are flat and lack cytoatypia (**B**).

whereas combined lesions have both superficial and deep components. Clinically, lymphangiomas have been described as soft, upraised lesions that may present a blue-black hue due to intralesional hemorrhage.[156] Histologically, these lesions are defined by thin-walled endothelial lined channels containing eosinophilic, amorphous lymph. Because hemorrhage into lymphangiomas is common, fresh blood or hemosiderin may be observed. Septae are composed of loose connective tissue, and smooth muscle cells are variably present. If cosmetically unacceptable, superficial lymphangiomas may be surgically excised.

The glomus tumor is a hamartoma arising from the Sucquet-Hoyer canal, a specialized arteriovenous anastomosis surrounded by smooth muscle cells. These shunts, known as the glomus apparatus, give rise to the glomus tumor. Uncommon on the eyelid, lesions appear blue and elevated. Some lesions may be tender, and they may occur singly or multiply.[158,159] Histologically, glomus tumors are composed of tangled vascular chan-

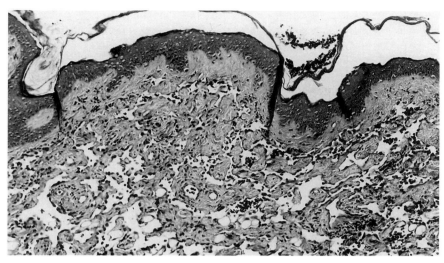

FIG. 2.76—In contrast with a hemangioma, an angiosarcoma is composed of anastamosing vascular channels lined by atypical endothelial cells showing hyperchromasia and tufting or projection into the vascular lumen.

nels lined by a single layer of endothelial cells surrounded by several layers of round to oval cells with central nuclei. Encapsulated lesions may be easily excised, but those lacking a capsule may be difficult to completely ablate.[158]

Among the malignant vascular tumors are Kaposi's sarcoma and angiosarcoma. Usually related to acquired immune-deficiency syndrome, Kaposi's sarcoma involving the eyelid is now being more frequently reported. Prior to the AIDS epidemic, only a few cases involving the eyelid had been documented.[160] Now, ocular involvement occurs in about 20% of patients with AIDS-associated Kaposi's sarcoma. Clinically, lesions are raised and violaceous. Histologically, Kaposi's sarcoma has been divided into three stages with increasing morphologic aggressiveness. Stage I lesions consist of thin vascular channels lined by flattened endothelial cells. Stage II lesions have plump, fusiform endothelial cells, and Stage III lesions have aggregates of hyperchromatic, mitotically active spindle cells.[161] Treatment may include chemotherapy, surgical excision, radiotherapy, or cryotherapy.

Angiosarcoma is a rare malignant neoplasm that may involve the eyelid. Seen most commonly in the elderly, angiosarcoma first presents as erythematous plaques, which may evolve into nodules. Under the microscope, these poorly delineated lesions are composed of atypical vascular structures lined by neoplastic endothelial cells that bulge or tuft into the lumen, a feature helpful in distinguishing angiosarcoma from Kaposi's sarcoma (Figure 2.76).

Other Mesenchymal Tumors. Other mesenchymal tumors that may involve the eyelid include tumors of fibroblast, histiocytic, and muscle origin. Rarely, fibromatosis will present as a firm, painless, nontender mass.[162] These tumors are composed of interlacing bundles of spindle-shaped fibroblasts with infiltrating margins. Often they invade adjacent muscle and fascia. Lesions are treated primarily by surgery, and recurrence rates are high.

Fibrous histiocytoma or fibroxanthoma is an uncommon lesion that tends to occur after minor trauma. It is uncommonly reported on the eyelid[163–165] and is composed of spindle and xanthoma cells arranged in a nodular pattern. Multinucleated cells may be scattered throughout the lesion. Atypical fibroxanthomas exhibit increased mitoses and cellular atypia.[166] The atypical lesions maybe locally aggressive and may recur.

Myxoma, which is a very rare, benign mesenchymal lesion of the eyelid,[167] is composed of stellate cells in a clear background. Although rare, a complex showing Mendelian dominant inheritance has been reported in which eyelid myxomas and ocular pigmentation are associated with cardiac, skin, and mammary myxomas and endocrine dysfunction.[168] The benign ocular manifestations may therefore prompt investigation for the potentially lethal cardiac myxoma.

Among the malignant mesenchymal lesions are fibrosarcoma[169] and rhabdomyosarcoma.[170] The former is a tumor composed of immature fibroblastic cells arranged in a herringbone pattern showing hypercellularity and mitotic activity. Immunohistochemical studies to exclude muscle and neural origin of the cells are required.

Rhabdomyosarcoma is a lesion presenting predominantly in children. Variable histologic types are described, including a diffuse lesion of small, basophilic, round cells and cells arranged in an alveolar pattern. Immunohistochemical studies may be performed, and electron microscopy may be particularly helpful in identifying actin and myosin filaments and cross-striation.

Nervous Tissue Tumors. Neural tumors that may involve the eyelid include neurofibroma, neurilemoma, ectopic meningioma, and granular cell tumor, a lesion of possible neural origin.

NEUROFIBROMAS. Neurofibroma is a lesion thought by some to be derived of Schwann cells. It may occur singly and sporadically or as part of von Recklinghausen syndrome, a hereditary condition characterized by cutaneous pigmented lesions (café-au-lait spots) and neurofibromatosis. Neurofibromatosis is an example of a phakomatoses, a hereditary hamartomatous condition involving peripheral nerves. Inherited in an autosomal dominant fashion with incomplete penetrance and variable expression, neurofibromatosis occurs in approximately one in 3000 live births.[171]

These small, well-defined, non-encapsulated spindle cell lesions may present with a mass effect of ptosis[172] and/or glaucoma due to infiltration of the angle with subsequent obstruction of aqueous outflow channels (Figure 2.77).[173] The latter is usually associated with a larger variant of the lesion thought to be characteristic of neurofibromatosis—plexiform neurofibroma—which is composed of hypertrophied nerve trunks that ramify in a vermiform manner.[69] When involving the lid, plexiform neurofibromas have been described as resembling a "bag of worms."[172] Surgical excision of these lesions is difficult, but successful approaches have been described.[174]

NEURILEMOMAS. Neurilemoma (schwannoma) is a benign tumor that usually occurs as a solitary lesion[175] or as a manifestation of neurofibromatosis.[172] Microscopically, lesions are composed of Antoni A and Antoni B patterns. The former is a fusiform proliferation of spindle cells, and the latter is a microcystic, mucinous network of round cells with pale cytoplasm.

GRANULAR CELL TUMORS. Granular cell tumor is a rare neoplasm of the eyelid with controversial histogenesis. Once thought to be of muscle origin, the name granular cell myoblastoma was applied.[176] Now, because of immunohistochemical characteristics, the lesion is thought to have Schwann cell derivation.[110] Affecting patients usually between decades 3 and 6, granular cell tumor presents as a slowly progressing mass.[177,178] Histologically, granular cell tumors are composed of round to oval, fairly uniform cells with small nuclei and abundant granular eosinophilic cytoplasm. Immunohistochemical staining is positive for S-100 protein. Ultrastructurally, the presence of a basement membrane, intracytoplasmic myelin figures, and ungulate bodies further supports the theory of Schwann cell origin.[177]

MENINGIOMAS. Ectopic (extradural) meningioma is extremely rare, but lid involvement has been reported.[179] Lesions are firm and slow growing. The most common histologic pattern is a whorl of spindle cells with occasional psammoma bodies. In the foregoing case with lid involvement, the tumor appeared to originate from the orbital roof.

Pigmented Tumors

NEVI. Melanocytic lesions are lesions composed of proliferative melanocytes. Normally, melanocytes reside in the basal layer of the epidermis. These dendritic cells exhibit contact inhi-

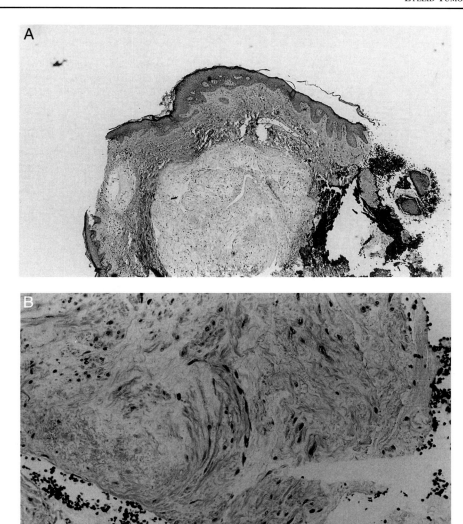

FIG. 2.77—This particular neurofibroma presented as a subcutaneous mass. **A:** On low power, a well-defined mass is seen in the dermis. **B:** High-power observation identifies benign spindle cells with elongated nuclei, confirming the diagnosis of neurofibroma.

bition for one another and tend to be separated by about 10 keratinocytes. They function to synthesize melanin and then transfer it to adjacent keratinocytes. Nevus cells differ from normal melanocytes by the following: loss of dendritic shape, loss of contact inhibition, tendency to retain pigment, and tendency to migrate from the basal epidermis to the papillary dermis.[69] Clinically, lesions are usually small with well-defined borders. Because of pigment retention, they may

be brown, black, or tan. Some lesions may be nonpigmented or amelanotic. The clinical characteristics that suggest malignancy are large size, irregular pigmentation, irregular borders, ulceration, or change in appearance.

The histologic classification of nevi is based primarily on architecture. The location of the nevocytes and their distribution readily classify most lesions. A contiguous linear proliferation of melanocytes in the basal layer without nests is

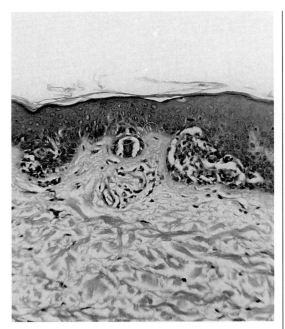

FIG. 2.78—The nevocytes in this junctional nevus are present at the dermal-epidermal junction only. The lack of cytoatypia and pagetoid spread of nevus cells is characteristic of a benign nevus.

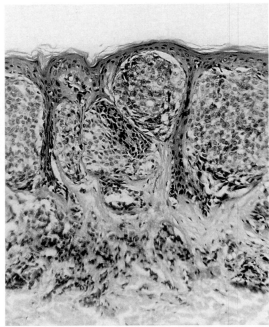

FIG. 2.79—Nevus cells arranged in nests occupying both the dermal-epidermal junction and the dermis are characteristic of this compound nevus.

called a lentigo. Once nests form at the dermal-epidermal junction, the lesion must be classified as a junctional nevus (Figure 2.78). If nests are present both at the dermal-epidermal junction and within the dermis, the lesion is termed a compound nevus (Figure 2.79). Finally, if all nevus cells are located within the dermis, the term intradermal nevus (Figure 2.80) is applied. Most nevi are acquired, but some are congenital. Of particular interest in the eyelid is the congenital divided or kissing nevus, a lesion that presumably arises in utero during stages of eyelid fusion.[180] Divided nevi are usually pigmented lesions occurring on opposing upper and lower lids. When the lids are closed, a single lesion is appreciated. Rarely, divided nevi lack pigmentation.[181]

MELANOMAS. Malignant melanoma of the eyelid skin is rare. One of the largest studies included 32 patients ranging in age from 23 to 93, with an average age of 60.[182] In general, three categories of melanoma of the eyelid skin are described: lentigo maligna, superficial spreading melanoma, and

nodular melanoma.[182–185] Common to all three types is the diagnostic requirement of pagetoid spread of atypical melanocytes into the dermis (Figure 2.81). Of particular interest are the striking differences between melanomas of the lids and conjunctiva and intraocular melanomas.[186] For example, melanoma of the lid, similar to that of skin elsewhere, tends to metastasize via lymphatics, whereas uveal and other orbital melanomas do not.

Lentigo maligna is a lesion most commonly located on sun-damaged skin. Also known as Hutchinson's melanocytic freckle, this lesion has a characteristic clinical appearance as a flat brown-black asymmetric macule with an irregular border. Histologically, it is recognized as a lentiginous proliferation of atypical melanocytes in the basal layer of the epidermis. Pigmentation may be extensive. Near the center of the lesion, pagetoid spread of atypical cells may be observed. It is characteristic for the lentiginous proliferation to extend downward along skin appendages.[187] Once the basement membrane has been invaded, the lesion is called lentigo

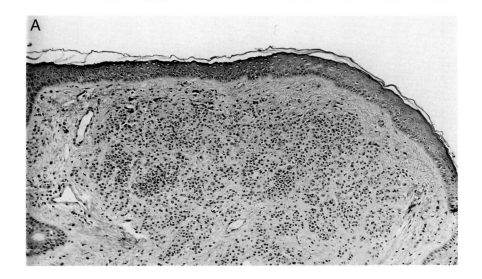

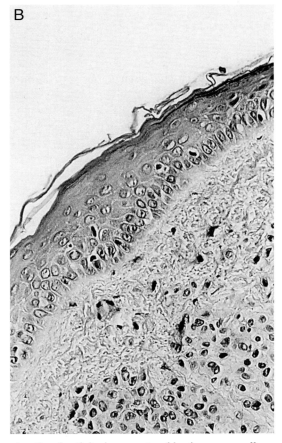

FIG. 2.80A and B—When no junctional activity is present and benign nevus cells are confined to the dermis, the lesion is designated as an intradermal nevus. Although the lesion is cellular, clues to benignity are the lack of pagetoid spread and cytoatypia, as well as the appropriate maturation of nevus cells toward the deeper dermis.

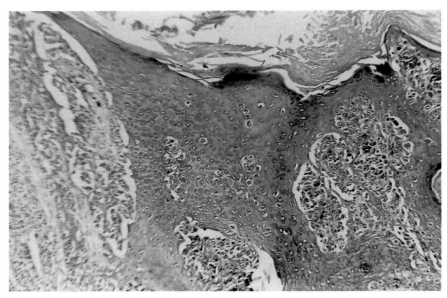

FIG. 2.81—Diagnostic features of this melanoma are the large hyperchromatic, atypical melanocytes and the prominent pagetoid spread of individual and nested neoplastic cells.

maligna melanoma. Associated with a very good prognosis, lentigo maligna and lentigo maligna melanoma rarely metastasize.[183] Treatment is surgical excision with clear margins.

Superficial spreading melanoma occurred in seven of 32 patients in a study by Grossniklaus and McLean,[182] in nine of 24 patients in the study by Garner et al.,[185] in three of six patients in the study by Naidoff et al.,[183] and in three of four patients in the study by Collin et al.[184] Clinically, the lesions are palpable plaques or papules with irregular borders exhibiting color variegation. Histologically, these lesions are characterized by their radial (horizontal) growth phase with or without a vertical phase. By definition, lesions exhibit pagetoid proliferation of atypical melanocytes into the epidermis, sometimes as single cells and sometimes in nests. The radial growth phase, which is always present, extends horizontally, parallel with the epidermis. A vertical or downward growth phase is variably present. Prognostically, depth of invasion is the most important parameter, with local recurrence and metastases to lymph nodes and distant sites common patterns of disease recurrence or progression. Therapy is by surgical excision with clear margins. Adjuvant therapy for advanced disease may be indicated.

Nodular melanoma has the poorest prognosis of all three types: 19 of 32 patients in the study by Grossniklaus and McLean,[182] 12 of 24 patients in the study by Garner et al.,[185] no patients in the study by Naidoff et al.,[183] and 1 of 4 patients in the study by Collin et al.[184] were diagnosed with nodular melanoma. Clinically, nodular melanoma presents as an irregular, raised, variably pigmented lesion. Histologically, it is characterized by the presence of malignant melanocytes in a vertical growth phase only. An interesting variant that may be difficult to diagnose histologically is the desmoplastic melanoma in which spindle and epithelioid cells are surrounded by a desmoplastic stroma.[188] In these cases, melanin pigment or atypical junctional activity may aid in establishing the diagnosis. The poor prognosis of nodular melanoma is related to the vertical growth phase and the resultant depth of invasion. In the study by Grossniklaus and McLean, two patients developed metastatic disease. One died and the other was lost to follow-up. Again, the lesion must be completely excised, and adjuvant therapy may be required.

Although most melanomas are pigmented, those that lack pigment—amelanotic melanomas—have been reported to involve the eyelid.[189] In such cases, the consideration of melanoma may be in the differential diagnosis of a poorly differentiated tumor. Immunoperoxidase staining for S-100 protein and HMB-45 is helpful in establishing the diagnosis of melanoma. Also, electron microscopy may identify the presence of premelanosomes and melanosomes.

The association of malignant melanoma with preexisting nevi has been explored. Grossniklaus and McLean[182] report finding nevi adjacent to melanoma in 38% of cases. Worrisome signs in a pigmented lesion include ulceration, hemorrhage, growth of the lesion, irregular borders, and variegated coloring. Like many skin tumors, sun exposure has been implicated as a risk factor for the development of melanoma, with histologic evidence of solar elastosis found in 41% of melanomas.[182]

Metastatic Tumors. Metastases to the eyelid are rare, with only a few large studies and scattered case reports in the literature. One of the largest studies of metastatic disease to the eyelid included 31 patients.[190] Metastases predominated in females, breast carcinoma being the most common primary tumor. The median age was 69 years, and only 17 of the 31 patients had a known primary malignancy. Although most lesions were adenocarcinoma, metastatic malignant melanoma, clear cell carcinoma, leiomyosarcoma, carcinoid tumor, and adnexal carcinoma were also observed. Besides the breast, other primary tumor sites included skin, kidney, gastrointestinal tract, ocular choroid, lung, hip, and hand. Additional cases reported in the literature include lymphoma,[191] osteogenic sarcoma of the leg,[192] lumbosacral chordoma,[193] choroidal melanoma,[194] malignant teratoma of the testis,[195] lung carcinoma,[1,196] stomach carcinoma,[197,198] and, of course, breast carcinoma.[198,199] Clinically, presentation is variable: a solitary painless or tender nodule; diffuse, nontender induration; or an ulcerative lesion.[196] Although, in some cases, the distinction between a primary tumor and metastatic disease is clear, it is occasionally difficult. Histologic features found to favor metastasis are neo-

plastic cells inside blood vessels, single-file cell arrangement suggesting lobular carcinoma of the breast, subcutaneous tumor location, prominent sclerosis around malignant cells, a relative absence of inflammatory response, and an absence of connections between neoplastic cells and skin structures.[190] In some cases, immunohistochemical staining for site-specific antigens like prostate-specific antigen may help to elucidate a primary focus. Irradiation may be palliative. According to a review of the literature,[196] mean survival after presentation with eyelid metastasis was 9.7 months. For those patients with breast carcinoma, mean survival was longer: 22 months.

Nonneoplastic Lesions That May Mimic Neoplasms. Inflammatory and other nonneoplastic conditions may produce mass lesions, mimicking tumor. Among these are granulomatous lesions, commonly associated with sarcoidosis or infectious processes, particularly fungus and tuberculosis (Figure 2.82). Viral processes such as molluscum contagiosum and verrucae vulgaris may also produce mass lesions, resulting in biopsy (Figure 2.83). Infiltration of lipid-laden histiocytes seen in xanthomatous lesions produce yellow nodules on the eyelid (Figure 2.84).

Additionally, primary localized amyloidosis may present as a margin tumor. These smooth, yellow to purple nodules contain deposition of amorphous eosinophilic material. This lesion has been reported both with or without systemic involvement.[200]

Pseudoepitheliomatous hyperplasia is a downward proliferation of epidermis into the dermis, mimicking low-grade squamous cell carcinoma. It is associated with chronic inflammatory processes and may be seen at the edges of chronic ulcers. It has been reported overlying granular cell tumor of the lid.[201] Although the invasion of the dermis is irregular, and keratin pearl formation and mitoses may be prominent, the keratinocytes lack atypia, such as individual cell keratinization and hyperchromasia. Frequently, the dermis and epidermis are infiltrated by inflammatory cells. In addition to the lack of cytoatypia and the inflammatory infiltrate, additional biopsies to exclude adjacent malignancy and clinical history may be helpful in establishing the diagnosis.

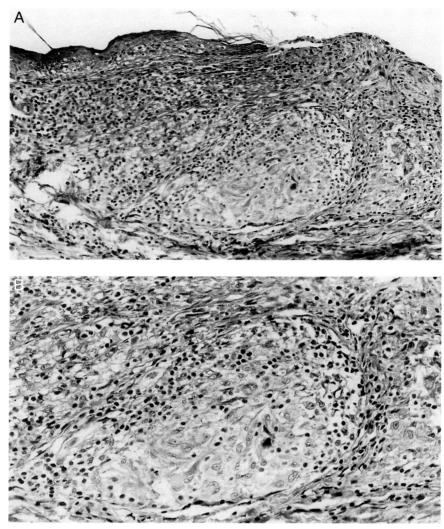

FIG. 2.82A and B—Granulomatous inflammation may mimic neoplasia by producing a mass. Histologically, granulomas composed of epithelioid histiocytes, multinucleated giant cells, and lymphocytes may be observed. A variety of infectious processes (tuberculosis and fungi) and noninfectious processes (sarcoidosis and foreign-body reactions) may cause granulomas.

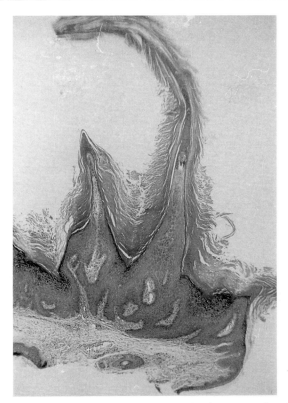

FIG. 2.83—Most likely secondary to viral infection, a verrucae vulgaris, commonly called a wart, may mimic a neoplasm. Histologically, note the hyperkeratosis, acanthosis, and mounds of parakeratosis overlying projections of the lesion. The elongated rete pointing toward the center of the lesion is a classic feature.

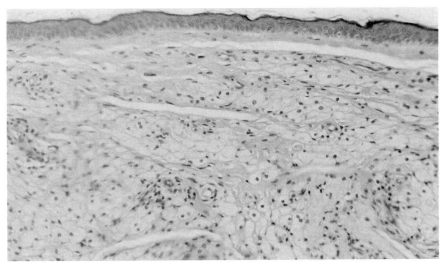

FIG. 2.84—Grossly an elevated, yellow papule, xanthoma is histologically composed of foamy histiocytes that infiltrate the dermis.

ACKNOWLEDGMENTS

R.C.R. is indebted to the wonderful contributions of skill and art by the following people: Mary Lou Norman for the histosections and Alexis Wenski-Roberts for the gross photomicrographs.

REFERENCES

1. Bevier DE, Goldschmidt MH. Skin tumors in the dog: I. Epithelial tumors and tumor-like lesions. *Compend Continuing Educ* 3:389, 1981.
2. Peiffer RL, Gelatt KN, Karpinski LG. The canine eyelids. In: Gelatt KN, ed. *Veterinary Ophthalmology*. Philadelphia: Lea and Febiger, 1981:277.
3. Madewell BR, Theilen GH. Tumors and tumor-like conditions of epithelial origin: Part I. In: *Veterinary Cancer Medicine*, 2d ed. Philadelphia: Lea and Febiger, 1987:223.
4. Bonney CH, Koch SE, Dice PF, Confer AW. Papillomatosis of conjunctiva and adnexa in dogs. *J Am Vet Med Assoc* 176:48, 1980.
5. Krehbiel JD, Langham RF. Eyelid neoplasms of dogs. *Am J Vet Res* 36:115, 1975.
6. Barrie KP, Gelatt KN, Parshall CP. Eyelid squamous cell carcinoma in 4 dogs. *J Am Anim Hosp Assoc* 18:123, 1982.
7. Lavach JD, Snyder SP. Squamous cell carcinoma of the third eyelid in a dog. *J Am Vet Med Assoc* 184:975, 1984.
8. Smith JS, Bistner SI, Riis RC. Infiltrative corneal lesions resembling fibrous histiocytoma: clinical and pathologic findings in 6 dogs and 1 cat. *J Am Vet Med Assoc* 169:722, 1976.
9. Gwin R, Gelatt KN, Peiffer RL Jr. Ophthalmic nodular fasciitis in the dog. *J Am Vet Med Assoc* 170:611, 1977.
10. Stannard AA, Pulley LT. Tumors of the skin and the soft tissues. In: Moulton JE, ed. *Tumors in Domestic Animals*, 2d ed. Berkeley: University of California Press, 1978:16.
11. Runnells RA, Benbrook EA. Epithelial tumors in horses. *Am J Vet Res* 3:176, 1942.
12. Blodi FC, Ramsey FK. Ocular tumors in domestic animals *Am J Ophthalmol* 64:627, 1967.
13. Hacker DV, Moore PF, Buyukmihci NC. Ocular angiosarcoma in 4 horses. *J Am Vet Med Assoc* 189:200, 1986.
14. Morgan G. Ocular tumors in animals. *J Small Anim Pract* 10:563, 1969.
15. Lavach JD. Ocular neoplasia. In: Robinson NE, ed. *Current Therapy in Equine Medicine*. Philadelphia: WB Saunders, 1992:604.
16. Kerr KM, Alden CL. Equine neoplasia, a 10-year survey. *Am Assoc Lab Diagn* 17:183, 1974.
17. Gelatt KN. Meibomian adenoma in a dog. *Vet Med Small Anim Clin* 10:962, 1975.
18. Holmberg DL. Cryosurgical treatment of canine eyelid tumors. *Vet Clin North Am Small Anim Pract* 10:831, 1980.
19. Roberts SM, Severin GA, Lavach JD. Prevalence and treatment of palpebral neoplasms in the dog: 200 cases. *J Am Vet Med Assoc* 189:1355, 1986.
20. Hargis AM, Thomassen RW. Solar keratosis and solar keratosis with squamous cell carcinoma. *Am J Pathol* 94:193, 1979.
21. Hargis AM, Thomassen RW, Phemister RD. Chronic dermatosis and cutaneous squamous cell carcinoma in the beagle dog. *Vet Pathol* 14:218, 1997.
22. Goldschmidt MH, Shafer FS. Squamous cell carcinoma. In: *Skin Tumors of the Dog and Cat*. Tarrytown, NY: Pergamon, 1992:37.
23. Klein MK, Roberts WG, Bems MW. Photodynamic therapy of cutaneous squamous cell carcinoma of cats using a phthalocyanine photosensitizer. *Proc Vet Cancer Soc* 3:24, 1989.
24. Himsel CA, Richardson RC, Craig JA. Cisplatin chemotherapy for metastatic squamous cell carcinoma in two dogs. *J Am Vet Med Assoc* 189:1575, 1986.
25. Muller GH, Kirk RW, Scott DW. Squamous cell carcinoma. In: *Small Animal Dermatology IV*. Philadelphia: WB Saunders, 1989:855.
26. Helper LC. Diseases and surgery of the lid and conjunctiva. In: *Magrane's Canine Ophthalmology*, 4th ed. Philadelphia: Lea and Febiger, 1989:99.
27. Dugan SJ, Curtis CR, Roberts SM, Severin GA. Epidemiologic studies on ocular/adnexal squamous cell carcinoma in horses. *J Am Vet Med Assoc* 198:251, 1991.
28. Dugan SJ, Roberts SM, Curtis CR, Severin GA. Prognostic factors and survival of horses with ocular/adnexal squamous cell carcinoma: 147 cases (1978–1988). *J Am Vet Med Assoc* 198:298, 1991.
29. Lavach JD, Severin GA. Neoplasia of the equine eye, adnexa, and orbit: a review of 68 cases. *J Am Vet Med Assoc* 170:202, 1977.
30. Lavach JD. Ocular neoplasia. In: Robinson NE, ed. *Current Therapy in Equine Medicine*. Philadelphia: WB Saunders, 1992:604.
31. Kainer RA. Bovine ocular squamous cell tumors. In: Howard JL, ed. *Current Veterinary Therapy, Food Animal Practice II*. Philadelphia: WB Saunders, 1986:833.
32. Russell WO, Wynne ES, Loguvan GS, Mehl DA. Studies on bovine ocular squamous carcinoma ("cancer eye"): I. *Pathol Anat Hist Rev Cancer* 9:1, 1956.
33. Monlux AW, Anderson WA, Davis CL. The diagnosis of squamous cell carcinoma of the eye ("cancer eye") in cattle. *Am J Vet Res* 18:5, 1957.
34. Bonney CH, Koch SE, Dice PF, Confer AW. Papillomatosis of conjunctiva and adnexa in dogs. *J Am Vet Med Assoc* 176:48, 1980.
35. Ford JN, Jennings PA, Spradbrow PB, et al. Evidence of papilloma viruses in ocular lesions in cattle. *Res Vet Sci* 32:257, 1982.
36. Vanselow BA, Spradbrow PB, Jackson AR B. Papilloma viruses, papillomas, and squamous cell carcinomas in sheep. *Vet Rec* 110:561, 1982.
37. Syverton JT. The pathogenesis of the rabbit papillomas-to-carcinoma sequence. *Ann NY Acad Sci* 54:1126, 1952.
38. Rudolph RL. Neoplasien der Haut bei einem wildfarbenen Inzuchtstamm von *Mastomys natalensis* (WSA Giessen). *Vet Pathol* 17:600, 1980.

39. Paulsen ME, Lavach JD, Snyder SP, Severin GA, Eichenbaum JD. Nodular granulomatous episclerokeratitis in dogs: 19 cases. *J Am Vet Med Assoc* 190:1581, 1987.

40. Gwin RM, Alsaker RD, Gelatt NK. Melanoma of the lower eyelid of a dog. *Vet Med Small Anim Clin* 9:929, 1976.

41. Dugan SJ. Ocular neoplasia. *Vet Clin North Am Equine Pract* 8:609, 1992.

42. Gelatt KN. Basal cell carcinoma of the eyelid in a dog. *Vet Clin North Am Small Anim Clin* 8:799, 1971.

43. Fretz DB, Barber SM. Prospective analysis of cryosurgery as the sole treatment for equine sarcoids. *Vet Clin North Am Equine Pract* 10:847, 1980.

44. Hoffman KC, Kainer RA, Shideler RK. Radiofrequency current-induced hyperthermia for the treatment of equine sarcoid. *Equine Pract* 5:24, 1983.

45. Trenfield K, Spradbrow PB, Vanselow B. Sequences of papillomavirus DNA in equine sarcoids. *Equine Vet J* 17:449, 1985.

46. Cheevers WP, Roberson SM, Brassfield AL. Isolation of a retrovirus from cultured equine sarcoid tumor cells. *Am J Vet Res* 43:804, 1982.

47. Owen RR, Hagger DW. Clinical observations on the use of BCG cell wall fraction for treatment of periocular and other equine sarcoids. *Vet Rec* 120:548, 1987.

48. Lane JG. The treatment of equine sarcoids by cryosurgery. *Equine Vet J* 9:127, 1977.

49. Herd RP, Donham JC. Efficacy of ivermectin against cutaneous *Draschia* and *Habronema* infection (summer sores) in horses *Am J Vet Res* 42:1953, 1981.

50. Rebhun WC. Diseases of the ocular system. In: Colahan PT, Mayhen IG, Merritt AM, eds. *Equine Medicine and Surgery,* 4th ed. Galeta, IL: American Veterinary Publications, 1991:1083.

51. Barrie KP, Parshall CJ Jr. Eyelid pyogranulomas in four dogs. *J Am Anim Hosp Assoc* 14:433, 1979.

52. Harvey CE, Koch SA, Rubin LF. Orbital cyst with conjunctival fistula in a dog. *J Am Vet Med Assoc* 153:1432, 1968.

53. Latimer CA. Membrana nictitans gland cyst in a dog. *J Am Vet Med Assoc* 183:1003, 1983.

54. Playter RF, Adams LG. Lacrimal cyst in 2 dogs. *J Am Vet Med Assoc* 171:736, 1977.

55. Rebhun WC, Edwards NJ. Two cases of orbital adenocarcinoma of probably lacrimal gland origin. *J Am Vet Med Assoc* 13:691, 1977.

56. Davidson HJ, Blanchard GL. Periorbital epidermal cyst in the medial canthus of 3 dogs *J Am Vet Med Assoc* 198:271, 1991.

57. Johnson BW, Brightman AH, Whiteley HE. Conjunctival mast cell tumor in two dogs. *J Am Anim Hosp Assoc* 24:439, 1988.

58. Saunders LH, Rubin LF. *Ophthalmic Pathology of Animals.* Basal: S Karger, 1975:236.

59. Hallstrom M. Mastocytomas in the third eyelid of a dog. *J Small Anim Pract* 11:469, 1970.

60. Kern TJ. Orbital neoplasms in 23 dogs *J Am Vet Med Assoc* 186:489, 1985.

61. Patnaik AK, Ehler WJ, MacEwin EG. Canine cutaneous mast cell tumor: morphologic grading and survival time. *Vet Pathol* 21:469, 1984.

62. Calvert CA. Canine viral and transmissible neoplasias. In: Greene CE, ed. *Clinical Microbiology and Infectious Diseases of the Dog and Cat.* Philadelphia: WB Saunders, 1984:461.

63. Perman V. Personal communication, 1970.

64. Howell RM, Alexander VG. Keratoacanthoma on the eyelid of a beagle dog. *Vet Med Small Anim Clin* 11:1022, 1968.

65. Rebhun WC, Berton A. Equine lymphosarcoma. *J Am Vet Med Assoc* 184:720, 1984.

66. Murphy CJ, Lavoic JP, Groff J. Bilateral eyelid swelling attributable to lymphosarcoma in a horse. *J Am Vet Med Assoc* 194:939, 1989.

67. Fawcett J, Altman N, Demaray SY. Multiple xanthomatosis in a cat. *Feline Pract* 7:32, 1977.

68. Aurora A, Blodi F. Lesions of the eyelids: a clinicopathological study. *Surv Ophthalmol* 15:94, 1970.

69. Murphy GF, Elder MB. *Atlas of Tumor Pathology: Non-Melanocytic Tumors of the Skin,* 3d ed. Washington, DC: AFIP, 1991.

70. Holdiness MR. The sign of Leser-Trélat. *Int J Dermatol* 25:564, 1986.

71. Ellis DL, Kafka SP, Chow JC, et al. Melanoma, growth factors, acanthosis nigricans, the sign of Leser-Trélat, and multiple acrochordons. *N Engl J Med* 317:1582, 1987.

72. Ni C, Merriam J, Abert DM. Irritated seborrheic keratosis of eyelid and its differential diagnosis: an electron microscopic and light microscopic study. *Chin Med J [Engl]* 101:555, 1988.

73. Sassani JW, Yanoff M. Inverted follicular keratosis. *Am J Ophthalmol* 87:810, 1979.

74. Mathur A, Mehrotra ML, Gupta A. Pigmented squamous cell papilloma: a case report. *Indian J Ophthalmol* 35:158, 1987.

75. Brauninger GE, Hood CI, Worthen DM. Sebaceous carcinoma of lid margin masquerading as cutaneous horn. *Arch Ophthalmol* 90:380, 1973.

76. Scott KR, Kronish JW. Premalignant lesions and squamous cell carcinoma. In: Woog JJ, Jakobiec FA, eds. *Principles and Practice of Ophthalmology: Clinical Practice.* Philadelphia: WB Saunders, 1994:1733.

77. McCallum DI, Kinmont PD, Williams DW, et al. Intraepidermal carcinoma of the eyelid margin. *Br J Dermatol* 93:239, 1975.

78. Gaasterland DE, Rodrigues MM, Moshell AN. Ocular involvement in xeroderma pigmentosum. *Ophthalmology* 89:980, 1982.

79. McDonnell JM, McDonnell PJ, Stout WC, et al. Human papillomavirus DNA in a recurrent squamous carcinoma of the eyelid. *Arch Ophthalmol* 107:1631, 1989.

80. Loeffler M, Hornblass A. Characteristics and behavior of eyelid carcinoma (basal cell, squamous cell sebaceous gland, and malignant melanoma). *Ophthalmic Surg* 21:513, 1990.

81. Reifler DM, Hornblass A. Squamous cell carcinoma of the eyelid. *Surv Ophthalmol* 30:349, 1986.

82. Doxanas MT, Iliff WJ, Iliff NT, et al. Squamous cell carcinoma of the eyelids. *Ophthalmology* 94:538, 1987.

83. Beyer-Machule CK, Riedel KG. Basal cell carcinoma. In: Woog JJ, Jakobiec FA, eds. *Principles and Practice of Ophthalmology: Clinical Practice.* Philadelphia: WB Saunders, 1994:1724.

84. Nerad JA, Whitaker DC. Periocular basal cell carcinoma in adults 35 years of age and younger. *Am J Ophthalmol* 106:723, 1988.

85. Wiggs EO. Morphea-form basal cell carcinomas of the canthi. *Trans Am Acad Ophthalmol Otolaryngol* 79:649, 1975.

86. Weshler Z, Leviatan A, Peled J, et al. Spinal metastases of basal cell carcinoma. *J Surg Oncol* 25:28, 1984.

87. Aldred WV, Ramirez VG, Nicholson DH. Intraocular invasion by basal cell carcinoma of the lid. *Arch Ophthalmol* 98:1821, 1980.

88. Chalfin J, Putterman AM. Frozen section control in the surgery of basal cell carcinoma of the eyelid. *Am J Ophthalmol* 87:802, 1979.

89. Older JJ, Quickert MH, Beard C. Surgical removal of basal cell carcinoma of the eyelids utilizing frozen section control. *Trans Am Acad Ophthalmol Otolaryngol* 79:658, 1975.

90. Frank HJ. Frozen section control of excision of eyelid basal cell carcinomas: 8 years' experience. *Br J Ophthalmol* 73:328, 1989.

91. Morley M, Finger PT, Perlin M, et al. Cis-platinum chemotherapy for ocular basal cell carcinoma. *Br J Ophthalmol* 75:407, 1991.

92. Simpson W, Garner A, Collin JR. Benign hair-follicle derived tumours in the differential diagnosis of basal-cell carcinoma of the eyelids: a clinicopathological comparison. *Br J Ophthalmol* 73:347, 1989.

93. Carreras B Jr, Lopez-Marin I Jr, Mellado VG, et al. Trichofolliculoma of the eyelid. *Br J Ophthalmol* 65:214, 1981.

94. Rodgers IR, Jakobiec FA, Hidayat AA. Eyelid tumors of apocrine, eccrine, and pilar origin. In: Woog JJ, Jakobiec FA, eds. *Principles and Practice of Ophthalmology: Clinical Practice.* Philadelphia: WB Saunders, 1994:1770.

95. Hidayat AA, Font RL. Trichilemmoma of eyelid and eyebrow: a clinicopathologic study of 31 cases. *Arch Ophthalmol* 98:844, 1980.

96. Reifler DM, Ballitch JA II, Kessler DL, et al. Tricholemmoma of the eyelid. *Ophthalmology* 94:1272, 1987.

97. Bardenstein DS, McLean IW, Nerney J, et al. Cowden's disease. *Ophthalmology* 95:1038, 1988.

98. Malherbe A, Chenantais J. Note sur l'epithéliome calcifié des glandes sébacées. *Prog Med (Paris)* 8:826, 1880.

99. Kleener J. Pilomatrixoma (epithelioma calcificans Malherbe): a clinical and histopathological survey of Danish material from 1954 to 1971. *Acta Ophthalmol* 51:692, 1973.

100. Ni C, Kimball GP, Craft JL, et al. Calcifying epithelioma: a clinicopathological analysis of 67 cases with ultrastructural study of 2 cases. *Int Ophthalmol Clin* 22:63, 1982.

101. Perez RC, Nicholson DH. Malherbe's calcifying epithelioma (pilomatrixoma) of the eyelid: Clinical features [clinical conference]. *Arch Ophthalmol* 97:314, 1979.

102. O'Grady RB, Spoerl G. Pilomatrixoma (benign calcifying epithelioma of Malherbe). *Ophthalmology* 88:1196, 1981.

103. Hashimoto K, Blum D, Fukaya T, et al. Familial syringoma: case history and application of monoclonal antieccrine gland antibodies. *Arch Dermatol* 121:756, 1985.

104. Ni C, Dryja TP, Albert DM. Sweat gland tumors in the eyelids: a clinicopathological analysis of 55 cases. *Int Ophthalmol Clin* 22:1, 1982.

105. Saornil MA. Ophthalmic pathology, pathology of the lids. In: Albert DM, Dryja TR, Jakobiec FA, eds. *Principles and Practice of Ophthalmology: Clinical Practice.* Philadelphia: WB Saunders, 1994:2288.

106. Levine MR, Grossniklaus H. Sclerosing syringoma. *Ann Ophthalmol* 22:110, 1990.

107. Bilroth T. Beobachturgen: Uber Geschwulste der Speicheldrusen. *Virchows Arch Pathol Anat* 17:357, 1859.

108. Grossniklaus HE, Knight SH. Eccrine acrospiroma (clear cell hidradenoma) of the eyelid: immunohistochemical and ultrastructural features. *Ophthalmology* 98:347, 1991.

109. Ahluwalia BK, Khurana AK, Chugh AD, et al. Eccrine spiradenoma of eyelid: case report. *Br J Ophthalmol* 70:580, 1986.

110. Netland PA, Townsend DJ, Albert DM, et al. Hidradenoma papilliferum of the upper eyelid arising from the apocrine gland of Moll. *Ophthalmology* 97:1593, 1990.

111. Jakobiec FA, Streeten BW, Iwamato T, et al. *Syringocystadenoma papilliferum* of the eyelid. *Ophthalmology* 88:1175, 1981.

112. Langer K, Konrad K, Smolle J. Multiple apocrine hidrocystomas on the eyelids. *Am J Dermatopathol* 11:570, 1989.

113. Bures FA, Kotynek J. Differentiating between apocrine and eccrine hidrocystoma. *Cutis* 29:619, 1982.

114. Font RL, Stone MS, Schwanzer MC, et al. Apocrine hidrocystomas of the lids, hypodontia, palmar-plantar hyperkeratosis, and onychodystrophy: a new variant of ectodermal dysplasia. *Arch Ophthalmol* 104:1811, 1986.

115. Rodgers IR, Jakobiec FA, Hornblass A, et al. Papillary oncocytoma of the eyelid: a previously undescribed tumor of apocrine gland origin. *Ophthalmology* 95:1071, 1988.

116. Thaller VT, Collin JR, McCartney AC. Oncocytoma of the eyelid: a case report. *Br J Ophthalmol* 71:753, 1987.

117. Wright JD, Font RL. Mucinous sweat gland adenocarcinoma of eyelid. *Cancer* 44:1757, 1979.

118. Khalil M, Brownstein S, Codere F, et al. Eccrine sweat gland carcinoma of the eyelid with orbital involvement. *Arch Ophthalmol* 98:2210, 1980.

119. Boi S, De Concini M, Detassis C. Mucinous sweat-gland adenocarcinoma of the inner canthus: a case report. *Ann Ophthalmol* 20:189, 1988.

120. Snow SN, Reizner GT. Mucinous eccrine carcinoma of the eyelid. *Cancer* 70:2099, 1992.
121. Ni C, Wagoner M, Kieval S, et al. Tumours of the Moll's glands. *Br J Ophthalmol* 68:502, 1984.
122. Futrell JW, Krueger GR, Chretien PB, et al. Multiple primary sweat gland carcinomas. *Cancer* 28:686, 1971.
123. Cooper PH. Carcinomas of sweat glands. *Pathol Annu* 1:83, 1987.
124. Sanke RF. Primary mucinous adenocarcinoma of the eyelid. *Ophthalmic Surg* 20:668, 1989.
125. Jakobiec FA, Austin P, Iwamoto T, et al. Primary infiltrating signet ring carcinoma of the eyelids. *Ophthalmology* 90:291, 1983.
126. Glatt HJ, Proia HJ, Tsoy EA, et al. Malignant syringoma of the eyelid. *Ophthalmology* 91:987, 1984.
127. Finan MC, Connolly SM. Sebaceous gland tumors and systemic disease: a clinicopathologic analysis. *Medicine (Baltimore)* 63:232, 1984.
128. Tillawi I, Katz R, Pellettiere EV. Solitary tumors of meibomian gland origin and Torre's syndrome. *Am J Ophthalmol* 104:179, 1987.
129. Jakobiec FA. Sebaceous adenoma of the eyelid and visceral malignancy. *Am J Ophthalmol* 78:952, 1974.
130. Wright P, Collin RJ, Garner A. The masquerade syndrome. *Trans Ophthalmol Soc UK* 101:244, 1981.
131. Kass LG, Hornblass A. Sebaceous carcinoma of the ocular adnexa. *Surv Ophthalmol* 33:477, 1989.
132. Doxanas MT, Green WR. Sebaceous gland carcinoma: review of 40 cases. *Arch Ophthalmol* 102:245, 1984.
133. Ni C, Searl SS, Kuo PK, et al. Sebaceous cell carcinomas of the ocular adnexa. *Int Ophthalmol Clin* 22:23, 1982.
134. Lemos LB, Santa Cruz DJ, Baba N. Sebaceous carcinoma of the eyelid following radiation therapy. *Am J Surg Pathol* 2:305, 1978.
135. Schlernitzauer DA, Font RL. Sebaceous gland carcinoma of the eyelid. *Arch Ophthalmol* 94:1523, 1976.
136. Wagoner MD, Beyer CK, Gonder JR, et al. Common presentations of sebaceous gland carcinoma of the eyelid. *Ann Ophthalmol* 14:159, 1982.
137. Condon GP, Brownstein S, Codere F. Sebaceous carcinoma of the eyelid masquerading as superior limbic keratoconjunctivitis. *Arch Ophthalmol* 103:1525, 1985.
138. Epstein GA, Putterman AM. Sebaceous adenocarcinoma of the eyelid. *Ophthalmic Surg* 14:935, 1983.
139. Margo CE, Lessner A, Stern GA. Intraepithelial sebaceous carcinoma of the conjunctiva and skin of the eyelid. *Ophthalmology* 99:227, 1992.
140. Russell WG, Page DL, Hough AJ, et al. Sebaceous carcinoma of meibomian gland origin: the diagnostic importance of pagetoid spread of neoplastic cells. *Am J Clin Pathol* 73:504, 1980.
141. Sakol PJ, Simons KB, McFadden PW, et al. DNA flow cytometry of sebaceous cell carcinomas of the ocular adnexa: introduction to the technique in the evaluation of periocular tumors. *Ophthalmic Plast Reconstr Surg* 8:77, 1992.
142. Harvey JT, Anderson RL. The management of meibomian gland carcinoma. *Ophthalmic Surg* 13:56, 1982.
143. Kluka E, David S Jr, Lyons GD. Meibomian gland adenocarcinoma of the eyelid metastasizing to parotid lymph nodes. *Ear Nose Throat J* 70:502, 1991.
144. Colak A, Akkurt C, Ozcan OE, et al. Intracranial extension of meibomian gland carcinoma. *J Clin Neuro Ophthalmol* 11:39, 1991.
145. Bryant J. Meibomian gland carcinoma seeding intracranial soft tissues. *Hum Pathol* 8:455, 1977.
146. Folberg R, Whitaker DC, Tse DT, et al. Recurrent and residual sebaceous carcinoma after Mohs' excision of the primary lesion. *Am J Ophthalmol* 103:817, 1987.
147. Kivela T, Tarkkanen A. The Merkel cell and associated neoplasms in the eyelids and periocular region. *Surv Ophthalmol* 35:171, 1990.
148. Mamalis N, Medlock RD, Holds JB, et al. Merkel cell tumor of the eyelid: a review and report of an unusual case. *Ophthalmic Surg* 20:410, 1989.
149. Magrini SM, Bianchi S, Mungai V, et al. Merkel cell carcinoma: report of two cases and clinical considerations. *J Surg Oncol* 49:131, 1992.
150. Fawcett IM, Lee WR. Merkel cell carcinoma of the eyelid. *Graefes Arch Clin Exp Ophthalmol* 224:330, 1986.
151. Truong L, Font RL. Intravenous pyogenic granuloma of the ocular adnexa: report of two cases and review of the literature. *Arch Ophthalmol* 103:1364, 1985.
152. Stigmar G, Crawford JS, Ward CM, et al. Ophthalmic sequelae of infantile hemangiomas of the eyelids and orbit. *Am J Ophthalmol* 85:806, 1978.
153. Deans RM, Harris GJ, Kivlin JD. Surgical dissection of capillary hemangiomas: an alternative to intralesional corticosteroids. *Arch Ophthalmol* 110:1743, 1992.
154. Hobby LW. Further evaluation of the potential of the argon laser in the treatment of strawberry hemangiomas. *Plast Reconstr Surg* 71:481, 1983.
155. Goble RR, Frangoulis MA. Lymphangioma circumscriptum of the eyelids and conjunctiva. *Br J Ophthalmol* 74:574, 1990.
156. Pang P, Jakobiec FA, Iwamoto T, et al. Small lymphangiomas of the eyelids. *Ophthalmology* 91:1278, 1984.
157. Rootman J, Hay E, Graeb D, et al. Orbital-adnexal lymphangiomas: a spectrum of hemodynamically isolated vascular hamartomas. *Ophthalmology* 93:1558, 1986.
158. Charles NC. Multiple glomus tumors of the face and eyelid. *Arch Ophthalmol* 94:1283, 1976.
159. Saxe SJ, Grossniklaus HE, Wojno TH, et al. Glomus cell tumor of the eyelid. *Ophthalmology* 100:139, 1993.
160. Kalinske M, Leone C Jr. Kaposi's sarcoma involving eyelid and conjunctiva. *Ann Ophthalmol* 14:497, 1982.

161. Dugel PU, Gill PS, Frangieh GT, et al. Treatment of ocular adnexal Kaposi's sarcoma in acquired immune deficiency syndrome. *Ophthalmology* 99:1127, 1992.

162. Hidayat AA, Font RL. Juvenile fibromatosis of the periorbital region and eyelid: a clinicopathologic study of six cases. *Arch Ophthalmol* 98:280, 1980.

163. Jakobiec FA, DeVoe AG, Boyd J. Fibrous histiocytoma of the tarsus. *Am J Ophthalmol* 84:794, 1977.

164. John T, Yanoff M, Scheie HG. Eyelid fibrous histiocytoma. *Ophthalmology* 88:1193, 1981.

165. Jordan DR, Addison DJ, Anderson RL. Fibrous histiocytoma: an uncommon eyelid lesion. *Arch Ophthalmol* 107:1530, 1989.

166. Boynton JR, Markowitch W Jr, Searl SS. Atypical fibroxanthoma of the eyelid. *Ophthalmology* 96:1480, 1989.

167. Bolcs S, Juhos P. A case of palpebral myxoma. *Ophthalmologica* 171:488, 1975.

168. Kennedy RH, Waller RR, Carney JA. Ocular pigmented spots and eyelid myxomas. *Am J Ophthalmol* 104:533, 1987.

169. Weiner JM, Hidayat AA. Juvenile fibrosarcoma of the orbit and eyelid: a study of five cases. *Arch Ophthalmol* 101:253, 1983.

170. Schuster SA, Ferguson E, Marshall RB. Alveolar rhabdomyosarcoma of the eyelid: diagnosis by electron microscopy. *Arch Ophthalmol* 87:646, 1972.

171. Kobrin JL, Blodi FC, Weingeist TA. Ocular and orbital manifestations of neurofibromatosis. *Surv Ophthalmol* 24:45, 1979.

172. Woog JJ, Albert DM, Solt LC, et al. Neurofibromatosis of the eyelid and orbit. *Int Ophthalmol Clin* 22:157, 1982.

173. Brownstein S, Little JM. Ocular neurofibromatosis. *Ophthalmology* 90:1595, 1983.

174. Tenzel RR, Boynton JR, Miller GR, et al. Surgical treatment of eyelid neurofibromas. *Arch Ophthalmol* 95:479, 1977.

175. Shields JA, Guibor P. Neurilemoma of the eyelid resembling a recurrent chalazion. *Arch Ophthalmol* 102:1650, 1984.

176. Rubenzik R, Tenzel RR. Granular cell myoblastoma of the lid: case report. *Ann Ophthalmol* 8:421, 1976.

177. Jaeger MJ, Green WR, Miller NR, et al. Granular cell tumor of the orbit and ocular adnexae. *Surv Ophthalmol* 31:417, 1987.

178. Friedman Z, Eden E, Neumann E. Granular cell myoblastoma of the eyelid margin. *Br J Ophthalmol* 57:757, 1973.

179. Wolter JR, Benz SC. Ectopic meningioma of the superior orbital rim. *Arch Ophthalmol* 94:1920, 1976.

180. Ehlers N. Divided nevus. *Acta Ophthalmol* 47:1004, 1969.

181. De Pietro WP, Sweeney EW, Silvers DN. Divided nevi: pigmented and achromatic. *Cutis* 27:408, 1981.

182. Grossniklaus HE, McLean IW. Cutaneous melanoma of the eyelid: clinicopathologic features. *Ophthalmology* 98:1867, 1991.

183. Naidoff MA, Bernardino VB, Clark WH. Melanocytic lesions of the eyelid skin. *Am J Ophthalmol* 82:371, 1976.

184. Collin JR, Allen LH, Garner A, et al. Malignant melanoma of the eyelid and conjunctiva. *Aust NZ J Ophthalmol* 14:29, 1986.

185. Garner A, Koornneef L, Levene A, et al. Malignant melanoma of the eyelid skin: histopathology and behaviour. *Br J Ophthalmol* 69:180, 1985.

186. Zimmerman LE. Melanocytic tumors of interest to the ophthalmologist. *Ophthalmology* 87:497, 1980.

187. Rodriguez-Sains RS, Jakobiec FA, Iwamoto T. Lentigo maligna of the lateral canthal skin. *Ophthalmology* 88:186, 1981.

188. Sutula FC, Dortzbach RK, Bolles JC. Desmoplastic malignant melanoma of the upper eyelid. *Ann Ophthalmol* 14:141, 1982.

189. Lessner A, Sexton M, Margo CE. Amelanotic malignant melanoma of the eyelid. *Arch Ophthalmol* 109:1166, 1991.

190. Mansour AM, Hidayat AA. Metastatic eyelid disease, *Ophthalmology* 94:667, 1987.

191. Morgan LW, Linberg JV, Anderson RL. Metastatic disease first presenting as eyelid tumors: a report of two cases and review of the literature. *Ann Ophthalmol* 19:13, 1987.

192. Newman NM, DiLoreto DA. Metastasis of primary osteogenic sarcoma to the eyelid. *Am J Ophthalmol* 104:659, 1987.

193. Malone TJ, Folberg R, Nerad J. Lumbosacral chordoma metastatic to the eyelid. *Ophthalmology* 94:966, 1987.

194. Shields JA, Shields CL. Sebaceous carcinoma of the glands of Zeis. *Ophthalmic Plast Reconstr Surg* 4:11, 1988.

195. Ham JA, Carr NJ. Testicular cancer presenting as a red swollen lid. *Br J Ophthalmol* 72:868, 1988.

196. Arnold AC, Bullock JD, Foos RY. Metastatic eyelid carcinoma. *Ophthalmology* 92:114, 1985.

197. Kuchle M, Holbach L, Schlotzer-Schrehardt U. Gastric adenocarcinoma presenting as an eyelid and conjunctival mass. *Eur J Ophthalmol* 2:3, 1992.

198. Rodrigues MM, Font RL, Shannon GM. Metastatic mucus-secreting mammary carcinoma in the eyelid: report of two cases. *Br J Ophthalmol* 58:877, 1974.

199. Nelson CC, Kincaid MC. Breast carcinoma metastatic to the eyelids. *Arch Ophthalmol* 105:1724, 1987.

200. Fett DR, Putterman AM. Primary localized amyloidosis presenting as an eyelid margin tumor. *Arch Ophthalmol* 104:84, 1986.

201. Ferry AP. Granular cell tumor (myoblastoma) of the palpebral conjunctiva causing pseudoepitheliomatous hyperplasia of the conjunctival epithelium. *Am J Ophthalmol* 91:234, 1981.

3

TUMORS OF THE CONJUNCTIVA

Brian Wilcock, Pearl S. Rosenbaum, and Jonathan Boniuk

Tumors arising from the conjunctiva demonstrate prominent similarities when comparing animals and humans; most commonly arising from the epithelium, the vasculature, or the melanocytes that populate the epithelium, biologic behavior appears to be similar, but, in a trend that will be evident throughout this chapter, the human diseases are documented in both greater numbers and detail, providing a sounder foundation for prediction of biologic behavior and management guidelines.

ANIMALS

Vascular Tumors

TERMINOLOGY. Vascular tumors of the conjunctiva represent a continuum of histologic appearance from telangiectasia to hemangioma, angiokeratoma and hemangiosarcoma. Technically, *telangiectasia* refers to a localized dilatation of veins or venules and is distinguished from hemangioma on the basis of the retention, in telangiectasia, of a structurally normal vessel wall that may include smooth muscle and pericytes. A diagnosis of *hemangioma* is warranted if there is a localized accumulation of dilated, thin-walled vascular channels lined by morphologically normal endothelial cells but without any smooth muscle or pericytes. These distinctions are easier to express on paper than they are to apply to the actual tissues. In practice, we diagnose hemangioma if the vascular proliferation creates a lump that has obliterated the resident architecture, which is preserved in simple telangiectasia. *Hemangiosarcoma* shares the same general features as hemangioma, except that the growth habit tends to be more invasive, and the endothelial cells show much more hyperchromasia, anisokaryosis, and even a few mitotic figures. As is true of these vascular tumors elsewhere, there is

considerable overlap between hemangioma and hemangiosarcoma, with many specimens occupying a middle ground in which there is hyperchromasia but virtually no observed mitotic activity.

Angiokeratoma is a term borrowed from human pathology and is used to describe the hemangioma-like proliferation of thin-walled vessels in the very superficial conjunctival lamina propria, the proliferation of which is accompanied by pseudocarcinomatous hyperplasia of the overlying epithelium. Since such hyperplasia is very commonly seen overlying a variety of benign eyelid or conjunctival tumors, there is reason to doubt that this epithelial hyperplasia should be used to justify a separate classification.

EPIDEMIOLOGY. Conjunctival vascular tumors probably occur in all domestic species but are reported only in dogs and horses. In dogs, they virtually always occur either along the leading edge of the third eyelid or in the bulbar conjunctiva at the lateral limbus. Most cases are initially unilateral, but it is not unusual to have bilateral or sequential lesions.[1–6] There is no sex predilection. The average age of affected dogs is 8½ years, but the range is quite broad and corresponds to the general "tumor-bearing" years in dogs.[6] The strong site predilections point to ultraviolet radiation as a predisposing factor, as is true for cutaneous hemangiosarcomas in this species.[2]

In horses, hemangiosarcomas are usually found on the bulbar surface of the third eyelid, near the free margin. It is likely that sunlight is a risk factor, but too few cases have been described to allow any useful epidemiologic inference about causation or to allow any generalizations about breed or sex predilection.[7–9]

MACROSCOPIC APPEARANCE. In dogs, conjunctival vascular tumors initially appear as a focal, well-circumscribed area of reddening of the limbal bulbar conjunctiva or of the palpebral surface of the third eyelid. Over the ensuing weeks or months, there is proliferation to form a smooth or multilobulated, red, exophytic nodule.

In horses, the appearance is more variable depending on whether the tumor is forming vascularized channels or, as is quite common, remains a primitive spindle cell tumor with only rudimentary channel formation. In the former instance, its appearance resembles that described for dogs. In the latter instance, it presents as a poorly circumscribed, firm, pink-to-tan plaque or nodule involving the bulbar aspect of the third eyelid or bulbar conjunctiva.[8,10]

HISTOPATHOLOGY. In dogs, conjunctival vascular tumors have considerable variation even within the same specimen, providing good evidence that they represent a continuum, which may include telangiectasia, hemangioma, angiokeratoma, and hemangiosarcoma. The archetypal specimen consists of a poorly circumscribed subepithelial proliferation of thin-walled vascular channels lined by an inconspicuous endothelium. The confluence of vessels obliterates all preexistent architectural features (Figures 3.1–3.3). At the other end of the spectrum (hemangiosarcoma), the endothelial cells are variable in their size, are hyperchromatic, and may form solid bundles of nondescript spindle cells with only focal formation of the typical vascular channels (Figure 3.4). Mitotic figures vary from few to many, and their absence does not weigh heavily against the diagnosis of malignancy. In those variants described as angiokeratomas, there is pseudocarcinomatous hyperplasia of the overlying conjunctival epithelium, separating the vascular proliferations into multiple subepithelial nodules.[3,5] Although immunohistochemical examination is not necessary for identification, and does not help separate hemangioma from hemangiosarcoma or angiokeratoma (if one should wish to bother!), these tumors are routinely positive for factor VIII-related antigen. Ultrastructural features have not been reported but are expected to resemble those reported for vascular tumors elsewhere.

In horses, the most typical histologic appearance is that of a pleomorphic plump spindle cell tumor that only focally develops the appearance of coalescing, flattened vascular channels that allows it to be identified as a vascular tumor (Figure 3.5).[10] Those not familiar with the existence of this mor-

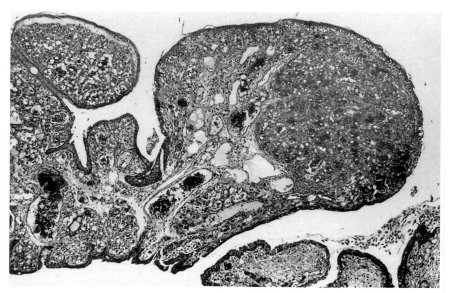

FIG. 3.1—This multilobulated, exophytic, red conjunctival nodule is made up of a coalescence of thin-walled, dilated vascular channels. Some normal lamina propria is still between the vascular channels, and this tumor could be classified as focal telangiectasia or hemangioma, depending on the exact microscopic field examined.

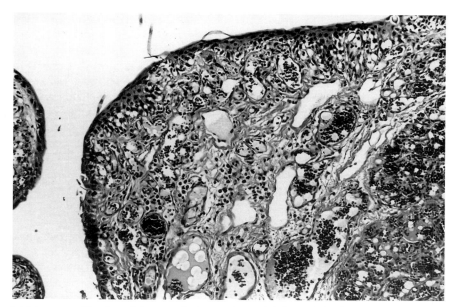

FIG. 3.2—A higher magnification of the same lesion as shown in Figure 3.1, with the blood-filled dilated channels separated by a lymphocyte-rich edematous lamina propria. This lesion was classified as telangiectasia.

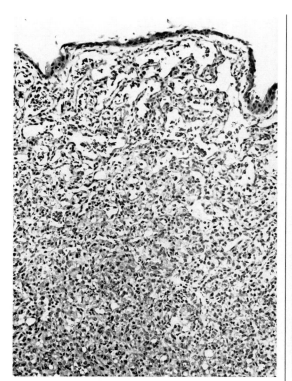

FIG. 3.3—A proliferation of thin-walled vascular channels has obliterated the preexistent tissue architecture, thus qualifying as hemangioma.

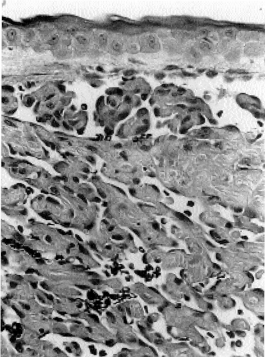

FIG. 3.4—Collapsed vascular channels are formed by hyperchromatic, slightly pleomorphic endothelium supported by an abundant, cell-poor collagenous connective tissue in this lesion diagnosed as hemagiosarcoma.

phologic variant will frequently misdiagnose the tumor as undifferentiated sarcoma, fibrosarcoma, or even fibrous histiocytoma. Most of these solid tumors also have abundant lymphocytic interstitial inflammation, a feature not seen in the canine tumors or in those equine tumors that look like more traditional capillary hemangiomas or hemangiosarcomas. Compared with the tumors in dogs, these solid equine hemangiosarcomas have a more infiltrative growth habit and frequently extend almost to the base of the third eyelid. Whether this reflects a fundamentally more aggressive behavior or just a longer interval between tumor occurrence and veterinary examination is not known. The few tumors tested have been positive for factor VIII-related antigen.[10]

TREATMENT AND PROGNOSIS. The treatment of choice for conjunctival vascular tumors is excision with or without ancillary procedures such as cryotherapy. The efficacy of laser surgery has not been established. Of the 22 cases followed by this author, there have been no recurrences and no metastases after simple excision or excision followed by cryotherapy.[6] Those tumors arising in bulbar conjunctiva might be expected to have a greater risk of recurrence because of the greater likelihood of initially incomplete excision. In the retrospective series reported by Hargis et al.,[2] two of 14 affected dogs had recurrence of tumor or development of a de novo tumor adjacent to the original site. No metastases were recorded.

In horses, solid hemangiosarcomas of the third eyelid frequently recur because of incomplete excision and will eventually undergo metastasis to local lymph nodes.[8] Presumably, greater recognition of these tumors and their infiltrative growth habit will result in more radical initial surgery (removal of the entire third eyelid), which should avert metastatic disease. The postoperative behavior of more typical capillary hemangiomas and hemangiosarcomas in horses has not been documented. In the only published report that included follow-up information on a single case, there were no complications 8 months after excision of a limbal capillary hemangioma.[7]

Adenocarcinoma of the Gland of the Third Eyelid

TERMINOLOGY. Adenocarcinoma of the gland of the third eyelid is an uncommon, slowly progressive carcinoma derived from the lacrimal gland on

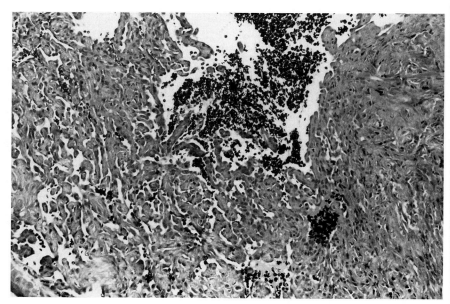

FIG. 3.5—As is typical for many of the equine conjunctival hemangiosarcomas, this one shows variation from solid spindle cells reminiscent of fibrosarcoma to areas in which the vascular channel formation is quite obvious.

the inferior bulbar aspect of the third eyelid. It is not to be confused with the much more common prolapse of the gland of the third eyelid, to which it bears some superficial clinical resemblance.

EPIDEMIOLOGY. This rare tumor occurs almost exclusively in very old dogs, with a mean age of approximately 10½ years. This may reflect only its typically slow growth, so the tumor may actually begin at a much younger age but not be noticed because of its occurrence on the bulbar aspect of the third eyelid. There is no breed or sex predilection, but the number of described cases is very small.[11]

They occur in cats, but there are no published reports.

MACROSCOPIC APPEARANCE. The lesion presents as a tan or pink, smooth, proliferative nodule on the bulbar aspect of the third eyelid. Large tumors, which presumably have grown for years before being noticed, may protrude past the free margin of the third eyelid (Figure 3.6).

HISTOPATHOLOGY. These tumors vary from well-differentiated adenocarcinomas to more

primitive solid carcinomas. In general, they exhibit considerable squamous metaplasia and have a moderately invasive growth habit.[11] They seldom present a diagnostic challenge, and exhibit the same range of morphologic appearance as would be appropriate to other glandular tumors (Figure 3.7). Considering the location,

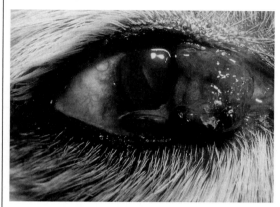

FIG. 3.6—Adenocarcinoma of the gland of the third eyelid, which is seen here as a multilobulated fleshy mass that originates within the bulbar aspect of the third eyelid and extends beyond its free margin.

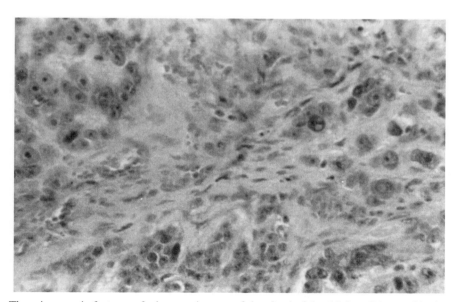

FIG. 3.7—The microscopic features of adenocarcinomas of the gland of the third eyelid resemble those of lacrimal or salivary tumors, varying from well-differentiated acinar and tubular carcinomas to those that are more solid and invasive.

there are no alternative diagnoses other than the occasional case of postinflammatory reparative dysplasia of the gland, which may simulate carcinoma. No immunohistochemical or ultrastructural studies have been reported.

TREATMENT AND PROGNOSIS. When first described, these tumors virtually always recurred because of incomplete initial excision. Now that that behavior is more widely understood, it is recommended that the entire third eyelid be excised right to its base; under these circumstances, the tumor should not recur. Even though in some cases tumors recurred two or three times, there have been no confirmed metastases.[11] This may reflect the advanced age of most of the dogs affected; death due to other causes may have intervened before any metastatic disease was likely to become clinically apparent.

Conjunctival Melanoma

TERMINOLOGY. As is true for melanomas in other tissues, veterinary pathologists have wisely decided not to embrace the complex terminology of human melanomas, which is burdened more with the weight of tradition than with biologic validity! At the moment, it seems quite adequate to determine that the lesion is indeed a melanoma and then to simply apply the adjective malignant or benign as indicated by the presence or absence of various prognostic variables. The most important variable seems to be site of origin, in that preliminary evidence suggests that those originating in the conjunctiva are much more dangerous than their counterparts arising in the anterior uvea, limbic sclera, or haired skin of the lid.[12–16]

EPIDEMIOLOGY. Primary conjunctival melanomas have been described in dogs and cats,[12–16] but there is no reason why they should not also occur in other species. Compared with the rather frequent observation of melanomas within the uveal tract, at the limbus, or involving the haired skin of the eyelid, primary conjunctival melanomas are distinctly uncommon.

In dogs, there is a strong predilection for the tumors to arise from the bulbar surface of the third eyelid.[16] Cases are too few to reveal any age, breed, or sex predilection, although most of the reported cases have been in dogs over 10 years of age.

MACROSCOPIC APPEARANCE. Not surprisingly, the typical macroscopic appearance is of a brown mass arising from the bulbar surface of the third eyelid or, less frequently, from elsewhere within the conjunctiva (Figures 3.8 and 3.9). Multiple adjacent tumors may occur, particularly when dealing with postoperative recurrences.

Even fewer examples have been described in cats. In one report, a pigmented tumor extensively infiltrated the dorsal and inferotemporal bulbar and palpebral conjunctiva of a 6-year-old spayed female black cat. The exact site of origin could

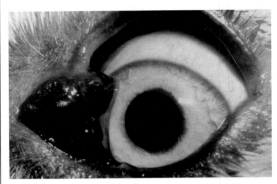

FIG. 3.8—A well-pigmented conjunctival melanoma. By the time they are this large, pinpointing the exact site of origin may be impossible. It is prognostically important to distinguish conjunctival from skin origin with caruncular and third eyelid involvement.

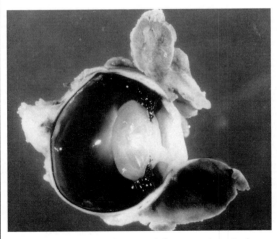

FIG. 3.9—A lightly pigmented, large conjunctival melanoma distends the third eyelid. Surgical cure seems to require excision of the entire third eyelid.

not be determined.[13] In a second report, three of 19 ocular melanomas arose from the palpebral conjunctiva (exact site not reported).[14]

HISTOPATHOLOGY. The microscopic appearance of primary conjunctival melanomas is very similar to what has been described for melanomas involving other mucous membranes, notably those involving the mouth and lips. Because the number of described cases is so small, it is premature to attempt to subclassify these melanomas in the hope of predicting subsequent behavior. It is well recognized that the cell type, mitotic index, or degree of pigmentation has no predictive value for the behavior of canine oral or lip melanomas, for which site alone seems to carry most of the prognostic weight.[17,18]

In both species, the conjunctival tumors consist primarily of epithelioid cells, spindle cells, or a mixture of the two. Formation of intraepithelial nests of pigmented tumor cells (junctional activity) is extremely common (Figure 3.10), and such junctional nests frequently are found 1 mm or more beyond what otherwise seems to be the tumor margin.[16] This growth habit probably explains the frequent recurrence of these tumors

following what seems, at first, to be adequate excision (see below). In contrast to melanomas found elsewhere in the canine eye, mitotic figures are relatively frequent, averaging between two and three per high power (40×) field.[16] Because all of the described tumors have had at least some pigmentation to facilitate histologic diagnosis (even if not as abundant as in melanomas elsewhere in the eye), no immunohistochemical or ultrastructural studies have been reported.

TREATMENT AND PROGNOSIS. No study has documented the treatment of choice for these rare tumors, but local tumor recurrence has been described in six of 11 dogs in which simple excision was the chosen treatment. In five of the six, the recurrence was predicted by the observation of neoplastic cells growing right at the edge of the excisional biopsy, suggesting that the surgery was unsuccessful in capturing all of the tumor.[16] There is too little information to comment about postoperative behavior other than local recurrence. Metastasis to local lymph nodes and orbital recurrence has been described in several dogs, but adequate follow-up postmortem investigation has not been done. Pending additional information, our current recommendation is for

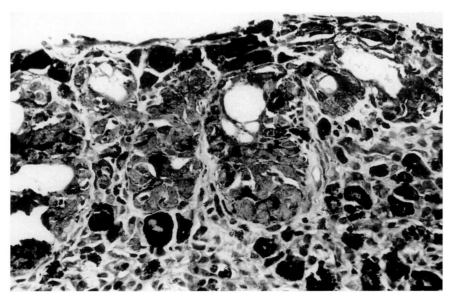

FIG. 3.10—Typically, conjunctival melanomas exhibit abundant junctional activity (intraepithelial tumor nests), but the prognostic importance of this or other histologic features has not yet been established.

wide surgical excision to prevent local metastasis. There are no reports of alternative therapeutic approaches such as diode laser surgery or cryotherapy.

All three cats in the one study that reported postoperative behavior were killed because of metastatic disease. Mean postoperative survival ranged from 99 to 108 days.[14] The two unpublished cases (B.W.) recurred within 3 months of initial excision but were cured by exenteration.

Papilloma

EPIDEMIOLOGY. Papillomas occur commonly on the canine conjunctiva, less commonly in other species; in young dogs, the lesions are likely to be multiple, associated with viral papillomatosis. In older dogs, solitary lesions involving the bulbar conjunctiva or palpebral surface of the third eyelid are seen.

Squamous Cell Carcinoma

EPIDEMIOLOGY. Although squamous cell carcinomas are occasionally described as affecting the periorbital tissues of various domestic and free-living species, most cases occur in three species: cattle, horses, and cats. In cats, the great majority of the tumors arise from the nonpigmented, haired skin of the eyelid margin and are considered in detail in the section on eyelid tumors. The disease in cattle and horses is very similar in almost all respects, although the therapeutic approaches are different because of the economic factors influencing the medical care in these two species. A great deal of what we know about this syndrome stems from a classic series of papers published by a group of American researchers between 1956 and 1964, and their conclusions remain valid today.[19–22] The disease has been subjected to numerous reviews, the most useful of which are those by Spradbrow and Hoffman[23] and, more recently, by Heeney and Valli.[24]

Ocular squamous cell carcinoma is the most common neoplasm of cattle and may reach a prevalence of as high as 5% of the cattle population in those climates characterized by abundant sunlight and high altitude.[21,25] The prevalence is even higher (25%–35%) if the data are restricted to Hereford cattle, which are particularly suscep-

tible (see below).[26,27] In the United States, ocular squamous cell carcinoma was reported to account for almost 80% of all carcass condemnations attributed to neoplasia.[25]

Approximately 70% of bovine ocular squamous cell carcinomas involve the bulbar conjunctiva at the limbus, particularly at the lateral canthus, which receives the greatest exposure to sunlight. Lesions involving the medial limbus, palpebral conjunctiva, and nictitating membrane are substantially less frequent. The distribution of the lesions and the overall prevalence are positively correlated with mean hours of sunlight, with altitude, with degree of periocular pigmentation, and with age.[19–24] Interpreting all of these data, it would appear that the only real variable is the cumulative amount of ultraviolet radiation that impacts upon lightly pigmented (and therefore unprotected) conjunctival epithelial cells.

The role of viruses, specifically bovine papillomavirus, in the pathogenesis of bovine ocular squamous cell carcinoma remains controversial. Although papilloma-like particles have been seen in some plaques and papillomas, neither viral antigen nor viral deoxyribonucleic acid (DNA) has been detected in outright carcinomas.[28,29]

In horses, the most common sites for squamous cell carcinoma are the leading edge of the third eyelid or at the limbus (accounting for about 40% and 30%, respectively), but it can also occur virtually anywhere in the bulbar or palpebral conjunctiva. Approximately 15% of horses have concurrent or sequential involvement of both eyes. The risk factors for horses appear to be virtually the same as with cattle, with positive correlations between tumor prevalence and age of affected animals, the amount of periocular pigmentation, and mean solar radiation.[30–34]

MACROSCOPIC APPEARANCE. The clinical appearance of squamous cell carcinoma varies with the stage of the disease, but early lesions appear as slightly raised white-pink granular plaques. Over time, this plaquelike lesion becomes more proliferative, forming a sessile or pedunculated papilloma. The full-fledged carcinoma is a white, granular, proliferative, and invasive plaque that frequently is ulcerated and inflamed (Figures 3.11–3.13).[22,35]

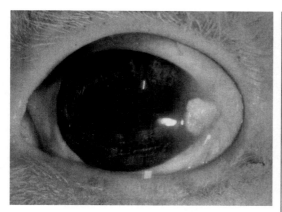

FIG. 3.11—A small gray-white proliferative plaque protrudes from the temporal limbus of this Hereford cow. With this appearance, it is probably an early squamous cell carcinoma.

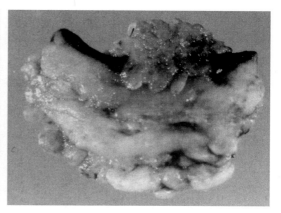

FIG. 3.13—An excised third eyelid from a horse with a papillated squamous cell carcinoma along its free margin.

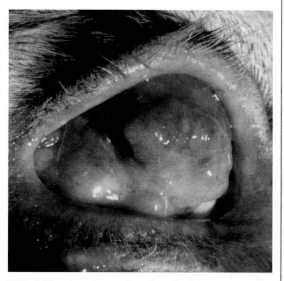

FIG. 3.12—An advanced conjunctival squamous cell carcinoma has filled the palpebral fissure in this Hereford cow. Despite its extent, intraocular invasion is very unlikely.

MICROSCOPIC APPEARANCE. The early lesion—squamous plaque—consists of abrupt focal epithelial hyperplasia with acanthosis and hyperkeratosis (Figure 3.14). The proliferation and hyperkeratosis occasionally are so severe as to form a structure similar to a cutaneous horn. Those examples that proliferate to form an exophytic papillated mass are termed *squamous*

papillomas, somewhat of a misnomer in that they have none of the cytopathic ballooning or inclusion bodies typical of true viral papillomas. Within either the plaque or the papilloma-like lesion, development of cytologic atypia heralds the onset of neoplastic transformation. Jumbling within the basal layer, anisokaryosis, hyperchromasia, dyskeratosis, and the formation of squamous pearls justify a diagnosis of carcinoma in situ. Full-fledged squamous cell carcinoma is diagnosed on the basis of unequivocal invasion by islands and cords of tumors cells, most of them resembling stratum spinosum cells, across the basement membrane.[22,25] Many tumors develop a lichenoid lymphocytic-plasmacytic infiltrate, perhaps in response to the acquisition of novel antigens as the tumor progresses from plaque to papilloma and, eventually, carcinoma (Figures 3.15 and 3.16).

The progression from plaque to outright carcinoma may take as little as 3 months or as long as several years. A substantial number of precancerous lesions spontaneously regress, and it is estimated that only 50%–75% of plaques eventually become squamous cell carcinomas.[22,26,35]

PROGNOSIS AND THERAPY. The prognosis for ocular squamous cell carcinoma is difficult to establish from the numerous reports in the literature, mostly because these reports span almost 40 years, reflect a wide range in economic and husbandry environments that influence the timing of

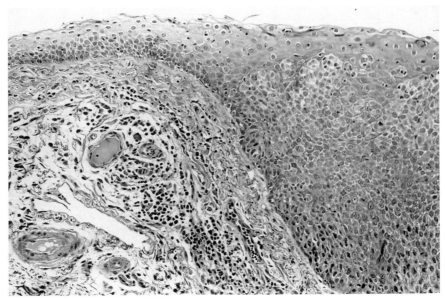

FIG. 3.14—This biopsy specimen from the limbus of a horse shows abrupt transition from normal stratified squamous epithelium into a thickened, jumbled plaque. If no evidence of invasion or greater cytologic atypia were found elsewhere in the section, the diagnosis would be of precancerous squamous plaque.

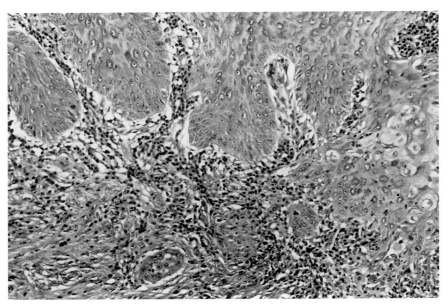

FIG. 3.15—Papillated epithelial hyperplasia with unequivocal invasion typical of squamous cell carcinoma. The presence of a lymphocytic-plasmacytic inflammatory infiltrate near the dermal-epidermal junction is a very common feature that may reflect the altered antigenicity of the full-fledged neoplasm.

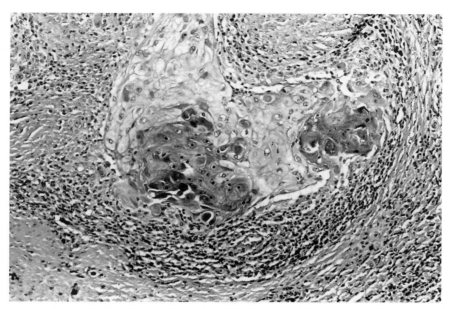

FIG. 3.16—An invasive cord of atypical, dyskeratotic epithelium resembling stratum spinosum is typical of squamous cell carcinomas in almost any location. Note, again, the lymphocytic-plasmacytic inflammation adjacent to the tumor.

tumor detection and its subsequent management, and almost never consider the stage of disease in reporting the success of therapy.[25–27,30–34] As a general conclusion, early lesions that are small and minimally invasive should be cured by local excision (although tumor may recur from adjacent sites that were similarly subjected to solar irradiation). Particularly in range cattle, however, surgical excision may not be economically feasible and early detection of lesions is a problem. Large lesions may not permit complete excision if one wishes to salvage the globe. These factors have stimulated considerable investigation of the efficacy of alternative therapies that include cryotherapy, radiotherapy using strontium 90, radioactive gold, or radon needles, hyperthermia using battery-powered probes, tumor ablation with carbon dioxide laser, and various types of immunotherapy. The extensive literature related to such diverse therapies has been reviewed by Davidson[36] and by Miller and Gelatt.[37]

In two more recent retrospective studies in horses, recurrence rates of 30% and 42% were reported following various protocols involving excision, irradiation, cryotherapy, and immunother-apy with autologous vaccine.[32,34] In each study, however, the uncontrolled variations in therapy and in the stage of tumor progression at the time of therapy make any accurate estimate of overall tumor behavior impossible. Nonetheless, there is abundant evidence that aggressive treatment of early and small tumors in either species should result in cure, and that only the most neglected cases represent life-threatening disease.

Incomplete excision of lesions results in local recurrence and invasion to involve orbit and even orbital bones. In both horses and cattle, metastasis is a very late event, with spread first to regional lymph nodes (parotid lymph node) and then to lung and other viscera. Much more common is local invasion into cornea, eyelids, and orbit. Intraocular penetration is uncommon in cattle and rare in horses, and probably occurs only in the most neglected of cases.[23,26,27,30–34]

Nodular Granulomatous Episcleritis

HISTORICAL PERSPECTIVE AND TERMINOLOGY. A nodular proliferative subconjunctival limbal lesion with histologic similarities to human nodular fasciitis was first described by Bellhorn and Henkind in 1967.[38] Since then, there have been numerous other individual and collected case reports of this syndrome, proposing a variety of names that all claim to draw parallels to various human conditions.[39–42] In surveying the 35 or so cases described in detail in the literature, one cannot help but notice that the clinical and histologic similarities among these lesions are much stronger than the few differences, and it is current practice by virtually all veterinary ophthalmic pathologists to lump all such cases together as one disease. There is still no consensus as to what name should be used, although nodular granulomatous episcleritis is perhaps the one most widely employed.

EPIDEMIOLOGY. Lesions of nodular granulomatous episcleritis are most commonly encountered in young to middle-aged dogs (mean and median age, 3½ years). There is no sex predilection, but collies and related breeds (Shetland sheepdogs, border collies, and collie-cross mongrels) are greatly overrepresented. In one study of 19 cases, for example, every affected dog was either purebred collie or collielike.[42] In collies and related breeds, lesions are usually bilateral but are not necessarily symmetrical or simultaneous in onset. In other breeds, lesions are more often unilateral.

The most common ocular site affected is the lateral subconjunctival limbus and the palpebral surface of the third eyelid. Limbic lesions tend to infiltrate the peripheral cornea but do not actually arise within the cornea.[38–42]

MACROSCOPIC APPEARANCE. The typical lesion is a smooth gray-pink nodule arising in the subconjunctival tissue of the third eyelid or limbus. The nodule is covered by a smooth, intact conjunctival epithelium. Those lesions that infiltrate the cornea are preceded by a haze of corneal edema, and old lesions may be complicated by corneal lipidosis. The size of the lesion at first presentation, and its rate of growth subsequent to diagnosis, are both highly variable. Most reports have described lesions from 0.5 to 1.5 cm in diameter (Figure 3.17).

HISTOLOGIC FEATURES. The classic lesion consists of a relatively well-circumscribed, nonencapsulated mass made up of plump fibroblasts, histiocytes, immature capillaries, and a variety of lymphocytes and plasma cells (Figure 3.18).

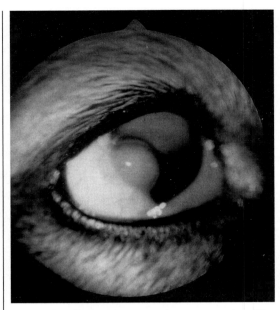

FIG. 3.17—The location, smooth contour, and mobility of this small nodule are typical for nodular granulomatous episcleritis.

There is a general tendency for the lymphocytes and plasma cells to concentrate around the periphery of the tumor. Many tumors seem to consist of a coalescence of smaller nodules. The proportions of fibroblasts versus histiocytes vary widely, and some lesions look very "inflammatory" whereas others look more "neoplastic." Cytologic atypia, however, is never seen, and mitotic figures usually are sparse. Although the lesions are certainly granulomatous, discrete granulomas never form, and one has no impression that the lesion is forming around any kind of discrete particulate foreign material. Collagenolysis is not a feature. Almost always, a thin zone of undisturbed normal lamina propria separates the lesion from the overlying conjunctiva (Figure 3.19). In large nodules, the conjunctiva may have undergone squamous metaplasia or even keratinization, but this is secondary to chronic irritation rather than a specific affect of the underlying tumor.

There is considerable variation among different areas of the same mass, or among different masses in the same dog (Figures 3.20 and 3.21). Until there is evidence that those lesions dominated by fibroblasts are prognostically or therapeutically distinct from those dominated by histiocytes, there seems little point in debating

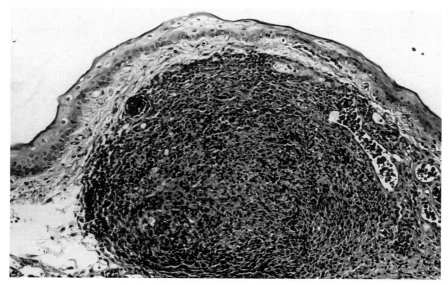

FIG. 3.18—An early lesion of nodular granulomatous episcleritis, with a relatively well-circumscribed mixture of various mononuclear leukocytes, in this instance not intimately associated with the overlying conjunctiva.

whether all of these lesions represent one disease with variable expression or several distinct diseases with histologic similarities.

TREATMENT AND PROGNOSIS. The first-described cases were successfully treated by surgical excision,[38,39,41] but many subsequent cases proved difficult to control with simple excision, which often would be followed by local recurrence of tumor. Currently, the vast majority of cases are successfully managed with topically applied corticosteroids, supplemented or replaced by azothioprine in stubborn cases. Cryotherapy is an alternative, but many dogs require at least periodic immunosuppressive therapy to control the lesion.[42]

HUMANS

Benign Epithelial Tumors. *Squamous cell papillomas* are benign and self-limited, may occur at any age, and may be either polypoid or sessile, depending on their location on the bulbar, fornical, or tarsal conjunctiva.

Infectious papillomas (Figure 3.22) are grayish red, soft, pedunculated masses usually located in the inferior fornix of children and young adults. Occasionally, the interpalpebral bulbar conjunctiva, the semilunar fold, the caruncle, or the limbal conjunctiva may be

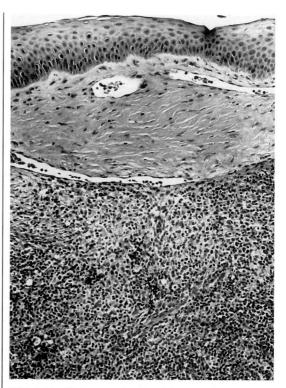

FIG. 3.19—This example of nodular granulomatous episcleritis is infiltrating the peripheral cornea. Note the variation from predominantly lymphocytic areas to more pale-staining cells that are probably macrophages. The formation of discrete granulomas is not seen, but the growth habit usually remains well circumscribed.

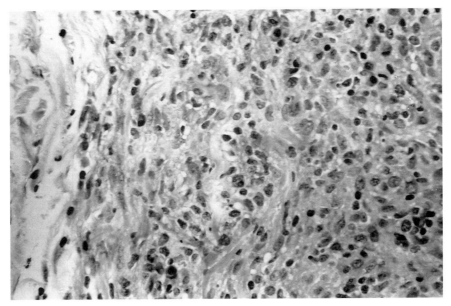

FIG. 3.20—Nodular granulomatous episcleritis. In this particular example, loosely interwoven macrophages predominate.

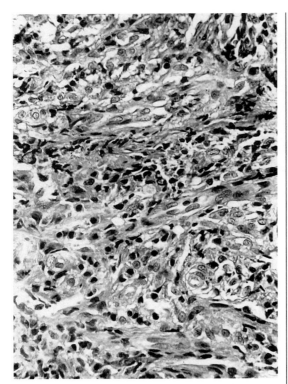

FIG. 3.21—In this example of nodular granulomatous episcleritis, fibroblast-like cells and macrophages predominate.

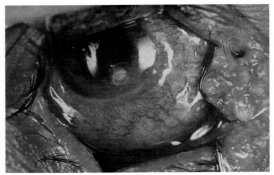

FIG. 3.22—A flesh-colored, pedunculated, papillomatous caruncular mass protrudes through the interpalpebral zone of an HIV-positive woman. An inferonasal corneal ulcer was caused by pressure from the large conjunctival tumor.

involved. Lesions may be multiple and bilateral. Infection by the human papillomavirus types 6 and 11 has been implicated in the pathogenesis of infectious papillomas of the conjunctiva[43,44] by the detection of both papillomavirus common antigen and papillomavirus DNA sequences in these lesions.

Limbal papillomas usually affect older adults. Occurring as single, unilateral growths, these

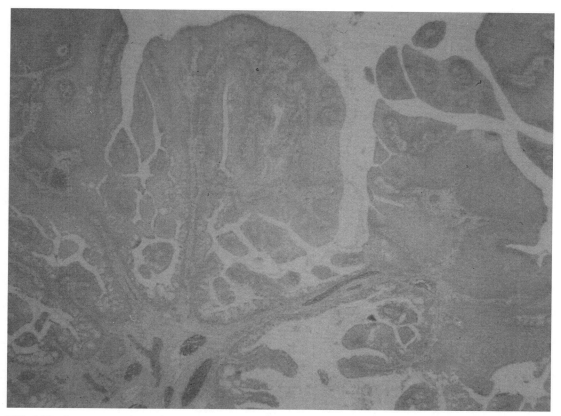

FIG. 3.23—Low-power photomicrograph shows papillomatosis and acanthosis of the conjunctival epithelium. Hematoxylin-eosin, ×6.3.

appear as flat, sessile lesions on the limbal conjunctiva, which may slowly enlarge toward the center of the cornea, thereby interfering with vision.

Histopathologically, the mass consists of papillomatous, fingerlike projections of acanthotic, nonkeratinizing, stratified squamous epithelium overlying an intact basement membrane and thin fibrovascular cores (Figures 3.23 and 3.24). Keratinization and epidermalization of the epithelium may occur if the papilloma is large and exposed through the interpalpebral fissure. There may be mild dysplasia as well as epidermalization of the exposed epithelium.

The *inverted papilloma* may develop on the conjunctiva (or in the lacrimal sac) as a slowly growing lesion that tends to invaginate into the underlying stroma rather than growing in an exophytic fashion. These papillomas more often occur in the nose and paranasal sinuses, where

they frequently recur after excision and may show malignant transformation to transitional cell, squamous cell, or mucus-secreting adenocarcinoma. On the conjunctiva, these lesions are less aggressive and without serious sequelae. Histopathologically, invasive lobules of benign-appearing acanthotic epithelium are present within the underlying connective tissue. As a result of mucus-secreting cells within these lobules, there may be cystic areas that stain for mucopolysaccharide. Jakobiec et al. suggested that this lesion be descriptively referred to as "benign mucoepidermoid of the conjunctiva."[45]

Recommended treatment of papillomas is by surgical excision, but, in cases with multiple recurrences, adjunctive cryotherapy may be required.

Epithelial cysts of the conjunctiva are generally acquired. These may become so large and tense

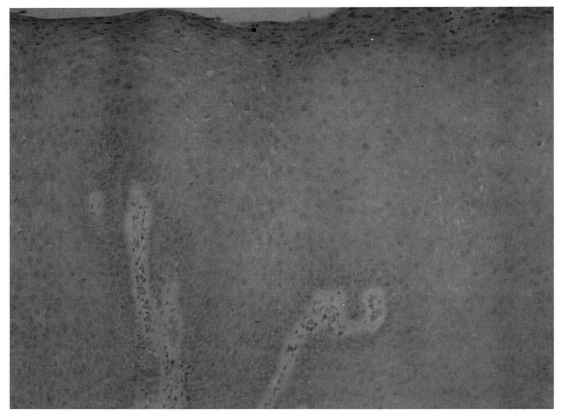

FIG. 3.24—High-power view of an infectious papilloma demonstrates an acanthotic epithelium with intracyto-plasmic vacuolization in the stratum spinosum. Hematoxylin-eosin, ×25.

that they protrude through the interpalpebral fissure, or they may be a source of ocular irritation or cosmetic concern to patients.

Implantation of surface epithelium in the bulbar conjunctival stroma may occur during accidental or surgical trauma or inflammation. Thin-walled *epithelial inclusion cysts* (Figure 3.25) develop as a result of proliferation of the implanted epithelium.

The cyst contains mucinous secretion, cellular debris and, occasionally, chronic inflammatory cells. The wall of the cyst is comprised of a flattened conjunctival epithelium containing scattered goblet cells (Figure 3.26). Surgical excision of the cyst wall is curative.

Conjunctival retention cysts (Figures 3.27 and 3.28) lie deep within the substantia propria and may arise as a result of obstruction of the outflow channels of the accessory lacrimal glands of Krause and Wolfring.[44] The cyst contains periodic

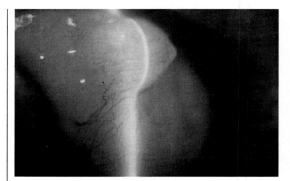

FIG. 3.25—Thin-walled bulbar conjunctival inclusion cyst subsequent to trauma. (Courtesy of Dr. Martin Mayers.)

acid-Schiff (PAS)-positive material and is lined by a single or double layer of cuboidal (ductal) epithelium. Often, chronic pericystic inflammatory charges are seen in the substantia propria.

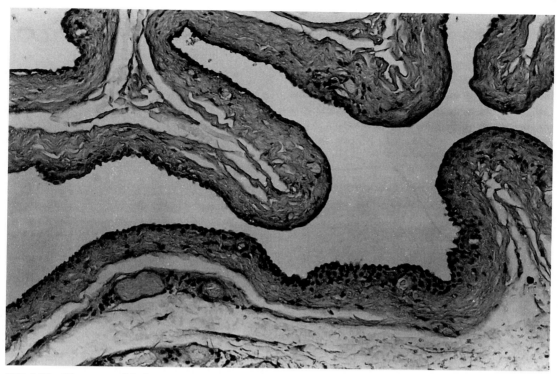

FIG. 3.26—The cyst wall is lined by conjunctival epithelium containing scattered goblet cells (periodic acid-Schiff, ×40.

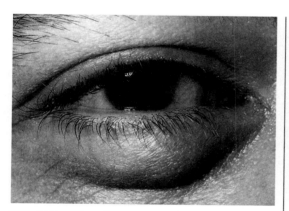

FIG. 3.27—Clinical appearance of right lower lid mass. (Courtesy of Dr. Donald Morris.)

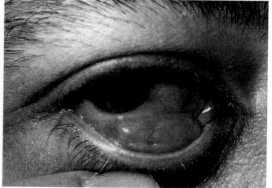

FIG. 3.28—Eversion of the right lower lid reveals a conjunctival cyst within the inferior fornix. (Courtesy of Dr. Donald Morris.)

Keratotic plaques of the conjunctiva result in a clinically well-demarcated, leukoplakic area of conjunctival thickening most often located on the limbal conjunctiva or on the bulbar conjunctiva in the interpalpebral zone. These lesions, which carry little or no malignant potential, may occur in simple degenerative conditions such as pingueculae or, less commonly, in the Bitot spot of hypovitaminosis A.

Keratotic plaques are often biopsied to exclude the presence of a conjunctival intraepithelial neoplasia.

Pseudoepitheliomatous hyperplasia is a nonspecific epithelial reaction to chronic irritation or inflammation of the conjunctiva. Clinically, this lesion is often associated with a preexisting pinguecula or pterygium that develops a thickened, leukoplakic appearance. Biopsy is performed to rule out the presence of a conjunctival intraepithelial neoplasia.

Histopathologically, there is acanthosis, parakeratosis, and hyperkeratosis of the conjunctival epithelium.

Keratoacanthoma and *inverted follicular keratosis* affect the skin of the eyelid more commonly than the bulbar conjunctiva and represent a variant of pseudoepitheliomatous hyperplasia.

Hereditary benign intraepithelial dyskeratosis (HBID) is an autosomal dominant trait with a high degree of penetrance. It occurs in descendants of an inbred isolate of Caucasian, American, Indian, and black origin in northeastern North Carolina, known as the Haliwa Indians because they reside in Halifax and Washington counties.[46–49] This disease is characterized by dyskeratosis of the conjunctival, corneal, and oral epithelium. Bilateral involvement of the nasal and temporal limbal conjunctiva appears clinically as elevated, vascularized plaques that may extend onto the cornea (Figure 3.29). Although mild cases may be asymptomatic, extensive involvement of the bulbar conjunctiva and cornea results in visual impairment.

Histopathologic examination of superficial keratectomy and conjunctivectomy specimens reveals prominent dyskeratosis of individual cells within an acanthotic epithelium, as well as overlying keratinization (Figure 3.30). The underlying stroma may contain chronic inflammatory cells.

Precancerous Epithelial Lesions. Precancerous bulbar conjunctival lesions most frequently arise in the interpalpebral fissure, consistent with ultraviolet radiation as a pathogenetic mechanism. There is a tendency for circumferential limbal spread, as well as for extension more peripherally along the bulbar conjunctiva and centrally along the corneal epithelium. Surgical management of these lesions is required, as these precancerous lesions can

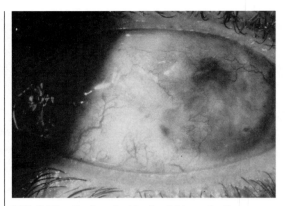

FIG. 3.29—Conjunctival leukoplakia and adjacent corneal scarring in a 33-year-old woman. The patient previously underwent multiple superficial excisions for recurrent benign intraepithelial dyskeratosis complicated by corneal stromal scarring and vascularization. (Courtesy of Dr. Kenneth Goldman.)

evolve into squamous cell carcinoma. Varying degrees of cellular atypia are often observed within a single lesion; these lesions are therefore diagnosed histopathologically according to the features observed in the most severely affected areas.

Conjunctival intraepithelial neoplasia (CIN) comprises a broad category of epibulbar squamous neoplasms, previously termed *intraepithelial epithelioma, Bowen's disease conjunctival dysplasia,* and *dyskeratosis.* The etiology of CIN is unclear. The epibulbar intraepithelial neoplasm typically is unilateral and affects fair-skinned men in their sixth decade.[50–52]

Risk factors for the development of CIN include exposure to ultraviolet radiation,[53] heavy smoking, exposure to petroleum derivatives, and human papillomavirus (HPV).[50,54–56] HPV types 6 and 8 have been identified in benign CIN, whereas types 16 and 18 have been identified in malignant conjunctival epithelial growths.[50,56–63]

It is recognized that conjunctival intraepithelial neoplasias represent a spectrum of epithelial alteration, both among different lesions as well as different areas of the same lesion. Clinically, however, all of these lesions may appear similarly as a gelatinous thickening of the conjunctiva (Figure 3.31), occasionally with areas of vascularization, papillomatosis, and leukoplakia (Figure 3.32).

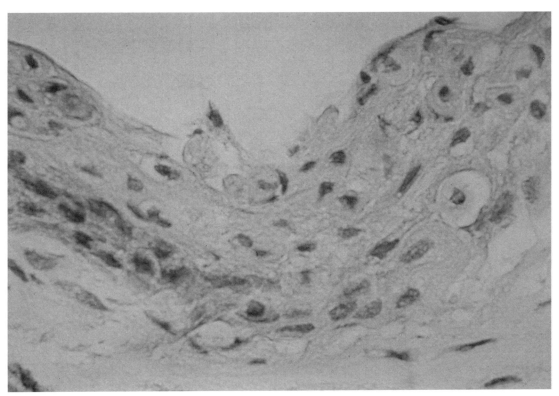

FIG. 3.30—The conjunctival epithelium is acanthotic and contains several dyskeratotic cells. Additionally, there is subepithelial fibrosis. Hematoxylin-eosin, ×80.

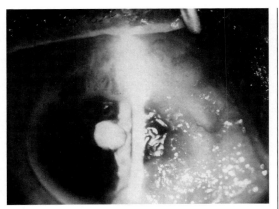

FIG. 3.31—Conjunctival and corneal intraepithelial neoplasia involving approximately 270° of the epibulbar surface. Note the grayish white, gelatinous clinical appearance as well as the fimbriated margins.

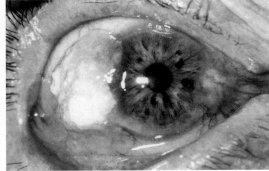

FIG. 3.32—A thickened, leukoplakic lesion is present on the limbal conjunctiva and cornea, temporally. A nasal pterygium on the same eye shows surrounding vascular dilatation and areas of leukoplakia. (Courtesy of Dr. Martin Mayers.)

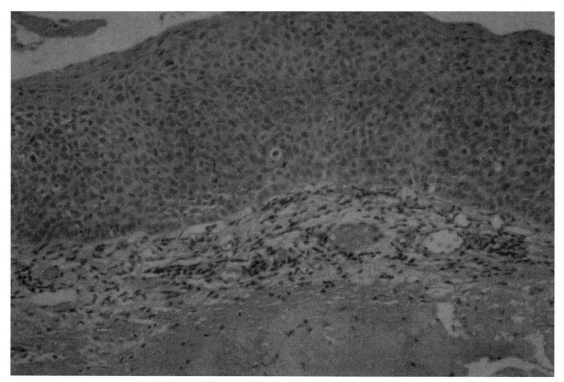

FIG. 3.33—Histopathology of the limbal conjunctiva nasally reveals severe dysplasia overlying an inflamed pterygium. Hematoxylin-eosin, ×40.

Epithelial dysplasia is diagnosed histopathologically as mild, moderate, or severe according to the degree of cellular atypia and disturbance of the normal maturation sequence observed within the conjunctival epithelium. Thus, in mild dysplasia, the atypical changes involve the basal third of the epithelium whereas, in severe dysplasia (Figures 3.33 and 3.34), the lower two-thirds or more of the epithelium may be involved.

Carcinoma in situ (Figure 3.35) is a full-thickness intraepithelial neoplasia characterized by an intact basement membrane. The World Health Organization considers this lesion to be a malignant, spreading intraepithelial neoplasm. In fact, the clinical behavior of carcinoma in situ is less aggressive and only infrequently evolves into invasive squamous cell carcinoma. Complete surgical resection with adjunctive cryotherapy is recommended to decrease the likelihood of local recurrence. Recurrence following excisional biopsy usually remains confined to the epithelium.

Actinic keratosis presents clinically as an insidious, leukoplakic lesion within the interpalpebral zone or overlying a pterygium or pinguecula. This lesion results from chronic exposure of the conjunctiva to ultraviolet irradiation. Histopathologic features of actinic keratosis of the conjunctiva are analogous to those observed in the skin and include acanthosis, parakeratosis, and hyperkeratosis of the epithelium, varying degrees of intraepithelial cellular atypia, and chronic non-granulomatous inflammation of the underlying substantia propria.

The prognosis for patients with this lesion is favorable subsequent to excision.[64–67]

Xeroderma pigmentosum is an autosomal recessive disease that occurs with an incidence of approximately 1 in 250,000, affecting all races worldwide.[68] Affected individuals inherit an impaired ability to repair DNA damage induced by ultraviolet light. Studies of the rate of DNA repair synthesis subsequent to ultraviolet exposure of conjunctival epithelial cells of a patient

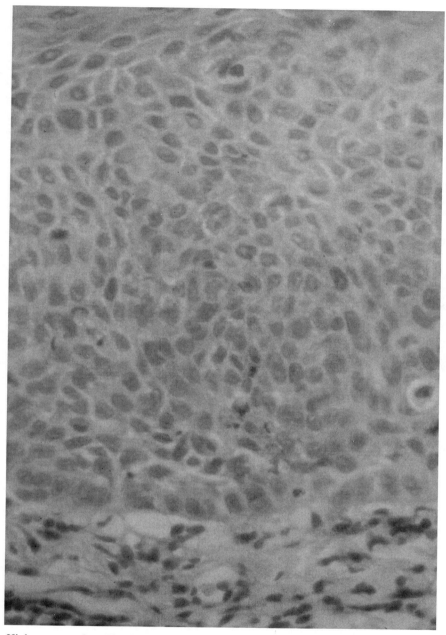

FIG. 3.34—Higher-power view. The dysplastic epithelial changes involve nearly the entire thickness of the conjunctiva. There are numerous mitotic figures. Hematoxylin-eosin, ×100.

with xeroderma pigmentosum showed a slower rate of tritiated thymidine incorporation compared with normal cadaver conjunctiva.[69] It is likely that defective DNA repair is present in all nucleated cells of affected individuals, but only those tissues exposed to ultraviolet light are at risk for the development of tumors.[46] Specifically, reduced rates of DNA repair have been documented in peripheral blood lymphocytes and in cutaneous epithelial cells and fibroblasts.[70–72]

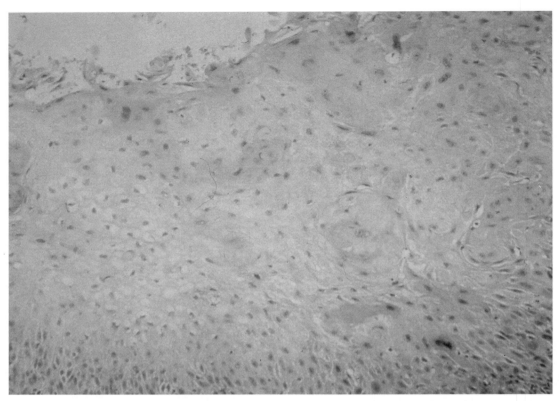

FIG. 3.35—Histopathology of the limbal conjunctiva temporally reveals squamous carcinoma in situ. Note the marked acanthosis, full-thickness dysplasia with vertical spindling of atypical basaloid cells, and whorls of cells showing squamous differentiation. The basement membrane is intact. Hematoxylin-eosin, ×40.

Clinical manifestations of this disease appear in the first decade of life with the development of focal areas of atrophy, hyperpigmentation, and telangiectasia of the skin. Later, because of the development of a variety of benign, premalignant, and malignant neoplasms on sun-exposed skin and mucous membranes, close clinical observation of these patients is required. Ophthalmologic complications of xeroderma pigmentosum affect the eyelids, conjunctiva, and cornea. The lid changes mirror those involving the skin, and ultimately may result in cicatricial entropion or ectropion. Corneal drying, inflammation, vascularization, ulceration, opacification, and intraepithelial neoplasias have been described.[69,73,74] The conjunctival manifestations of this disease include chronic inflammation, edema, telangiectasia, scarring and symblepharon, xerosis, irregular pigmentation, and a variety of conjunctival intraepithelial neoplasias as well as invasive carcinoma.

Malignant Epithelial Tumors. *Squamous cell carcinoma* of the conjunctiva characteristically arises in the interpalpebral region of the perilimbal conjunctiva; less commonly, the tumor is located in the fornix or on the palpebral conjunctiva. The degree of differentiation of the neoplastic cells, as well as the associated inflammation, vascularity, and chronicity of the tumor, influence the clinical appearance of these lesions. The tumor may be sessile, pedunculated, or papillomatous (Figures 3.36–3.38). Well-differentiated squamous cell carcinomas grow slowly and display surface leukoplakia as a result of keratin production. In contrast, poorly differentiated tumors progress more rapidly as a gelatinous, opalescent lesion with ill-defined borders. Limbal carcinomas can spread onto the adjacent cornea. Neglected lesions can enlarge massively, resulting in an exophytic mass that covers the cornea and protrudes through the interpalpebral fissure.[75–78] Pigmented squamous cell carcinomas occur predominantly in black patients as a result of the presence of melanocytes interspersed among the neoplastic squamous cells.[79–81]

Squamous cell carcinomas of the conjunctiva tend to have a relatively benign clinical course as they usually are only superficially invasive.[82–84] Intraocular invasion is uncommon as a result of the natural barrier provided by the scleral lamellae, Bowman's layer, and the corneal lamellae against tumor penetration.[44] Secondary intraocular invasion may result from neoplastic extension along the scleral emissaria.[44] Iliff et al.[84] reviewed 27 cases and found three with deep corneal invasion, two with intraocular extension, four with orbital invasion, and two with metastasis to regional lymph nodes. One patient's death in this

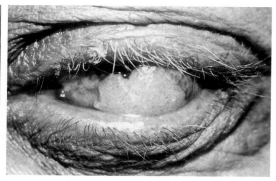

FIG. 3.36—A broad-based vascularized and papillomatous bulbar conjunctival and corneal mass, inferotemporally. The tumor is prominent in the interpalpebral zone.

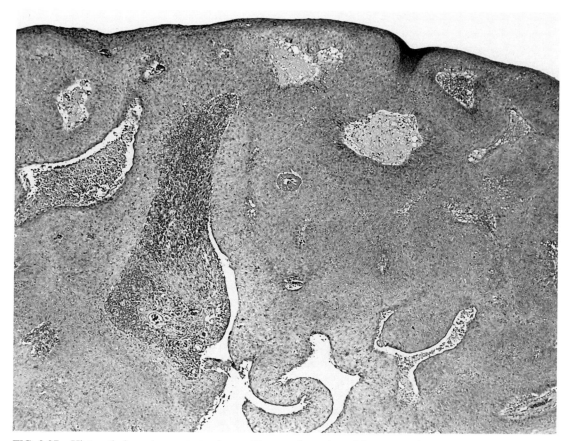

FIG. 3.37—Histopathology demonstrates the papillary configuration of the tumor. Hematoxylin-eosin, ×10.

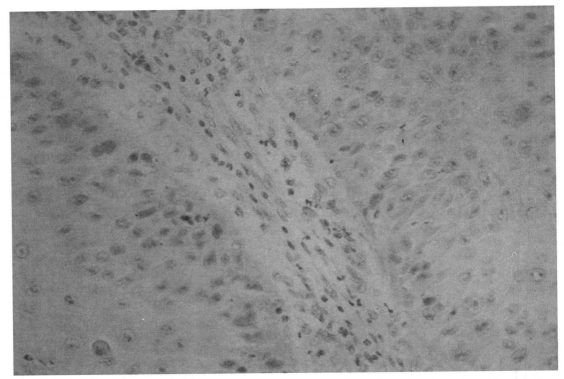

FIG. 3.38—Higher-power view. There is an abnormal maturation sequence involving the entire thickness of the conjunctival epithelium (squamous carcinoma in situ) as well as chronic inflammation of the adjacent substantia propria. Note the individual cell dyskeratosis. Hematoxylin-eosin, ×63.

series was tumor related. In another review of 87 cases of conjunctival squamous carcinoma with follow-up of at least 5 years, Zimmerman[83] found metastasis in four cases and tumor-related death in only one case.

Histopathologically, the conjunctival basement membrane is interrupted and neoplastic squamous cells infiltrate the underlying substantia propria (Figure 3.39). Most lesions are well differentiated and thus display surface keratinization. Keratin pearl formation and individually keratinized cells are observed within the tumor.

Management of conjunctival squamous cell carcinoma includes complete surgical excision of the lesion (Figure 3.40) with adjunctive cryotherapy. Limbal lesions may require superficial lamellar dissection. Lesions involving the corneal epithelium are best removed without violating the Bowman's layer,[64] which is considered to provide an anatomic barrier against deeper penetration. More extensive surgical procedures, such as enucleation or orbital exenteration, are reserved for cases with intraocular and orbital invasion. Adjunctive radiotherapy may be required in recurrent cases.[64]

Mucoepidermoid carcinoma is a variant of squamous carcinoma and usually affects individuals in the seventh decade of life. It typically is more locally aggressive than is squamous cell carcinoma and exhibits a tendency for invasion of the globe and orbit as well as for early recurrence after incomplete surgical excision. The tumor consists of an admixture of malignant mucus-secreting cells, squamous cells, and intermediate cells (basal cells).

Adnexal Tumors. The caruncle is lined by conjunctival epithelium rich in goblet cells. The subepithelial tissue of the caruncle contains adnexal structures of the eyelid, including hair follicles, sebaceous glands, sweat glands, and accessory lacrimal glands. Thus, tumors from

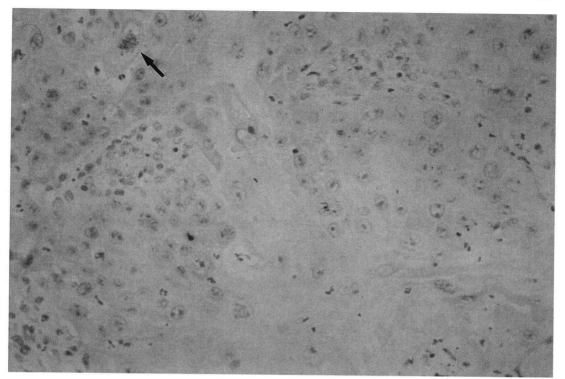

FIG. 3.39—Neoplastic squamous cells focally infiltrate the substantia propria. The nuclei are pleomorphic and contain prominent nucleoli. Dyskeratotic cells and mitotic figures (arrow) are present. Hematoxylin-eosin, ×63.

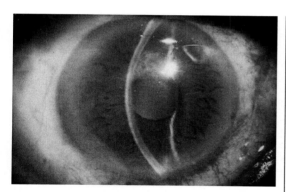

FIG. 3.40—Same patient as in Figure 3.11. Postoperative appearance 4 days subsequent to conjunctivectomy and superficial lamellar keratectomy with adjunctive application of 95% ethyl alcohol to the surgical bed.

the adnexal structures of the eyelid (pleomorphic adenoma; sweat gland carcinoma, adenoma, or cyst; oncocytoma; and sebaceous gland carcinoma) may primarily originate in the caruncle. The incidence of these tumors is relatively uncommon as compared with their incidence in the skin. The histopathologic features of these conjunctival tumors mimic those that occur in the skin; additionally, there may be papillomatosis and keratinization of the overlying caruncular epithelium.[44,85]

Oncocytoma, also referred to as *oxyphil cell adenoma, oxyphilic granular cell adenoma,* and *eosinophilic cyst adenoma* is a benign tumor. This lesion most commonly involves the caruncle as an asymptomatic, slow-growing, reddish blue, solid or cystic mass;[86] the lacrimal gland, lacrimal sac, and other glandular and mucosal tissues may also be involved.[46] Oncocytoma is considered to arise as an aging phenomenon in individuals (predominantly women)[87] older than age 60.[86–92] Most oncocytic lesions arise from oncocytic metaplasia of ductal and acinar cells of lacrimal or salivary gland elements of the ocular adnexae.[46]

Microscopically, sheets, cords, nests, or ductular and cystic glandular structures are comprised of benign epithelial cells displaying abundant

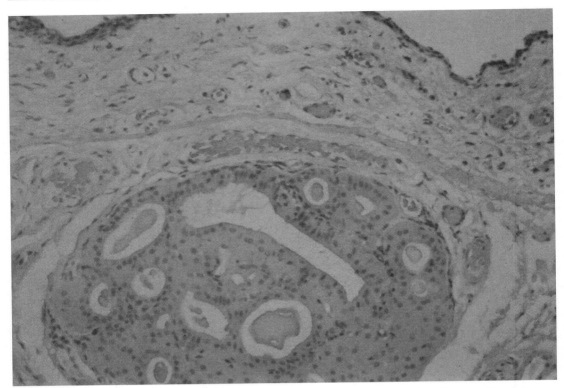

FIG. 3.41—A nodular aggregate of cystic spaces lined by a double layer of oncocytic cells and goblet cells is within the substantia propria of the conjunctiva. The cystic spaces contain sparse seromucinous secretion. The preoperative clinical diagnosis was pterygium. Hematoxylin-eosin, ×40.

eosinophilic cytoplasm (Figure 3.41).[46] Ultrastructurally, the cytoplasm of these cells contains abundant mitochondria.

Benign Melanocytic Tumors. Congenital epithelial melanosis, also described as an *ephelis* or *freckle,* presents at birth or childhood as a flat, irregularly shaped, brown patch on the bulbar conjunctiva. Histopathologically, this lesion results from excessive melanotic pigmentation of the basal epithelium. There is no associated cytologic atypia or malignant potential.

Melanocytic nevi of the conjunctiva are common lesions that may occur at the limbus (Figure 3.42), eyelid margin, caruncle (Figure 3.43), plica, or on the tarsal conjunctiva. These hamartomas are usually flat or minimally thickened and vary in pigmentation according to the degree of melanization of the nevus cells. Often, amelanotic or lightly pigmented conjunctival nevi become darker during puberty or pregnancy as a result of hormonal influences.

Conjunctival nevi may increase in size and raise clinical concern that malignant transformation has taken place. In fact, in many cases, enlargement of the lesion can be attributed to either an increase in melanotic pigmentation of the constituent nevus cells, to the formation of pseudocysts, or to associated inflammation. Pseudocyst formation within the nevus results from cystic inclusions of conjunctival epithelium containing goblet cells that slowly enlarge due to the accumulation of mucin. Clinical identification of pseudocysts within the lesion by slit-lamp biomicroscopy is useful in differentiating the nevus from a malignant melanoma, as their presence is seen in over 50% of conjunctival nevi[44] and not in acquired melanosis or malignant melanoma.

Melanocytic nevi of the conjunctiva are classified histopathologically in a scheme used for nevi

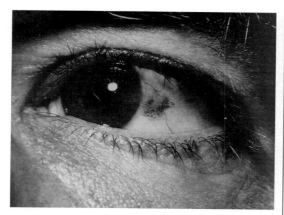

FIG. 3.42—Flat, brown conjunctival pigmentation on the limbal conjunctiva.

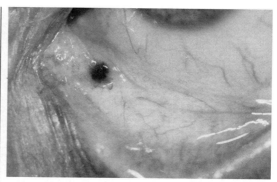

FIG. 3.43—Flat, brown conjunctival pigmentation on the caruncle.

of the skin. These include *junctional (intraepithelial), subepithelial, compound, spindle* or *epithelioid cell (Spitz nevus), blue,* and *cellular blue nevus.* Of note, the subepithelial nevus is the conjunctival analog of the intradermal nevus of the skin. The *balloon cell nevus* is an uncommon variant[44] predominantly consisting of large cells with small, round, centrally located nuclei and finely granular cytoplasm.[93] The vast majority of conjunctival nevi are subepithelial (Figures 3.44 and 3.45); or compound junctional nevi are observed only in very young patients.

The histopathologic differential diagnosis of a junctional nevus and acquired melanosis of the conjunctiva can be difficult, particularly on a small biopsy specimen, when basilar nests of nevoid melanocytes are seen. Often, in these cases, the clinical history must be relied upon.[46]

Reese[94] first described *acquired melanosis* of the conjunctiva. This entity consists of excessive melanotic pigmentation of the conjunctival epithelium as a result of accumulation of melanin within the intraepithelial melanocytes.

Acquired epithelial melanosis, in the *bilateral* form, carries no malignant potential. It occurs most often as a racial phenomenon due to normal aging changes in the limbal or perilimbal conjunctiva of blacks and other nonwhite individuals. Less commonly, metabolic or toxic factors result in bilateral acquired melanosis of the conjunctiva.[46]

Unilateral acquired melanosis of the conjunctival epithelium may be idiopathic or secondary.

Secondary acquired melanosis most often occurs in nonwhite patients as a result of irritation of the conjunctival epithelium by some other primary conjunctival epithelial or subepithelial lesion. Thus, excessive melanization of the conjunctival epithelium can occur in association with such entities as conjunctival cyst, papilloma, or squamous cell carcinoma. In these cases, the primary conjunctival lesion may appear pigmented and lead to the erroneous clinical diagnosis of malignant melanoma.[46]

Primary acquired melanosis (PAM) of the conjunctival epithelium is always an idiopathic, unilateral condition, generally affecting white patients over the age of 40. It begins insidiously as a freely mobile, flat area of golden-brown stippling (Figure 3.46). Limbal lesions often spread onto the contiguous corneal epithelium (Figure 3.47), whereas those located on the palpebral conjunctiva or caruncle may involve the adjacent epidermis of the eyelid. The clinical course of PAM is highly variable over many years. Typically, the lesion "waxes and wanes"; that is, pigmentation spontaneously resolves in some areas while increased pigmentation occurs in others. In some cases, there is total spontaneous resolution of the pigmentation whereas, in others, there is malignant degeneration. Reese approximated that 17% of cases of PAM of the conjunctiva progress to malignant melanoma.[95,96] Zimmerman proposed and later modified an objective histologic classification of idiopathic primary acquired melanosis of the conjunctiva[46,97] in order to provide a clinical

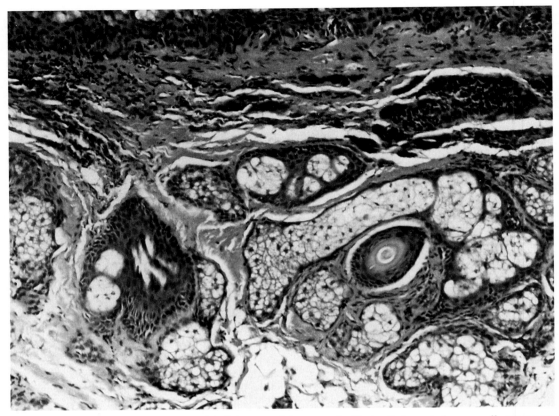

FIG. 3.44—Photomicrograph of a subepithelial nevus of the caruncle. Nests of pigmented nevus cells are superficial to unremarkable pilosebaceous units. Hematoxylin-eosin, ×32.

prognosis subsequent to biopsy of the most suspicious areas of the lesion. The classification scheme appears as follows:[46]

Stage I: Benign acquired melanosis
    A. With minimal melanocytic hyperplasia
    B. With atypical melanocytic hyperplasia
       1. Mild to moderately severe
       2. Severe (in situ malignant melanoma)
Stage II: Malignant acquired melanosis
    A. With superficially invasive melanoma (tumor thickness less than 1.5 mm)
    B. With more deeply invasive melanoma (tumor thickness greater than 1.5 mm)

In this classification scheme, tumor thickness of 1.5 mm was chosen to differentiate stages IIA and IIB based on series that have shown that tumors greater than 1.8 mm thick were lethal whereas those less than 1.5 mm thick carried a more favorable prognosis.[98] Jakobiec et al.[99] showed that PAM composed of epithelioid cells or PAM exhibiting intraepithelial pagetoid extension (Figure 3.48) have, respectively, a 75% or 90% chance of eventuating in invasive melanoma. Folberg et al.[100] found that approximately 50% of PAM cases with atypical melanocytic hyperplasia (Stage IB) develop into invasive melanoma. Thus, incisional biopsy of the clinically most suspicious areas in PAM is not only useful prognostically but also guides the clinical management of patients.

PAM of the conjunctiva can be managed conservatively with close clinical observation. However, any areas that display vascularization, thickening,

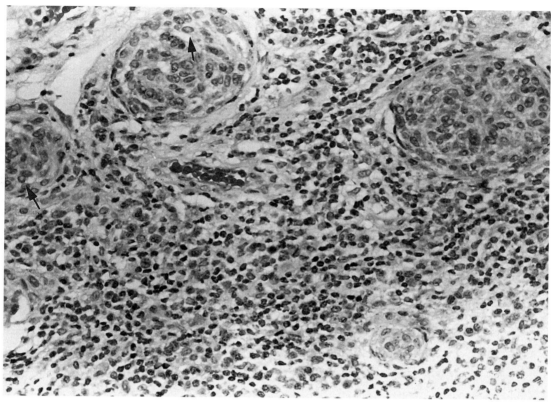

FIG. 3.45—Nests of nevus cells within the substantia propria of the conjunctiva. The nevus cells have uniform, ovoid nuclei that occasionally demonstrate intranuclear sequestration of cytoplasm (arrows). There is a surrounding lymphocytic infiltrate. Hematoxylin-eosin, ×63.

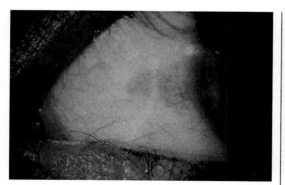

FIG. 3.46—Primary acquired melanosis of the limbal conjunctiva nasally and of the caruncle. Note the flat, golden-brown speckled pigmentation of the bulbar conjunctiva.

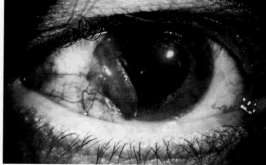

FIG. 3.47—An elevated, brown, vascularized limbal conjunctival mass extending onto the adjacent cornea. Note the dilated episcleral vessels temporally.

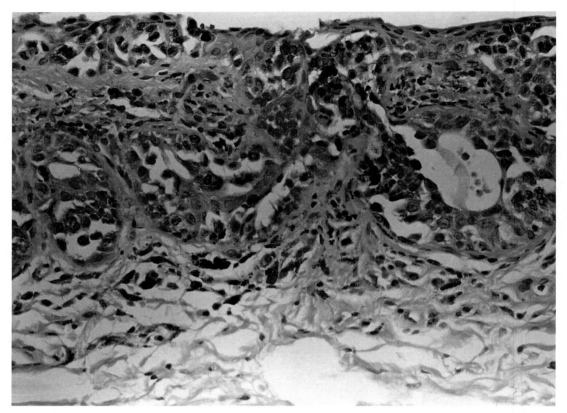

FIG. 3.48—Photomicrograph of primary acquired melanosis of the tarsal conjunctiva shows pagetoid spread of atypical melanocytes as well as intraepithelial nests of atypical melanocytes along pseudoglands of Henle. The basement membrane is intact throughout. Hematoxylin-eosin, ×63.

inflammation, or spread of diffuse disconnected pigment may represent malignant transformation and should be biopsied (Figure 3.49).[101]

Malignant Melanoma. *Primary malignant melanoma* of the conjunctiva is an uncommon tumor, comprising fewer than 2% of all ocular melanomas and fewer than 1% of malignant tumors of the eye.[102,103] The conjunctival melanoma can arise from preexisting acquired melanosis (Figure 3.50), from preexisting nevi, or de novo. In many cases, the lack of clinical information regarding preexisting conjunctival pathology as well as a conjunctival biopsy of small size preclude definitive histopathologic assessment pertaining to the origin of the tumor. Thus, this pathogenetic classification is often more of con-

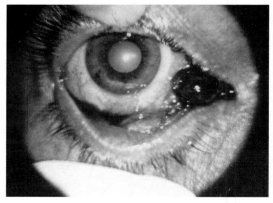

FIG. 3.49—Areas of thickening in extensive primary acquired melanosis of the fornical and tarsal conjunctiva and in the caruncle represent malignant transformation into conjunctival melanoma.

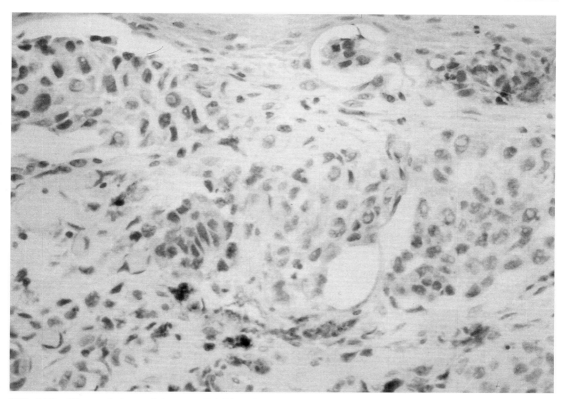

FIG. 3.50—Histopathology of the superficial lamellar keratectomy and conjunctivectomy show conjunctival melanoma arising in primary acquired melanosis. Variably pigmented epithelioid melanoma cells are within the substantia propria and limbal corneal stroma. Nests of atypical melanocytes are within the overlying conjunctival epithelium. Hematoxylin-eosin, ×100.

ceptual than of practical value.[46] Histopathologically, neoplastic melanocytes comprised of small polyhedral cells, large epithelioid cells, spindle cells, and/or balloon cells invade the substantia propria. A tendency toward maturation, as would be expected in nevus, is absent in melanoma.[46,104] Conjunctival melanoma typically affects adults between decades 4 and 7. There is no sex predilection, and its occurrence in nonwhite patients and in children has been reported only rarely.[44,102,105–107] Clinically, malignant melanoma of the conjunctiva presents as a variably pigmented limbal mass usually located in the interpalpebral region. The fornical, palpebral, and caruncular conjunctiva are less commonly involved.[97,106,108,109] Conjunctival melanoma can spread locally to adjacent ocular and adnexal structures, including the cornea, eyelid, lacrimal drainage apparatus, and orbital soft

tissues. Some studies relate tumors of the caruncle, palpebral conjunctiva, or fornix, diffuse melanomas, the presence of marked cytologic atypia, and pagetoid spread to high metastatic risk.[97,98,101,104,105,107,110–116] Reese[94] showed that, in cases of conjunctival melanoma with at least 5 years of follow-up, tumors derived from acquired melanosis or de novo had a mortality rate of approximately 40%, whereas those derived from preexisting nevi had a mortality rate of approximately 20%.[46] Other series fail to demonstrate a relationship between metastatic risk and tumor extent, its anatomic location, or its pathogenetic derivation.[101,117] In a series of 131 cases of conjunctival melanoma, Folberg et al.[118] found an overall mortality rate of 26%. The mortality rate was 25.5% and 27.3% in melanoma without and with PAM, respectively. In this series, the presence or absence of preexisting nevi had no effect on the prognosis.

Even minimally invasive conjunctival melanoma may result in lymphatic, and ultimately hematogenous, dissemination. The substantia propria of the conjunctiva is rich in lymphatics, some of which are located superficially. Lymphatic invasion and subsequent neoplastic spread to the regional lymph nodes dictate that attention be directed to the preauricular, intraparotid, submandibular, and cervical lymph nodes in the clinical evaluation of these patients. The incidence of local recurrence of conjunctival melanoma ranges from approximately 20% to 56%.[119]

The appearance of one or more subepithelial nodules of melanoma subsequent to excision of a conjunctival melanoma that histopathologically demonstrated evidence of lymphatic invasion may represent local lymphatic metastasis. The conjunctiva, eyelid, or lacrimal gland can thusly be involved by local lymphatic metastatic melanoma. Tumor seeding of the surgical bed at the time of excision of the melanoma can also result in subsequent recurrent conjunctival melanoma. Alternatively, apparent local recurrence of conjunctival melanomas may simply represent multifocal primary conjunctival melanomas arising in preexisting acquired melanosis.[46]

Excisional biopsy of conjunctival melanoma with adjunctive cryotherapy to the remaining surgical margins is currently the most commonly employed treatment.[105,108,116,120–123] There is both clinical and ultrastructural evidence that double freeze-thaw cryotherapy at temperatures below $-20°C$ is selectively destructive to melanocytes.[116,121,122] Other therapeutic modalities include combined surgical excision and radiotherapy,[105] local excision alone,[111] and various forms of radiation therapy.[105,124–126] Orbital exenteration is reserved for extensive, unresectable conjunctival melanomas that show orbital or intraocular invasion, extensive involvement of the fornix, or recurrence after irradiation.[101,127] However, it has never been proven that orbital exenteration improves patient survival in these cases.[98,120]

Stromal Tumors

MESENCHYMAL TUMORS. Primary soft tissue tumors of the conjunctiva are rare[44] and include

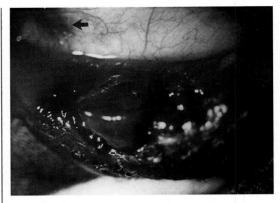

FIG. 3.51—Nodular, reddish purple conjunctival Kaposi's sarcoma on the tarsal conjunctiva of the right lower lid of a 42-year-old HIV+ black man. Flat, bulbar conjunctival Kaposi's sarcoma is also present laterally (arrow).

the full spectrum of benign and malignant fibrous, xanthomatous, histiocytic, mesenchymal, vascular, and neural tumors. The tumor, if extensive, often affects the adjacent orbit and eyelids;[46] conversely, the conjunctiva may be secondarily involved by local extension of these lesions from the orbit or eyelid. These soft tissue tumors are more comprehensively considered in sections dealing with the pathology of the orbit or eyelid.

Conjunctival *Kaposi's sarcoma* (KS) (Figure 3.51) is worth emphasizing as it is observed and diagnosed with increasing frequency in young individuals with acquired immunodeficiency syndrome (AIDS). In 1872, Moritz Kaposi (a Hungarian dermatologist) first described this cutaneous neoplasm in five patients who had multiple pigmented sarcomas of the skin. Currently, four categories of KS are recognized. *Classic KS* afflicts patients of Eastern-European Jewish and Mediterranean descent between the ages of 50 and 80 years. There is a male predominance with a male-to-female ratio of 10–15:1. *Endemic KS* affects black African men between the ages of 25 and 40 years, with a male-to-female ratio of 17:1. *Iatrogenic immunosuppression KS* occurs subsequent to organ transplantation. *Epidemic AIDS-related KS* occurs in approximately 30% of patients with AIDS and in 20% of patients with AIDS-associated systemic KS.[123,124] Infection by retrovirus has been implicated in the pathogenesis of conjunctival KS in patients with AIDS.[128–130]

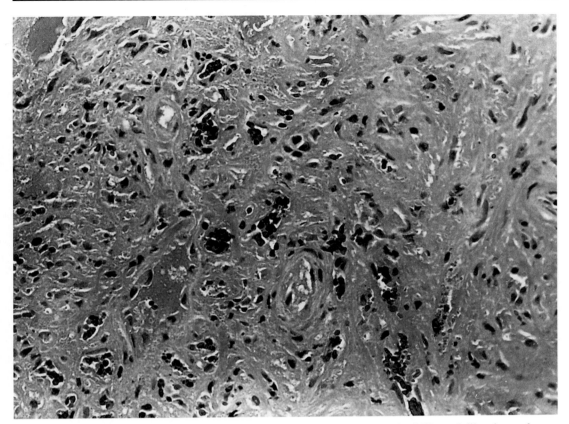

FIG. 3.52—Histopathology of Kaposi's sarcoma of the tarsal conjunctiva reveals slitlike and dilated vascular spaces amid a proliferation of spindle cells. Hematoxylin-eosin, ×63. (Courtesy of Dr. Alan H. Friedman.)

In general, the clinical appearance of a reddish blue, diffuse vascular conjunctival lesion is almost pathognomonic of KS in a patient with AIDS.[131–133] Dugel et al.[133] classified 18 cases of ocular adnexal KS lesions related to AIDS into three clinical and histologic types. Clinically, Type I and II tumors are flat (less than 3 mm elevation) and patchy and of less than 4 months' duration. Type III KS lesions are nodular (greater than 3 mm elevation). Histopathologically, type I lesions consist of thin, dilated, and blood-filled vascular channels lined by flat endothelial cells (Figure 3.52). Type II lesions display plump, fusiform endothelial cells, often with hyperchromatic nuclei, immature spindle cells, and slit spaces. Type III KS is comprised of large aggregates of densely packed spindle cells with hyperchromatic nuclei, occasional mitotic figures, and slit spaces containing erythrocytes.

KS is a slow-growing, rarely invasive tumor, so, in a patient with AIDS, surgical intervention is reserved for lesions resulting in cosmetic defects or functional impairment. The tumor is radiosensitive,[130,134] so radiation therapy can be instituted in place of surgical excision, particularly in cases where excision of large KS lesions would require extensive conjunctival surface reconstruction. Successful resolution of KS treated with cryotherapy or chemotherapy has been reported.[135–142]

Congenital Epibulbar Choristomas. Choristomas are congenital tumors comprised of displaced, histologically normal, tissue elements. Choristomas have little or no growth potential.[46] Epibulbar choristomas may occur as an isolated finding or as one of the clinical manifestations of a systemic syndrome.

DERMOIDS AND DERMOLIPOMAS. Dermoids and dermolipomas may occur as one of the systemic manifestations of Goldenhar's syndrome (oculoauriculovertebral dysplasia), Treacher Collins syndrome or Franceschetti's syndrome (mandibulofacial dysostosis), and Solomon's syndrome or linear nevus sebaceous of Jadassohn (bandlike cutaneous nevus and central nervous system dysfunction).[50]

Conjunctival dermoids are most often *limbal,* located inferotemporally. These appear as well-circumscribed, solid, firm, tan masses, varying in size from 2 to 15 mm. Small dermoids usually present only a cosmetic problem,[46] but larger tumors may protrude through the interpalpebral fissure and result in corneal astigmatism. Occasionally, fine hairs are evident along the surface of the dermoid. Biomicroscopic examination of the adjacent corneal epithelium may reveal an iron line or an arc of lipid deposited in the superficial corneal stroma.[46,143]

Histopathologically, the limbal dermoid is covered by stratified squamous epithelium that may display keratinization. The stroma consists of dense collagenous connective tissue containing scattered hair follicles and sweat and sebaceous glands.

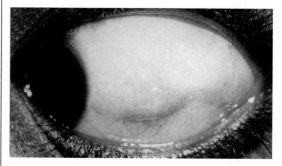

FIG. 3.53—Clinical appearance of a dermolipoma located temporally on the eye of a 6-year-old boy. Note the yellowish fusiform mass covered by a smooth conjunctival surface.

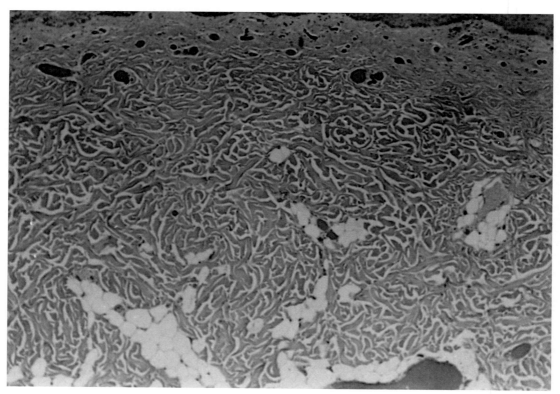

FIG. 3.54—Conjunctival epithelium lines abnormally thickened and variably oriented bundles of collagen as well as lobules of adipose tissue. No pilosebaceous units are present in this section. Hematoxylin-eosin, ×16.

Surgical excision by lamellar dissection is performed in selected cases. The morbidity associated with the surgery includes decreased ocular motility, corneal astigmatism, and corneal perforation.[50,144]

Dermolipomas of the conjunctiva are yellowish tan, soft, fusiform tumors,[46] typically located temporally near the insertion of the lateral rectus muscle (Figure 3.53). The tumor often extends posteriorly and superiorly, between the lateral and superior recti muscles, into the orbit. This choristoma is histopathologically similar to the dermoid except for a paucity of pilosebaceous units and abundant adipose tissue (Figure 3.54).

Complex choristomas of the conjunctiva clinically resemble the limbal dermoid or the dermolipoma but histopathologically contain other ectopic tissues such as cartilage, lacrimal gland, and smooth muscle.[46]

Osseous choristomas are solitary episcleral nodules that also clinically resemble conjunctiva dermoids. The mass is either freely mobile or adherent to the bulbar conjunctiva and sclera. The typical location of the episcleral osseous choristoma, 5–10 mm posterior to the limbus superotemporally, helps to differentiate it clinically from a dermoid.[50] This lesion may be considered a variant of a complex choristoma, since it contains mature, compact bone as well as other choristomatous elements within connective tissue.

REFERENCES

1. Peiffer RL, Terrell T. Episcleral hemangioma in a dog. *J Am Vet Med Assoc* 173:1338, 1978.
2. Hargis AM, Lee AC, Thomassen RW. Tumor and tumor-like lesions of perilimbal conjunctiva in laboratory dogs. *J Am Vet Med Assoc* 173:1185, 1978.
3. Buyukmihci NC, Stannard AA. Canine conjunctival angiokeratomas. *J Am Vet Med Assoc* 178:1279, 1981.
4. Murphy CJ, Bellhorn RW, Buyukmihci NC. Bilateral conjunctival masses in two dogs. *J Am Vet Med Assoc* 195:225, 1989.
5. George C, Summers BA. Angiokeratoma: a benign vascular tumour of the dog. *J Small Anim Pract* 31:390, 1990.
6. Wilcock BP. Conjunctival vascular tumors in dogs: histologic-behavioural correlation, presented at the Midwest Association of Veterinary Ophthalmologists, Madison, 5 February 1994.
7. Vestre WA, Turner TA, Carlton WW. Conjunctival hemangioma in a horse. *J Am Vet Med Assoc* 180:1481, 1982.
8. Hacker DW, Moore PF, Buyukmihc NC. Ocular angiosarcoma in four horses. *J Am Vet Med Assoc* 189:200, 1986.
9. Crawley GR Bryan GA, Gogolewski RP. Ocular hemangioma in a horse. *Equine Pract* 9:11, 1987.
10. Moore PF, Hacker DV, Buyukmihci NC. Ocular angiosarcoma in the horse: morphological and immunohistochemical studies. *Vet Pathol* 23:240, 1986.
11. Wilcock B, Peiffer RL. Adenocarcinoma of the gland of the third eyelid in seven dogs. *J Am Vet Med Assoc* 193:1549, 1988.
12. Levene A. Precancerous and cancerous melanosis of the canine conjunctiva. *J Comp Pathol* 83:253, 1973.
13. Cook CS, Rosenkrantz W, Peiffer RL, MacMillan A. Malignant melanoma of the conjunctiva in a cat. *J Am Vet Med Assoc* 186:505, 1985.
14. Patnaik AK, Mooney S. Feline melanoma: a comparative study of ocular, oral, and dermal neoplasms. *Vet Pathol* 25:105, 1988.
15. Croxatto JO, Herrera HD, Lightowler CH. A case report: malignant melanoma arising from primary acquired melanosis in a dog. *Canine Pract* 17:22, 1992.
16. Collins BK, Collier LL, Miller MA, Linton LL. Biologic behavior and histologic characteristics of canine conjunctival melanoma. *Prog Vet Comp Ophthalmol* 3:135, 1994.
17. Todoroff RJ, Brodey RS. Oral and pharyngeal neoplasia in the dog: a retrospective survey of 361 cases. *J Am Vet Med Assoc* 175:567, 1979.
18. Harvey HJ, MacEwen EG, Braun D, Patnaik AK, Withrow SJ, Jongeward S. Prognostic criteria for dogs with oral melanoma. *J Am Vet Med Assoc* 178:580, 1981.
19. Anderson DE, Chambers D, Lush JL. Heritability of lid pigmentation and cancer eye susceptibility in cattle. *J Anim Sci* 15:1224, 1956.
20. Anderson DE, Lush JL, Chambers D. Studies on bovine ocular squamous cell carcinoma ("cancer eye"): II. Relationship between eyelid pigmentation and occurrence of cancer eye lesions. *J Anim Sci* 16:739, 1957.
21. Anderson DE, Skinner PE. Studies on bovine ocular squamous cell carcinoma ("cancer eye"): XI. Effects of sunlight. *J Anim Sci* 20:474, 1961.
22. Monlux AW, Anderson DE, Davis CL. The diagnosis of squamous cell carcinoma of the eye in cattle. *J Vet Res* 18:5, 1957.
23. Spradbrow PB, Hoffman D. Bovine ocular squamous cell carcinoma. *Am J Vet Res* 36:115, 1975.
24. Heeney JL, Valli VEO. Bovine ocular squamous cell carcinoma: an epidemiological perspective. *Can J Comp Med* 49:21, 1985.
25. Russel WO, Wynne ED, Loquvan GS. Studies on bovine ocular squamous cell carcinoma ("cancer eye"). *Cancer* 9:1, 1956.
26. French GT. A clinical and genetic study of eye cancer in Hereford cattle. *Aust Vet J* 35:474, 1959.
27. Anderson DE. Cancer eye in cattle. *Mod Vet Pract* 51:43, 1970.

28. Sundberg JP, Junge RE, Lancaster WE. Immunoperoxidase localization of papillomaviruses in hyperplastic and neoplastic epithelial lesions of animals. *Am J Vet Res* 45:1441, 1984.

29. Rutten VPM, Klein WR, De Jong MAC, Quint W, Den Otter W, Ruitenberg EJ, Melchers WJG. Search for bovine papilloma virus DNA in bovine ocular squamous cell carcinomas (BOSCC) and BOSCC-derived cell lines. *Am J Vet Res* 53:14, 1992.

30. Gelatt KN, Meyers VS, Perman V, Jessen C. Conjunctival squamous cell carcinoma in the horse. *J Am Vet Med Assoc* 165:617, 1974.

31. Lavach JD, Severin GA. Neoplasia of the equine eye, adnexa and orbit: a review of 68 cases. *J Am Vet Med Assoc* 170:202, 1977.

32. Schwink K. Factors influencing morbidity and outcome of equine ocular squamous cell carcinoma. *Equine Vet J* 19:198, 1987.

33. Dugan SJ, Curtis CR, Roberts SM, Severin GA. Epidemiologic study of ocular/adnexal squamous cell carcinoma in horses. *J Am Vet Med Assoc* 198:251, 1991.

34. Dugan SJ, Roberts SM, Curtis CR, Severin GA. Prognostic factors and survival of horses with ocular/adnexal squamous cell carcinoma: 147 cases (1978–1988). *J Am Vet Med Assoc* 198:298, 1991.

35. Taylor RL, Hanks MA. Developmental changes in precursor lesions of bovine ocular carcinoma. *Vet Med Small Anim Clin* 67:669, 1972.

36. Davidson MG. Equine ophthalmology. In: Gelatt KN, ed. *Veterinary Ophthalmology,* 2d ed. Philadelphia: Lea and Febiger, 1991:chap 15.

37. Miller TM, Gelatt KN. Food animal ophthalmology. In: Gelatt KN, ed. *Veterinary Ophthalmology,* 2d ed. Philadelphia: Lea and Febiger, 1991:chap 16.

38. Bellhorn RW, Henkind P. Ocular nodular fasciitis in a dog. *J Am Vet Med Assoc* 150:212, 1967.

39. Lavignette AM, Carlton WW. A case of ocular nodular fasciitis in a dog. *J Am Anim Hosp Assoc* 10:503, 1974.

40. Smith JS, Bistner S, Riis R. Infiltrative corneal lesions resembling fibrous histiocytoma: clinical and pathologic findings in six dogs and one cat. *J Am Vet Med Assoc* 169:722, 1976.

41. Gwin RM, Gelatt KN, Peiffer RL. Ophthalmic nodular fasciitis in the dog. *J Am Vet Med Assoc* 170:611, 1977.

42. Paulsen ME, Lavach JD, Snyder SP, Severin GA, Eichenbaum JD. Nodular granulomatous episclerokeratitis in dogs: 19 cases (1973–1985). *J Am Vet Med Assoc* 190:1581, 1987.

43. Lass JH, Jenson AB, Papale JJ, Albert DM. Papillomavirus in human conjunctival papillomas. *Am J Ophthalmol* 95:364, 1983.

44. Völcker HE, Naumann GOH. Conjunctiva. In: Naumann GOH, Apple DJ, eds. *Pathology of the Eye.* New York: Springer-Verlag, 1986:chap 6.

45. Jakobiec FA, Harrison W, Aronian D. Inverted mucoepidermoid papillomas of the epibulbar conjunctiva. *Ophthalmology* 94:283, 1987.

46. Spencer WH, Zimmerman LE. Conjunctiva. In: *Ophthalmic Pathology: An Atlas and Textbook,* vol 1. Philadelphia: WB Saunders, 1985:chap 2.

47. Von Salliman L, Paton D. Hereditary dyskeratosis of the perilimbal conjunctiva. *Trans Am Ophthalmol Soc* 57:53, 1959.

48. Von Salliman L, Paton D. Hereditary benign intraepithelial dyskeratosis. *Arch Ophthalmol* 63:421, 1960.

49. Witkop CJ, Shankle DH, Graham JB, et al. Hereditary benign intraepithelial dyskeratosis: II. Oral manifestations and hereditary transmission. *Arch Pathol* 70:696, 1960.

50. Conlon MR, Alfonso EC, Starck T, Albert DM. Tumors of the cornea and conjunctiva. In: Albert DM, Jakobiec FA, eds. *Principles and Practice of Ophthalmology.* Philadelphia: WB Saunders, 1994:276.

51. Jakobiec FA. Corneal tumors. In: Kaufman H, Barron B, McDonald M, Waltman SR, eds. *The Cornea.* New York: Churchill Livingstone, 1988:chap 21.

52. Erie JC, Campbell RJ, Liesigang TJ. Conjunctival and corneal intraepithelial and invasive neoplasia. *Ophthalmology* 93:176, 1986.

53. Clear AS, Chirambo MC, Hutt MSR. Solar keratosis, pterygium and squamous cell carcinoma of the conjunctiva in Malawi. *Br J Ophthalmol* 63:102, 1979.

54. Napora C, Cohen EJ, Genvert GL, et al. Factors associated with conjunctival intraepithelial neoplasia: a case control study. *Ophthalmic Surg* 21:27, 1990.

55. McDonnell JM, Mayr AJ, Martin WJ. DNA of human papillomavirus type 16 in dysplastic and malignant lesions of the conjunctiva and cornea. *N Engl J Med* 320:1442, 1989.

56. Lauer SA, Malter JS, Meier AJ. Human papillomavirus type 18 in conjunctival intraepithelial neoplasia. *Am J Ophthalmol* 110:23, 1990.

57. Lass JH, Grove AS, Papale JJ, et al. Detection of human papillomavirus DNA sequences in conjunctival papilloma. *Am J Ophthalmol* 96:670, 1983.

58. Pfiser II, Fuchs PG, Völcker HE. Human papillomavirus DNA in conjunctival papilloma. *Graefes Arch Clin Exp Ophthalmol* 223:169, 1985.

59. Naghashfar Z, McDonnell PJ, McDonnell JM, et al. Genital tract papilloma type 6 in recurrent conjunctival papilloma. *Arch Ophthalmol* 104:1814, 1986.

60. McDonnell PJ, McDonnell JM, Kessis T. Detection of human papillomavirus type 6/11 DNA in conjunctival papillomas by in situ hybridization with radioactive probes. *Hum Pathol* 18:115, 1987.

61. McDonnell JM, Carpenter JD, Jacobs P, et al. Conjunctival melanocytic lesions in children. *Ophthalmology* 98:986, 1989.

62. Odrich MG, Jakobiec FA, Lancaster WD, et al. A spectrum of bilateral squamous conjunctival tumors associated with human papillomavirus type 16. *Ophthalmology* 98:626, 1991.

63. McDonnell JM, Wagner D, Ng ST, et al. Human papillomavirus type 16 DNA in ocular and cervical swabs of women with genital tract condylomata. *Am J Ophthalmol* 112:61, 1991.

64. Ash JE, Wilder HC. Epithelial tumors of the limbus. *Am J Ophthalmol* 33:1203, 1950.

65. Divine RD, Anderson RL. Nitrous oxide cryotherapy for intraepithelial epithelioma of the conjunctiva. *Arch Ophthalmol* 101:782, 1983.

66. Pierse D, Steele ADMcG, Garner A, Tripathi RC. ("Bowen's disease") of the cornea. *Br J Ophthalmol* 55:664, 1971.

67. Tripathi R, Garner C. The ultrastructure of preinvasive cancer of the corneal epithelium. *Cancer Res* 32:90, 1972.

68. Robbins JH, Kraemer KH, Lutzner MA, et al. Xeroderma pigmentosum: an inherited disease with sun sensitivity, multiple cutaneous neoplasms and abnormal DNA repair. *Ann Intern Med* 80:221, 1974.

69. Newsome DA, Kraemer KH, Robbins JH. Repair of DNA in xeroderma pigmentosum conjunctiva. *Arch Ophthalmol* 93:660, 1975.

70. Burk PG, Lutzner MA, Clark DD, et al. Ultraviolet-stimulating thymidine incorporation in xeroderma pigmentosum lymphocytes. *J Lab Clin Med* 77:759, 1971.

71. Robbins JH, Kraemer KH, Lutzner MA, et al. Xeroderma pigmentosum: an inherited disease with sun sensitivity, multiple cutaneous neoplasms and abnormal DNA repair. *Ann Intern Med* 80:221, 1974.

72. Robbins JH, Moshell AN. DNA repair processes protect human beings from premature solar skin damage: evidence from studies on xeroderma pigmentosum. *J Invest Dermatol* 73:102, 1979.

73. Bellows RA, Lahay M, Lepreau FJ, Albert DM. Ocular manifestations of xeroderma pigmentosum in a black family. *Arch Ophthalmol* 92:113, 1974.

74. Gaasterland DE, Rodrigues MM, Moshell AN. Ocular involvement in xeroderma pigmentosum. *Ophthalmology* 89:980, 1982.

75. Cha SB, Shields JA, Shields LL, Wang MX. Squamous cell carcinoma of the conjunctiva. *Int Ophthalmol Clin* 33:19, 1993.

76. Spencer WH, Zimmerman LE. Conjunctiva. In: Spencer WH, ed. *Ophthalmic Pathology: An Atlas and Textbook*, vol 1, 3d ed. Philadelphia: WB Saunders, 1985:chap 2.

77. Ni C, Searl SS, Kriegstein HJ, Wu BF. Epibulbar carcinoma. *Int Ophthalmol Clin* 22:1, 1982.

78. Tabbara KF, Kersten R, Daouk N, Blodi FC. Metastatic squamous cell carcinoma of the conjunctiva. *Ophthalmology* 95:318, 1988.

79. Cha SB, Shields JA, Shields LL, Wan MX. Squamous cell carcinoma of the conjunctiva. *Int Ophthalmol Clin* 33:19, 1993.

80. Jauregui HO, Klintworth GK. Pigmented squamous cell carcinoma of the cornea and conjunctiva: a light microscopic, histochemical, and ultrastructural study. *Cancer* 38:778, 1976.

81. Salisbury JA, Szpak CA, Klintworth GK. Pigmented squamous cell carcinoma of the conjunctiva: a clinicopathologic ultrastructural study. *Ophthalmology* 90:1477, 1976.

82. Zimmerman LE. Squamous cell carcinoma and related lesions of the bulbar conjunctiva. In: Boniuk M, ed. *Ocular and Adnexal Tumors: New and Controversial Aspects*. St Louis: CV Mosby, 1964:49.

83. Zimmerman LE. The cancerous, precancerous, and pseudocancerous lesions of the cornea and conjunctiva. In: Rycroft CV, ed. *Corneoplastic Surgery: Proceedings of the Second International Corneaoplastic Conference*. Oxford: Pergamon, 1969:547.

84. Iliff WJ, Marback R, Green WR. Invasive squamous cell carcinoma of the conjunctiva. *Arch Ophthalmol* 93:119, 1975.

85. Lever WF, Schaumbert-Lever G. *Histopathology of the Skin*, 7th ed. Philadelphia: JB Lippincott, 1990:chap 27.

86. Cha SB, Shields JA, Shields LL, Wang MX. Squamous cell carcinoma of the conjunctiva. *Int Ophthalmol Clin* 33:35, 1993.

87. Biggs SL, Font RL. Oncocytic lesions of the caruncle and other ocular adnexa. *Arch Ophthalmol* 94:474, 1977.

88. Radnot M, Lapis K. Ultrastructure of the caruncular oncocytoma. *Ophthalmologica* 63:161, 1970.

89. Noguchi TT, Lonser ER. Oncocytoma of the caruncle and eyelid. *Arch Pathol* 69:516, 1960.

90. Deutsch AR, Duckworth JK. Oncocytoma (oxyphilic adenoma) of the caruncle. *Am J Ophthalmol* 64:458, 1967.

91. Hamperl H. Benign and malignant oncocytoma. *Cancer* 15:1019, 1962.

92. Geer CH. Oxyphil cell adenoma of the lacrimal caruncle. *Br J Ophthalmol* 53:198, 1969.

93. Lever WF, Schaumberg-Lever G. *Histopathology of the Skin*, 7th ed. Philadelphia: JB Lippincott, 1990:chap 33.

94. Reese AB. Precancerous and cancerous melanosis of the conjunctiva. *Am J Ophthalmol* 39:96, 1966.

95. Reese AB. Precancerous and cancerous melanosis. *Am J Ophthalmol* 61:1272, 1966.

96. Zimmerman LE. Criteria for management of melanosis. *Arch Ophthalmol* 76:307, 1966.

97. Zimmerman LE. The histogenesis of conjunctival melanomas: the First Algernon B. Reese Lecture. In: Jakobiec FA, ed. *Ocular and Adnexal Tumors*. Birmingham, AL: Aesculapius, 1967:600.

98. Silvers D, Jakobiec FA, Freeman T, et al. Melanoma of the conjunctiva: a clinicopathologic study. In: Jakobiec FA, ed. *Ocular and Adnexal Tumors*. Birmingham, AL: Aesculapius, 1978:583.

99. Jakobiec FA, Folberg R, Iwamoto T. Clinico-pathologic characteristics of premalignant and malignant melanocytic lesions of the conjunctiva. *Ophthalmology* 96:147, 1989.

100. Folberg R, McLean IW, Zimmerman LE. Malignant melanoma of the conjunctiva. *Hum Pathol* 16:136, 1985.

101. Char DH. *Clinical Ocular Oncology,* 1st ed. New York: Churchill Livingstone, 1989:chap 4.

102. Cha SB, Shields JA, Shields LL, Wang MX. Squamous cell carcinoma of the conjunctiva. *Int Ophthalmol Clin* 33:25, 1993.

103. Grossniklaus HE, Green WR, Luckenbach M, Chan CC. Conjunctival lesions in adults: a clinical and histopathologic review. *Cornea* 6:78, 1987.

104. Folberg R, McLean IW, Zimmerman LE. Malignant melanoma of the conjunctiva. *Hum Pathol* 16:36, 1985.

105. Lommatzsch PK, Lommatzsch RE, Kirsch J, Fuhrmann P. Therapeutic outcome of patients suffering from malignant melanomas of the conjunctiva. *Br J Ophthalmol* 74:615, 1990.

106. Liesigang TJ, Campbell J. Mayo Clinic experience with conjunctival melanomas. *Arch Ophthalmol* 98:1385, 1980.

107. Croxatto JO, Iribarren G, Ugrin C, et al. Malignant melanoma of the conjunctiva: report of a case. *Ophthalmology* 94:1281, 1987.

108. Cha SB, Shields JA, Shields LL, Wang MX. Squamous cell carcinoma of the conjunctiva. *Int Ophthalmol Clin* 33:27, 1993.

109. Jakobiec FA. The ultrastructure of conjunctival melanocytic tumors. *Trans Am Ophthalmol Soc* 82:599, 1984.

110. Jay B. Naevi and melanomata of the conjunctiva. *Br J Ophthalmol* 49:169, 1965.

111. Guillen KJ, Albert DM, Mihm MC Jr. Pigmented melanocytic lesions of the conjunctiva: a new approach to their classification. *Pathology* 17:275, 1985.

112. Jeffrey IJM, Lucas DR, McEwan C, Lee WR. Malignant melanoma of the conjunctiva. *Histopathology* 10:3638, 1986.

113. Crawford JB. Conjunctival melanomas: prognostic factors—a review and an analysis of a series. *Trans Am Ophthalmol Soc* 78:467, 1980.

114. Fuchs U, Kivela T, Liesto K, Tarkkanen A. Prognosis of conjunctival melanomas in relation to histopathological features. *Br J Cancer* 59:261, 1989.

115. Folberg R, McLean IW, Zimmerman LE. Conjunctival melanosis and melanoma. *Ophthalmology* 91:673, 1984.

116. Jakobiec FA, Rini FJ, Fraunfelder FT, Brownstein S. Cryotherapy for conjunctival primary acquired melanosis and malignant melanoma: experience with 62 cases. *Ophthalmology* 95:1058, 1988.

117. Cha SB, Shields JA, Shields LL, Wang MX. Squamous cell carcinoma of the conjunctiva. *Int Ophthalmol Clin* 33:26, 1993.

118. Folberg R, McLean IW, Zimmerman LE. Conjunctival malignant melanoma. *Hum Pathol* 16:136, 1985.

119. Cha SB, Shields JA, Shields LL, Wang MX. Squamous cell carcinoma of the conjunctiva. *Int Ophthalmol Clin* 33:28, 1993.

120. Collin JRO, Garner A, Allen LH, Hungerford JL. Malignant melanoma of the eyelid and conjunctiva. *Aust NZ J Ophthalmol* 14:29, 1986.

121. Jakobiec FA, Brownstein S, Wilkinson RD, et al. Combined surgery and cryotherapy for diffuse malignant melanoma of the conjunctiva. *Arch Ophthalmol* 18:1390, 1980.

122. Jakobiec FA, Iwamoto T. Cryotherapy for intraepithelial conjunctival melanocytic proliferations: ultrastructural effects. *Arch Ophthalmol* 101:904, 1983.

123. Shields JA, Shields CL, Augsburger JJ. Current options of management of conjunctival melanoma. *Orbit* 6:25, 1986.

124. Lederman M, Wybar K, Busby E. Malignant epibulbar melanoma: natural history and treatment by radiotherapy. *Br J Ophthalmol* 68:605, 1984.

125. Lederman M. Radiotherapy of malignant melanomata of the eye. *Br J Radiol* 34:21, 1961.

126. Lederman M. Discussion of pigmented tumors of the conjunctiva. In: Boniuk M, ed. *Ocular and Adnexal Tumors.* St Louis: CV Mosby, 1964:24.

127. Gow JA, Spencer WH. Intraocular extension of an epibulbar malignant melanoma. *Arch Ophthalmol* 90:57, 1973.

128. Shuler JD, Holland GN, Miles SA, et al. Kaposi's sarcoma of the conjunctiva and eyelids associated with the acquired immunodeficiency syndrome. *Arch Ophthalmol* 107:858, 1989.

129. Friedman AH. Massive Kaposi's sarcoma of the eyelid in an aids patient. Presented at Verhoeff Society Meeting, 22–25 April, Coral Gables, FL, 1993.

130. Dugel PV, Gill PS, Frangieh GT, et al. Particles resembling retrovirus and conjunctival Kaposi's sarcoma. *Am J Ophthalmol* 110:86, 1990.

131. Macher AM, Palestine A, Masur H, et al. Multicentric Kaposi's sarcoma of the conjunctiva in a male homosexual with the acquired immunodeficiency syndrome. *Ophthalmology* 90:879, 1983.

132. Weiter JJ, Jakobiec FA, Iwamoto T. The clinical and morphologic characteristics of Kaposi's sarcomas of the conjunctiva. *Am J Ophthalmol* 89:546, 1980.

133. Dugel PV, Gill PS, Frangieh GT, Rao NA. Ocular adnexal Kaposi's sarcoma in acquired immunodeficiency syndrome. *Am J Ophthalmol* 89:546, 1990.

134. Ghabria R, Quivey JM, Dun JP Jr, Char DH. Radiation therapy of acquired immunodeficiency syndrome-related Kaposi's sarcoma of the eyelids and conjunctiva. *Arch Ophthalmol* 110:1423, 1992.

135. Dugel PU, Gill PS, Frangieh GT, Rao NA. Treatment of ocular adnexal Kaposi's sarcoma in acquired immunodeficiency syndrome. *Ophthalmology* 99:1127, 1992.

136. Ghyka G, Alecu M, Halalau F, Coman G. Intralesional human leukocyte interferon treatment alone or associated with IL-2 in non-AIDS related Kaposi's sarcoma. *J Dermatol* 19:35, 1992.
137. Evans LM, Itri LM, Campion M, et al. Interferon-alpha 2a in the treatment of acquired immunodeficiency syndrome-related Kaposi's sarcoma. *J Immunol* 10:39, 1991.
138. Schaart FM, Bratzke B, Ruszczak Z, et al. Long-term therapy of HIV-associated Kaposi's sarcoma with recombinant interferon alpha-2a. *Br J Dermatol* 124:62, 1991.
139. Paredes J, Krown SE. Interferon-alpha therapy in patients with Kaposi's sarcoma and the acquired immunodeficiency syndrome. *Int J Immunopharmacol* 13:77, 1991.
140. Krone SE. Interferon and other biologic agents for the treatment of Kaposi's sarcoma. *Hematol Clin North Am* 5:311, 1991.
141. Scadden DT, Bering HA, Levine JD, et al. Gm-csf as an alternative to dose modification of the combination zidovudine and interferon-alpha in the treatment of AIDS-associated Kaposi's sarcoma. *Am J Clin Oncol* 14:540, 1991.
142. Mitsuyasu RT. Interferon alpha in the treatment of AIDS-related Kaposi's sarcoma. *Br J Haematol* 79:69, 1991.
143. Elsas FJ, Green WR. Epibulbar tumors in childhood. *Am J Ophthalmol* 79:1001, 1975.
144. Grove AS. Dermoid. In: Fraunfelder FT, Roy FH, eds. *Current Ocular Therapy 2.* Philadelphia: WB Saunders, 1985:192.

4

NEOPLASMS OF THE LACRIMAL DRAINAGE SYSTEM

Harry H. Brown

Neoplasms involving the lacrimal drainage system in humans are rare; virtually every publication on the subject begins with some minor variation of that statement. The majority of cases are described in single case reports or small series; various authors have, at differing times, reviewed the world literature and added personal experiences that, in toto, number over 300 cases. The majority of primary neoplasms are epithelial in origin, but the list of tumor types is diverse and includes tumors of mesenchymal, neural crest, and hematopoietic derivation as well (Table 4.1). The lacrimal sac is the most common site of involvement; neoplasms arising in, or confined to, the canaliculi or nasolacrimal duct rarely have been reported. Secondary involvement of the lacrimal drainage system by neoplasms arising in adjacent tissues, such as the overlying skin, nasal cavity and paranasal sinuses, conjunctiva and orbit, occurs more frequently than primary neoplasms

Due to their rarity, few clinicians encounter more than a handful of cases of primary neoplasms. Difficulties in management are common since patient symptoms early in the disease may be indistinguishable from dacryocystitis, and, when overtly clinically malignant by virtue of size and invasion of surrounding tissues, surgical extirpation results in severe cosmetic deformity. Likewise, few institutions acquire sufficient numbers of cases to develop significant statistical analyses of treatment and prognosis for specific tumor types.

Likewise, the incidence of nasolacrimal drainage apparatus neoplasms is extremely uncommon in animals. Congenital cystic lesions, presumably derived from ectopic ductal derivatives, have been observed in dogs and cats. All of the material presented in this chapter has been gleaned from literature on humans.

HISTORICAL PERSPECTIVES

According to Duke-Elder and MacFaul,[1] reports of tumors of the lacrimal sac date as far back as Janin's *Memoires* in 1772. Penman and Wolff,[2] however, stated that that tumor was actually a polyp and did not include Janin's case in their review and compilation of the world literature of lacrimal drainage system neoplasms. In their 1938 publication, they listed 64 cases, 32 (50%) of which were epithelial in origin, and 24 (75%) of those were malignant The benign epithelial tumors included seven papillomas and one adenoma. Twenty cases (31%) were sarcomas (although two were described as "melanotic"), and the remainder included five cases (8%) of lymphomas, four cases (6%) of endotheliomas, two cases (3%) of fibromas, and a single plasmacytoma.

Subsequent cases included in reviews by Duke-Elder in 1952 and Radnot and Gall[3] in 1966 increased the number of accumulated cases in the world literature to 138, of which 86 (62%) were epithelial [22 (26%) benign and 64 (74%) malignant], 31 (22%) mesenchymal [5 (16%) benign and 26 (84%) malignant], 15 (11%) reticuloses, five (4%) melanomas, and one (1%) nevus. Several additional individual case reports and series have been published since their series.

Ryan and Font[4] collected 27 case reports of primary epithelial neoplasms of the lacrimal sac from the archives of the Armed Forces Institute of Pathology (AFIP) and the Wilmer Institute: 18 (67%) were papillomas, three of which subsequently evolved into invasive carcinoma and four of which showed microscopic foci of carcinoma in the original pathological specimen. The remainder were carcinomas from the outset. Thus, 16 (59%) of the 27 cases either initially or eventually were judged to be malignant.

Table 4.1—Neoplasms of the lacrimal drainage system

	Age range (yr.)	Median age (yr.)	Mean age (yr.)	Sex M:F	Recurrence (%)	Metastasis (%)	Death from disease (%)
Papilloma[2,4,9-22,24-28]	1–89	36	38	3:2	46	6	0
Oncocytoma[3,5,9,29-35]	40–88	67	68	6:5	20	0	0
Carcinoma[2-4,9,10,18,43-67 a]	10–85	56	54	2:1	47	19[b]	14[b]
Melanoma[7,8,68-72]	38–80	59	60	1:1	67	31	20
Lymphoma[2-3,6,7,10,73-81 c]	1–82	64	61	2:3	33[d]	56[d,e]	19[d]
Fibrous Histiocytoma[7,82-84]	9–60	38	37	1:1	7	0	0
Hemangiopericytoma[5,7,91-96]	27–48	34	37	2:5	38	0	0

a: Cases reported as squamous cell carcinoma, transitional cell carcinoma, epidermoid carcinoma, and basal cell carcinoma are included.

b: Ni et al.[5] reported lymph node metastases in 28%, visceral metastases in 8%, and death from disease in 37.5% of 74 malignant neoplasms (71 of which were carcinomas); data from this series are not included.

c: Data include cases with either prior, concurrent, or subsequent systemic hematopoietic malignancy.

d: Data include early reports; more recent cases reflect a lower rate of recurrence, systemic involvement, and mortality.

e: Data refer to systemic involvement.

The largest series of lacrimal sac neoplasms from a single institution, 82 cases from the Shanghai First Medical College, was reported by Ni et al.[5] in 1982. Their study included 77 epithelial neoplasms (71 carcinomas, five cysts, and one oncocytoma), two "malignant granulomas," and one each reticulum cell sarcoma, neurilemoma, and hemangiopericytoma.

The findings of Ni et al. are significantly different from the accumulated literature both in the high percentage of epithelial tumors (94%) and in the high incidence of malignancy (90% of cases). Of the 71 carcinomas, however, 31 (44%) histologically demonstrated a papillary architecture. Assuming that others might interpret some, if not all, of these neoplasms to be papillomas, the adjusted percentage of malignant neoplasms would drop to as low as 52%, a figure more in keeping with the previous reports. The high proportion of epithelial neoplasms is likely a more accurate reflection of the distribution of types of lacrimal sac neoplasms, since it is an accumulation of all cases seen at one institution over a period of time, rather than a compilation of selected cases at multiple institutions.

The most recent series and/or reviews of the literature to date are those by Bartley,[6] Pe'er et al.[7] and Stefanyszyn et al.[8] Bartley, who compiled the most complete listing of histologic types of neoplasms causing acquired lacrimal drainage obstruction, added several vignettes of cases from his experience at the Mayo Clinic, including unusual entities such as lymphomatoid granulomatosis, metastatic carcinoma of the breast, and metastatic malignant melanoma from the opposite nasal cavity. Pe'er et al. reported the findings on 35 nonepithelial neoplasms gathered over 24 years at the AFIP, whereas Stefanyszyn et al. included both epithelial and nonepithelial tumors from the AFIP files for a total of 115 cases (82 epithelial and 33 nonepithelial).

CLINICAL FINDINGS

The clinical symptoms of neoplasms of the lacrimal drainage pathway are difficult to distinguish from dacryocystitis. Both usually present with epiphora of weeks' to months' duration and the development of swelling in the inner canthal region (Figures 4.1 and 4.2). Hornblass et al.[9]

listed some qualities that may help in the differentiation of inflammation from neoplasia: abrupt onset of tearing and a compressible mass below the medial canthal tendon, with tenderness, warmth, and erythema in the former; and insidious

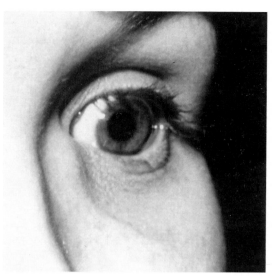

FIG. 4.1—Medial canthal mass in a 26-year-old white woman with a history of papilloma of the superior canaliculus, now presenting with epiphora and blood-tinged tears.

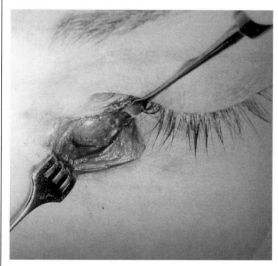

FIG. 4.2—Intraoperative appearance of a pink-white, firm mass distending the lacrimal sac of the patient described in Figure 4.1.

onset of tearing and a noncompressible, nontender mass with a bloody discharge in the latter.

In general, neoplasms should be suspected if (1) there is a bloody discharge either spontaneously or during probing; (2) the mass, if present, is not compressible or extends above the medial canthal tendon; or (3) there is patency of the drainage system to irrigation. Clinical clues that may be useful in discriminating benign from malignant processes include the larger size of the mass, and the presence of telangiectasia overlying the mass, in malignant neoplasms.

Jones[10] categorized four clinical stages in the development of a lacrimal sac neoplasm: Stage I, epiphora; Stage II, simulating dacryocystitis; Stage III, firm, nonreducible swelling; and Stage IV, extension beyond the confines of the sac. As he so succinctly stated, "It is apparent nothing in Stage I or II suggests tumor, and Stage III is by no means diagnostic."

Ancillary studies may help in detecting neoplasms within the lacrimal drainage system. Dacryocystography is advantageous in delineating defects in the shape of the lacrimal sac, due to either an intraluminal mass or an extrinsic compression. Distention of the drainage system by the injection pressure of the contrast material may overcome a functional obstruction and cause a false-negative interpretation. Radionuclide scanning of the lacrimal drainage system (Figure 4.3) offers a more physiologic assessment of the patency of the drainage system, since the labeled isotope is instilled into the conjunctival fornix rather than directly into the canaliculi.

Computed tomography (Figure 4.4) and magnetic resonance imaging are now the most widely used methods in assessing bone changes and soft tissue densities, respectively, in the nasolacrimal drainage system and adjacent sinuses.

Histopathologic examination of tissue is necessary to determine the particular type of neoplasm present and to guide the clinician in the therapeutic management of the patient. Frozen-section interpretation at the time of dacryocystorhinostomy, or planned dacryocystectomy if a neoplasm is suspected, may be indicated in order to determine (1) whether a mass is inflammatory or neoplastic; (2) if neoplastic, whether benign or malignant; and (3) if malignant, to ascertain the

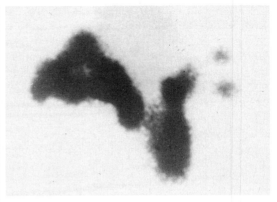

FIG. 4.3—Dacryoscintigram of a lacrimal sac neoplasm obstructing the nasolacrimal duct in a 33-year-old patient with hemangiopericytoma. (Courtesy of Sanford I. Roth, MD. Case presented at the 1989 Georgiana Theobald Eye Pathology Society Meeting, Oklahoma City, OK.)

extent of involvement and adequacy of the margins of excision.

BENIGN EPITHELIAL NEOPLASMS

Papilloma

HISTORICAL PERSPECTIVE. Papillomas of the canaliculi and lacrimal sac have been described by numerous authors over the past 2 centuries; according to Duke-Elder and MacFaul,[1] the earliest report of a lacrimal sac tumor, that by Janin, was a papilloma. Considering all cases of neoplasms of the canaliculi and lacrimal sac reported, the lacrimal sac is the more common site of origin, by a factor of 2:1; in 10% of cases, both sites are involved, either synchronously or metachronously. The greatest number of cases in a single publication is 32, collected by Stefanyszyn et al.[8] Interestingly, the largest series of neoplasms of the lacrimal drainage system, by Ni et al.,[5] do not list any cases diagnosed as papillomas, although 31 of the 71 carcinomas are described as papillary.

TERMINOLOGY. A confusing and conflicting terminology has arisen when applied to benign epithelial proliferations of the lacrimal drainage pathway. Names such as papilloma, squamous

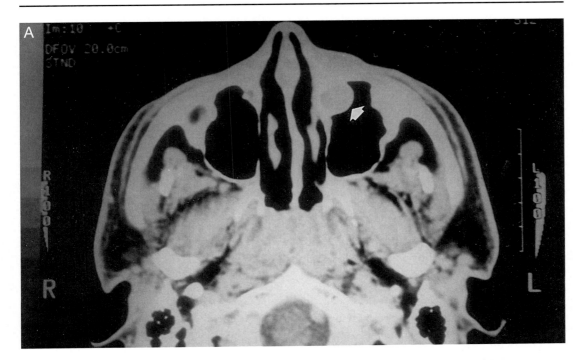

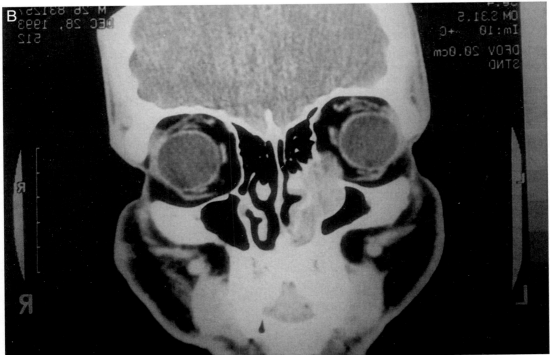

FIG. 4.4—Axial (**A**) and coronal (**B**) computed tomographic scans of a carcinoma in the lacrimal sac (**A, arrow**) and involving the nasolacrimal duct and nasal cavity in a 26-year-old white man. Foci within the neoplasm demonstrate histologic evidence of a preexisting inverted papilloma.

papilloma, transitional cell papilloma, inverted papilloma, Schneiderian papilloma, and benign epithelioma have been used by various authors.[11]

Perhaps the most practical classification is that by Ryan and Font,[4] who categorized papillomas by architecture as exophytic, inverted, or mixed, and by morphologic cell type as squamous cell, transitional cell, or mixed. Architectural patterns may demonstrate frondlike proliferations of epithelial-lined fibrovascular papillae into the lumen of the lacrimal drainage system, invaginations of surface epithelium deep into the submucosa, or some mixture of both. Ryan and Font[4] termed the former pattern exophytic and the latter inverted, whereas Ni et al.[5] labeled the first endophytic and the second exophytic, or infiltrating.

Karcioglu et al.[11] prefer the appellation Schneiderian papilloma to emphasize the embryonic origin of lacrimal drainage epithelium from the Schneiderian membrane and the common features of papillary neoplasms from the lacrimal drainage system with those of the lateral wall of the nasal cavity and paranasal sinuses, also Schneiderian derivatives. They consider the term transitional cell misleading, since there is no epithelial lining in the lacrimal drainage system equivalent to urothelium.

CLINICAL FINDINGS. Clinical information was compiled from 50 cases reported in the literature (Table 4.1). Papillomas of the lacrimal drainage system have occurred in patients from infancy to the ninth decade. The youngest person reported is an 8-month-old with a raspberry-like mass protruding from the right lower punctum, who, after excision, proceeded to have a dozen recurrences over a 5-year span involving the canaliculi, conjunctiva, and eyelids.[15] Of 46 cases where age was stated, the average age of onset was 38, and the median age was 36. Males outnumbered females 27 to 18. The right side was involved in 17 cases and the left in 10.

The lacrimal sac was the primary site of involvement in 29 cases, the canaliculi in 13 cases, and in 4 cases both sites were affected, either at presentation or during recurrences. Those in the canaliculi often presented as polypoid masses protruding from the puncta (Figure 4.5); lacrimal sac papillomas were occasionally clinically occult and discovered only at the time of surgery to relieve

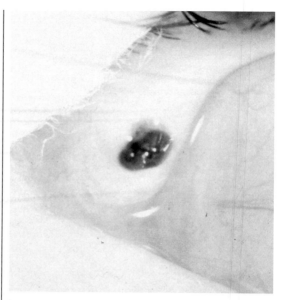

FIG. 4.5—Papilloma protruding from the superior punctum, when pressure is applied to the lacrimal sac, in the 26-year-old white woman described in Figures 4.1 and 4.2.

epiphora, but more often caused a swelling in the medial canthal region.

In 17 of 37 cases where follow-up was available, papillomas recurred, usually in the nasolacrimal drainage system but also in the conjunctiva, caruncle, eyelids, and in two cases as submandibular nodules. Multiple recurrences were documented in 9 of the 17 cases. The majority of recurrences were detected within 1 year of initial diagnosis and histologically were of the inverted type.

PATHOLOGIC FINDINGS. Papillomas are benign neoplastic proliferations of the epithelial cells lining the nasolacrimal drainage system. They may assume a growth pattern whereby papillary fronds of fibrovascular tissue lined by acanthotic epithelium protrude into the lumen of the sac or duct, or one in which acanthotic epithelium forms invaginations into the stroma, the so-called inverted or inverting papilloma (Figure 4.6). Not infrequently there may be a mixture of the two patterns within a given neoplasm. In Ryan and Font's[4] series of 11 papillomas, six were exophytic (i.e., the first pattern), three were inverting, and two were

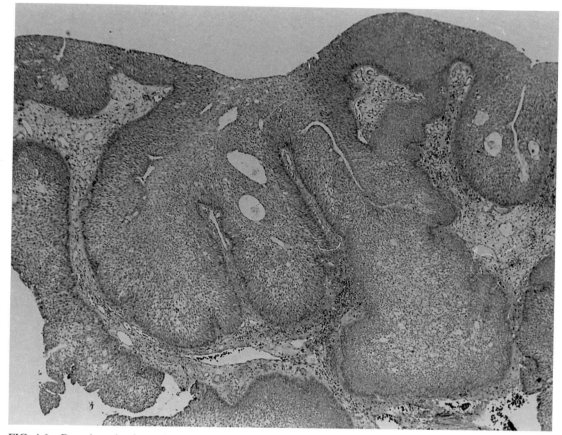

FIG. 4.6—Deep invaginations of surface epithelium characterize an inverted papilloma. Despite the pseudoinvasive pattern, the basement membrane surrounding the invaginations is intact. Hematoxylin-eosin, original magnification ×10.

mixed. In all types, there is a smooth and distinct demarcation of the epithelium from the underlying stroma by a basement membrane

As stated previously, Ryan and Font[4] also classified papillomas according to the morphology of the neoplastic cells: seven were termed transitional cell due to the histologic similarity to transitional epithelium of the genitourinary tract, three were squamous cell, and in one case there was an admixture of the two cell types. Often seen in papillomas of either cell type are entrapped clusters of mucin-producing goblet cells (Figure 4.7), sometimes resulting in mucus-filled cystic spaces within the epithelium. Also frequently observed are acute inflammatory cells interspersed within the epithelium, as well as acute and chronic inflammatory cells within the stroma.

Although human papilloma virus (HPV) was identified in all three lacrimal sac papillomas examined by in situ hybridization, and specifically as HPV types 6 and 11 in two cases by polymerase chain reaction and slot-blot analysis, in a study by Madreperla et al.,[23] histologic evidence of viral infection (i.e., koilocytosis) is not usually present. HPV has also been identified by in situ hybridization.[25,27]

Ultrastructural studies demonstrate typical findings for epithelial cells: specialized intercellular junctional structures (desmosomes) and interdigitating cell membranes between adjacent tumor cells.

TREATMENT/PROGNOSIS. Treatment of papillomas is complete excision, often coupled with

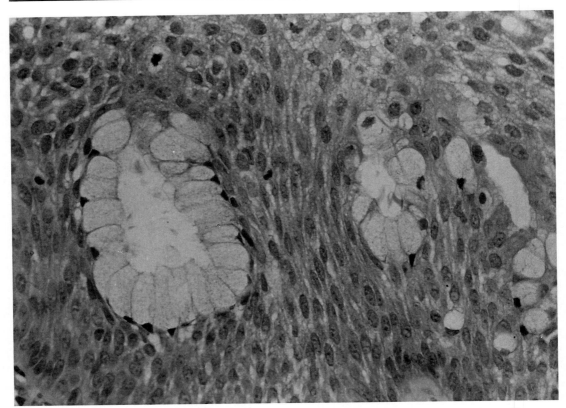

FIG. 4.7—Aggregates of mucin-producing goblet cells form microcysts within an inverted papilloma. Hematoxylin-eosin, original magnification ×80.

cryotherapy. In spite of this, as already stated, recurrences are not uncommon, and in particular the inverting types of papillomas are prone to recur. The risk of malignant transformation is low, but again more likely to occur in papillomas with inverting architecture: in the report by Ryan and Font,[4] three cases of papillomas (two inverting and one mixed) evolved into carcinoma over periods ranging from 1 to 4 years, and in four other cases microscopic foci of invasive carcinoma were present in the initial excision of the papilloma (one inverting and three mixed). One of the seven cases resulted in death due to local invasion of the carcinoma, 3 years after presentation.

Oncocytoma

HISTORICAL PERSPECTIVE/TERMINOLOGY. Oncocytic transformation of epithelial cells within pro-liferations of the lacrimal sac was first described by Bock[29] in 1940, followed by Radnot[30] in 1941. More than a dozen cases of oncocytomas of the lacrimal drainage system are found in the world literature; almost all involve the lacrimal sac. Diagnostic terminology has varied, including oncocytoma, oxyphil cell adenoma, oncocytic metaplasia, and oncocytic adenomatous hyperplasia.

CLINICAL FINDINGS. From information compiled from 11 case reports (Table 4.l), the median age of patients with oncocytoma is 67, and the average age is 68. The series by Stefanyszyn et al.[8] includes four cases of oncocytoma [three men and one woman; age range, 66–80 (mean, 72)]. Only one case has been reported in a patient less than age 60, that by Ni et al.[5] of a 40-year-old Chinese man, also included in the publication by Lamping et al.[33] Sexes were almost equally affected (male/female, 1.2:1), in contrast to the

2.4:1 female/male ratio reported by Biggs and Font[32] in their series of oncocytic lesions of the entire ocular adnexa. The left side was involved more often than the right. Signs and symptoms of lacrimal drainage obstruction were typically present for a number of years. Concomitant or previous episodes of dacryocystitis were not uncommon.

PATHOLOGIC FINDINGS. Oncocytic transformation refers to a distinctive alteration whereby the epithelial cells exhibit cytomegaly, with a strikingly granular eosinophilic cytoplasm. Cells may be polygonal or columnar in shape, and architecturally may form acini, trabeculae, or line papillae (Figure 4.8). The nuclear characteristics are usually quite regular, with centrally placed nuclei, smooth chromatin, and often a single, prominent nucleolus. Mitotic figures are rare. The unique cytoplasmic appearance by light microscopy is due to the presence of numerous, variably sized mitochondria packing the cytoplasm at the ultrastructural level (Figure 4.9). The mitochondria may be normal in internal architecture or display derangement of cristae.[4]

TREATMENT/PROGNOSIS. Surgical excision is the treatment of choice. One recurrence has been reported of a benign oncocytoma, 7 months after excision, without further recurrences in 4 years of follow-up.[32] However, five cases of oncocytic adenocarcinoma are on record,[4,8,36,37] two of which were initially histologically diagnosed as oncocytic adenoma, and only after multiple recurrences over a 7-year span did the tumors transform to a low-grade adenocarcinomas.[36,37] No distant metastases or death from malignancy were reported in any case.

Pleomorphic Adenoma. Only two cases of pleomorphic adenoma of the lacrimal sac have been reported in detail, by White et al.[38] in 1938 and by McCool[14] in 1939. McCool's single case report outlined the occurrence of a mixed-cell tumor in a 54-year-old man who presented with a 6-month history of epiphora and a mass in the left medial canthus. Irrigation of the drainage system was unsuccessful. The mass was firm, nontender, and noncompressible. Excision was followed by a radium implant, and at 10 months following surgery no recurrence was detected.

Interestingly, White et al.[38] reported the subsequent development of a pleomorphic adenoma of the parotid gland 4 months after extirpation of the lacrimal sac neoplasm. Stefanyszyn et al.[8] mention two men with pleomorphic adenomas (ages 55 and 80). For a detailed description of the pathologic findings and treatment, see the discussion of pleomorphic adenoma in tumors of the lacrimal gland.

MALIGNANT EPITHELIAL NEOPLASMS
Carcinoma

HISTORICAL PERSPECTIVE. Carcinomas constitute the majority of reported cases of neoplasms of the lacrimal drainage system. Early reports date back to the late 1800s, and by the end of the first half of this century Duke-Elder listed 39 cases in the literature, supplemented by Radnot and Gall's[3] additional 25 cases through 1964. Including the largest series from a single institution (Ni et al.,[5] 71 cases), the total number now exceeds 150. The vast majority have been categorized as either squamous cell carcinoma or cylindrical cell (transitional cell) carcinoma. Rare types include mucoepidermoid carcinoma, adenocarcinoma (mucus secreting and oncocytic), adenoid cystic carcinoma, and basal cell carcinoma.

TERMINOLOGY. Most malignancies originating from the epithelial lining of the lacrimal drainage system are variably termed cylindrical cell, transitional cell, basal cell, or epidermoid carcinoma,[7] unless the neoplastic cells exhibit unequivocal squamous differentiation, in which case the terminology squamous cell carcinoma is obviously appropriate. Use of the term transitional cell has been challenged, since the normal lining of the lacrimal sac, while similar histologically, bears no embryologic connection to that of the transitional mucosa of the urinary tract; others have used the term transitional only to indicate cells intermediate in appearance between squamous and columnar epithelium.[3]

A more pragmatic approach may be to think of carcinomas of the lacrimal drainage system as representing a continuum from basaloid or cylindrical epithelial cells to more polygonal cells,

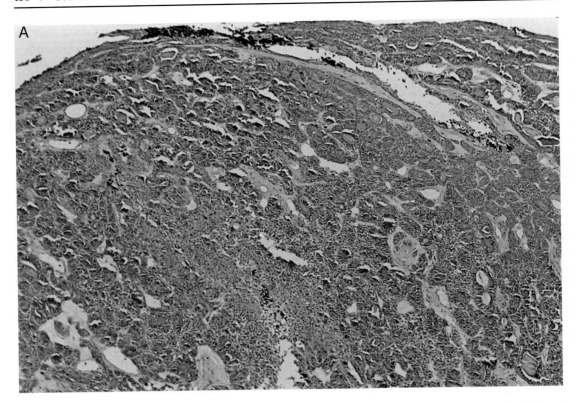

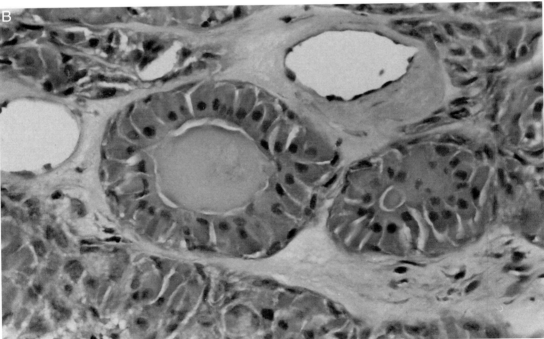

FIG. 4.8—Oncocytoma of the lacrimal sac in a 67-year-old white man, characterized histologically by columnar to polygonal cells with prominent eosinophilic granular cytoplasm forming glands and trabeculae. Hematoxylin-eosin; **A,** original magnification ×10; **B,** original magnification ×80.

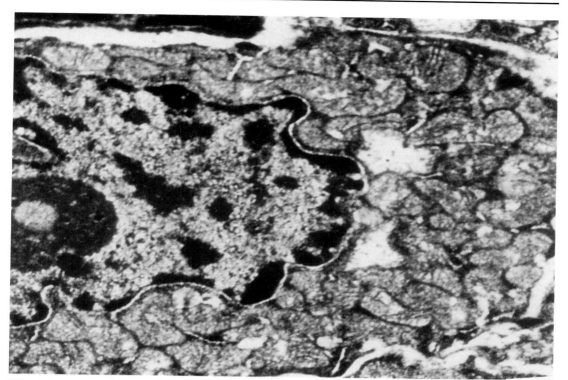

FIG. 4.9—Innumerable mitochondria pack the cytoplasm of the neoplastic epithelial cell in an oncocytoma. Original magnification ×2500.

often with squamous characteristics. No significant differences in the clinical presentation or epidemiologic data was observed between transitional cell carcinoma and squamous cell carcinoma when information from individual cases are summarized.[3]

CLINICAL FINDINGS. From 91 individual cases where information was available (Table 4.1), the following data are compiled: median age of diagnosis, 56 (range, 10–85; average, 54); 2.1:1 male/female ratio; and 0.8:1 left-side/right-side involvement. These data are very similar to those presented by Ni et al.[5] in their compilation of 71 cases of carcinoma at a single institution: age range, 14–74; peak incidence, sixth decade; and 2.3:1 male/female ratio. Duration of signs and symptoms ranged from 1 month to 10 years, with the vast majority of cases manifesting within 1 year.

No clinical findings are specific for a diagnosis of malignancy: Hornblass et al.[3] proposed that certain criteria—namely, large size of a medial canthal mass, and telangiectasia of the overlying skin—to be distinguishing features for a malignant neoplasm, but supporting evidence for these characteristics has not often been reported by others. Radiographic studies, including computed tomography and magnetic resonance imaging, may demonstrate an infiltrative process with bone destruction in malignant conditions. Accurate diagnosis, of course, is possible only with pathologic examination of excised or aspirated tissue.

PATHOLOGIC FINDINGS. As might be expected from the variety of names given to carcinomas of the lacrimal drainage system, histologic appearances are variable. Squamous cell carcinomas are identified by polygonal cells with eosinophilic cytoplasm forming infiltrating nests to solid sheets of cells (Figure 4.10). Intercellular bridges are present linking contiguous cells. Keratinization may be evident either as individual cell

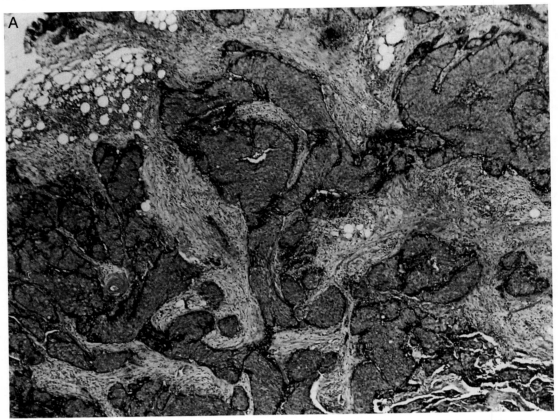

FIG. 4.10—Squamous cell carcinoma of the lacrimal sac in a 70-year-old white woman. Note the infiltrative pattern of epithelial nests at low power **(A)** (continued)

dyskeratosis or keratin pearl formation in more differentiated neoplasms. Carcinomas without obvious squamous features contain smaller, often more elongate cells with higher nucleus/cytoplasm ratios (Figure 4.11).

Human papilloma virus has been identified by in situ hybridization within three of six neoplasms studied and, by polymerase chain reaction amplification of DNA by using primers specific for HPV subtypes, HPV type 18 was identified in one case of squamous cell carcinoma.[23]

The rare cases of adenocarcinoma are diagnosed by the presence of glandular architectural configuration and/or intracytoplasmic mucin, and are presumed to have originated from serous gland acini or ducts normally present in the wall of the lacrimal sac. At least five cases of oncocytic adenocarcinoma have been reported,[4,8,36,37]

as mentioned in the prior discussion of oncocytomas. Other carcinomas, primarily occurring in salivary glands (mucoepidermoid carcinoma[8,39–41] and adenoid cystic carcinoma[8,42]), have also been described in the lacrimal sac.

Mucoepidermoid carcinomas are typified by the admixture of cells with squamous differentiation and mucin-positive cells, as well as cells intermediate in appearance between the two. Those neoplasms exhibiting little mucin positivity or glandular architecture are difficult to distinguish from squamous cell carcinoma, and misdiagnosis may occur if the presence of mucin is not investigated.

Adenoid cystic carcinoma classically demonstrates a cribriform or "Swiss cheese" architecture of basaloid epithelial cells, often with perineural involvement. These neoplasms are more

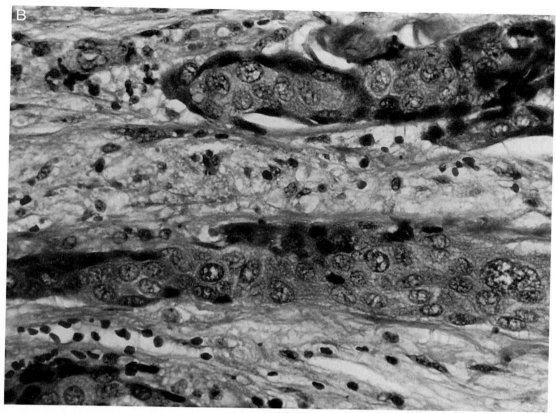

FIG. 4.10 (continued)—and the polygonal nature of the neoplastic epithelium, with occasional anaplastic nuclei **(B)** Hematoxylin and eosin; **A,** original magnification ×10; **B,** original magnification ×80. (Courtesy of Morton E. Smith, MD. Case presented at the 1993 Georgiana Theobald Eye Pathology Society Meeting, Lake of the Ozarks, MO.)

common in the lacrimal gland than the lacrimal sac, and are discussed more fully in the chapter on orbital neoplasms.

TREATMENT/PROGNOSIS. Wide surgical excision is recommended for carcinomas of the lacrimal drainage system, with frozen-section diagnosis if necessary to ensure adequate margins. Adjuvant therapy in the form of radiation has been advocated, and Ni et al.[5] stated that papillary squamous cell carcinoma is more responsive to radiation than are other types of lacrimal sac carcinomas.

Stage at the time of presentation is the greatest prognostic indicator. Neoplasms that have infiltrated beyond the confines of the lacrimal sac into bone and adjacent tissue (nasal cavity, paranasal sinuses, orbit) are associated with higher morbid-ity and mortality rates. No prognostic differences between squamous and transitional carcinomas were reported in the review by Ni et al.,[5] of the cases in which those diagnoses were rendered. Stefanyszyn et al.,[8] however, reported an increased risk of recurrence and metastasis in transitional cell carcinomas.

Compilation of follow-up information in cases reported individually in the literature demonstrated an increased likelihood of death due to either local spread or metastasis in cases diagnosed as squamous cell carcinoma or epidermoid carcinoma (6 of 29 cases), when compared with cases diagnosed as transitional cell carcinoma, cylindrical cell carcinoma, basal cell carcinoma, or epithelioma [2 of 18 cases (odds ratio, 2.087:1)]. The majority of mucoepidermoid carcinomas were low-grade neoplasms, one of which

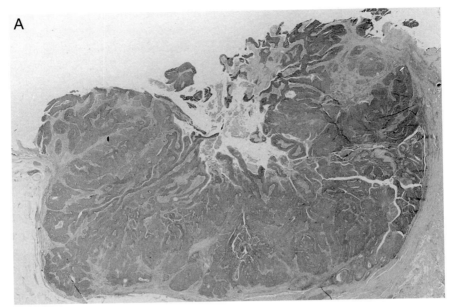

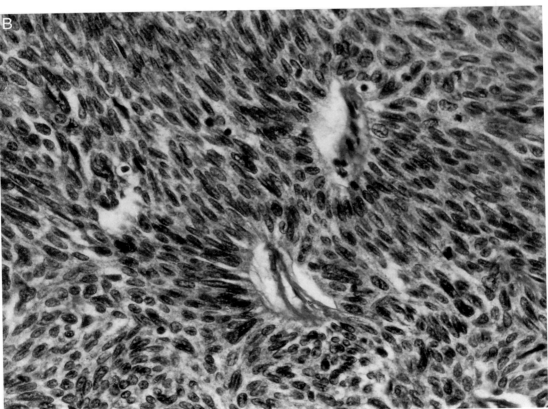

FIG. 4.11—Carcinoma of the lacrimal sac demonstrating papillary and inverting architecture, but with foci of invasion into the surrounding tissues **(A).** Neoplastic cells are histologically similar to those of transitional cell carcinoma of the urothelium: tightly packed ovoid to elongate cells with high nucleus/cytoplasm ratios and minimal nuclear atypia. Hematoxylin-eosin; **A,** original magnification ×4; **B,** original magnification ×80. (Courtesy of Alan D. Proia, MD. Case presented at the 1990 Georgiana Theobald Eye Pathology Society Meeting, Philadelphia, PA.)

recurred as a high-grade carcinoma. Only one tumor caused death by local invasion.

MELANOMA

Historical Perspective. Lloyd and Leone[68] in 1984 described a case and summarized 12 cases in the literature of primary malignant melanoma of the lacrimal sac, dating from the first report from Russia by Muravleskin in 1926. Since that time, additional cases[7,8,68–72] have been reported or presented, bringing the total number of cases to over 25.

Clinical Findings. Melanomas of the lacrimal drainage system have been reported in patients ranging in age from 38 to 80 (Table 4.1). The median age at diagnosis is 58, and the average age is 60. Males and females are equally affected.

Clinical signs and symptoms are indistinguishable from other lacrimal sac neoplasms: epiphora is usually present, but a visible mass may not be. Bloody discharge from the punctum or nose, either spontaneous or following compression or irrigation, is often reported. Despite the presence of epiphora, the drainage system may be patent by irrigation. The diagnosis may be suspected at the time of surgery by the dark brown color on visual examination of the neoplasm.

Pathologic Findings. Melanomas of the lacrimal sac, as elsewhere, may display varied morphology and, in the absence of identifiable melanin pigment, be difficult to classify histologically. Malignant cells may be spindled or polygonal, the cytoplasm may be vacuolated or eosinophilic and may or may not contain melanin pigment; and the nuclei may be bland or anaplastic. Helpful, but not specific, nuclear features include the presence of single, prominent, centrally placed eosinophilic nucleoli and intranuclear cytoplasmic invaginations (nuclear pseudoinclusions). Hemorrhage, necrosis, and admixed chronic inflammatory cells may obscure the neoplastic cells.

Histochemical demonstration of melanin by using Fontana-Masson stain may be useful. However, immunohistochemical documentation of antibody reactivity to antigens S-100 protein, HMB-45 and Mart-1 are the usual markers utilized in differentiating melanoma from other neoplasms.

Treatment/Prognosis. Complete surgical excision is the recommended treatment; postoperative radiation and chemotherapy have been used in some instances as well. Of 16 cases where follow-up was available, 10 cases recurred and six developed metastases. Four deaths, all within 2 years of diagnosis, have been reported due to visceral and bone metastases.

LYMPHOMA/LEUKEMIA

Historical Perspective. Hematopoietic malignancies involving the lacrimal drainage system, particularly those either presenting in or isolated to that area, are rare. Penman's[2] review of the literature in 1938 identified seven cases of lacrimal sac neoplasms classified as lymphoma, lymphosarcoma, lymphoblastoma, or plasmacytoma. Radnot and Gall[3] included those cases among 15 categorized as reticuloses. Ni et al.[5] reported only one case of reticulum cell sarcoma in their series of 82 lacrimal sac neoplasms. Pe'er et al. reported an additional eight cases of lymphoma and two of atypical lymphoid hyperplasia.[7]

With the technological advancement in diagnosis, and evolution of diagnostic terminology and classification schemes, it is difficult to determine the accuracy of diagnosis and categorization of early reports. More recent reports include those by Saccogna et al.,[78] Kheterpal et al.,[79] Erickson et al.,[80] Ferry et al.,[81] and Nakamura et al.[82]

Terminology. As previously mentioned, terminology has changed considerably and often in the classification of malignant lymphoma. Currently, categorization of lymphomas is usually performed according to the Revised European-American Lymphoma (REAL) Classification, combining cell type, morphology, and architectural pattern into low-, intermediate-, and high-grade groups. Extrapolation of criteria to extranodal lymphoid proliferations is sometimes difficult. Immunophenotyping aids in classifying neoplasms as either T-cell or B-cell populations, and, if B-cell, as κ or λ light chain restricted. Leukemias are categorized by cell type as lymphoid, myeloid, monocytoid, erythroid, or megakaryocytic. Molecular studies may delineate monoclonal rearrangement within immunoglobulin or T-cell receptor genes. Sophisticated techniques such as polymerase chain reaction are employed to detect abnormal gene sequences within neoplastic cells, such as the t14:18 BCL2 rearrangement often found in follicular lymphoma.

Clinical Findings. Hematopoietic malignancies involving the lacrimal drainage system have been reported in patients ranging from 4 months[3] to 82 years of age[79] (Table 4.1). Carlin and Henderson[74] reported an average age of 48 in summarizing reported cases of malignant lymphoma of the lacrimal sac, whereas Pe'er et al.[7] reported a mean age of 60 and a median age of 64 in eight cases of lymphoma from the AFIP files. Compilation of data from more recent reports[74–82] shows a similar median age (63) and an equal sex distribution.

Signs and symptoms do not differ significantly from other lacrimal sac neoplasms, although lymphomas may not always produce a mass effect. Secondary inflammation and fistula formation have been described. Although some reported lymphomas of the lacrimal drainage system are primary and remain localized, more often they are associated with either prior, concurrent, or subsequent systemic involvement.

Pathologic Findings. Lymphomatous involvement of the lacrimal sac usually produces either a pink, fleshy mass bulging into the lumen or a diffusely thickened gray wall of the sac. Bone destruction is distinctly uncommon.

Microscopic examination reveals infiltration of the mucosa and submucosa by lymphoid cells, with little or no desmoplastic reaction. The majority of cases have been low grade, composed of small, well-differentiated or cleaved lymphocytes. Intermediate- and high-grade neoplasms can also occur, with larger cells displaying nuclear hyperchromasia, nucleoli, nuclear membrane irregularities, and increased mitotic activity. Distinction of low-grade lymphoma, and particularly lymphomas of the mucosa-associated lymphoid tissue type (MALT), from a reactive inflammatory process may be problematic on routine histologic preparations, and obtaining sufficient tissue for immunophenotypic studies is desirable, if possible. Certainly, in any patient with a known systemic

lymphoid malignancy presenting with epiphora, the pathologist should be alerted prior to biopsy in order to optimally handle the specimen for maximum diagnostic information. Immunophenotypic studies by flow cytometry of fresh-tissue or immunohistochemical studies on frozen or paraffin-embedded sections may be beneficial in typing any suspicious lymphoid proliferation.

Treatment/Prognosis. Treatment consists of a surgical procedure (incisional biopsy alone or during dacryocystorhinostomy) to obtain tissue for diagnosis and postoperative radiation. Patients with localized disease may be cured by local irradiation, with no subsequent recurrence or systemic involvement.[75,76] Chemotherapy may be indicated in patients with localized but histologically high-grade lymphomas. However, a significant number of cases are associated with either synchronous or metachronous systemic disease. All newly diagnosed patients, of course, should be evaluated for the presence of systemic disease, and, if it is present, referred for appropriate management.

BENIGN MESENCHYMAL NEOPLASMS

Historical Perspective. A number of individual case reports describe various benign neoplasms of mesenchymal origin involving the lacrimal drainage system. These include fibrous histiocytoma,[83–85] fibroma,[86] neurofibroma,[87] neurilemoma (schwannoma),[88] hemangioma,[89] granular cell tumor, glomus tumor,[6] and solitary fibrous tumor.[90] The most extensive collection of cases was reported by Pe'er et al.,[7] who found 15 cases of benign mesenchymal neoplasms over a 24-year span in the files of the AFIP (13 fibrous histiocytomas, one lipoma, and one neurofibroma).

Fibrous Histiocytoma

HISTORICAL PERSPECTIVE. Fibrous histiocytoma involving the lacrimal drainage system was first described by Cole and Ferry[83] in 1978. Few case reports followed until the number of occurrences nearly quadrupled with the series by Pe'er et al.[7] in 1994.

TERMINOLOGY. Since the cell of origin is thought to be a pluripotential primitive mesenchymal cell, the morphologic appearances of these neoplasms may be diverse and the pathologic appellations reflective of the predominant cell type. Thus, other terms used include fibroma, histiocytoma, fibrohistiocytoma,[7] and fibroxanthoma.[3]

CLINICAL FINDINGS. Fibrous histiocytomas have occurred in patients ranging from ages 9 to 75, with the average age 39 (Table 4.1). Males and females are equally affected. Symptoms are usually long-standing epiphora, with a shorter duration of an enlarging medial canthal mass. Radiographic studies show a soft tissue density without bone destruction.

PATHOLOGIC FINDINGS. Examination of excised specimens reveals a gray-white to yellow, firm mass, often circumscribed. Microscopic appearances vary from spindle cells in storiform arrays to more plump, polygonal cells with foamy cytoplasm. Individual cells display little nuclear pleomorphism or mitotic activity. Myxoid areas and zones of necrosis have been described. Myxoid change, vascularization, and/or sclerosis may be focally accentuated, causing diagnostic confusion with other entities such as neurofibroma, hemangiopericytoma, or sclerosing hemangioma.

Immunohistochemical markers and electron microscopy may be used to aid in differentiating fibrous histiocytomas from other spindle cell neoplasms. Fibrous histiocytomas are vimentin positive, but negative for markers of specific intermediate filaments. Ultrastructurally, neoplastic cells have rough endoplasmic reticulum but few other cytoplasmic organelles, and no intercellular junctions or basal lamina. Thus, the diagnosis of fibrous histiocytoma by these specialized techniques is based primarily on the absence of any specific immunohistochemical or ultrastructural characteristics of fibrous histiocytomas (diagnosis of exclusion) rather than any distinguishing features.

TREATMENT/PROGNOSIS. In all cases, the neoplasms were excised. Of the 13 cases reported by Pe'er et al.,[7] 10 were classified on histologic criteria as benign and three as locally aggressive, and one local recurrence was reported. No malignant fibrous histiocytomas have been reported involving the lacrimal drainage system.

MALIGNANT MESENCHYMAL NEOPLASMS

Historical Perspective. Sarcomas of the lacrimal drainage system comprised up to one-third of neoplasms in the earlier literature (22 of 64 cases compiled by Penman[2] in 1938). Since that time, relatively few reports have surfaced so that sarcomas now account for a small percentage of malignant neoplasms of the lacrimal sac. Ni et al.[5] reported only one sarcoma in their series of lacrimal sac neoplasms spanning 25 years (1955–80).

Many of the earlier reports did not further specify the histologic type of sarcoma. Of the more recent cases, virtually the only type of sarcoma reported is hemangiopericytoma.[7,91–96]

Terminology. Early reports of sarcomas often described neoplasms comprised of round cells, which in modern parlance would fall into the general category of small blue cell tumors, e.g., neuroblastoma, Ewing sarcoma, embryonal rhabdomyosarcoma, lymphoma, and small cell undifferentiated carcinoma. Thus, it is likely that some of the early cases reported may not, in fact, have been sarcomas at all, but rather epithelial or hematopoietic in origin.

Clinical Findings. Sarcomas in the lacrimal drainage system have been described as occurring in a younger population than epithelial neoplasms. Review of clinical information, where available, was collated in 29 cases reported in the literature.[2,5,7,10,18,45,55,91–97] The average age at diagnosis for 23 cases of sarcoma was 37, with the median age 39. Patient ages ranged from 5 months to 84 years. Type and duration of clinical signs and symptoms did not differ from other types of neoplasms involving the lacrimal drainage system. Recurrences and/or metastatic disease occurred in 44% (8 of 18 cases); deaths were reported in five cases.

Hemangiopericytoma

CLINICAL FINDINGS. Several cases of hemangiopericytoma have been reported since 1971[91–96] (Table 4.1). Patients ranged in age from 27 to 48 (seven cases), with a median age of 34. Five of the seven patients were women.

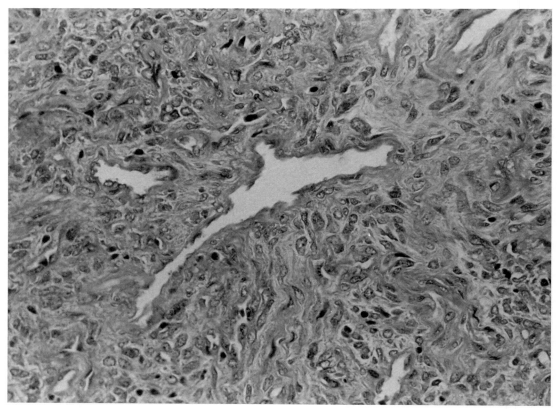

FIG. 4.12—Plump spindle cells surrounding irregularly branching vascular channels are the histologic features of hemangiopericytoma. Hematoxylin-eosin, original magnification ×80. (Courtesy of Sanford I. Roth, MD. Case presented at the 1989 Georgiana Theobald Eye Pathology Society Meeting, Oklahoma City, OK.)

Symptoms, as with other neoplasms in this region, included epiphora and a mass in the medial canthal area. In one case,[91] a dacryocystorhinostomy had been performed 5 years previously, and recurrent neoplasms diagnosed as schwannomas were excised 3 and 2 years, respectively, prior to the time of the third excision and diagnosis of hemangiopericytoma. No further recurrences were reported in this case in 3½ years of follow-up. Recurrences in other cases were detected, ranging from 4 months[95] to 15 years.[93] No metastatic spread has been reported.

PATHOLOGIC FINDINGS. Hemangiopericytomas in the lacrimal sac and nasolacrimal duct are circumscribed neoplasms, often with a dense fibrous rim. No distinguishing macroscopic features are characteristic: the neoplasms are variably pink-tan to gray-white, soft to firm, and polypoid to nodular.

The microscopic appearance of hemangiopericytoma is characterized by a plump, spindle cell proliferation surrounding irregularly branching, thin-walled, endothelial-lined vascular channels, often described as "staghorn" (Figure 4.12). Nuclei are generally round or oval, without significant dysplasia. Mitotic activity is often undetectable. The cytoplasm is without distinguishing features, and cell borders are indistinct. Necrosis and hemorrhage are not typical findings in this neoplasm.

As with most other sarcomas, hemangiopericytomas are vimentin positive and cytokeratin negative. Weak positivity for actin and myoglobin has been reported in one case. Perhaps the most important immunohistochemical application is S-100 protein; it is uniformly negative in hemangiopericytoma as opposed to strong positivity in melanoma. The endothelial cells of the vascular channels, but not the neoplastic spindle cells, demonstrate reactivity to factor VIII. Hemangiopericytomas are often positive for CD34.

At the ultrastructural level, hemangiopericytomas are characterized by a discontinuous, focally redundant basal lamina separating individual spindle cells. Intercellular junctions are sparse and poorly formed. No cytoplasmic or nuclear findings are distinctive for this neoplasm.

TREATMENT/PROGNOSIS. Complete surgical excision is the treatment of choice for hemangiopericytoma. Recurrences are not uncommon and in particular may occur many years after the initial episode. The potential for metastatic spread is present in these neoplasms, but has not been reported in the cases involving the lacrimal sac.

SECONDARY NEOPLASMS

The lacrimal drainage system may be compromised by either contiguous spread or metastasis of neoplasms originating in other sites. Involvement of the lacrimal drainage region by direct spread of cutaneous neoplasms, particularly basal cell carcinoma, is much more common than is the development of a primary neoplasm. Rare examples of basal cell carcinoma have demonstrated direct contiguity with the epithelium of the lacrimal drainage system, and may represent a potential avenue of spread not apparent clinically.[64,67]

Far less likely, but also reported, is secondary involvement from neoplasms arising in the nasal cavity, paranasal sinuses, and orbit. In these cases, the type of neoplasm is usually either carcinoma or lymphoma, although Baron et al.[97] described an embryonal rhabdomyosarcoma of the inferonasal eyelid and orbit secondarily involving the nasolacrimal duct of a 5-month-old boy. Metastasis to the lacrimal sac is extremely rare: the only reported primary neoplasms include prostate[98] and breast[6] carcinomas, and melanoma arising in the uveal tract and in the nasal cavity.[6]

REFERENCES

1. Duke-Elder S, MacFaul PA. Diseases of the lacrimal passages. In: Duke-Elder S, ed. *System of Ophthalmology,* vol 13, part 2. St Louis: CV Mosby, 1974:735.
2. Penman GG, Wolff E. Primary tumours of the lacrimal sac. *Lancet* 1:1325, 1938.
3. Radnot M, Gall J. Tumoren des Tranensackes. *Ophthalmologica* 151:1, 1966.
4. Ryan SJ, Font RL. Primary epithelial neoplasms of the lacrimal sac. *Am J Ophthalmol* 76:73, 1973.
5. Ni C, D'Amico DJ, Fan CQ, Kuo PK. Tumors of the lacrimal sac: a clinicopathological analysis of 82 cases. *Int Ophthalmol Clin* 22:121, 1982.
6. Bartley GB. Acquired lacrimal drainage obstruction: an etiologic classification system, case reports, and a review of the literature: part 3. *Ophthalmic Plast Reconstr Surg* 9:11, 1993.
7. Pe'er JJ, Stefanyszyn M, Hidayat AA. Nonepithelial tumors of the lacrimal sac. *Am J Ophthalmol* 118:650, 1994.
8. Stefanyszyn MA, Hidayat AA, Pe'er JJ, Flanagan JC. Lacrimal sac tumors. *Ophthalmic Plast Reconstr Surg* 10:169, 1994.
9. Hornblass A, Jakobiec FA, Bosniak S, Flanagan J. The diagnosis and management of epithelial tumors of the lacrimal sac. *Ophthalmology* 87:476, 1980.
10. Jones IS. Tumors of the lacrimal sac. *Am J Ophthalmol* 42:561, 1956.
11. Karcioglu ZA, Caldwell DR, Reed HT. Papillomas of lacrimal drainage system: a clinicopathologic study. *Ophthalmic Surg* 15:670, 1984.
12. Hird RB. Papilloma of the lachrymal sac. *Br J Ophthalmol* 16:416, 1932.
13. Burke JW. Papilloma lying within lower canaliculus. *Am J Ophthalmol* 21:189, 1938.
14. McCool JL. Mixed-cell tumor of the lacrimal sac. *Am J Ophthalmol* 22:734, 1939.
15. Walker JD. Recurrent juvenile papilloma of the conjunctiva. *Am J Ophthalmol* 28:751, 1945.
16. Crawford JS. Papilloma of the lacrimal sac. *Am J Ophthalmol* 51:1303, 1961.
17. Anderson RR. Unilateral epiphora caused by a papilloma of the lower canaliculus. *Arch Ophthalmol* 78:618, 1967.
18. Harry J, Ashton N. The pathology of tumours of the lacrimal sac. *Trans Ophthalmol Soc UK* 88:19, 1968.
19. Schoub L, Timme AH, Uys CJ. A well-differentiated inverted papilloma of the nasal space associated with lymph node metastases. *S Afr Med J* 47:1663, 1973.
20. Fechner RE, Sessions RB. Inverted papilloma of the lacrimal sac, the paranasal sinuses and the cervical region. *Cancer* 40:2303, 1977.
21. Nunziata BR, Horbeek JH, Gombos GM. Lacrimal sac papilloma: presentation of an unusual case. *Ophthalmic Surg* 13:919, 1982.
22. Williams R, Ilsar M, Welham RAN. Lacrimal canalicular papillomatosis. *Br J Ophthalmol* 69:464, 1985.
23. Madreperla SA, Green WR, Daniel R, Shah KV. Human papillomavirus in primary epithelial tumors of the lacrimal sac. *Ophthalmology* 100:569, 1993.
24. Rubin PA, Bilyk JR, Shore JW, Sutula FC, Cheng HM. Magnetic resonance imaging of the lacrimal drainage system. *Ophthalmology* 101:235, 1994.

25. Nakamura Y, Mashima Y, Kameyama K. Human papilloma virus DNA detected in case of inverted squamous papilloma of the lacrimal sac [letter]. *Br J Ophthalmol* 79:392, 1995.

26. Buchwald C, Skoedt V, Tos M. An expansive papilloma of the nasolachrymal drainage system harbouring human papilloma virus. *Rhinology* 34:184, 1996.

27. Nakamura Y, Mashima Y, Kameyama K, Mukai M, Oguchi Y. Detection of human papillomavirus infection in squamous tumours of the conjunctiva and lacrimal sac by immunohistochemistry, in situ hybridization, and polymerase chain reaction. *Br J Ophthalmol* 81:308, 1997.

28. Hung SL, Ma L. Recurrent lacrimal sac papilloma: case report. *Chang-Keng I Hsueh Tsa Chih* 23:113, 2000.

29. Bock I. Eine eigenartige Geschwulst des Tranensackes. *Klin Monatsbl Augenheilkd* 105:367, 1940.

30. Radnot M. Uber eine aus Onkocyten bestehende adenomartige Geschwulst des Tranensackes. *Ophthalmologica* 101:95, 1941.

31. Aurora AL. Oncocytic metaplasia in a lacrimal sac papilloma. *Am J Ophthalmol* 75:466, 1973.

32. Biggs SL, Font RL. Oncocytic lesions of the caruncle and other ocular adnexa. *Arch Ophthalmol* 95:474, 1977.

33. Lamping KA, Albert DM, Ni C, Fournier G. Oxyphil cell adenomas: three case reports. *Arch Ophthalmol* 102:263, 1984.

34. Brown HH. Lacrimal sac oncocytoma. Presented at the Georgiana Theobald Eye Pathology Society Meeting, Lake of the Ozarks, MO, 20–22 May 1993.

35. Fukuo Y, Hirata H, Takeda N, Hayami H, Katayama T. A case of oncocytoma in the eyelid. *Ophthalmologica* 208:54, 1994.

36. Peretz WL, Ettinghausen SE, Gray GF. Oncocytic adenocarcinoma of the lacrimal sac. *Arch Ophthalmol* 96:303, 1978.

37. Perlman JI, Specht CS, McLean IW, Wolfe SA. Oncocytic adenocarcinoma of the lacrimal sac: report of a case with paranasal sinus and orbital extension. *Ophthalmic Surg* 26:377, 1995.

38. White JP, Michaelson IC, Heggie JF. Tumour of lachrymal sac of cellular mixed parotid type associated later with tumour of parotid region of same histological character. *Trans Ophthalmol Soc UK* 58:159, 1938.

39. Ni C, Wagoner MD, Wang WJ, Albert DM, Fan CO, Robinson N. Mucoepidermoid carcinomas of the lacrimal sac. *Arch Ophthalmol* 101:1572, 1983.

40. Bambirra EA, Miranda D, Rayes A. Mucoepidermoid tumour of the lacrimal sac. *Arch Ophthalmol* 99:2149, 1981.

41. Blake J, Mullaney J, Gillan J. Lacrimal sac mucoepidermoid carcinoma. *Br J Ophthalmol* 70:681, 1986.

42. Kincaid MC, Meis JM, Lee MW. Adenoid cystic carcinoma of the lacrimal sac. *Ophthalmology* 1989.96:1655,

43. Spratt CN. Primary carcinoma of the lacrimal sac. *Arch Ophthalmol* 18:267, 1937.

44. Spratt CN. Carcinoma of the lacrimal sac: report of a second case. *Arch Ophthalmol* 24:1237, 1940.

45. Ashton N, Choyce DP, Fison LG. Carcinoma of the lacrimal sac. *Br J Ophthalmol* 35:366, 1951.

46. Locke JC. Primary carcinoma of the nasolacrimal sac. *Arch Ophthalmol* 46:229, 1951.

47. Davis RJ. Epidermoid carcinoma of the lacrimal sac. *Arch Ophthalmol* 55:21, 1956.

48. Spaeth EB. Carcinomas in the region of the lacrimal sac. *Arch Ophthalmol* 57:689, 1957.

49. Brown OA. Tumor of the lacrimal sac. *Am J Ophthalmol* 49:1420, 1960.

50. Farrior RT. Carcinoma of inner canthus and lacrimal apparatus. *Arch Otolaryngol* 77:48, 1963.

51. Griffith BH. Squamous cell carcinoma of the lacrimal sac. *Plast Reconstr Surg* 40:332, 1967.

52. Milder B, Smith ME. Carcinoma of lacrimal sac. *Am J Ophthalmol* 65:782, 1968.

53. Jones HM, Thornhill CW. Transitional celled carcinoma of the lacrimal sac. *J Laryngol Otol* 83:397, 1969.

54. Paxton BR, Davidorf FH, Makley TA Jr. Carcinoma of the lacrimal canaliculi and lacrimal sac. *Arch Ophthalmol* 84:749, 1970.

55. Schenck NL, Ogura JH, Pratt LL. Cancer of the lacrimal sac: presentation of five cases and review of the literature. *Ann Otol Rhinol Laryngol* 82:153, 1973.

56. Schindler R, Watson TA, Oliver G. Carcinoma of the lacrimal sac. *Can J Ophthalmol* 8:161, 1973.

57. Flanagan JC, Stokes DP. Lacrimal sac tumors. *Ophthalmology* 85:1282, 1978.

58. Khalil MK, Lorenzetti DWC. Epidermoid carcinoma of the lacrimal sac: a clinicopathological case report. *Can J Ophthalmol* 15:40, 1980.

59. Kohn R, Nofsinger K, Freedman SI. Rapid recurrence of papillary squamous cell carcinoma of the canaliculus. *Am J Ophthalmol* 92:363, 1981.

60. Bonder D, Fischer MJ, Levine MR. Squamous cell carcinoma of the lacrimal sac. *Ophthalmology* 90:1133, 1983.

61. Spira R, Mondshine R. Demonstration of nasolacrimal duct carcinoma by computed tomography. *Ophthalmic Plast Reconstr Surg* 2:159, 1986.

62. Proia AD. Transitional cell carcinoma of the lacrimal sac. Presented at the Georgiana Theobald Eye Pathology Society Meeting, Philadelphia, PA, 10–12 May 1990.

63. Smith ME. Cancer of the lacrimal sac. Presented at the Georgiana Theobald Eye Pathology Society Meeting, Lake of the Ozarks, MO, 20–22 May 1993.

64. Garrett AB, Dufresne RG Jr, Ratz JL, Berlin AS. Basal cell carcinoma originating in the lacrimal canaliculus. *Ophthalmic Surg* 24:197, 1993.

65. Anderson KK, Lessner AM, Hood I, Mendenhall W, Stringer S, Warren R. Invasive transitional cell carcinoma of the lacrimal sac arising in an inverted papilloma. *Arch Ophthalmol* 112:306, 1994.

66. Rahangdale SR, Castillo M, Shockley W. MR in squamous cell carcinoma of the lacrimal sac. *Am J Neuroradiol* 16:1262, 1995.
67. Fosko SW, Gibney MD, Holds JB. Basal cell carcinoma involving the lacrimal canaliculus: a documented mechanism of tumor spread. *Dermatol Surg* 23:203, 1997.
68. Lloyd WC, Leone CR Jr. Malignant melanoma of the lacrimal sac. *Arch Ophthalmol* 102:104, 1984.
69. Glaros D, Karesh JW, Rodrigues MM, Hirsch DR, Zimmerman LE. Primary malignant melanoma of the lacrimal sac. *Arch Ophthalmol* 107:1244, 1989.
70. Torczynski E. Malignant melanoma of the lacrimal sac. Presented at the Georgiana Theobald Eye Pathology Society Meeting, Philadelphia, PA, 10–12 May 1990.
71. Levine MR, Dinar Y, Davies R. Malignant melanoma of the lacrimal sac. *Ophthalmic Surg Lasers* 27:318, 1996.
72. Kuwabara H, Takeda J. Malignant melanoma of the lacrimal sac with surrounding melanosis. *Arch Pathol Lab Med* 121:517, 1997.
73. Cant JS. Dacryocystitis in acute leukaemia. *Br J Ophthalmol* 47:57, 1963.
74. Carlin R, Henderson JW. Malignant lymphoma of the nasolacrimal sac. *Am J Ophthalmol* 78:511, 1974.
75. Benger RS, Frueh BR. Lacrimal drainage obstruction from lacrimal sac infiltration by lymphocytic neoplasia. *Am J Ophthalmol* 101:242, 1986.
76. Jordan DR, Nerad JA. Diffuse large-cell lymphoma of the nasolacrimal sac. *Can J Ophthalmol* 23:34, 1988.
77. Karesh JW, Perman KI, Rodrigues MM. Dacryocystitis associated with malignant lymphoma of the lacrimal sac. *Ophthalmology* 100:669, 1993.
78. Saccogna PW, Strauss M, Bardenstein DS. Lymphoma of the nasolacrimal drainage system. *Otolaryngol Head Neck Surg* 111:647, 1994.
79. Kheterpal S, Chan SY, Batch A, Kirkby GR. Previously undiagnosed lymphoma presenting as recurrent dacryocystitis. *Arch Ophthalmol* 112:519, 1994.
80. Erickson BA, Massaro BM, Mark LP, Harris GJ. Lacrimal collecting system lymphomas: integration of magnetic resonance imaging and therapeutic irradiation. *Int J Radiat Oncol Biol Phys* 29:1095, 1994.
81. Ferry JA, Yang W, Zukerberg LR, Wotherspoon AC, Arnold A, Harris NL. CD5+ extranodal marginal zone B-cell (MALT) lymphoma. *Am J Clin Pathol* 105:31, 1996.
82. Nakamura K, Uehara S, Omagari J, et al. Primary non-Hodgkin's lymphoma of the lacrimal sac. *Cancer* 80:2151, 1997.
83. Cole SH, Ferry AP. Fibrous histiocytoma (fibrous xanthoma) of the lacrimal sac. *Arch Ophthalmol* 96:1647, 1978.
84. Marback RL, Kincaid MC, Green WR, Iliff WJ. Fibrous histiocytoma of the lacrimal sac. *Am J Ophthalmol* 93:511, 1982.
85. Choi G, Lee U, Won NH. Fibrous histiocytoma of the lacrimal sac. *Head Neck* 19:72, 1997.
86. Howcroft MJ, Hurwitz JJ. Lacrimal sac fibroma. *Can J Ophthalmol* 15:196, 1980.
87. Milder B. Neurofibroma of the lacrimal sac. *Am J Ophthalmol* 53:1016, 1962.
88. Sen DK, Mohan H, Chatterjee PK. Neurilemmoma of the lacrimal sac. *Eye Ear Nose Throat Mon* 50:179, 1971.
89. Ferry AP, Kaltreider SA. Cavernous hemangioma of the lacrimal sac [letter]. *Am J Ophthalmol* 110:316, 1990.
90. Woo KI, Suh YL, Kim YD. Solitary fibrous tumor of the lacrimal sac. *Ophthalmic Plast Reconstr Surg* 15:450, 1999.
91. Gurney N, Chalkley T, O'Grady R. Lacrimal sac hemangiopericytoma. *Am J Ophthalmol* 71:757, 1971.
92. Carnevali L, Trimarchi F, Rosso R, Stringa M. Haemangiopericytoma of the lacrimal sac: a case report. *Br J Ophthalmol* 72:782, 1988.
93. Roth SI, August CZ, Lissner GS, O'Grady RB. Hemangiopericytoma of the lacrimal sac. *Ophthalmology* 98:925, 1991.
94. Lim KH, Kim YD, Kim YI. Hemangiopericytoma of the lacrimal sac. *Korean J Ophthalmol* 5:88, 1991.
95. Rubin PA, Shore JW, Jakobiec FA, To K. Hemangiopericytoma of the lacrimal sac. *Ophthalmic Surg* 23:562, 1992.
96. Charles NC, Palu RN, Jagirdar JS. Hemangiopericytoma of the lacrimal sac. *Arch Ophthalmol* 116:1677, 1998.
97. Baron EM, Kersten RC, Kulwin DR. Rhabdomyosarcoma manifesting as acquired nasolacrimal duct obstruction. *Am J Ophthalmol* 115:239, 1993.
98. Kaden IH, Shields JA, Shields CL, Rose LJ. Occult prostatic carcinoma metastatic to the medial canthal area: diagnosis by immunohistochemistry. *Ophthalmic Plast Reconstr Surg* 3:21, 1987.

TUMORS OF THE CORNEA AND SCLERA

Craig A. Fischer, Denise M. Lindley, William C. Carlton, and Holly Van Hecke

SMALL ANIMALS

Compared with neoplasia of the eyelids and conjunctiva, neoplasia of the cornea and sclera is less common in dogs and cats. Most neoplasia involving the cornea and sclera is secondary to extension of conjunctival, limbal, or intraocular neoplasia; these lesions are discussed in detail in other chapters. Primary neoplasia (without limbal or conjunctival involvement) of the cornea is uncommon, whereas primary neoplasia of the sclera is rare compared with the much more common proliferative inflammatory disorders. Papillomas, epitheliomas, squamous cell carcinomas (SCCs), hemangiomas, hemangiosarcomas, lymphosarcomas, limbal or intraocular melanomas, mast cell tumors, fibrosarcomas, angiosarcomas, and sarcomas are examples of neoplasia that can affect the cornea and sclera.

Papillomas. Papillomas are probably the most common primary corneal neoplasia in young dogs[1] and resemble papillomas found on eyelid skin, conjunctiva, and oral mucosa. Histologically, this neoplasia is described as having hyperplastic epithelium that does not show local infiltration. Chronic superficial keratitis characterized by corneal pigmentation, neovascularization, and inflammatory cell infiltration can be associated with corneal papillomas in older animals (Figures 5.1–5.3).[2] Superficial keratectomy is the treatment of choice.

Squamous Cell Carcinoma

INCIDENCE. SCC of the cornea occurs more frequently in cattle and horses than in small animals.[3–12] The majority of cases represent extension of primary conjunctival, third eyelid, or eyelid neoplasia.

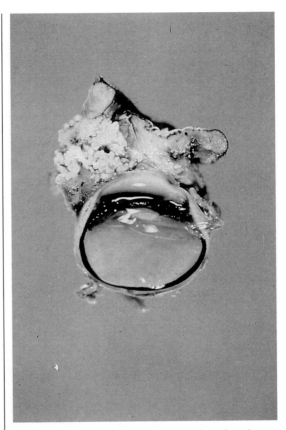

FIG. 5.1—Gross pathology of an enucleated canine globe hemisected through the optic nerve, demonstrating severe corneal papillomatosis.

Primary corneal SCC without limbal involvement is rare, but has been reported in dogs,[2,13] occurring in eyes with pigmentary keratitis. SCC involving the lateral aspect of the cornea in a cheetah has been described.[14]

PATHOLOGIC FEATURES. Corneal SCC appears as a placoid white (leukoplakic) to fleshy pink

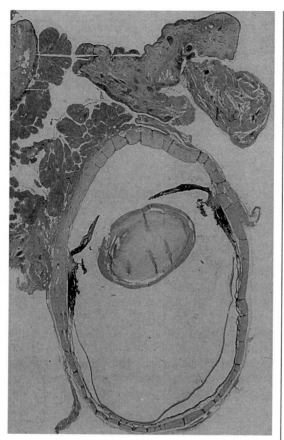

FIG. 5.2—Histopathologic section of the enucleated globe (see Figure 5.1). Hematoxylin-eosin, ×5.

multilobulated mass. Superficial corneal vascularization and haziness associated with corneal edema often surround the lesion (Figure 5.4). SSC involving the cornea and sclera tends to be less inwardly invasive, possibly because of the density of the underlying connective tissue, than similar lesions involving skin and mucus membrane.[15] Tissue necrosis, ulceration, inflammatory cell infiltration, and hemorrhage appear in more than 40% of invasive SCCs[16] (Figures 5.5–5.7).

In dogs, corneal SCC has been described as consisting of acanthotic squamous epithelium with deep rete pegs, keratin pearl formation, prominent intercellular bridges, anisocytosis, anisokaryosis, and dyskeratosis. Vesicular nuclei with one or more prominent nucleoli are common. Most cells are epithelioid, with occasional spindle cells.[13]

TREATMENT. Treatment of SCC of the cornea usually involves lamellar keratectomy, cryosurgical ablation, β irradiation, and/or radiofrequency hyperthermia. The prognosis is improved when surgical debulkment and a second treatment modality are combined.[11]

BIOLOGIC FEATURES. The long-term prognosis for recurrence and metastasis varies with the extent

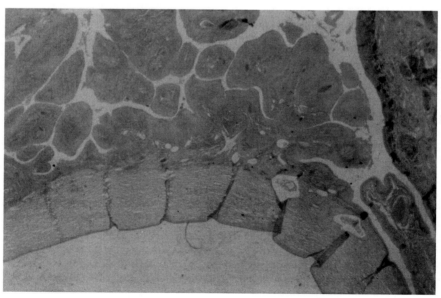

FIG. 5.3—Corneal papilloma and keratitis (see Figures 5.1 and 5.2). Hematoxylin-eosin, ×10.

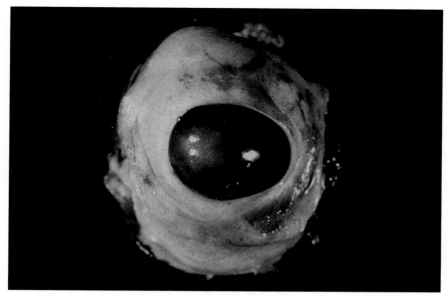

FIG. 5.4—Enucleated bovine globe with squamous cell carcinoma involving the temporal one-half of the cornea.

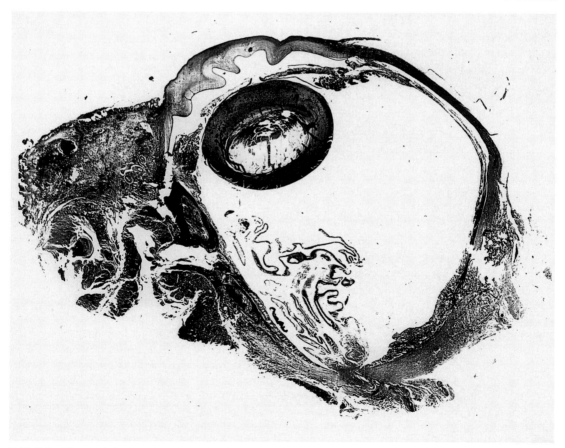

FIG. 5.5—Histopathologic section of a bovine globe with squamous cell carcinoma invading the cornea, subconjunctival space, and sclera. Hematoxylin-eosin, ×4.

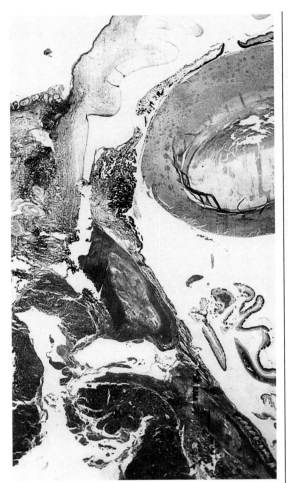

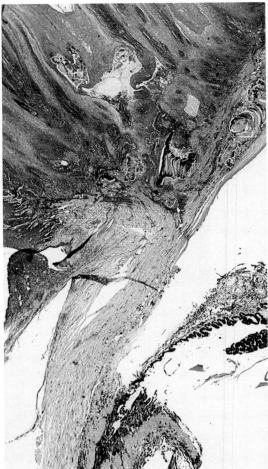

FIG. 5.6—Histopathologic section of a bovine globe with squamous cell carcinoma invading the cornea, subconjunctival space, and sclera. Hematoxylin-eosin, ×10.

FIG. 5.7—Deep invasion and destruction of the bovine corneal stroma by squamous cell carcinoma. Hematoxylin-eosin, ×10.

of adnexal and periocular tissue involvement. In cattle, metastasis from tumors of the limbus and cornea is less likely than from conjunctiva and adnexa.[16] The relative avascularity of the corneal stroma and sclera has been suggested as offering impediments to metastasis.[17]

Melanoma

INCIDENCE. Two types of melanoma have been reported to involve or invade the fibrous tunics of the eye: limbal or epibulbar melanocytomas[18–21] (Figure 5.8) and intraocular melanomas (those that arise from the uvea and ex-

tend through cornea and sclera)[22–25] (Figures 5.9 and 5.10).

PATHOLOGIC FEATURES. Limbal melanocytomas are smooth and darkly pigmented neoplasms that arise from the melanocytes normally encountered in the corneoscleral junction of dogs and cats, and extend both anteriorly and posteriorly to involve the corneal stroma and/or sclera. In young dogs (2–4 years of age), the tumors may grow rapidly. In older dogs (8–11 years of age) and cats, tumors are typically more stationary. The superior quadrants are most commonly affected. The German shepherd, Labrador

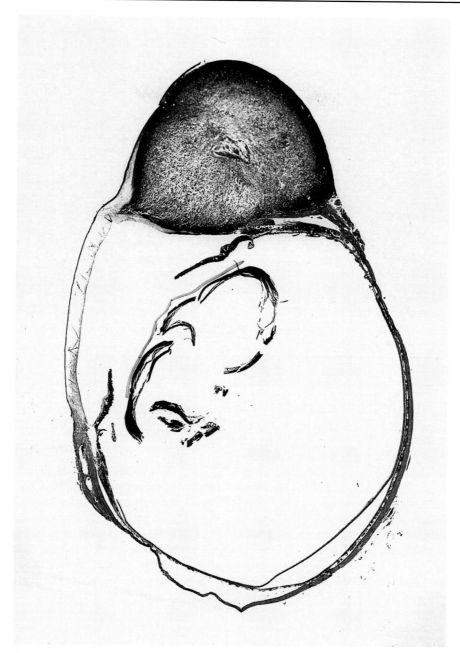

FIG. 5.8—Limbal melanocytomoma with associated corneal invasion in an enucleated cat globe. Hematoxylin-eosin, ×5.

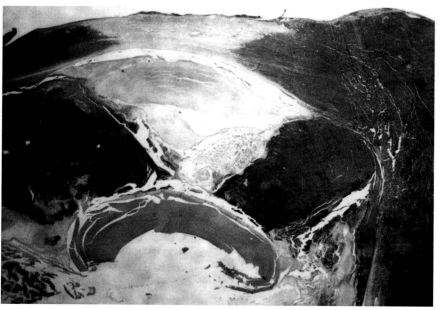

FIG. 5.9—Extensive intraocular melanoma in a dog. Extension of the pigmented neoplasm obliterated fibrous tunic architecture. Hematoxylin-eosin, ×5.

retriever, and schnauzer breeds are examples of heavily pigmented dogs that tend to be more commonly predisposed.[18–21]

Histologically, limbal melanocytomas are composed of mostly large, round or polyhedral, non-cohesive, heavily pigmented cells with bland nuclear features; single nucleoli are the rule. There is a small percentage of stellate-to-spindle lightly pigmented cells that are more easily seen on bleached histologic sections.

TREATMENT. Excision of the neoplastic tissue with corneoscleral or third-eyelid cartilage grafts to fill the fibrous tunic defect has been recommended to maintain a functional eye.[26] Cryosurgical[21] and laser[27] ablation offer effective treatment options as well.

BIOLOGIC FEATURES. Limbal melanocytoma may uncommonly extend into the anterior uvea and filtration angle and jeopardize the eye. Limbal melanocytomas and the great majority of uveal melanomas (many of which have identical cellular populations) are benign and the prognosis for general health is excellent.

Hemangiomas and Hemangiosarcomas

PATHOLOGIC FEATURES. Hemangiomas and hemangiosarcomas of the cornea and sclera are considered uncommon[28] and are described only in dogs. Histologically, hemangiomas are characterized by clear-cut vascular differentiation. Plump endothelial cells lining interconnecting vascular channels are subdivided by trabeculae of fibrous connective tissue. As the cornea is avascular, the neoplasm originates at the limbus and extends into the fibrous tunic, obliterating normal architecture (Figure 5.11).

Equine angiomas can extend from the conjunctiva into the adjacent cornea (Figure 5.12).

TREATMENT. Clinically, hemangiosarcomas are more aggressive than hemangiomas. Treatment consists of excision and cryosurgical or CO_2 laser ablation or β irradiation.

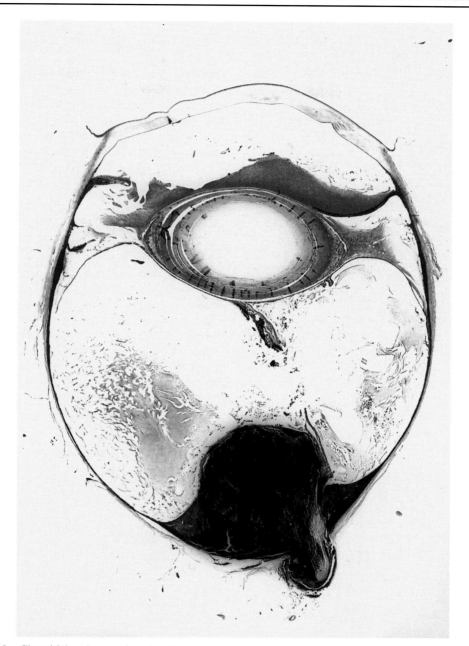

FIG. 5.10—Choroidal melanoma in a dog that extends into the adjacent posterior sclera and optic nerve. Hematoxylin-eosin, ×5.

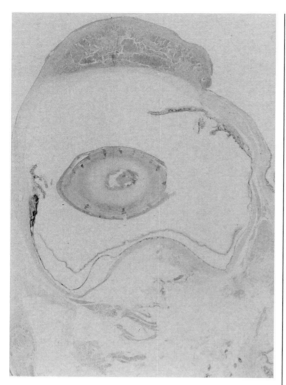

FIG. 5.11—Hemangiosarcoma involving the cornea of a 10-year-old collie. Hematoxylin-eosin, ×12.

Sarcomas. Feline intraocular sarcomas can invade the cornea and sclera[29,30] (Figure 5.13).

Miscellaneous Fibrous Tunic Neoplasms. A primary epithelioma of the cornea was excised from a 10-year-old German shepherd;[1] no description of the neoplasm was noted. Likewise, corneal fibrosarcomas in dogs are mentioned as being rare.[1] Because of the invasive nature of fibrosarcoma, enucleation is recommended as the treatment of choice.

Experimental Corneal Neoplasia. Corneal tumors can be produced in rats, mice, hamsters, and opossums by chronic exposure to ultraviolet radiation.[31–35] Ultraviolet radiation-induced corneal tumors arising in the central cornea rather than at the limbus are almost always derived from keratocytes rather than epithelial cells. These neoplasms are fibrosarcomas and more rarely hemangiosarcomas.

Clinically, in the opossum, corneal neovascularization and cloudiness involving the entire corneal surface precedes tumor development. The cloudiness is due to proliferation of corneal fibroblasts (keratocytes) in a zone immediately underneath the corneal epithelium. Eventually,

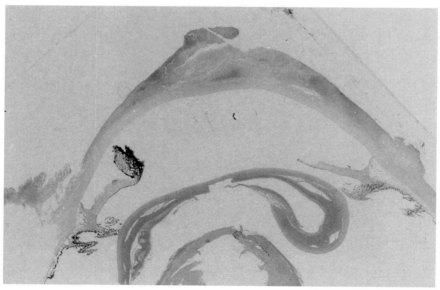

FIG. 5.12—Anterior one-half of an enucleated globe from a 6-year-old Arabian horse. The entire superficial corneal is covered by a vascular neoplasm diagnosed as angiosarcoma. Hematoxylin-eosin, ×6.

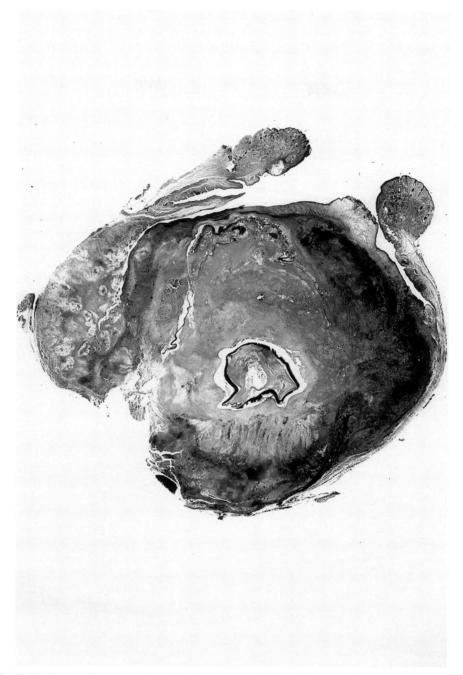

FIG. 5.13—Feline intraocular sarcoma invading the cornea and sclera. Hematoxylin-eosin, ×4.

neoplastic cells completely replace the corneal stroma, penetrate Descemet's membrane, and invade the intraocular structures. Grossly, the corneal fibrosarcomas appear as a thickened cornea or a discrete white or reddish mass located on an opaque cornea. In two opossum eyes, SCC was described overlying the stromal neoplasm.[34]

Pyrimidine dimers are involved in tumorigenesis. Opossums uniquely possess the ability to remove pyrimidine dimers in DNA (the chromophore) by photoreactivation. When photoreactivation (exposure to UVA/visible light) is prevented after an opossum has been exposed to chronic, low-dose ultraviolet radiation, primary corneal fibrosarcomas develop. When photoreactivation after ultraviolet radiation occurs, induction of the corneal neoplasia is suppressed.[35]

LARGE ANIMALS

Epithelial neoplasms, especially of the squamous epithelium, are the most common neoplasms of the cornea and sclera of large domestic animals; of the epithelial neoplasms, SCCs account for most of the cases in cattle and horses.[7,36,37] Corneal and scleral neoplasms are rare in sheep and goats. Mesenchymal neoplasms have been described in the cornea and sclera, but all are uncommon to rare.

Bovine Ocular Squamous Cell Carcinoma

INCIDENCE. Bovine ocular SCC is of economic importance only in the Hereford breed, although the neoplasm has been described in other breeds of cattle.[38] The prevalence of the neoplasm has been estimated at about 5% in Hereford cattle, but much less (about 1%) in the non-Hereford cattle population. In the Hereford breed, ocular SCC is the most common malignant neoplasm.[3]

The incidence is greatest at the lateral (temporal) corneoscleral junction (limbus) of the globe within the palpebral fissure, but the neoplasm also commonly develops in the bulbar conjunctiva and cornea and less frequently on the palpebral surface of the third eyelid.[3,15] Bovine ocular SCC occurs primarily in older cattle, with peak age incidence between 7.4 and 9 years.[3,5,38]

ETIOLOGY. Exposure to the ultraviolet radiation of sunlight is a factor in the development of ocular SCC. Exposure to greater intensity and increased duration of sunlight has been associated with a greater prevalence of bovine ocular SCC. The incidence of ocular SCC is greatest in those geographic areas characterized by high levels of sunlight (ultraviolet radiation).[39,40] Thus, the incidence increases significantly with (1) an increase in average annual hours of sunshine, (2) a decrease in average latitude, and (3) an increase in average altitude. Cattle at higher altitudes are exposed to a greater intensity of ultraviolet radiation, whereas cattle at lower latitudes are exposed to a greater intensity and longer duration of ultraviolet radiation. Also, SCC has a marked predilection for development on the medial and lateral aspects of the globe, areas not generally protected by the eyelids. The precursor and neoplastic lesions develop in those regions of the globe that lack pigment.[41,42]

PATHOLOGIC FEATURES. The continuum of lesions observed include plaque, benign squamous cell papillomas, in situ SCC, and invasive SCC. In most surveys, the majority of the lesions are the latter.[3,7,15]

Plaque is considered the initial lesion in the development of bovine ocular SCC. These lesions are gray to pearly white, slightly elevated projections, with flattened surfaces. They are opaque with circular or oblong to irregular shapes and are firm to hard, depending on the amount of keratinization, and are located on the globe at sites where SCC is common, especially the temporal limbus. Microscopically, plaque is composed of hyperplastic corneal epithelium (Figure 5.14) without extension through the basal epithelium (Figures 5.15 and 5.16). The amount of thickening is variable, and a plaque may be 2–15 times the normal thickness of the epithelium. Other lesions in the plaque include dyskeratosis, cellular atypia, and keratinization of varying severity. These lesions are akin to those encountered in actinic keratosis.

Squamous cell papillomas are epithelial outgrowths located most commonly at the temporal corneoscleral junction (Figure 5.17) and consist of fronds of hyperplastic squamous epithelium

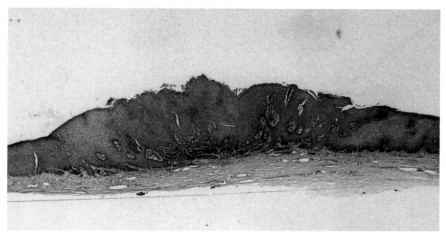

FIG. 5.14—Globe, cornea; cow. Squamous corneal plaque. The lesion consists of a focus of marked thickening of the corneal epithelium. Hematoxylin-eosin, ×35.

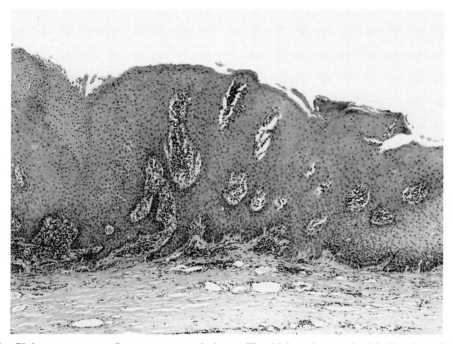

FIG. 5.15—Globe, cornea; cow. Squamous corneal plaque. The thickened corneal epithelium is well organized and confined by the basal epithelium. The stroma has blood vessels and infiltrates of inflammatory cells. Hematoxylin-eosin, ×56.

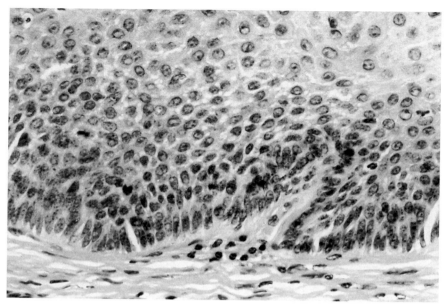

FIG. 5.16—Globe, cornea; cow. Squamous corneal plaque. The hyperplastic corneal epithelium is confined by an orderly basal epithelium without invasion into the underlying stroma. Hematoxylin-eosin, ×350.

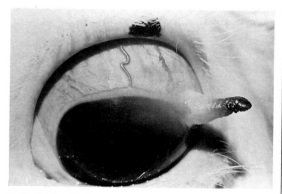

FIG. 5.17—Globe, cornea; cow. Squamous cell papilloma. A papilloma has arisen at the corneal-conjunctival junction and protrudes from the cornea and has keratinized.

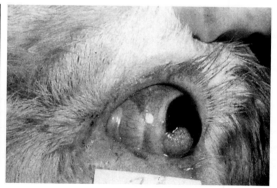

FIG. 5.18—Globe, cornea; cow. Squamous cell carcinoma. A small, plaquelike lesion has arisen at the corneal-conjunctival junction and extends over the surface of the cornea. (Slide provided by Dr. Lynn F. James.)

about cores of connective tissue. Other lesions consist of small rounded protuberances from a large confluent basal attachment to the globe. Some are markedly keratinized, but none invade through the basement membrane.

Clinically, SCCs may resemble either a plaque (Figure 5.18) or a squamous cell papilloma (Figure 5.19) or appear distinctly different from these lesions, with variability in size and the extent of both exophytic growth and invasion into cornea and adjacent tissues (Figure 5.20). Early carcinomas may resemble either a plaque (Figure 5.21) or papilloma microscopically, but have nests of neoplastic cells, or squamous eddies, at the base of the epithelium (Figures 5.22 and 5.23). These nests penetrate the basal layer of the proliferated

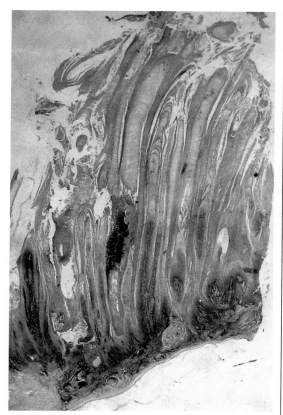

FIG. 5.19—Globe, cornea; cow. Squamous cell carcinoma. Most of this lesion consists of elongated columns of keratin and resembles a squamous cell papilloma. Hematoxylin-eosin, ×16.

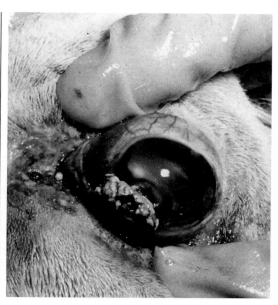

FIG. 5.20—Globe, cornea; cow. Squamous cell carcinoma. A lesion located at the limbus extends from the cornea and has a roughened surface. (Slide provided by Dr. Lynn R. James.)

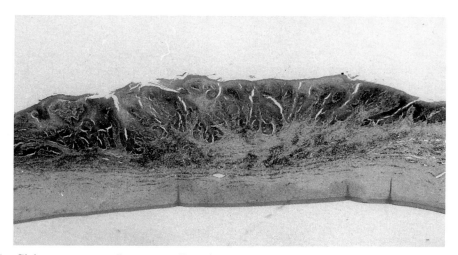

FIG. 5.21—Globe, cornea; cow. Squamous cell carcinoma. This plaquelike lesion has nests and cords penetrating the underlying corneal stroma. Hematoxylin-eosin, ×35.

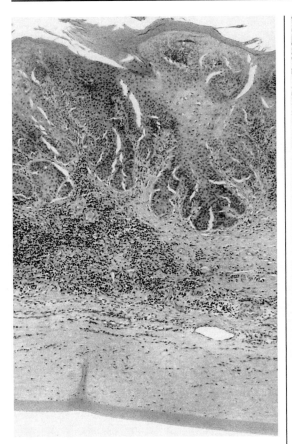

FIG. 5.22—Globe, cornea; cow. Squamous cell carcinoma. Thickened, keratinized corneal epithelium has multiple, papillary ingrowths into the underlying cornea stroma containing vessels and infiltrates of inflammatory cells. Hematoxylin-eosin, ×56.

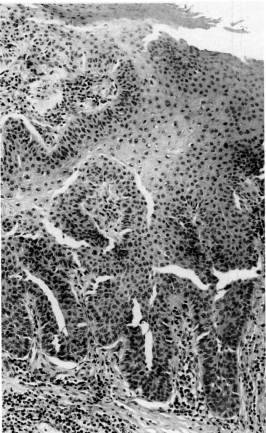

FIG. 5.23—Globe, cornea; cow. Squamous cell carcinoma. Pegs of neoplastic squamous epithelium extend into the corneal stroma infiltrated by inflammatory cells. Hematoxylin-eosin, ×140.

epithelium to invade the underlying stroma (Figure 5.24). Some nests have central cornified areas to form epithelial pearls. Large untreated SCCs are hemorrhagic and ulcerated, have areas of necrosis, and may protrude through the palpebral fissure and invade deeply into corneal stroma (Figure 5.25).

In carcinoma in situ, the bovine equivalent of corneal intraepithelial neoplasia (CIN), malignant transformation in a plaque is manifested by nests of pleomorphic, hyperchromatic cells with increased mitotic activity, double nuclei, and loss of epithelial polarity. Invasive SCCs extend from the basal region of the neoplasm. Invasive cords of anaplastic cells may extend into the cornea to

Descemet's membrane and replace much of corneal stroma (Figure 5.26). Lateral extension can occur under an intact corneal, conjunctival, or cutaneous epithelium. The neoplasm may invade and obliterate the anterior chamber, but the sclera is rarely invaded. The infiltrating cords of cells may have central keratinization (Figure 5.27) and are composed of large cells with a well-defined nuclear membrane, large prominent nucleoli with mitotic activity (Figure 5.28), and a moderately abundant eosinophilic cytoplasm.

BIOLOGIC FEATURES. SCCs arising on the cornea or corneoscleral junction have less tendency to metastasize than those originating from

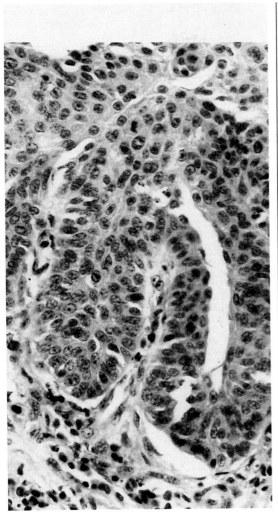

FIG. 5.24—Globe, cornea; cow. Squamous cell carcinoma. Pegs of neoplastic squamous epithelium extend into the corneal stroma. Hematoxylin-eosin, ×350.

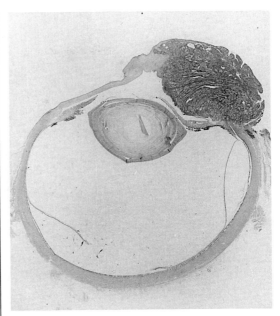

FIG. 5.25—Globe, cornea; cow. Squamous cell carcinoma. The large neoplasm extends above the surface of the cornea, has replaced much of the cornea, and extends into the anterior chamber. Hematoxylineosin, ×5.

the conjunctival surfaces (bulbar, palpebral, and third eyelid).[3,15] However, a few do metastasize to regional nodes late in the disease.

TREATMENT. The treatment of bovine ocular SCC can be grouped into five principal categories: surgery, cryotherapy, radiation, hyperthermia, immunotherapy, and various combinations of the above.[36]

Surgical excision is the most frequently utilized modality for the neoplasm in cattle and is the most successful. The surgical procedures vary depending on the size and extent of invasion of ocular structures by neoplastic tissue.

Cryotherapy is an effective method of treatment for SCC in cattle when the lesions are small (less than 2.5 cm). Larger lesions (greater than 5 cm) do not respond as well to cryotherapy, and the recurrence rate is high. Cryotherapy is not recommended for large, invasive lesions or neoplasms that have metastases.

Radiation from such β-ray emitters as strontium 90 has been used to treat small lesions (less than 5 cm). For larger lesions, cesium or cobalt needles are implanted for periods of time to deliver approximately 5000 rad. Radioactive gold [^{198}Au] as small seeds have been used to treat SCCs in cattle, especially small lesions of the medial canthus and third eyelid.

Hyperthermia produced by radiofrequency electric current is an effective treatment for small lesions, but is not recommended for SCCs larger than 5 cm and those that have invaded deeply into ocular/adnexal tissues.

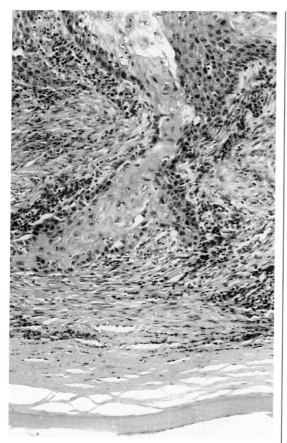

FIG. 5.26—Globe, cornea; cow. Squamous cell carcinoma. This invasive squamous cell carcinoma has pegs of neoplastic epithelium extending deep into the corneal stroma, reaching near Descemet's membrane. Reactive fibrosis and cellular infiltrates involve the corneal stroma. Hematoxylin-eosin, ×140.

Immunotherapy includes the injection of an allogeneic saline extract of SCC and the intralesional injection of emulsified cell walls of *Mycobacterium bovis*. The best response with this therapy modality has been obtained with small lesions (less than 2.5 cm).

Equine Squamous Cell Carcinoma

INCIDENCE. SCC is the most common neoplasm of the equine cornea,[5,43,44] but occurs with greater frequency on the third eyelid and the eyelid. The prevalence of SCC increases with age. The globe and ocular adnexa accounted for about 43% in a series of SCCs in horses.[3]

ETIOLOGY. As in Hereford cattle, ultraviolet radiation and the associated physical variables such as latitude and altitude modify the prevalence of ocular SCC in horses. Periocular pigmentation is one of several factors affecting the prevalence of ocular SCC.

PATHOLOGIC FEATURES. SCCs in horses vary greatly in size, shape, and extent of local invasion. Small (early) lesions may be white raised masses with flattened surfaces (Figure 5.29). Larger (older) lesions may be papillary with varying keratinization and extent of involvement of the corneoscleral and bulbar conjunctival regions. Neglected neoplasms may reach large proportions and present as ulcerated, necrotic, fungating masses (Figure 5.30) that have essentially replaced the anterior segment or much of the globe and involve the third eyelid. Such neoplasms may be infected, have areas of inflammation, and have an associated copious mucopurulent discharge from the affected eye. Involvement of the third eyelid by SCC can vary in extent, but the neoplasm may replace much of involved portion of membrana nictitans (Figure 5.31). The neoplasm may extend to the cartilage (Figure 5.32).

Microscopically, equine ocular SCC varies from well-differentiated neoplasms with minimal pleomorphism and mitotic activity, to anaplastic neoplasms with cellular and nuclear pleomorphism, increased mitotic activity, and local tissue and vascular invasion (Figure 5.33). Pegs of neoplastic epithelium extend into the substantia propria of the cornea and may have varying extensions along and into the cornea and adjoining bulbar conjunctiva. Invasion of the sclera is rarely observed, as the sclera appears to act as a barrier to the spread of SCC.

BIOLOGIC FEATURES. Equine ocular SCCs are locally aggressive and may metastasize to regional lymph nodes. These neoplasms recur, with the risk of recurrence increasing with the larger neoplasms and with multiple neoplasms. Incidence of recurrence has varied from 30.4% in one study to 42.4% in another.

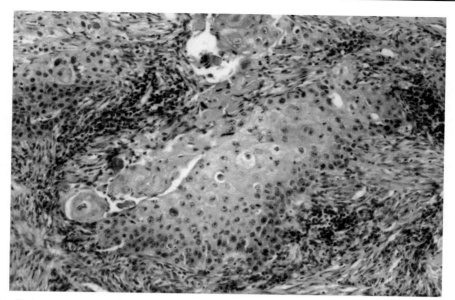

FIG. 5.27—Globe, cornea; cow. Squamous cell carcinoma. This island of keratinizing neoplastic squamous epithelium is surrounded by reactive fibrous tissue and infiltrated by inflammatory cells. Hematoxylin-eosin, ×224.

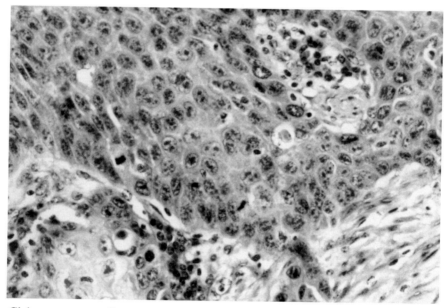

FIG. 5.28—Globe, cornea; cow. Squamous cell carcinoma. A cord of neoplastic squamous epithelium is composed of large cells with round-to-oval nuclei that have well-defined nuclear membranes, prominent nuclei, and mitotic figures. Hematoxylin-eosin, ×350.

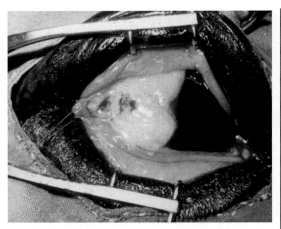

FIG. 5.29—Globe, cornea; horse. Squamous cell carcinoma. A flattened mass is present at the medial canthus and extends over the cornea.

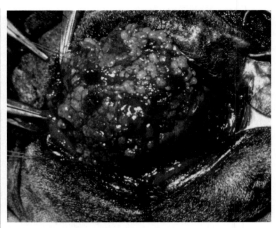

FIG. 5.30—Globe, cornea; horse. Squamous cell carcinoma. A mass with a roughened, nodular surface has replaced most of the cornea.

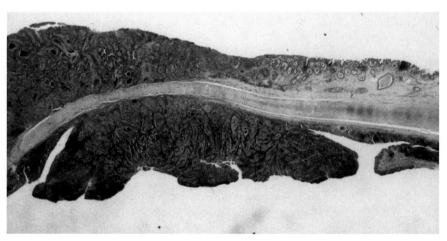

FIG. 5.31—Third eyelid; horse. Squamous cell carcinoma. This neoplasm has replaced most of the tip of the third eyelid. Hematoxylin-eosin, ×20.

TREATMENT. Horses with ocular/adnexal SCC are treated with various procedures, including enucleation/exenteration, removal of third eyelid, cytoreductive surgery, ^{90}Sr β irradiation, cryotherapy, cesium interstitial radiotherapy, and immunotherapy. The results of treatment have been modified by such factors as the size of the neoplasm (greater survival with small lesions), the number of neoplasms (multiple neoplasms increase risk of recurrence), and the treatment modality.

Other Ocular Neoplasms in Horses. Other neoplasms of the cornea and sclera are rare and are represented by only a few cases. These reported neoplasms include hemangioma,[45,46] mastocytoma,[47,48] and melanocytoma.[49] Hemangiosarcomas arising in the conjunctiva have been

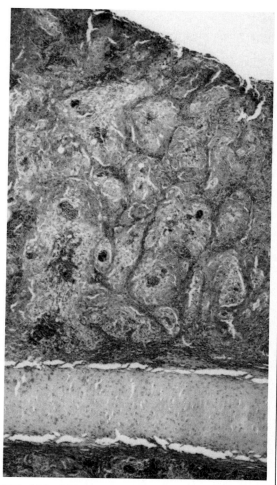

FIG. 5.32—Third eyelid; horse. Squamous cell carcinoma. Neoplastic tissue extends from the surface to the cartilage plate. Hematoxylin-eosin, ×35.

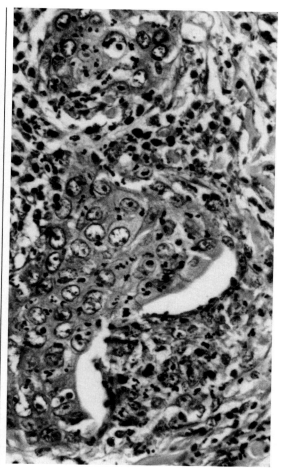

FIG. 5.33—Globe, cornea; horse. Squamous cell carcinoma. Nests of pleomorphic neoplastic squamous epithelium are surrounded by inflammatory granulation tissue. Hematoxylin-eosin, ×350.

described,[45,50] but no reports of hemangiosarcoma of the cornea and sclera were found.

A hemangioma of the temporal limbus in a thoroughbred gelding had morphologic features that were similar to this neoplasm elsewhere and was composed of areas of well-differentiated endothelial cells lining vascular channels of varying dimensions. These channels contained blood, and some were thrombosed. The flattened endothelial cells were uniform with oblong nuclei.[45] In a second report of ocular hemangioma, a highly vascular, irregularly shaped lesion occupied 80% of the cornea and was raised about 4 mm above the corneal surface. This lesion in a 26-year-old mare was a circumscribed, focally ulcerated mass that microscopically involved nearly the full thickness of the cornea and was composed of endothelial-lined vascular channels filled with blood.

Of the two corneal mastocytomas described, one was observed in a 12-year-old quarter horse as a pink-white mass with roughened surface located on the peripheral cornea at about the limbus.[47] The nonencapsulated mass involved both peripheral cornea and bulbar conjunctiva and was composed of nodules and broad sheets of neoplastic mast cells mixed with eosinophils. Neoplastic round-to-oval cells had basophilic granular cytoplasm and round-to-oval nuclei with deep basophilic nucleoli. Cytoplasmic granules were metachromatic with toluidine blue stain.

The second ocular mastocytoma, removed from a 5-year-old mare, was a flat, irregular gray-white friable lesion at the corneoscleral junction. Microscopically, the well-demarcated lesion was composed of densely packed, uniform, round-to-oval cells with basophilic granular cytoplasm and round-to-oval nuclei. The lesion had abundant eosinophils scattered throughout. Foci of necrosis and calcification were present in the lesion.[48]

The prolonged exposure of ocular tissue to ultraviolet radiation may play a role in the development of vascular neoplasms involving the ocular and adnexal tissues. For example, in the case of corneal hemangioma described by Crawley et al.,[46] the mare had been pastured in Utah for more than 20 years at an elevation of more than 5000 feet above sea level. Also, ultraviolet radiation was considered a likely factor in the development of conjunctival hemangiomas and hemangiosarcomas.[49] The conjunctiva lacks pigment and would likely be very susceptible to the oncogenic effects of solar radiation.

PROLIFERATIVE INFLAMMATORY DISORDERS OF THE SCLERA AND EPISCLERA IN ANIMALS

Primary inflammation of the episclera, in the form of a regional area of clinical reddening and mild thickening of the tissue between the overlying conjunctiva and underlying sclera, has been described in dogs and has been rarely seen in cats and horses. A more distinct episcleral inflammatory entity, nodular granulomatous episcleritis (NGE), has been well documented in dogs.[51–53] Reports of a similar ocular entity is noted in a cat[54] and in a bear.[55]

Clinically, in dogs, the anterior sclera is more commonly involved than is the posterior sclera.[56–60] In more long-standing cases, panscleritis with or without uveal extension has been seen.[51,56] An aggressive variant involves a bilateral necrotizing process.

Episcleritis

ANATOMY. The episclera is a rather ill-defined area made up of mainly Tenon's capsular tissue and is bordered by the limbus anteriorly and the extraocular muscle attachments posteriorly. The external confines of the episclera is made up of the superficial episcleral layer that is the parietal layer of Tenon's capsule. The superficial branch of the anterior ciliary artery courses through this tissue layer. The internal border of the episcleral layer is the visceral layer of Tenon's capsule in which the deep episcleral vascular plexus courses. Between these two layers is a potential space with loosely joined connective tissue (Figure 5.34).

The superficial episcleral vascular plexus anastomoses anteriorly with the conjunctival vasculature. In simple localized episcleritis, it is the superficial episcleral vascular plexus that becomes congested and in which the early stages of inflammation are first seen. Edema and inflammatory exudates tend to accumulate in the space between the superficial and deep layers of the episclera. The deep episcleral vascular plexus is an extension of a deep branch of the anterior ciliary artery and vein and has penetrating vascular branches that course through the sclera and into the anterior uvea. The deep episcleral vascular plexus is involved in active inflammation of the sclera and only limitedly in true episcleritis (Figure 5.34).

PATHOLOGY

SIMPLE EPISCLERITIS. This rather ill-defined entity appears regional clinically and histopathologically is characterized by accumulation of lymphocytes and plasma cells. It is self-limiting and responds well to intralesional corticosteroid injections. Etiologic factors have not been defined.

NODULAR GRANULOMATOUS EPISCLEROKERATITIS. On the other hand, another type of episcleritis seen mainly in dogs is now most popularly termed nodular granulomatous episclerokeratitis (NGE) and is clinically and histopathologically distinct.

Terms used earlier in the literature for this entity include fibrous histiocytoma,[53,61] ocular nodular fasciitis,[62–65] and proliferative keratoconjunctivitis. It arises typically at or near the

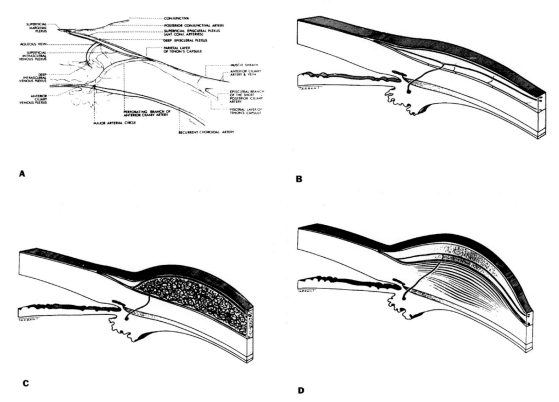

FIG. 5.34—Normal anatomy and pathologic anatomy as they relate to episcleritis and scleritis. **A:** Major vascular networks of the episclera and sclera. **B:** The two major vascular networks include superficial episcleral plexus and deep episcleral plexus. **C:** Episcleritis. Inflammatory components originate principally from the superficial and deep episcleral vascular plexuses. **D:** Scleritis. Inflammatory components originate principally from the deep episcleral vascular plexus and underlying uveal vasculature. From Watson,[126] with permission.

limbus and is raised and may be multifocal, occurring on the palpebral surface of the third eyelid and/or the cornea. Lipid degeneration of adjacent cornea is a common association (Figure 5.35). There is a tendency to be bilateral and a predilection for the collie breed. The behavior of NGE is rather benign and usually is quite responsive to surgical excision, cryodestruction, and intralesional injection of corticosteroids as well as oral azathiaprine.[61]

Histopathologically, NGE is characterized by lymphocyte, plasma cell, histiocyte, and epithelioid cell accumulations. In addition, neovascularization with polymorphonuclear inflammatory cell infiltration, as well as immature fibroblastic cells and abundant reticulum fiber formation are seen (Figure 5.35).

Scleritis

ANATOMY. Anatomically, the outer protective coat of the globe consists of irregularly arranged collagen and elastic fibers admixed within a fully hydrated ground substance. The sclera's main source of nourishment originates from the small vessels within the episclera and the uvea, and little comes from the larger vessels that transverse through it. There are numerous sensory nerve endings in the sclera, where the extraocular muscles attach, and it is damage and/or stimulation of

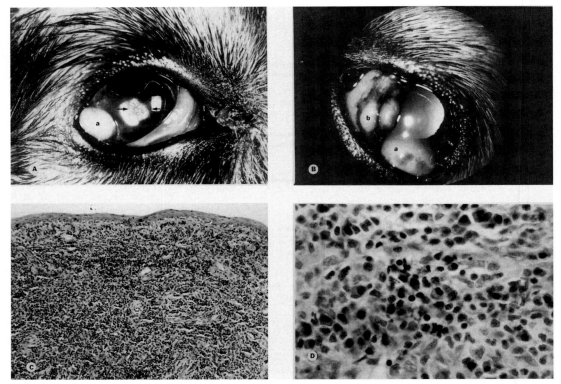

FIG. 5.35—One form of canine episcleritis: nodular granulomatous episclerokeratitis. **A:** Clinical ocular findings include focal or multifocal raised masses at the corneoscleral junction and extending into the adjacent cornea (a) and nodular thickenings in the nictitating membrane (b) in a 5-year-old beagle. **B:** In addition to the raised corneoscleral masses (a) and thickened nictitating membrane, focal granular subepithelial corneal opacities (arrow) representing focal corneal degeneration are often seen. Camera flash reflections are present on either side of the corneal lesion in a 6-year-old collie mix. **C:** Partial excisional biopsy specimen of the corneoscleral mass in **A** reveals marked thickening associated with intense inflammatory cell infiltrate within the corneal stroma. Hematoxylin-eosin, ×100. **D:** Magnified view of an area within the corneal stroma in **C** revealing collections of lymphocytes, plasma cells, histiocytes, and epithelioid cells. Hematoxylin-eosin, ×400. (Original magnification factors.)

these that causes the characteristic pain associated with scleritis (Figure 5.34).

CLINICAL AND LABORATORY FEATURES. Clinically, dogs with scleritis are usually presented with brawny tan sector lesions arising near but posterior to the limbus, and there may be some adjacent corneal edema. If present, anterior uveitis is nongranulomatous, and gonioscopic evaluation of the iridocorneal angle may reveal congestion of the peripheral iris in the area of the affected scleral sector. In advanced canine scleritis, there may be diffuse corneal stroma infiltration as well as posterior scleral and uveal tract progression with secondary retinal involvement.

These fundus changes may be seen ophthalmoscopically and can be presented as focal or regional areas of retinochoroidal degeneration with supra-adjacent preretinal and vitreous exudates (Figures 5.36–5.38).

In dogs, clinical laboratory parameters used to define systemic collagen diseases, such as canine rheumatoid factor, anti-DNA antibody, L.E. cell identification, and other methods, are usually normal in cases of canine scleritis. The author (C.A.F.) has seen, however, in a line of closely bred American cocker spaniels, dogs with scleritis as well as autoimmune hemolytic anemia and rheumatoid arthritis with positive canine rheumatoid factors.

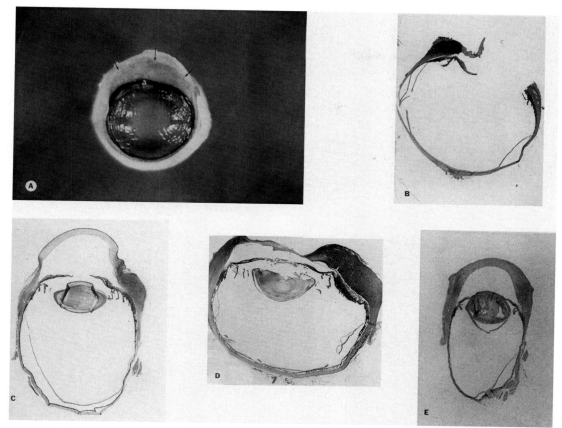

FIG. 5.36—Scleritis. **A:** Gross specimen showing regional thickening and discoloration of the sclera in a 6-year-old American cocker spaniel. **B:** Scleritis. Histopathologic appearance of the scleral inflammatory mass seen in Figure 5.37A. Hematoxylin-eosin, ×5. **C:** Scleritis. Multifocal anterior scleral thickenings and associated uveitis in a 5-year-old collie. Hematoxylin-eosin, ×5. **D:** Scleritis: diffuse anterior scleral inflammation and associated uveitis in a 5-year-old Airedale terrier. Hematoxylin-eosin, ×5. **E:** Scleritis. Diffuse anterior scleritis with diffuse corneal inflammation in a 9-year-old standard poodle. Hematoxylin-eosin, ×4. (Original magnification factors.)

A family of collies was also noted to have multifocal arthritic changes along with scleritis. Recently, the author (C.A.F.) managed a case of scleritis in an Akita with Rocky Mountain spotted fever. In one eye, the inflammation affected both the anterior and posterior sclera; in the fellow eye, only the posterior sclera was involved. We have also seen focal dermal lesions on the face of some dogs that, when biopsied, appear microscopically similar to the scleral lesions (Figure 5.37).

PATHOLOGY

NONNECROTIZING SCLERITIS. Scleritis in dogs, as well as humans, has been subdivided as nonnecro-tizing and necrotizing. Nonnecrotizing scleritis is the most common form seen in dogs, and the microscopic character of a typical case is similar to the nonnecrotizing form in humans. These histologic changes include inflammation characterized by lymphocytes, plasma cells, and epithelioid cells; multinucleated giant cells are uncommon. Extension of the lesion into adjacent cornea is common (Figures 5.36–5.38).

Although collagenolysis may be observed, frequently within a cluster of epithelioid macrophages, necrosis of scleral collagen is not a common feature. In chronic cases, scleral fibrosis and the formation of cystic intrascleral cavities may be seen.

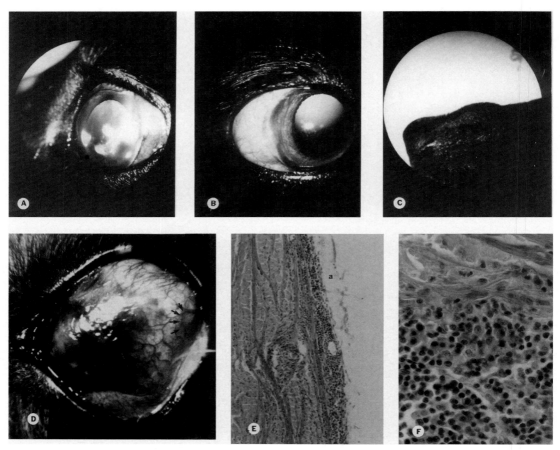

FIG. 5.37—Scleritis. This dog had recurrent episodes of scleritis that, when left untreated, eventually resulted in the loss of function in one eye. **A:** The left eye had multifocal areas of corneal opacification as a result of multiple episodes of scleritis. **B:** The right eye shows relatively mild and focal involvement of the anterior sclera and adjacent cornea during the first scleritis episode in this eye. **C:** During one of the scleritis episodes, this elevated mass that was noted on the bridge of the nose was biopsied, and the microscopic picture is seen in Figure 5.38E. **D:** This is the left eye from **A** 2 years after recurrent episodes of scleritis that were left essentially untreated. There is diffuse corneal infiltration. The arrows denote a focal area of scleral thinning (scleromalacia). **E:** Microscopic appearance of the biopsy specimen taken from the right eye in **B** during the first episode of scleritis in this eye. The mononuclear inflammatory response is mainly seen in the outer scleral region and has a distinct perivascular orientation. Hematoxylin-eosin, ×200. **F:** Microscopic appearance of a biopsy specimen taken from the bridge of the nose shown in **C.** The inflammation response consists of assorted mononuclear inflammatory cells similar to those seen in scleral biopsy of the same patient. Hematoxylin-eosin, ×200. (Original magnification factors.)

When present, the posterior segment alterations include a mononuclear choroiditis adjacent to the areas of scleral involvement, and there may be an associated focal retinal degeneration characterized by loss of outer retinal layers and hypertrophy, hyperplasia, and migration of retinal pigment epithelium. The vitreous exudate is nongranulomatous (Figures 5.36–5.38).

NECROTIZING SCLERITIS. This challenging clinical disease is fortunately rare and commonly bilateral when it does occur, although not always synchronously. The necrosis is seen in the most intensely inflamed areas of the sclera and is often perivascularly oriented. Granulomatous inflammation surrounds the areas of necrosis characterized by palisading epithelioid cells and multinucleated giant cells (Figure 5.39).

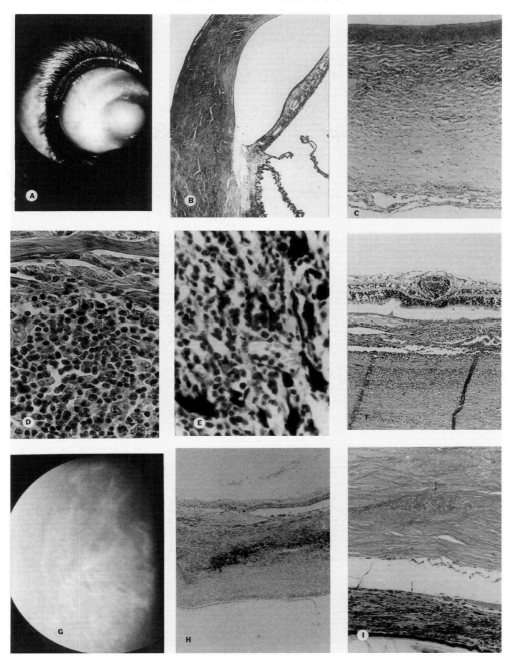

FIG. 5.38—Scleritis. **A:** A 9-year-old poodle with scleritis extension into the cornea. **B:** Diffuse inflammation in the anterior scleral, cornea, and anterior uvea. Hematoxylin-eosin, ×10. **C:** Corneal involvement in scleritis. Hematoxylin-eosin, ×50. **D and E:** Typical mononuclear inflammatory involvement seen in the sclera **(D)** and iris **(E).** Hematoxylin-eosin, ×400. **F:** Posterior scleritis in a dog. There is scleritis with inflammation of adjacent choroid. Perivascular inflammatory infiltrates surround this large retinal vessel. Hematoxylin-eosin, ×100. **G:** Fundus photograph of a dog with posterior scleritis. There are areas of retinal degeneration in the peripheral nontapetum. **H:** Microphotograph of the changes seen in posterior scleritis in the dog in **G.** There is diffuse scleritis with adjacent chorioretinitis. Hematoxylin-eosin, ×65. **I:** Focus of scleritis (arrow) and adjacent uveitis seen further anteriorly in the dog in **G.** Hematoxylin-eosin, ×65. (Original magnification factors.)

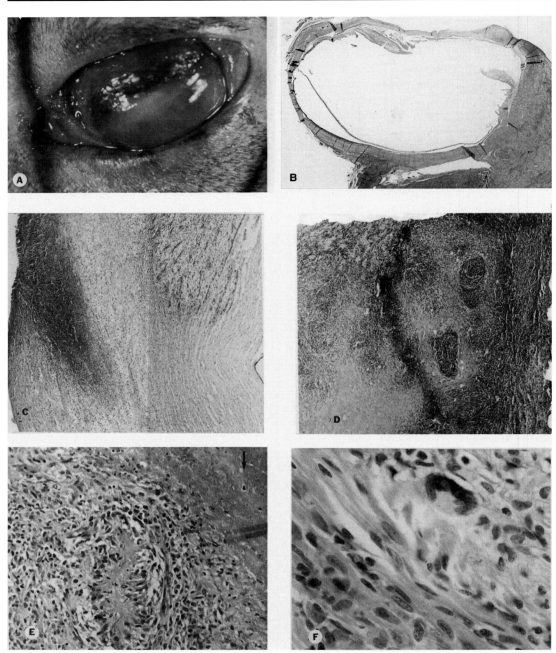

FIG. 5.39—Necrotizing scleritis. **A:** Necrotizing scleritis in a dog suspected of having systemic vasculitis disorder. A 6-year-old weimaraner had a chief complaint of progressive unilateral periorbital swelling and ocular pain. The eye was removed because of possible neoplasia, and the dog was lost to follow-up evaluation. **B:** There is diffuse anterior and posterior scleral involvement as well as extension of the inflammation into the adjacent uvea, corneal, and periorbital tissues. Hematoxylin-eosin, ×5. **C:** The keratitis is diffuse. Hematoxylin-eosin, ×75. **D:** Within the markedly inflamed sclera are multifocal areas, intense vasculitis, and perivascular necrosis. Hematoxylin-eosin, ×75. **E:** There is necrosis of the vessel wall with surrounding granulomatous inflammation and areas of scleral necrosis (arrow). Hematoxylin-eosin, ×400. **F:** In some areas, the inflammation is characterized by palisading epithelioid cells and multinucleated giant cells. Hematoxylin-eosin, ×900. (Original magnification factors.)

HUMANS

Choristoma

TERMINOLOGY. Choristoma, from the Greek *choristos,* meaning "separated," and *oma,* meaning "tumor,"[66] is a neoplasia of tissue not indigenous to the site of growth. The term can apply to solid or cystic growth and to varying combinations of tissue type. All tissues have the common origin of pluripotential cells that develop into tissue of a specific type or types. Depending on the predominant tissue, the mass can be classified; for example, a pilosebaceous structure with a predominance of collagen is a dermoid. If fat is a major component, it may be termed a lipodermoid or dermolipoid. Predominantly acinar tissue may be called an ectopic lacrimal gland, whereas bony tissue is an osseous choristoma or epibulbar osteoma. A purely fatty tumor is a lipoma, but most fatty tumors of conjunctiva are actually lipodermoids, and many other "tumors" are simply herniated orbital fat. Epibulbar fibroma is a neoplasm of fibrous tissue elements.

ORIGIN. Currently, it is felt that choristomas arise from early metaplasia of mesoblasts between the rim of the optic nerve and the surface ectoderm. A useful categorization breaks down the broad term *choristoma* into four entities: dermoid, lipodermoid, complex choristoma, and single-tissue choristoma, of which ectopic lacrimal gland and epibulbar osseous choristoma are examples. While it may be pointed out that a dermoid and a lipodermoid are *complex* in the sense that there is more than one tissue type involved, the term *complex choristoma* is often reserved for the rarer entities such as ectopic lacrimal tissue in association with muscle, cartilage, fat, or some other tissue.[67] Tissue derived from three germ layers represents *teratomas,* whereas tissue from two layers is termed *teratoid.* Teratomas, though choristomatous in the sense that they are derived from pluripotential cells and are of ectopic origin, in contrast to most choristomas, possess malignant potential. They are most commonly found in gonads. These, too, are technically complex, but generally warrant their own designation in the literature. Choristomas can contain far-ranging elements and be quite complicated aside from the semantic confusion they foster. Rudimentary teeth have been reported, as has respiratory epithelium in a limbal dermoid.[68]

HISTORY. The first historical references to choristomas came from Mauchard and from Samuels, who individually described epibulbar choristomas in 1742. In 1853, Ryba coined the term "dermoid," while Virchow, in 1860, defined metaplasia as "histologic substitution" to describe congenital anomalies of the dermoid type. Stargardt, in 1917, described a disorder of aberrant mesoblast behavior early in embryonic life. In 1926, Khan published an outstanding photographic example showing a pig eye with the anterior structures entirely replaced by hair-bearing epithelium in what was probably the first description of a porcine dermoid.

EPIDEMIOLOGY. Choristomas are the most common type of pediatric epibulbar and orbital tumor. The incidence of epibulbar choristomas is between 1/10,000 and 3/10,000, with decreasing incidence with increasing age. Most choristomas are clinically recognized before patients reach age 16.

LIMBAL DERMOID. The most common choristoma of ocular tissues is the dermoid, which often is found straddling the limbus to involve peripheral cornea. Reports of corneal choristomas replacing normal tissue completely with cutaneous, fatty, and fibrous tissue are not rare, though certainly a more extreme finding. A limbal dermoid is most often found in the inferotemporal quadrant (more than 90% are temporal and more than 80% are inferior), but can extend broadly, as mentioned. They vary greatly in size and range, from 2 to 15 mm in diameter. They are infrequently confined to conjunctiva and may not only replace the cornea and anterior chamber but extend into lacrimal ducts, surround extraocular muscles, and enter the orbit. The subject of orbital dermoids is beyond the scope of this chapter, but this is a frequent form of ocular choristoma. Choristomas in general can be found in almost any ocular tissue, including optic nerve, retina, and choroid. Usually a unilateral mass with a yellow-white smooth appearance, a dermoid is often noted at birth. The growth rate parallels that of the eye, but may accelerate with irritation, trauma, or at puberty (which is a time both irritating and traumatic). A rare bilateral annular form of limbal dermoid is well documented.[69] This form not only rings the limbus of both eyes, but can also extend broadly onto conjunctiva. Cystic nests in corneal tissue have also been found.

ASSOCIATIONS. The association of ocular dermoid and facial anomalies was first described in 1882 by Van Duyse, and many case reports were published in the following years.[66] In 1952, Goldenhar described the triad of epibulbar dermoids, pretragal fistulas, and auricular appendages that we call *Goldenhar's syndrome.*[70] In 1963, he noted the vertebral anomalies, including fusion of cervical vertebrae, platybasia, and occipitalization of the atlas. Gorlin described the microtia, mandibular, and vertebral anomalies. The syndrome is most accurately termed *Goldenhar-Gorlin syndrome.* One-third to one-half of the affected patients have dermoids, and most of these are limbal in location. They are frequently bilateral. Associated ocular anomalies include lid and retinal colobomas, aniridia, lacrimal system anomalies, strabismus, (including Duane's syndrome), tortuous retinal vessels, miliary aneurysms, macular hypoplasia, tilted discs, microphthalmos, and anophthalmos.

The facial findings range in severity from small ear tags to hemifacial microsomia and mandibular hypoplasia. There is clefting of lip and/or palate in about 15% and hearing loss in nearly 50% of all patients. Mental retardation is found in around 10%. Goldenhar-Gorlin syndrome occurs sporadically, but some autosomal dominant and autosomal recessive pedigrees have been established. The incidence is somewhere between 1/5600 and 1/26,500 live births.

Limbal dermoids are seen in association with other, rarer syndromes as well, including linear nevus of Jadassohn or organoid-nevus syndrome.[71] This syndrome, described in 1895 by Jadassohn, includes bandlike cutaneous nevi, central nervous system dysfunction, and dermoids. Another rare syndrome that bears mention is Benjamin-Allen syndrome, a cutaneous nevus syndrome that includes dermoids, alopecia, and growth and developmental delay. In 1962, Feuerstein and Mims[72] described the triad of midline facial linear nevus of Jadassohn, neurologic impairment, and

ocular abnormalities and termed this the *linear nevus sebaceous syndrome.* Histologically, these dermoids contain rudimentary pilosebaceous structures, cartilage, and lacrimal gland nests. They have been known to transform into malignant basal cell tumors. Although multiple congenital anomalies in association with limbal dermoids and other choristomas are not uncommon, the majority of these lesions occur without other evidence of further abnormal development.

HISTOLOGY. Histopathologically, these are among the most dramatic and fascinating neoplasms. Limbal dermoids are a variable mixture of collagenous tissue with pilosebaceous structures, including formed hair, glands, blood vessels, lymphatics, cartilage, muscle, bone, nerves, keratin, and fat (Figure 5.40). They are covered by stratified squamous epithelium that is usually thin and nonkeratinized, but which may take on a thickened, granular, keratin-producing layer. These are benign tumors with sometimes less than benign behavior. On the whole, malignant transformation of choristomatous tissues is rare. Both teratomas and lacrimal tissue have been known to become invasive, and the dermoids associated with cutaneous nevus syndromes have been described with this capability. Even a common, benign limbal dermoid however, is often treated.

TREATMENT. The major indication for treatment of a limbal dermoid is cosmesis. If the lesion is

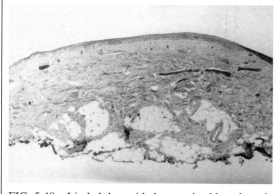

FIG. 5.40—Limbal dermoid characterized by adnexal structures and a compact collagenous stroma, as well as deeper adipose tissue.

amblyogenic, either by occlusion of the visual axis or by induction of astigmatism, surgical excision must be strongly considered. This is accomplished by shaving the elevated portion by lamellar keratoplasty, or occasionally by penetrating keratoplasty. Cornea and sclera may be quite unexpectedly thin beneath a lesion, making the excision at times quite difficult. Patch grafts may be necessary. Significant meridional change can persist after excision, and postoperative corneal leukoma may continue to present significant amblyogenic potential. Usually, however, visual acuity is not negatively affected by surgical excision.

In a series of 10 patients who underwent surgical treatment for limbal dermoids, Panton and Sugar[73] of the University of Illinois Eye and Ear Infirmary noted no significant visual change in eight of the patients, and all 10 had good cosmetic results. This was true despite the finding of 40% recurrent epithelial defects and 70% peripheral corneal vascularization. In the treatment of large lesions, muscle damage may occur if the tumor is unfortunately situated. The excision of other types of choristomas is more variable in indication, however; often this is done for diagnostic purposes.

The differential diagnosis of tumors of the conjunctiva, sclera, limbus, cornea, muscles, and glands of the eye is broad, and many times only histopathologic studies can determine the origin of the tissue.

ECTOPIC LACRIMAL GLAND. Ectopic lacrimal gland is a special type of choristoma for several reasons. It may be a simple choristoma, that is, consisting of only the acinar tissue, or it may be part of a complex choristoma. Pokorny et al.[74] of Manhattan Eye, Ear and Throat Hospital presented three cases of complex epibulbar choristomas containing lacrimal gland as well as smooth muscle and cartilage. They suggested that these were examples of aberrant migration of the palpebral lobe of the lacrimal gland. The first ectopic lacrimal gland was reported in 1877 by Peuch as a case of "adenoma of the choroid." Such tissue has since been reported in the orbit; on the lids, conjunctiva, and cornea; intraocularly; and in nasal mucosa as well. Although the concept of the palpebral lobe of the lacrimal gland migrating into the nose in embryonic development is an intriguing one, suffice it to say, the presence of this tumor in its varied locations gives credence to the concept of cellular pluripotentiality.

A lacrimal gland choristoma is usually present at birth, but may not become clinically obvious until it grows larger with growth of the eye. This pinkish, richly vascularized mass is nearly always benign, but adenocarcinomas have been documented to arise from this tissue. Even a benign lesion can extend deeply into surrounding tissue, making excision difficult. These tumors are usually unilateral, but may be bilateral and may have more than a single focus in one eye. They tend to grow slowly and usually are asymptomatic. The patient may present with a well-vascularized mass, often temporal in location. A malignancy could be missed if it is assumed the lesion is a benign choristoma and not excised or biopsied.

HISTOLOGY. Histologically, lacrimal tissue is found accompanied by inflammatory infiltrate, presumably secondary to stasis of glandular secretions. This stasis can also give rise to cystic lesions. When limbal in location, as may be the case either with a simple lesion or as part of a dermoid, significant corneal stromal sclerosis can ensue because of this inflammation. Pathologic examination can confirm the presence of complex tissues, such as muscle, cartilage, adipose, and other tissues, in addition to the gland, which, as discussed previously, are found in complex choristomas, including dermoids. Electron microscopy reveals acinar elements with myoepithelial cells and zymogen granules confirming the glandular origin of this tumor.

EPIBULBAR FIBROMA. Epibulbar fibroma is a rare congenital rest of primitive mesoderm that develops into connective tissue elements. Described in the early days of ophthalmology by Von Graefe in 1854 in association with the plica and caruncle, and in forniceal conjunctiva by Elschnig in 1889, these tumors are known to occur on any conjunctival, corneal, or limbal surface. They can be orbital in location as well. Occasionally, fibromas are found in association with mixed tissue. As with other choristomas, fat, bone, cartilage, blood vessels, or myxomatous tissue can be found with the fibrous element. When a simple fibromatous choristoma is found, it may be a keloid, which will be discussed in another section of this chapter. Excision is the treatment for large, suspicious, or visually significant lesions.

EPIBULBAR OSTEOMA. Epibulbar osteoma, also called episcleral osseous choristoma, is a benign, slow-growing tumor of bone. Often, this tumor is found as a small, single, firm, white mass of mature bone on the surface of the sclera. The usual locations are either the upper temporal quadrant or over the lateral rectus muscle within Tenon's capsule. It may also grow at the limbus, although bony tissue in this location is nearly always associated with a limbal dermoid or complex choristoma. It may also be found in the orbit and paranasal sinuses, may be mobile or adherent, and ranges in size from microscopic to several centimeters.

Hematopoietic marrow within a bony choristoma has been documented,[75] but the usual histologic finding is of a rudimentary haversian system. A rare finding at birth, perhaps because of its small size and white color, it grows and becomes apparent with growth of the eye. It is believed that this tumor develops from congenital nests of pluripotent mesoderm and, like all choristomas, can be found with a variety of tissue elements. Theories of development include three possible etiologies: developmental, traumatic, or infectious.[76] Interestingly, bone in the scleral tissues is a normal finding in many fish, reptiles, amphibians, and birds. Although calcium deposits are a well-known finding in patients with hypercalcemia, hyperphosphatemia, hyperparathyroidism, and hypervitaminosis D, it is not commonly deposited in the sclera.

Scleral cartilage has been reported as well, notably in association with nevus sebaceous of Jadassohn. Chondro-osteomatous growths are usually found in conjunction with complex choristomas or adjacent colobomatous structures. Ectopic retina in a scleral tissue bed has also been described in a premature neonate with triploidy by Fulton et al.[77]

Choristomas are perhaps so fascinating because of the glimpse they afford us into embryonic development and cell potential. The evolutionary link they may represent between humans and other life forms is intriguing. The challenge that these tumors present to clinicians and pathologists alike is another reason that choristomas are compelling.

Epithelial Tumors. Squamous epithelial tumors and tumor-like lesions are seen on the limbal conjunctiva and cornea. They may be classified as benign, dysplastic, precancerous, or malignant. The mitotically active epithelial stem cells at the palisades of Vogt may predispose the area to neoplasia.[69] Although limbal lesions frequently extend onto cornea, they rarely invade deeper than Bowman's layer; however, aggressive lesions, trauma, or infection can lead to the extension of epithelial neoplasia into the corneal stroma and beyond.

BENIGN LESIONS. Benign epithelial growths include papillomas and keratoses.

INFECTIOUS PAPILLOMA. Squamous cell papillomas or infectious papillomas, as they are also called, are benign, self-limited epithelial lesions of children and young adults. Associated with conjunctivitis or follicular reaction, they are usually found in the inferior conjunctival fornix, but may be found in interpalpebral areas, including the limbus.

Papillomas are verrucous, often pedunculated fibrovascular lesions that may be pigmented in darker individuals. They are often grayish red, soft, and lobulated. Bilateral papillomas are not unusual and may be diffusely distributed. These lesions have a predilection for recurrence after excision unless great care is taken to avoid spread by contact. They may also present as a fine, diffuse epithelial keratitis.

Origin. These infectious tumors are of human papilloma viral origin, with clinical findings similar to those of papovavirus lesions of skin. Although different serotypes of the virus are said to be responsible for verrucae of different bodily regions, cases have been reported of genital condyloma accuminatum isolate found in conjunctiva.[78] Conjunctival papillomas have also been observed in siblings and in association with verrucae of skin, with presumed transmission by direct contact. Immunospecific antigens have been employed in the isolation of human papilloma virus (HPV) and molecular hybridization techniques used to specifically type the viral DNA.[79] Using in vitro gene amplification and polymerase chain reaction testing, HPV types 16 and 18 have been demonstrated in conjunctiva in a number of dysplastic squamous cell lesions.[80] Their role in pathogenesis is not completely defined, but there is an accepted association between these serotypes and cervical dysplasia.

Treatment. Like warts on the skin, conjunctival papillomas may spontaneously resolve with or without intervention. This phenomenon is famous in folklore, and some of the management is quite whimsical. Of course, the authors would never go on record as denying the value of dead cats, moonlight, or raw bacon, but they would not apply many of these "cures" to the eye. Unless circumstances such as tumor bulk, visual impairment, or irritation warrant it, it is often best simply to observe these lesions for spontaneous regression for up to 2 years. At that point, surgical excision or cryotherapy is not unreasonable, if desired. When excision is performed, it is always advisable to use caution to avoid spread of the lesion by seeding viral particles. Minimal handling and adjunctive cryotherapy to the site often bring a good result. Even so, these papillomas can recur. If the cornea is involved, a lesion may be peeled off the surface, or a lamellar keratectomy may be required.

Histology. These lesions are usually readily identified histologically by their characteristic branching fronds with a central vascularized core of connective tissue. A nongranulomatous inflammatory cell infiltrate is present. The surface is covered by stratified squamous epithelium that is acanthotic and nonkeratinized and contains goblet cells. Viral inclusions can be identified in some sections. Viral papillomas can be found in the larynx and trachea and can reach proportions large enough to cause obstructive airway disease. For this reason, when a patient is undergoing surgical excision under anesthesia, a thorough examination of the airway is indicated in cases in which an obstructed airway is suspected.

LIMBAL PAPILLOMA. Limbal papillomas, or verrucoid squamous papillomas, as they are called,

are found in an older population. These tumors are usually more sessile in appearance and tend to spread laterally. When near the cornea, they can spread to occlude the visual axis. Limbal papillomas differ from the infectious variety in that they are rarely multiple or bilateral. They are also more commonly dysplastic or frankly malignant. The etiology is not known to be viral in this form of papilloma. The distinction between viral and limbal papillomas was first pointed out in the medical literature by Contino in 1911.

Histology. The folds of tissue are covered by squamous epithelium with variable degrees of cellular pleomorphism ranging from mild to frankly dysplastic. Usually, the basal membranes remain intact; however, invasive lesions occur. There is usually moderate keratinization of these sessile masses when located in the limbal area, but hyperkeratosis can occur when found on the lid. Biopsy should be performed to differentiate this type of lesion from a carcinomatous one especially in the case of a suspicious or rapidly enlarging lesion.

Treatment. This type of papilloma is amenable to excision by stripping or lamellar keratoplasty in most cases. Tissue should be sent for pathologic evaluation for the reasons previously mentioned.

INVERTED PAPILLOMA. A third form of papilloma, the inverted papilloma, is commonly found in the nose or sinuses. It rarely presents in the lacrimal sac or on the conjunctiva.[81] As the name implies, this is an inversion of exophytic squamous proliferation downward into mucosa or subconjunctiva. It is also called endophytic papilloma for this reason. Up to 13% of nasal, sinus, or lacrimal sac lesions have been found to transform into transitional cell, squamous cell, or adenocarcinomatous neoplasia. Conjunctival masses are less aggressive and have not been found on the cornea or limbus.

Histology. Like keratoacanthoma, this lesion is a rapidly growing entity in nasal mucosa, but growth is more indolent in the eye. It is considered to be a variant of pseudoepitheliomatous hyperplasia by some. Acanthosis, parakeratosis, and squamous eddies may be found. Lobules of benign squamous epithelium are seen interspersed with mucin-filled cysts and goblet cells.

PSEUDOEPITHELIOMATOUS HYPERPLASIA. Also known as pseudocarcinomatous hyperplasia, this is a benign reactive epithelial conjunctival lesion of acanthotic, parakeratotic, and hyperkeratotic tissue. It is felt to arise secondary to irritation and inflammation, and may develop on preexisting pterygia or pingueculae. Because the interpalpebral areas of limbal and bulbar conjunctiva are frequent sites of carcinoma, and this is a lesion of hyperplastic epithelium, excisional biopsy may be performed. The lack of pleomorphism and the extensive dyskeratosis differentiate this benign lesion from a carcinomatous one.

These lesions arise over a period of weeks to months. Some possess central umbilication, making the clinical differentiation from keratoacanthoma difficult. Most pseudocarcinomatous hyperplasias develop at the limbus, whereas keratoacanthoma is often found at the lid margin.

Histology. This tissue often grows on the surface of pterygia or pingueculae. Piled-up masses of epithelium are found that push down into underlying substantia propria. A zone of lymphocytic infiltrate can be seen in the uninvolved adjacent tissue. This lesion in epithelium has a gradual transition from uninvolved to hyperplastic tissue, in contrast to carcinomatous intraepithelial neoplasia and SCCs, where abrupt transition is the rule. These tumors are not considered precursors of carcinoma.

HEREDITARY BENIGN INTRAEPITHELIAL DYSKERATOSIS. A rare, benign disorder of autosomal dominant inheritance, this epithelial lesion is found in an isolate of Caucasian, Native American, and African-American origins.[81,82] This group from North Carolina is known as the Haliwa Indians because they reside in Halifax and Washington counties.

Patients have bilateral, raised, granular-appearing, semitransparent plaques on the perilimbal tissue. The injected appearance is due to dilated blood vessels. They may be nasal or temporal, are horseshoe shaped, and are found in the interpalpebral fissures. The lesions can extend onto cornea and become visually significant due to corneal vascularization and opacification. Patients may present with a foreign-body sensation, photophobia, tearing, iritis, rubeosis irides, and loss of vision. Oral lesions with a white, spongy appearance are also seen on the buccal and labial oral mucosa and tongue.

Histology. The growths are characterized by epithelial hyperplasia, acanthosis, and keratinization of cells of the conjunctiva and oral mucous membranes. The conjunctival epithelium may be quite thick and keratinization prominent in individual cells, but the basal layer is intact. There is a chronic, nongranulomatous stromal inflammatory infiltrate. These lesions are truly benign despite some dysplastic characteristics, and they lack malignant potential.

CIN. CIN, which stands for *carcinomatous, conjunctival, or corneal intraepithelial neoplasia,* is a term designed to unite the complex system of multiple designations used in the past under an umbrella that describes epithelial dysplastic processes. It encompasses the precancerous lesions, squamous dysplasia, and carcinoma in situ. Under the classification of squamous dysplasia, one can place actinic keratosis and the now somewhat outdated term, leukoplakia. Leukoplakia is also a term once applied to pseudoepitheliomatous hyperplasia, the aforementioned benign reactive epithelial lesion. It really is a description of the effect that keratinization has on an epithelial tumor. As cited in Duke-Elder,[83] this was first described in 1849 by Bowman. The term simply means "white plaque." Best in 1899 called such lesions cornifications, Mohr and Schein in 1899 called them keratoses, Lister and Hancock in 1903 referred to them as plaques, Saemisch in 1904 labeled them callosities, and Cickanova in 1929 called them leukoplakia. Carcinoma in situ, once known as Bowen's disease, was first recognized as a precancerous lesion in skin by an American dermatologist, John T. Bowen (1857–1940). It was first described as an ophthalmologic entity in 1942 by McGavic.

CIN, whether conjunctival, limbal, or corneal, occurs most often in elderly, fair-skinned individuals in interpalpebral locations, validating the belief that ultraviolet exposure plays a role in the pathogenesis.[84] These are slow-growing, reddish, raised, gelatinous tumors that develop in areas of inflammation, chemical or environmental exposure, radiation, or spontaneously. The potential for carcinomatous transformation exists. They may be found overlying a pterygium or pinguecula and be clinically impossible to distinguish from pseudoepitheliomatous hyperplasia or SCC.

On the cornea, they may be mistaken for keratitis, dystrophic lesions, or scar. While most often located on conjunctiva or in limbal regions, reports document primary corneal carcinomatous intraepithelial neoplasia with no known limbal or conjunctival involvement.[85] Elevated white dots may be seen in some cases of corneal intraepithelial neoplasia,[86] making the diagnosis all but impossible without tissue studies. The tissue may be peeled intact from the stroma and submitted for pathologic study. Although recurrences are common, invasion beyond Bowman's layer is rare in corneal lesions.

HISTOLOGY. Loss of the ordinarily orderly progressive maturation of epithelium is the hallmark of CIN. Varying degrees of cellular atypia can be found. The changes range from mildly thickened, acanthotic epithelium to parakeratotic, hyperkeratotic, and frankly pleomorphic epithelium with atypia, including a high nuclear-to-cytoplasmic ratio and atypical mitoses. Increased vascularity and inflammatory reaction are typically seen. When these changes occur to less than full thickness of the epithelial layer, squamous dysplasia is diagnosed. When the full extent of the epithelium is involved up to, but not through, the basal layer, carcinoma in situ is the designation (Figure 5.41). If the dysplastic changes break through the basal layer into subepithelial substantia propria, SCC is the diagnosis. CIN therefore possesses metastatic malignant potential.[87] CIN appears to have a preference for areas of epithelial transition; therefore, it is frequently limbal in location. In the cornea, keratinization is a rare finding, but has been reported masquerading as a calcific scar.[88]

TREATMENT. Treatment is excision with histologic tissue studies to define the presence and degree of dysplasia. Corneal lesions may be defined with rose Bengal and debrided. Conjunctival resection may be done with cryotherapy to

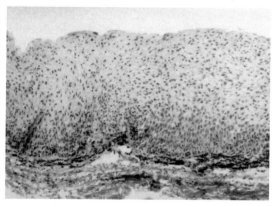

FIG. 5.41—Limbal carcinoma in situ. Note the marked thickening of the epithelium along with the underlying intact basement membrane. Hematoxylin-eosin, ×60.

margins and base. Although recurrences are common, CINs are slow-growing lesions and, unless malignancy ensues, prognosis is good, even with multiple recurrences. Even corneal clarity can be maintained in most cases, although a stromal haze may persist after debridement. There is seldom an indication for excision to involve corneal stroma, so scarring is minimized. The surgeon must excise normal-appearing tissue at times to obtain microscopic areas of dysplasia in order to minimize recurrences.[89] If the tumor is associated with pingueculae or pterygia, these should be removed as well. Following subtotal resection, many carcinomas in situ are known to regress, raising the possibility of a link with the clinical behavior of viral papillomas.[90] Nevertheless, observation is not the recommendation, and removal is still the treatment of choice.

Malignant Lesions. Epithelial malignancies of the conjunctiva, limbus, and cornea include SCC, spindle cell carcinoma, mucoepidermoid carcinoma, and sebaceous cell carcinoma.

SQUAMOUS CELL CARCINOMA. SCC, which is the most common of the epithelial malignancies of the eye, is usually found in the interpalpebral areas of perilimbus and presents a variable clinical appearance. The lesions may be exophytic, papillary, or leukoplakic or resemble pterygia or pingueculae. The well-differentiated lesions contain more keratin and therefore have a more leukoplakic appearance (Figure 5.42). The poorly differentiated lesions are a more rapidly growing neoplasm and have a translucent appearance. This is a tumor of older people in North America, but is found with increasing frequency and at younger ages in geographic areas with more sun exposure. Intraocular extension is rare and metastases even more uncommon. Once again, Bowman's membrane stands guard to prevent intracorneal extension in nearly all cases. Deep stromal invasion, intraocular spread, and regional lymph node extension are rare, but not unheard of. Vessels feed and grow into tumor tissue from adjacent conjunctiva, and fibrovascular pannus of the cornea can be seen at the edge of a limbal lesion. Sclera, likewise, seems to provide a barrier to intraocular invasion, but this can occur via emissary vessels.

Purely corneal SCCs are rare, and it is difficult to rule out a microscopic area of neoplasia at the limbus to explain the finding.[91] This parallels the situation with carcinoma in situ of the cornea. Daxecker et al.[85] reported a case they believed was a primary corneal carcinoma in 1989. This was an unexpected finding at pathologic examination of a corneal button from a penetrating keratoplasty performed for a presumed dystrophy. The graft failed and was removed. Stromal invasion was documented in the graft, and multiple limbal and conjunctival biopsies specimens were clean. This does not, of course, prove carcinoma was not there, but the case raises interesting questions about the etiology of malignant transformation.

HISTOLOGY. SCC is, by definition, an invasion of squamous dysplasia beyond the underlying basement membrane into subepithelial connective tissue stroma. Again, there is often an abrupt area of transition from the orderly arrangement of epithelial cell maturation to loss of organization and hyperplasia.

The hallmarks include acanthosis, parakeratosis, hyperkeratosis, mitotic figures, and cellular pleomorphism. There is a spectrum of cellular atypia from CIN to invasive carcinoma, as this malignancy is felt to arise from an in situ lesion. Papanicolaou-stained preparations may be helpful in establishing the diagnosis. If intraocular extension has occurred, a paracentesis specimen

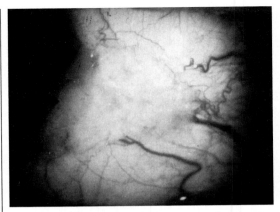

FIG. 5.42—External photograph of a squamous cell carcinoma. Note the gelatinous appearance with invasion of limbal cornea.

may be obtained for diagnosis. Otherwise, biopsy of affected tissue is performed.

TREATMENT. Treatment is wide local excision, including scleral lamellar resection or penetrating keratoplasty, if needed. Cryotherapy to the margins and base of limbal lesions is recommended. If the neoplasm is extensive, enucleation and even orbital exenteration may be lifesaving. As this is a slow-growing and visible tumor, this is rarely needed, and prognosis is good even if it recurs. Sometimes repeated excisions are required. Limbal autograft reconstruction has been successfully performed in two patients with extensive limbal and corneal SCC by Copeland and Char[92] as reported in 1990. Careful follow-up is mandatory in these patients, as it is in patients with CIN, because of the possibility of recurrence and invasion.

SPINDLE CELL CARCINOMA. Spindle cell carcinoma is a variant of SCC in which the cells of the tumor are spindle shaped and appear similar to fibroblasts. They are found in the cornea and limbal conjunctiva, and have also been found growing on skin and other mucous membranes of the body. In conjunctiva, these tumors behave aggressively with invasive capability and the tendency for recurrence after surgical excision. In a report of eight cases by Ni and Guo,[93] four tumors arose from sites of previous corneal ulcers. The meaning of this finding is unclear, but it makes one speculate as to the stimulus the injury may have provided for malignant transformation.

HISTOLOGY. These lesions may be confused pathologically with fibrosarcoma and have been called pseudosarcoma. They are, however superficial in location, and transition from squamous cell to malignant spindle cell has been documented. Histologic characteristics include pleomorphism and hyperchromatism of spindle-shaped cells.

Electron-micrographic studies reveal cells of epithelial origin, with desmosomes and tonofibril elements. Immunohistochemical staining is positive, with antikeratin antibodies providing further evidence of epithelial cell origin. Ni and Guo have classified these tumors into three categories—fibrosarcomatous, fibrohistiocytomatous, and rhabdomyosarcomatous—based on the histologic similarities with fibrosarcoma, histiocytoma, and rhabdomyosarcoma, respectively.[93]

MUCOEPIDERMOID CARCINOMA. Mucoepidermoid carcinoma is an aggressive, mucus-secreting malignancy of epithelial cell origin. Depending on the content of the tumor, it may exhibit more squamous cell characteristics or secretory behavior. This type of tumor is rare. It is usually found in the elderly in a limbal location, although lesions of the cul-de-sac are also found. In some cases, there has been documentation of transformation of an initially epidermal-type tumor to a predominantly mucin-secreting one, raising the question of environmental influence on tissue differentiation.

HISTOLOGY. Mucoepidermoid carcinoma is made up of varying proportions of squamous cells, mucin-secreting cells, and basal cells. The mucinous material stains with mucicarmine, Alcian blue, and colloidal iron. It contains acid mucopolysaccharide resistant to hyaluronidase digestion and may be found in a cystic structure with epithelial lining. These tumors are more likely than SCCs to invade the substantia propria, globe, and orbit and to metastasize. It is therefore important to obtain material for pathologic diagnosis. These tumors can be classified as high-grade or low-grade malignancies. Low-grade tumors contain a large number of mucin-producing cells and variable epidermoid elements.

High-grade lesions are dominated by epidermoid cells. Immunohistochemical stains are used to identify squamous and mucoid differentiation.

TREATMENT. Treatment of choice is wide local excision with cryotreatment to the margins and base. If the tumor is extensive, enucleation or exenteration is required.

SEBACEOUS CELL CARCINOMA. Also known as intraepithelial sebaceous epithelioma, this is not a tumor of cornea, limbus, or sclera, but deserves mention because of its tendency to spread into these regions. This tumor originates from sebaceous glands (meibomian or of Zeiss) or caruncle and spreads in a pagetoid manner into glandular ducts and across epithelium. Usually a tumor of older patients, it may present as a lid or conjunctival nodule, diffuse epithelial thickening, lid deformity, lash loss, chronic conjunctivitis, blepharoconjunctivitis, or keratoconjunctivitis with discharge.

This is therefore a formidable lesion, as it can appear in the form of routine ophthalmologic problems[94] and be overlooked. The incidence of spread is between 1.3% and 21.4%. The mortality rate is approximately 15% in a modern setting. Treatment of choice is surgical excision under frozen-section control. Multiple biopsies may be required to define the full extent of the lesion.

Melanogenic Tumors. In this section, melanocytic tumors and pigmentary changes that may give rise to, or be confused with, tumors are discussed. The limbus and epibulbar surfaces harbor many melanin-producing cells that give rise to a variety of pigmented and nonpigmented lesions. Melanocytes were described by Unna in 1893 as normal basal cells that convert into melanocytes. Neurogenic origin was proposed by Masson in 1926, who held these cells to be a Schwann's cell derivative. Currently, melanocytes are considered to be of neural crest origin. They are seen on hematoxylin-eosin stain as dendritic cells with delicate branching processes. The cells vary even in nonneoplastic tissue in size, number, and melanin content. Melanocytes are incontinent of their product and discharge melanin to surrounding tissue, where it is engulfed by histiocytes, fibroblasts, and epithelial cells.

CONGENITAL MELANOSIS. Melanosis, by definition, is an excess of melanin. Congenital melanosis of the epithelium, also known as benign epithelial melanosis, is the presence of melanin in the epithelium from birth or shortly thereafter. Seen more often in darker individuals, the pigment is located in the basal layers of epithelium. It appears as brown or black plaques and is not associated with atypia or malignant transformation. It may be considered a sort of ephelis or "freckle,"[95] the ubiquitous pigmented skin lesion of childhood and Norman Rockwell paintings. The melanin is located in basal keratinocytes, where the number of melanocytes and the melanin content within them are basically normal. The melanocytes may be slightly enlarged, but there are no atypical cells. Congenital melanosis may also be located deeper, in subepithelial, episcleral, or scleral tissues.

MELANOSIS OCULI AND NEVUS OF OTA. Melanosis oculi, also called ocular melanocytosis, is an increase in the number and size of melanocytes in subepithelial layers. This type of congenital melanosis is found in uveal tissue, sclera, and episclera. It is usually recognized as clinically obvious pigmentation on the globe, but may present as iris heterochromia. When found in association with ipsilateral pigment deposition in periocular skin, it is termed oculodermal melanocytosis or nevus of Ota. These subepithelial congenital melanoses are usually unilateral, but, when bilateral, are asymmetric. The lesions appear blue-gray on sclera and skin, attesting to their deeper location than the brown-black epithelial melanosis.

Nevus of Ota is found in all races, although it is more frequent in Asians and darker races than in Caucasians. Caucasians, on the other hand, are more predisposed to the purely ocular form of melanosis oculi. Both melanosis oculi and nevus of Ota have been associated with malignant transformation, although rarely.

ACQUIRED MELANOSIS. Acquired melanotic pigmentation of epithelium is common and found in the limbal and perilimbal areas of dark-skinned individuals. It is also termed *racial melanosis*. Acquired melanosis is also attributable to numerous toxic and metabolic factors.

Chemicals such as epinephrine, arsenic, and thorazine, to name a few, are capable of causing pigment deposition. Chronic conjunctival disorders such as trachoma and vernal conjunctivitis, and metabolic disorders such as alcaptonuria and vitamin A deficiency, can also do this. This kind of acquired melanosis does not predispose individuals to melanoma, but is occasionally confused with malignancy. This condition is simply the result of excess melanin production leading to its dispersal into substantia propria. Here, melanophages engulf the particles, becoming pigment laden. Because this is nearly always a bilateral finding, unilateral, spontaneous, acquired melanosis should be closely observed for atypical changes.

Melanosis can also be acquired secondary to any lesion that causes the surface of the globe to become irregular or inflamed. A scar, cyst, foreign body, or nerve loop may induce melanization by stimulating dormant melanocytes into action. First described by Axenfeld in 1902, Axenfeld's loops are a frequent cause for concern. They appear as nodular pigmented lesions deep to the conjunctiva. Although benign, epithelial melanosis along an intrascleral nerve loop is in the differential diagnosis of malignant melanoma. This may also provide a route of extension of melanoma or other intraocular neoplasms or infections to the surface of the globe. These lesions are therefore worthy of a careful slit-lamp examination. They vary in size from 4 to 7 mm and are found more often in dark-skinned people. They are usually nodular but may be cystic and are occasionally nonpigmented. Located between the rectus muscle insertions, these are extensions of the long posterior ciliary nerves looping out through the sclera in the area of the ciliary body. There is no potential for malignant transformation in these lesions, but their importance lies in their ability to cloud the diagnosis. It may be clinically difficult to distinguish them from melanoma, neurofibroma, or foreign body, and occasionally excision must be performed for histologic diagnosis.

Epithelial tumors such as SCC, papilloma, mucoepidermoid carcinoma, and actinic keratosis can acquire melanin pigment, making the distinction from melanoma difficult. Corneal epithelium can also acquire pigment from various toxic and inflammatory influences, and limbal epithelium can migrate onto the surface, leading to corneal pigmentation from melanin.

PRIMARY ACQUIRED MELANOSIS. Primary acquired melanosis (PAM) is a unilateral, idiopathic melanin deposition into conjunctival epithelium. It begins in the middle years with a faint stippling. Any conjunctival surface may be involved, including limbus. The cornea may become involved by extension from limbal tissue. This pigmentation can wax and wane, but gradual progressive pigment accumulation is the rule. This is a lesion with malignant potential. Up to 17% of these may undergo malignant transformation. The development of a nodular area, thickened plaque, or tumor must be investigated for malignant melanoma, even though in many cases inflammation is responsible. Biopsy should be performed to distinguish melanophages from epithelioid cells of melanoma.

A useful classification proposed by William Spencer and others[76] attempts to organize primary acquired melanoses into clinicopathologic categories for diagnostic and prognostic purposes. Although it refers to conjunctival lesions, it will be discussed with regard to limbal, conjunctival, corneal, and scleral extensions.

In *Stage IA,* there is pigment accumulation in normal tissue. There may be an increase in the number and size of melanocytes, and scattered nevoid cells may be found. Malignant potential is minimal.

In *Stage IB,* the pigmentation is accompanied by atypical melanocytic hyperplasia with large melanocytes in a palisade arrangement along the basal layer. There are also prominent foci of melanocytes at various levels of the epithelium. The nuclei are large, and there may be mitotic figures. There is, however, no invasion beyond the basal layer and, for this reason, a Stage IB lesion is considered benign.

Two features are useful in predicting malignant potential: the arrangement of the epithelium and the presence of epithelioid cells.[96] When the atypical melanocytes are found in nests or throughout the epithelium, the risk of melanoma is higher than if these cells are confined to the basal layer. Likewise, the presence of epithelioid cells carries a greater risk of melanoma. Therefore, biopsying

a PAM lesion is reasonable and excision of a Stage IB lesion prudent.

Stage II is malignant. Malignant melanoma has arisen from existing benign primary acquired melanosis with invasion beyond the basal lamina and atypical melanocytes. The cells are more heterogeneous and less cohesive. There is more nuclear material, and more mitotic figures are seen. Normal tissue architecture is compromised.

Stage IIA is malignant acquired melanosis that is superficially invasive. It refers to lesions less or equal to 1.5 mm thick.

Stage IIB is a more deeply invasive tumor greater than 1.5 mm thick. Although this is considered the most malignant category, it must be pointed out that even a thin, spreading tumor has lethal potential in the conjunctiva because of the rich lymphatics in this tissue.

Malignant acquired melanoses most likely to spread are those with pagetoid spread, scleral invasion, or recurrence after excision. Unusual nonpigmented amelanotic acquired melanoses exist in which diffuse, atypical, hyperplastic melanocytes are seen without melanin production. The area involved may advance subclinically to an advanced stage until biopsy reveals the diagnosis. There is an association of PAM and melanoma with nevi, although the presence of a nevus in the area of PAM does not appear to increase the risk of malignancy. Although inflammatory cells in the stroma are a frequent finding with PAM, the greater the degree, the greater the risk of malignancy. Increased vascularity may also lead diagnosticians to be suspicious of a high-risk lesion.

Treatment. In many cases, observation and photographic documentation are adequate. If change occurs or the lesion is large, deep, recurrent, or atypical, biopsy should be performed. Increased vascularity or rapid growth is also an indication for tissue studies. Specimens should be taken from multiple biopsy sites and, if the diagnosis of malignancy is established, wide excision with cryotherapy to the base and margins performed. All areas of atypia should be excised. Wood's lamp may help detect subtle areas of early pigmentation. If there is invasion beyond the margins, enucleation, exenteration, and radiation therapy may be necessary.

NEVUS. Nevi, from *noevus,* Latin for a "mark," of conjunctiva are included in this discussion because of their occasional appearance at the limbus and cornea, and because of their relationship to malignant melanoma. These are benign lesions of polyhedral cell nests, 50% of which appear in childhood and 75% of which are present by age 30. In older individuals, nevi may involute and disappear. These benign, hamartomatous, ocular lesions are classified like those of skin.

Junctional nevi or intraepithelial nevi are located in basal epithelium at the junction of epithelium and subepithelium and have the potential to invade deeper, becoming malignant. These are found in the first two decades of life. This may therefore be considered a juvenile stage of nevus development. These tend to be flat and diffuse, rather than nodular, as they are, by definition, confined to the epithelium unless undergoing invasive change. Cords and nests of nevus cells may reach up to the surface. The cells can be large and hard to distinguish from malignant melanoma cells.

Subepithelial nevi or dermal nevi, as they are called in skin, are very common lesions in conjunctiva that lie in the subepithelial tissue and involute with age. These do not undergo malignant transformation. Compound nevi are also called intraepithelial/subepithelial nevi, designating their location. This form, also common in conjunctiva, may appear cystic due to epithelial inclusions and possess qualities of both junctional and dermal nevi. Nests of conjunctival epithelium may be found as cystic structures lined with epithelium and mucus-secreting goblet cells in subepithelial or compound nevi. Cysts are found in half of all compound nevi and in many other types of nevi as well. These cysts may transilluminate, aiding in the clinical distinction of nevi from malignant melanomas, which do not. They may be considered a special form of complex choristoma. Subepithelial and compound nevi therefore may be cystic, nodular, or diffuse in form. The cells are large and may undergo a maturation in which they take on a neural appearance.

Spindle cell nevi, also called epithelioid nevi, juvenile melanoma, or Spitz nevi, are characterized by intra- or subepithelial nests of spindle-shaped cells. Rarely, epithelioid cells appear that often look like multinucleated giant cells. This type of nevus is found in children and has a benign course.

Blue nevi arise from congenital nests of melanocytes deep in dermis or substantia propria of conjunctiva. They appear blue because of their depth in tissue, but are freely mobile in tissue over the globe. Histopathologically, they are composed of spindle-shaped or dendritic cells in episclera. Malignant change has not been seen. Cellular blue nevi are actually brown-black and are also deep due to arrest of neural crest migration toward the surface epithelium. Other than their color, they are similar to blue nevi. In patients with nevus of Ota, episcleral pigmented lesions within areas of the melanosis are equivalent to cellular blue nevus.

There must always be a term for those lesions that defy categorization, and this is the combined nevus, a mixture of intraepithelial, subepithelial (therefore compound), blue, and cellular blue nevi.

A number of factors can predispose nevi to change. Growth of epithelial inclusions, inflammation, involution, or malignant transformation are all changes that nevi can undergo. Nevi have variable pigmentation from lesion to lesion and within a single nevus during its existence. They range from amelanotic to pink, yellow, brown, or black, depending on the amount of melanin the cells possess. Seventy percent are considered "fully melanized" and are dark.

Conjunctival nevi often occur at the limbus, but can appear almost anywhere, including plica, caruncle, fornix, lid margin, and bulbar and palpebral conjunctiva. Whether they can occur primarily on cornea is controversial.[97] Nests of nevus cells have been documented in corneal stroma with normal overlying epithelium and normal endothelium, but this is with adjacent limbal involvement. Some cases reported in the older literature do not stand up to scrutiny and are probably acquired melanosis.

Treatment. Although nevi do not often transform into melanomas, a quarter of all melanomas are said to arise from nevi. The standard of care demands observation with photographic documentation and careful measurements. Biopsy with excision for suspicious lesions is indicated.

However, because a benign nevus can also increase in size, growth is not always a malignant sign, especially in a cystic nevus. These lesions stem from melanocytes and, as such, stain for S-100 protein.

MALIGNANT MELANOMA. This malignancy is a much more common finding in uveal tissue than on conjunctiva, sclera, or cornea, at least primarily. Ocular tumors comprise 30%–79% of non-cutaneous melanomas, and only 2% of these are conjunctival. Melanomas account for 70% of all eye malignancies, with an incidence eight times greater in Caucasians than in blacks, and in blacks eight times greater than in Asians. The first limbal-corneal melanoma was documented in 1892 by Sgosso, and since then many cases have been described. Malignant melanoma may arise de novo, from a nevus, or from primary acquired melanosis. The de novo lesion is sometimes referred to as "nodular" for its tendency toward a vertical growth pattern without radial spread. Many de novo lesions, however, are not nodular, and many melanomas from preexisting pigmented lesions are. In general, it may be said that melanoma can appear in many forms, including nodular, diffuse, fungating, and ulcerative (Figure 5.43). Approximately 50% of primary malignant melanomas are said to arise de novo and 50% from PAM or nevi.

The behavior of conjunctival melanomas is variable, but metastatic disease is potentially deadly regardless of site of origin. Although uveal melanomas do not generally metastasize to regional lymphatics, conjunctival melanomas do. The most common routes include preauricular, intraparotid, submandibular, and cervical lymph nodes. Once into lymphatic channels, hematogenous spread is possible. Scleral involvement in melanomas is variable. It can be as a consequence of spread from overlying conjunctival or adjacent limbal structures or, more commonly, via uveal extension. The emissarial route may provide an early pathway to the external globe. A mucoid-type swelling of sclera overlying choroidal melanomas has been reported.[95] Hyaluronidase-resistant deposits of acid mucopolysaccharides have been found between scleral lamellae. Recurrence of conjunctival melanomas is a consequence of several things. It may be that the excision of a lesion was incomplete, or it may be a new primary occurrence. Melanomas are also well known for their satellite lesions, a form of local metastasis also common in cutaneous lesions. There may also be seeding of tumor cells during surgery. Corneal melanomas, like those of sclera, are not uncommonly the result of extension from intraocular structures.[98] Both iris and ciliary body lesions can break through the anterior chamber, and of course spread from the adjacent limbal tissues onto corneal epithelium is an even more common route.

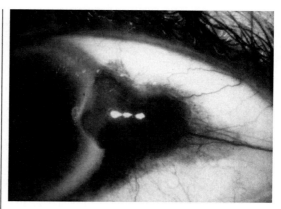

FIG. 5.43—External photograph of a limbal based, pigmented melanoma. Note that the tumor is extending onto and within the temporal cornea.

Histology. The amelanotic melanomas provide a special diagnostic challenge. Histologic stains that aid in the diagnosis include Fontana, Warthin-Starry, and immunoperoxidase stain for S-100 protein. Cytologic classifications are very important for prognostication of uveal melanomas, and therefore the Callender classification[99] system is employed for these tumors. The Armed Forces Institute of Pathology classification builds on the Callender classification.[100] Basically, they define the cell types, carefully differentiating between spindle cell and epithelioid cell content. Because this is not the system employed for conjunctival lesions, the author will forgo detailed discussion of the cell features. The conjunctival, limbal, and corneal primary melanomas are treated histologically like cutaneous lesions. The cell pattern is pleomorphic with epithelioid cells arranged in loose clumps.

Features to consider include the number of mitotic figures, melanin and reticulin content, regressive changes including necrosis, and invasion. Epithelioid cells are large plump cells, often multinucleated with hyperchromatism and prominent nucleoli. Large spaces between cells can be observed, as their cohesion is abnormal. The mitotic figures are more abundant in a more malignant lesion, but the prognostic value of melanin content is not clear (Figure 5.44). The better differentiated the cell, the more its ability to form normal cell products, so poorly differentiated epithelioid cells form little reticulin.

Necrosis is a common finding as the tumor outgrows its blood supply. There is often lymphocytic infiltrate in these areas, and cytotoxic antibodies have been demonstrated in patients with uveal melanomas. The fact that the incidence of these malignancies is greater in immunocompromised patients also lends credence to the concept of immune phenomena playing a role in their pathogenesis.

Treatment. The earliest treatment for melanoma was simple excision, which involved predictably frequent recurrences. In the 20th century, more aggressive management began with wide excision, enucleation, and exenteration as standard of care. The latter half of the century brought radiation therapy and chemotherapy into the armamentarium. The first line of treatment is removal, be it stripping a mass from the cornea, keratectomy, keratoplasty, or conjunctival or scleral resection with cryotherapy or patch graft. Unfortunately, exenteration for primary conjunctival disease is sometimes necessary.

It should also be pointed out that a scleral tumor is almost invariably a secondary extension, and, as this is a poor prognostic sign, these eyes are almost always removed. Corneal melanoma that has arisen via an extension from primary iris or ciliary body malignancies that have broken through the anterior chamber structures also carries a poorer prognosis.

Brachytherapy is sometimes used, and the Collaborative Ocular Melanoma Study is conducting clinical trials to assess the effectiveness of radiation versus enucleation for uveal melanomas. Perhaps their findings will be extrapolated to corneal and conjunctival lesions. Metastasis at the

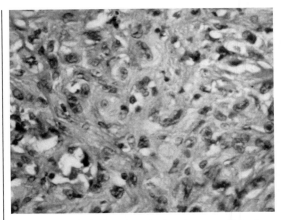

FIG. 5.44—Limbal conjunctival melanoma. Note the marked nuclear pleomorphism and prominent nucleoli. Hematoxylin-eosin, ×100.

time of diagnosis of an ocular melanoma is a finding in 2% of all cases, and this worsens the prognosis significantly. It is treated with palliative resection, radiation, and chemotherapy. It is said that de novo lesions carry a worse prognosis, with a mortality rate of 40% as compared with those tumors that arise from nevi or PAM, which have a mortality rate of 20%.

MELANOCYTOMA. Melanocytoma is a benign, melanocytic lesion famous for its jet-black appearance on the optic nerve and peripapillary structures. It has also been reported on sclera and episclera,[101] where its appearance is more blue than black, and it may be considered a special form of nevus. It is composed of normal dendritic melanocytes that are polyhedral, large, and packed with melanin. Their main importance is their frequent misdiagnosis as melanoma.

Lymphomatous Tumors. The conjunctiva is rich in lymphoid tissue; therefore, the limbus and cornea may be involved by extension in lymphomatous disease, including neoplasia. It is well known that the lacrimal gland, uvea, and adnexae of the eye are involved in lymphomatous tumors, but limbal findings are less well recognized. Lymphoid tissue, whether reactive proliferation or frank neoplasm, can be found at the limbus, assuming its contour as a single or multiple nontender, uniform, elevated mass of salmon color.

The border and overlying conjunctiva are smooth. Between 15% and 20% are bilateral. The tumors may be primary to the eye or as part of a systemic process. These lesions are often insidious in their growth pattern, but are important to recognize, as they may be the first clue to a treatable systemic disease.

The spectrum is broad. It ranges from non-neoplastic pseudotumors to malignancies, with gradations in between. They may be T or B cell predominant, polyclonal benign lesions, or mono-clonal malignant lymphomas. Whereas poly-clonal tumors and well-differentiated B-cell tumors carry a good prognosis, the risk of sys-temic disease and a poorer prognosis exist for monoclonal and poorly differentiated B-cell tumors. In either case, the growth is usually slow and survival long.

The most important characteristic of benign lymphoid hyperplasia is its cellular pleomor-phism. A mixed-cell infiltrate with lymphocytes, reticulum cells, eosinophils, polymorphonuclear neutrophils, plasma cells, and macrophages car-ries the benign diagnosis of reactive lymphoid hyperplasia. This is usually successfully treated with systemic steroids, and a dramatic response is the rule. Some additional histologic features include plasmacytoid cells, Russell bodies, and Dutcher bodies. If steroids fail to resolve the hyperplasia (which can be marked in orbital lesions), radiation is sometimes used in low doses.

The zone between benign and malignant lesions has cellular pleomorphism and atypia of malignancy with polymorphism of a benign entity. A systemic workup is performed to exclude systemic malignancy in this case, and the prognosis is not clear-cut.

Malignant lymphoma may be of the non-Hodgkin's or Hodgkin's variety. The latter is characterized by the presence of Reed-Sternberg cells, anaplastic, binucleate histiocytes. More commonly a malignancy of orbit, Hodgkin's dis-ease has been known to infiltrate limbus, cornea, and sclera. The cellular infiltrate is anaplastic and poorly differentiated. This is usually found in the eye in late systemic disease, and the workup includes radiology as well as bone marrow biopsy and ultrasound of liver and spleen. Serum studies are also performed.

TREATMENT. A localized conjunctival, limbal, or corneal lesion can be excised. For systemic involvement, radiation therapy is the treatment of choice.

LEUKEMIA. Leukemia is a hematogenous form of malignant lymphoma in which the malignant cells are released to circulation from bone mar-row. It is not considered a finding of conjunctiva, cornea, or sclera, except as manifested by hemor-rhages and inflammatory changes. A nodular myelogenous leukemic infiltrate has been described on sclera with the appearance of brawny scleritis or scleromalacia perforans. Meller in 1906 described a case of bilateral lym-phatic "leucoemia" of conjunctiva and all four lids presenting as a red, brawny, bloodless growth. He also described an eye with similar findings at the limbus, accompanied by corneal infiltrate and vascularization. Rollet in 1904 described brawny infiltrative nodules at the lim-bus histologically consistent with myelogenous leukemia. How these tumors would be classified today is not known, but, when nodular growth appears on the eye with atypical lymphocytosis, we tend to call it lymphoma.

MULTIPLE MYELOMA. This is a disorder of pro-liferation of plasma cells, with the production of homogeneous serum protein. This protein can then deposit onto many surfaces, including cornea, conjunctiva, and sclera. The systemic dis-ease may present with decreased visual acuity and corneal opacification. Multiple myeloma of the cornea was first documented in 1958 by Burki[102] in *Ophthalmologica.* Ocular findings also include orbital, scleral, and optic nerve dep-ositions,[103] crystalline deposits in conjunctiva and cornea,[104] and all the consequences of sludging of blood flow in the eye. The hyperviscosity is sec-ondary to massive production of immunoglobulin or a subunit of immunoglobulin, usually immu-noglobulin G (IgG). IgA and IgM proteins are also found. These are usually polyvalent light chains of the kappa type.

In cornea, an important site of involvement, bilateral deposits may appear as gray or yellow, with a punctate or linear shape.[103] They may be crystalline in appearance and are found at various depths of corneal tissue. The cornea may take on a fine stippled appearance. The epithelium and stroma are typically involved with sparing of limbus. Slit-lamp diagnosis of multiple myeloma affords the opportunity for the ophthalmologist to diagnose a potentially treatable systemic disease, although it is not straightforward. Interestingly, IgG gamma paraproteins have been found in tears.

A Kayser-Fleischer ring, a gold-green cuprous deposition in Descemet's membrane seen in Wilson's disease and other hepatic diseases, can also be seen in IgG monoclonal gammopathy. Kayser in 1902 noted a pigmented corneal deposition in association with "disseminated sclerosis," and Fleisher in 1903 associated this with "pseudo-sclerosis," which we now term hepatolenticular degeneration or Wilson's disease.

HISTOLOGY. Due to the variable manner of deposition, clinical recognition of ocular multiple myeloma can be difficult. It is occasionally a surprise finding in the examination of a corneal transplant button. By light microscope, non-birefringent crystals of varying lengths up to 32.5 μm and widths up to 7.5 μm can be seen. The corneal epithelium may appear elevated by an eosinophilic amorphous material. Deposits are found in and between cells and stain positive for periodic acid-Schiff (PAS) and red with Masson's trichrome. Electron-microscopic studies reveal an irregular to hexagonally shaped crystal in the epithelial cell cytoplasm. These deposits stain with immunohistochemical techniques for immunoglobulin as previously described.

TREATMENT. Treatment of the systemic disease may decrease the deposits, but visual acuity may remain unsatisfactory. In that case, penetrating keratoplasty may be required. Systemic treatment involves chemotherapy, and survival is variable. The finding of unusual corneal deposits may warrant a limited workup to rule out multiple myeloma. This might include a complete blood count and serum protein electrophoresis, and, if these raise suspicion, a bone marrow study is diagnostic in most cases. If protein remains in serum, redeposition in cornea and other ocular tissues can occur.

Fibrocytic Tumors

FIBROUS HISTIOCYTOMA. Also called fibroxanthoma, this heterogeneous group of tumors composed of fibrocytes and histiocytes is found in corneal, scleral, and conjunctival tissue. The cells are derived from primitive mesenchyme. The tissue has a broad range of histologic findings, ranging from a predominantly fibrous to predominantly cellular tissue. Often presenting as a yellow-white mass, these tumors may be locally invasive and recurrent, and may possess metastatic potential. Some consider them to be a reactive process and completely benign. One classification scheme places these tumors into three groups: benign, locally aggressive, and malignant, based on histopathologic criteria.

These tumors may be found anywhere in the orbit, cutaneous or subcutaneous tissue, sclera, or episclera. They are also found on conjunctiva and limbus, with or without corneal extension. They are the most common type of mesenchymal orbital tumor in adults[105] and, in fact, are the most common soft tissue tumor in adults overall. On the whole, they are a rare finding on conjunctiva, cornea, or sclera. In a series of 14 patients with corneal, scleral, and limbal fibrous histiocytomas by Lahoud et al.,[106] the median age was 24 years, with a range of 3–74. Male patients equaled female in number, and the median duration of symptoms was 9 months.

HISTOLOGY. The usual pattern is a storiform arrangement of fibroblasts with collagen and lipid-laden histiocytes interspersed. Multinucleated giant cells can also be found. Actually, variable histologic patterns are described, including myxoid, inflammatory, angiomatoid, pleomorphic, xanthomatous, and xanthogranulomatous. The malignant cases contain more anaplastic cells with large hyperchromatic and pleomorphic nuclei and atypical mitoses. Immunohistochemistry for lysozyme may be performed. Lysozyme is a histiocytic marker. This tumor is positive for α-antitrypsin, α-antichymotrypsin, and lysozyme, and is negative for keratin (a marker for carcinoma), desmin (a marker for leiomyosarcoma), and S-100 protein (a marker for melanoma and schwannoma). Thus, it is considered a separate entity from those previously mentioned.

TREATMENT. Simple excision with adjunct cryotherapy to the base and margins or radiation therapy may be performed for conjunctival lesions. Keratectomy, sclerectomy, or sclerokeratectomy may be performed for limbal, corneal, or scleral tumors. If malignancy is diagnosed, enucleation has been performed, as has exenteration. Recurrences are more frequent with the more malignant tumors. Since there are few reported cases of corneal, limbal, conjunctival, or scleral fibrous histiocytomas, it is difficult to make an accurate prognosis. They appear to be more benign in these locations than the orbital variety. Recognition is often earlier in anterior locations, and this improves the prognosis.

FIBROSARCOMA. On the spectrum of tumors stemming from fibrocytic cells, which broadly includes not only fibrous histiocytoma but also keloid, choristoma, fibroxanthoma, and granuloma, one can place fibrosarcoma of sclera. Primary fibrosarcomas of the eye are very rare tumors of mesenchymal cell origin and have not been described on limbus or cornea. Fibrosarcoma of sclera was described by Von Heydenreich[107] in 1964, but is also quite rare. The orbit is the most common site, but, in the past, tuberculoma, lymphoma, and syphilitic nodules have been mistakenly diagnosed as this tumor in the orbit. This is a very aggressive neoplasm and potentially lethal; therefore, when diagnosed, exenteration is often necessary.

CORNEAL MYXOMA. A rare primary subepithelial corneal mass of spindle-shaped cells in a collagenous ground substance was reported by Lo et al.[108] in 1990. A 44-year-old woman presented with a slow-growing gelatinous mass without antecedent ocular history or significant systemic abnormalities. The grayish, avascular, subepithelial mass measured 8×4 mm and was peeled from underlying tissue easily. Histology revealed intact epithelium, absent Bowman's membrane, and a mass of myxomatous tissue in a fibrillar matrix. It was Alcian blue positive only at pH 2.5 and sensitive to hyaluronidase digestion, and therefore composed of gycosaminoglycans. Masson trichrome stained the fibrillar collagenous tissue, whereas Congo red, Wilder reticulin, and mucicarmine stains were negative.

Electron-microscopic studies showed fusiform cells with elongated cytoplasmic processes. Nuclei were also elongated and possessed small nucleoli. The matrix contained collagen with a periodicity of 50–60 nm and a random orientation. Only two prior cases have been described, by Mitvalsky in 1984 and one by Bussy in 1925.

Myxomas are found in the heart, subcutaneous tissue, muscle, sinuses, neurovascular tissue, conjunctiva, orbit, and lid, but corneal myxomas are exceedingly rare. Their origin is uncertain; they probably arise from pluripotential mesenchymal nests, but may be from mature, though abnormal, fibroblasts. In the case of corneal myxomas, keratocytes might be the cell of origin.

TREATMENT. Local excision is sufficient. When a tumor is this rare, it is difficult to predict the prognosis accurately, but this is generally a growth with a benign outcome. The tumors are slow growing, painless, and do not metastasize. However, they have been known to recur.

Histiocytic Tumors

JUVENILE XANTHOGRANULOMA. Also called nevoxanthoendothelioma, this tumor is neither nevoid nor endothelial. It is a benign, idiopathic, inflammatory skin disease of children with dermatologic and ocular findings. This is found in all races, male and female equally, and is not hereditary. It is present at birth in 30%, but, if not, becomes apparent early in life and is only rarely diagnosed in an adult.[70] Skin and visceral lesions undergo spontaneous regression and disappear in 3–6 years. Most patients have self-limited skin lesions as the only manifestation. These are few to multiple in number, commonly on the upper body and of variable appearance. They may be flat, elevated, round, or oval, 1 to 20 mm in diameter, and grow before regressing to leave an occasional atrophic scar.[109]

Classic ocular findings include infiltration of iris and ciliary body with histiocytic masses with or without skin findings. Patients may present with iris heterochromia,[110] a red eye, a mass, or a spontaneous hyphema. Corneal clouding due to secondary glaucoma can also occur. The tumors can be single or multiple discrete masses, or a diffuse iris thickening can be seen. On or near the cornea, a yellowish or pink, epibulbar, phlyctenular-type growth, may be found. Ocular sites include iris, and ciliary body (common); cornea, extraocular muscles, conjunctiva, lids, and orbit (rare); and optic nerve, disc, and choroid (very rare).

Noncutaneous sites of involvement include lungs, pericardium, muscle, viscera, gonads, and bone. Obviously, the site determines the effect of the lesion on the patient, and clearly this disease is not always benign in its behavior.

HISTOLOGY. This granulomatous inflammatory disorder can be diagnosed by biopsy of a mass or, if in the classic location, Papanicolaou stain of aqueous fluid. Eosinophils and other inflammatory cells are seen along with the famous Touton giant cell, an orderly arrangement of nuclei in a circular fashion, with foamy peripheral cytoplasm. The tumor has thin-walled blood vessels, which leads to spontaneous bleeding at the site of involvement. The concept that this is a local tissue response to injury is supported by the finding of lipid vacuoles in smooth muscle cells, Schwann's cells, and mast cells.

TREATMENT. In patients with only cutaneous findings, observation alone will suffice. Likewise, with lid or epibulbar involvement, cases can be followed conservatively unless the lesion is amblyogenic. With uveal involvement, treatment with topical or oral steroids is recommended. Radiation or surgical treatment is usually not necessary, but, as glaucoma is a potential complication with the risk of visual loss, steroid treatment should be undertaken.

ASSOCIATIONS. An association with neurofibromatosis has been proposed. Many patients with juvenile xanthogranuloma (JXG) have café au lait spots or relatives with neurofibromatosis. Some patients have both JXG and neurofibromatosis. There is a further association with juvenile chronic myeloid leukemia, a rare childhood leukemia, and JXG.[111] Up to 20% of children with this leukemic disorder have café au lait spots and a positive family history for neurofibromatosis. There is a complex relationship among these three entities that is somewhat elusive. JXG has

also been rarely associated with Niemann-Pick disease and urticaria pigmentosa.

HISTIOCYTOSIS X. This is group of diseases involving proliferation of histiocytes causing cystic bone lesions filled with histiocytes, giant cells, and eosinophils.[112] It is a spectrum of diseases ranging from the most mild and local histiocytosis, eosinophilic granuloma, to the most malignant and lethal, Letterer-Siwe disease, a rapidly fatal disseminated form that strikes children under the age of 2. In between lies Hand-Schüller-Christian disease, which has an insidious onset and chronic course. This form, which usually presents as multifocal bone lesions with adjacent soft tissue findings, can cause a corneal infiltrate of yellow-white cells throughout all layers. The infiltrate is an abnormal deposition of lipid-laden histiocytes. There may be proptosis secondary to orbital involvement and choroidal infiltrate as well. Because of the painful and erythematous bone lesions and proptosis, a misdiagnosis of orbital cellulitis could be made. Radiology will usually clarify this. The corneal infiltrate is actually relatively rare, but the cornea may become secondarily involved if a limbal nodule extends over it. The xanthomata can be disseminated and occur almost anywhere in ocular and nonocular tissues. Diabetes insipidus may be the presenting sign if the pituitary gland is infiltrated.

HISTOLOGY. All of the histiocytoses involve abnormal proliferation of Langerhan's cells, a subset of histiocytes found in the skin, in the conjunctiva, and especially at the limbus. Early lesions may be predominantly histiocytes and, later, necrosis and eosinophilic infiltrate may be found. On electron microscopy, both tumor cells and normal-appearing Langerhan's cells have Birbeck's granules and stain strongly positive for S-100 on immunohistochemical studies.

TREATMENT. Diagnosis can be established by biopsy once clinical and radiologic evidence has been gathered. The bone lesions are radiographically distinctive with scalloped borders and adjacent tissue reaction. Surgical excision of masses may be performed, although some cases regress spontaneously. Radiation therapy may be necessary in some cases. Complications such as secondary glaucoma, iritis, scleritis, and corneal ulcers must be addressed. With widespread systemic histiocytosis X, chemotherapy is employed.

Vascular Tumors

KAPOSI'S SARCOMA. First described in 1872 by Kaposi as an aggressive angiosarcoma,[113] and felt to arise from tissues ranging from neural to reticuloendothelial, we now believe this tumor to be of vascular, endothelial cell, or pericyte origin. A previously rare tumor, there has been a surge of cases recently because of its frequency in AIDS patients. Kaposi's sarcoma occurs often in AIDS patients, and the eye is involved in nearly a quarter of these occurrences.

The lesions present as nodular or diffuse masses, often in the conjunctival fornices, although caruncle, bulbar conjunctiva, lids, and limbal tissue may be affected.[114] The tumors are usually associated with some inflammation, and patients may present with a red, itchy eye. These masses are reddish blue to deep brown and should be biopsied whenever suspect. Because AIDS patients often have subconjunctival hemorrhage for unrelated reasons, any red conjunctival lesion warrants a very careful slit-lamp evaluation. Any immunocompromised person can be affected, including those with leukemia or lymphoma in addition to AIDS, as previously mentioned. Alert ophthalmologists may again be in a position to diagnose a potentially fatal and treatable systemic disease. These tumors are slow growing and rarely invasive, but may possess considerable bulk and interfere with lid function or vision on that basis.

HISTOLOGY. This neoplasm is composed of elongated, spindle-shaped cells with oval nuclei, capillaries, and vascular slits without endothelial lining. A classification system proposed by Dugel et al.[115] defines three classes of malignancy.

Class I has thin dilated vascular channels lined by flat endothelial cells and filled with red blood cells. A moderate monocyte infiltrate is present.

Class II has plump fusiform endothelial cells lining dilated empty vascular channels. A varied inflammatory infiltrate is present.

Class III lesions contain large groups of densely packed spindle cells with hyperchromatic nuclei and occasional mitotic figures. Slit spaces are present between these spindle cells, and a few of them contain red blood cells. Inflammatory cells are scanty.

The prognostic value of this system is not completely established, but the observation has been made that Types I and II are patchy, flat tumors of less than 4 months duration, whereas Type III lesions are nodular and of longer than 4 months duration. The authors believe this to be a continuum, with only Type III being the classic spindle cell tumor. The three classes may represent a progressive involution of vascular and granulation tissue with the evolution of spindle cells.

TREATMENT. Excision of the tumor under local anesthesia with 2-mm margins where possible is performed if the patient's condition allows. Fluorescein angiography may be performed first to better define the margins of bulbar lesions by leakage.[115] Cryotherapy alone may be used for lid lesions to avoid extensive resections. Immunotherapy, chemotherapy, and radiation therapy all have been used with varying degrees of success. A lesion treated by any method can recur. Kaposi's sarcoma in AIDS patients is a more aggressive tumor than in non-AIDS patients, and one must weigh the risks and benefits of treatment carefully. As a rule, even in AIDS patients, this is a slow-growing tumor, and, unless bulky and causing interference with vision, lid function, or a cosmetic issue, one may elect to do nothing but observe. It may also require resection if ulceration or secondary infection becomes a problem. Radiation alone can be palliative even though there is a high rate of recurrence. The treatment of Kaposi's sarcoma with vascularization-inhibiting cytokines is currently under investigation. As the life expectancy of AIDS patients continues to increase thanks to the development of new treatment modalities, it becomes increasingly important to diagnose and treat even this slow-growing tumor.

Neural Tumors

SCHWANNOMA. Primary intrascleral schwannomas have been very rarely described. Cases published in 1943 by Szabo and Cseh[116] and in 1976 by Quintana and Lee[117] are the only two in the literature thus far. A schwannoma is a neoplasm of Schwann's cells. It is a well-defined, slow-growing, cellular tumor with pleomorphic spindle-shaped cells arranged in bundles. Usually a solitary mass in the head and neck region, these lesions generally present between ages 20 and 50. They are rarely found in the orbit.

HISTOLOGY. This tumor is a proliferation of Schwann's cells in a perineural capsule, a mixture of tight, ordered Schwann's cells, called Antoni A cells, or more loosely arranged components, called Antoni B cells.[118] Axons may be seen as eccentric nerve bundles in the capsule. On electron-microscopic studies, the Antoni A cells appear as stacks of processes surrounded by a well-defined basal lamina. The Antoni B cells have a less dense arrangement. One can also find lymphocytoid cells, hyalinized blood vessels, cyst formation, calcification, and hemorrhage.

In the case of the scleral tumor, the cells have long nuclei and prominent nucleoli. Atypical mitotic figures and some inflammatory reaction are seen on light microscopy. Head and neck schwannomas are only rarely associated with malignant transformation, although these mitotic figures can be seen. Electron-microscopic studies revealed the spindle-shaped cells with oval, indented nuclei, a clumped or dispersed nucleolemma, and prominent cytoplasmic processes. Axons were not identified, nor were melanocytic or myofibrillary structures. A notable finding was the presence of basement membrane around cytoplasmic processes. Thus, one can conclude that a schwannoma can occur on sclera, which does contain neural tissue, but is a very rare occurrence.

ASSOCIATIONS. There is an association of this tumor with neurofibromatosis, and the malignant tumors have this association 50% of the time.

Mysteries

AMYLOIDOSIS. Amyloidosis is a group of conditions of diverse etiologies characterized by the accumulation of fibrillar material in various tissues. It may be inflammatory, hereditary, or neoplastic; local or systemic; a benign process or a malignant one. Symptoms and prognosis depend largely on the site and amount of deposition.

This material has precursors of normal, soluble proteins, for example, intact immunoglobulin light chains.[119] What transforms these to pathologic amyloid deposition is not known. Various classification schemes have attempted to bring order to this complex subject. One, based on chemical composition, aids in clarifying the tissue of origin. Immunoglobulin light chains, procalcitonin, prealbumin, and gamma fragment polymers are all found in amyloidosis. Type AA is found in association with inflammatory processes such as tuberculosis, rheumatoid arthritis, and inflammatory bowel disease. The precursor fibril is termed *AA fibril prototype,* a less than enlightening designation. Type AL is the most common type in medical practice and is in the spectrum of diseases including multiple myeloma, previously discussed. It represents a plasmacytosis of light-chain proteins, κ or λ, with malignant outcome. A "senile" type amyloidosis has been found in heart, brain, and pancreas of asymptomatic elderly at routine autopsy. Certain forms have a predilection for certain areas of deposition.

In the eye, there is a localized, sometimes nodular salmon-pink to yellow-white mass found on cornea. It can also appear on the conjunctiva, the Tenon's capsule, the lacrimal gland, or in the orbit. On cornea, it is most often found in association with chronic inflammation such as trachoma, interstitial keratitis, uveitis, sarcoidosis, or Hansen's disease. It is also known to occur in association with trauma, glaucoma, retinopathy of prematurity, keratoconus, and corneal dystrophies, including lattice and gelatinous dystrophy. In fact, gelatinous dystrophy is also called familial subepithelial amyloidosis, a bilateral deposition of amyloid of autosomal recessive inheritance with systemic findings. Corneal amyloid deposition may present as small punctate elevations in central cornea and occasionally extends to the periphery and limbus. These can coalesce and enlarge, producing milky nodules in subepithelium and superficial stroma.

The site of amyloid production is believed to be the corneal epithelial cells, which contrasts with lattice dystrophy, where stromal fibroblasts are responsible. It is not the author's (H.V.H.) purpose to discuss the corneal dystrophies, but she includes gelatinous dystrophy as a "masquerade" because this dystrophy is capable of producing a mass lesion.

Amyloid can also deposit locally in the eye as part of primary systemic amyloidosis. The eye findings may be the first manifestation of systemic disease. Waxy infiltrations of glycoproteins produced by the reticuloendothelial system can be related to gammaglobulins, Bence Jones proteins, and other myeloma proteins, making this an important diagnosis.

HISTOLOGY. On hematoxylin-eosin stain, amyloid stains eosinophilic with a hyaline appearance. It is also PAS positive. With Congo red, it stains brown with a characteristic dichroism on examination with polarized light. It also displays birefringence and fluoresces apple green with thioflavin T stain. On electron microscopy, filaments of 80-angstrom length are the major component. A rodlike pentamer or *P component* makes up the minor component. This is known to be an acute-phase reactant.

TREATMENT. Corneal lesions may interfere with vision to the point where penetrating keratoplasty becomes necessary. Conjunctival or scleral lesions may be resected as needed for tissue evaluation. Refer to the section on lymphomatous tumors for a discussion of the treatment of multiple myeloma.

ICHTHYOSIS. From the Greek *ichthys,* meaning "fish," this is a heterogeneous group of genetic disorders of the skin.[109] It is inherited in an autosomal dominant, autosomal recessive, or X-linked recessive fashion and is characterized by thickened, scaly skin with loose, polyhedral scales, fissures, and poor sweat and sebaceous gland function. The Superficial, gray nodular corneal degenerative lesions are found. The nodules are opaque and appear along with stromal opacity, prominent corneal nerves, and band keratopathy. These nodular lesions are found only in the X-linked recessive form of the disease in affected males and, to a lesser extent, in female carriers.

The X-linked recessive form of ichthyosis has a prevalence of 1/6000 and is a metabolic disease of aryl sulfatase C and steroid sulfatase defi-ciency. The enzyme has been found to be encoded by a gene on the X chromosome and is thus congenital. Scales appear at birth or early in life on scalp, face, trunk, and limbs and impart a yellowish appearance to the areas involved.

The other forms of ichthyosis—ichthyosis vulgaris, lamellar ichthyosis, and epidermolytic hyperkeratosis—display the finding of scales on lashes and lids, but not the corneal nodules. Histologically, the corneal lesions are a mystery as to composition and etiology. Not truly a neoplasm, they are included here as a potential source of confusion in the diagnosis of corneal tumors. Notably, an ichthyosis-like presentation can occur as a manifestation of malignancy. It is seen in Hodgkin's disease, lymphosarcomatous tumors, multiple myeloma, and carcinoma of breast and lung.

Other Masses to Confuse You

PTERYGIUM. From the Greek *pteron,* meaning "wing," this is a winglike extension of elastotic degeneration that fans over from the conjunctiva to the cornea, crossing the limbus. It can extend across cornea to occlude vision, becoming a "kissing" lesion with its counterpart on the opposite side. The tissue is subepithelial in location, with the overlying epithelium variably thin, thick, normal, or dysplastic. In the case of a dysplastic lesion, carcinoma must be ruled out. Located in the interpalpebral fissure, there is an association with actinic exposure. The nasal side is usually affected before the temporal side. The term *pinguecula* refers to a lesion of the same origin and histology that is confined to the conjunctiva and does not cross over the limbus onto cornea to a large extent. Clinically, the pinguecula may appear more like an elevated button of pinkish or yellowish tissue at the limbus. As this tissue spreads, it is renamed a pterygium.

HISTOLOGY. Hematoxylin-eosin stain shows subepithelial limbal tissues, peripheral corneal stroma, and Bowman's membrane containing thick, degenerated connective tissue (Figure 5.45). The usually eosinophilic fibrous tissue is replaced by amorphous, basophilic tissue. Pterygia share some features of actinic exposure with skin. The tissue appears similar to elastic tissue, but does not

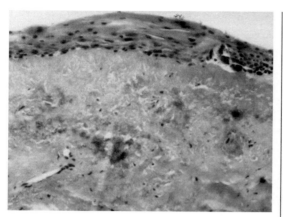

FIG. 5.45—Elastotic degeneration of the cornea. Note the disruption of the underlying collagen. Hematoxylin-eosin, ×50.

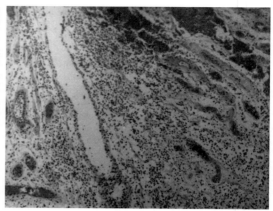

FIG. 5.46—Pyogenic granuloma. Note the marked, diffuse mixed inflammatory cell infiltrate along with the proliferating capillaries and edema. Hematoxylin-eosin, ×25.

contain elastin, so it is referred to as *elastotic* degeneration. Electron-microscopic studies reveal the basophilic material to contain elastic fiber precursors. Elastin secreted into the area by fibroblasts may be seen as part of a secondary repair process. CIN and nevi have been identified in the overlying tissues.

TREATMENT. Treatment is observation alone unless the visual axis is threatened or suspicious, or malignant-appearing changes occur. Simple surgical excision is followed by an annoying recurrence rate of up to 40%.[120] Topical mitomycin C or an intraoperative application has been tried by some with a better long-term result, but this technique is not favored by all. It causes considerable delay in healing and can result in significant corneal/limbal ectasia.[121] Radiation and conjunctival autografts have also been used to delay regrowth. Trials with antimetabolites in low concentrations probably are the best hope for reducing the recurrence rate along with our current surgical techniques.

PYOGENIC GRANULOMA. Pyogenic granulomas appear in the differential diagnosis of tumors of the eye and will be therefore briefly discussed. They are simply exuberant growth of granulation tissue that is stimulated by injury or infection (Figure 5.46). They may arise without known history of trauma, but even a seemingly minor event

could stimulate the growth of this mass. Injury is often iatrogenic, and these are fairly common following surgical disruption of conjunctiva. They may appear on the cornea, although rarely. They appear clinically as red, highly vascularized tissue with a lobulated, sometimes pedunculated appearance. Kaposi's sarcoma is in the differential diagnosis for this highly colored tumor. If there is clinical suspicion that a pyogenic granuloma may not be the diagnosis, or if the lesion interferes with vision or lid function, it should be excised and sent for histologic evaluation. This tumor may also cause a cosmetic problem and is often excised on that basis. Pyogenic granulomas can recur.

NODULAR FASCIITIS. This is a rare, benign, reactive fibroblast proliferation that results in a nodular, vascularized mass. Usually presenting as isolated, tender, rapidly growing nodules on the trunk and upper extremities, these masses are also found in the skin of the head and neck, Tenon's capsule, ligaments of the extraocular muscles, and orbital septum. Episcleral lesions present as painful nodules and can occur over the limbus or muscle insertions. The mass can arise in as little as a week to over a period of months. It may be present for years without being problematic, but this is unusual. There is rarely a known antecedent event prior to its appearance.

HISTOLOGY. The nodules range in size from 0.5 to 1.5 cm in diameter, and are round, nonencapsulated bundles of immature fibroblasts. Configurations vary from spindles to stellate cell arrangements. The interspersed ground substance is myxoid in nature, with blood vessels, lymphocytes, and mononuclear cells present. Mitotic figures may be present, making the differentiation from malignant sarcoma difficult. The differential diagnosis also includes benign fibromas, neurofibromas, and neurilemomas.

TREATMENT. The treatment is simple excision.

KELOID. Also called hypertrophic cicatrix, keloid is a posttraumatic, postinflammatory, or foreign-body reaction of fibroblastic proliferation over a focus of scar. There is a resemblance to both fibrocytic tumors and choristomas, making the classification of this lesion difficult. It is best left in a category of its own.

HISTORY. In 1849, Sir William Bowman, of membrane fame, devoted study to the healing of corneal stroma to learn the nature of tissue response to injury. Because of its convenient transparency, the cornea has often been the focus of observation of inflammatory and repair mechanisms. Bowman noted increased cellularity and ascribed this to fixed corneal "corpuscles." As cited in Duke-Elder,[83] Strube in 1851, Virchow in 1852, His in 1856, Weber in 1858, Rindfleisch in 1859, and Langhans in 1861, all pondered the mechanisms of corneal repair. Other investigators, including Von Recklinghausen and Cohnheim, noted the migration of cells and concluded that the theory of fixed corpuscular proliferation was not complete. Many interesting theories blossomed, including Grawitz's theory of *Schlummerzellen* (sleeping cells) that awoke to participate in repair when stimulated. From the contributions of these 19th-century pioneers and others on into the 20th century were formed the modern concepts of corneal healing with hematogenous, local, and limbal contributions.

APPEARANCE. Corneal keloids range from a denser-than-usual scar to a tumorlike mass with resemblance to a dermoid. As previously mentioned, they occur after an insult and can result in a leukoma, a white tumor-like mass on the corneal surface. A keloid can arise at the site of an ulcer perforation or a staphyloma. The whiteness is attributed to the loss of the usually orderly arrangement of collagen and a paucity of blood vessels. In the early stages of formation, the *fibroblastic stage,* these lesions may be quite vascular and full of inflammatory cells. Remodeling leads to opacification in any stromal injury, but the greater degree of response is what defines a keloid. The healing process can vary greatly from person to person. Those with keloid tendencies in skin are prone to heal with the same overly responsive scar formation on ocular tissues.

HISTOLOGY. Scar is composed of irregular arrangements of connective tissue and fibrocytes with a more eosinophilic cytoplasm and more deeply staining nuclei on hematoxylin-eosin stain than is usually found. This exuberant proliferation of tissue may have nodular whorls of collagen bundles in the matrix. The bundles eventually come to lie closer to the surface in a parallel fashion. The cornea is thick, and intraepithelial cysts may form. Electron-microscopic studies reveal fibers of variable thickness, and extracellular mucopolysaccharide microfilaments are present. Inflammatory cells and blood vessels can be found, and elastic elements are rarely seen.

ASSOCIATIONS. Keloids of the cornea may be congenital, secondary to intrauterine injury to the fetal cornea, birth trauma, or as part of a syndrome. Lowe's syndrome is an X-linked hereditary syndrome that includes congenital cataracts, meiosis, mental retardation, and decreased renal tubular function. Bilateral corneal keloids are the major cause of poor visual acuity in these children.[122] Corneal keloids in these children can extend the full corneal thickness, making treatment difficult. Although the etiology is unclear, it may be that minor trauma leads to a hyperplastic tissue response bilaterally, leading to the formation of exuberant scar. Many of these patients have a seizure disorder, and treatment with phenytoin may also enhance collagen formation. This is speculative. Renal acidosis may also play a role. Treatment is difficult, and recurrence in resected areas is common. Conjunctival flap and steroids have been tried to halt this progression.

TREATMENT. Over the years, many pharmacologic methods have been tried to treat and prevent keloid formation. Drugs used to promote resorption include yellow oxide of mercury, calomel powder, noviform ointment, jequirity, subconjunctival sodium chloride, intramuscular sodium, and magnesium sulfate and streptokinase. Wintergreen oil and sterilized animal vitreous have also been used. Massage with the fingers or electric devices, ultraviolet light, and radiation have also been tried. Dermatologists can use topical steroids and pressure patches, but ophthalmologists are forced to perform surgery or laser to reduce these lesions. Sometimes penetrating keratoplasty is needed, and excimer laser is enjoying some success in the treatment of corneal scars.

CYSTS. Scleral cysts may be seen at the limbus of infants. These are inclusion cysts of conjunctival epithelium or choristomas. They may be connected to the anterior chamber by a thin membrane, and collapse of the anterior chamber has occurred as fluid enters the cystic space.

Corneal intrastromal cysts can form after trauma. During incision of the cornea, epithelium gains entry into the stroma through a breech in Bowman's membrane. There the cells can proliferate and form an interlamellar cyst. They may appear clear or opaque on slit-lamp examination.

XERODERMA PIGMENTOSUM. This autosomal recessively inherited disease of extreme sun sensitivity was first described by Kaposi in 1870. Affecting 1 in 250,000 individuals, it is found in all races, but is less commonly found in the darker races. The etiology is defective DNA repair after ultraviolet damage of epidermal, lymphocytic, and fibroblastic cells.[109] A number of changes can ensue. Exposure to routine amounts of sun causes dry, erythematous skin with patches of alternating depigmentation and hyperpigmentation. Benign and malignant neoplasms can grow, including hyperkeratotic plaques, actinic keratoses, carcinoma in situ (CIS), SCC, basal cell carcinoma, and malignant melanoma. In the eye, blepharoconjunctivitis, corneal opacities and ulcers, iris atrophy, fundus changes, and symblepharon formation can also occur.

A slow rate of tritiated thymidine incorporation into DNA has been found in the conjunctiva of affected individuals. Patients may present with reactions to sun exposure early in life, ranging from severe sunburn to telangiectasias, atrophic patches, and pigmented lesions. The lids, conjunctiva, and cornea can be severely affected.[123] Pterygium-like masses may be found on the cornea, as well as epithelial neoplasms. With early recognition and scrupulous avoidance of ultraviolet exposure, the prognosis can be fairly good. When the case is severe, death usually results from malignancy. These patients undergo multiple surgical procedures during a lifetime, and the cosmetic issues are legion. They often take employment in the night to maintain as normal an existence as possible.

TREATMENT. The mainstay of treatment involves protection from the sun by whatever means possible. Frequent skin and ocular examinations are recommended so that neoplasms can be rapidly treated. Actinic keratoses should be treated with 5-fluorouracil, and melanomas and carcinomas should be excised. The corneal lesions may be stripped whenever possible, but extensive lesions require keratoplasty. Conjunctival masses are treated with excision. The sclera is affected by extension of conjunctival or corneal masses and should be treated with excision as well.

Metastasis. Previously discussed were local metastases in conjunction with malignant melanoma and carcinoma. Metastasis from distant sites to cornea, conjunctiva, and sclera is very rare. Breast carcinoma has been documented on the sclera by Reed as an elevated nodule. Prostate carcinoma was reported by Liu et al.[124] in 1992 to metastasize to choroid and sclera. Seeding tissue with malignant cells is a recognized route of local metastasis, whereas other routes such as hematogenous and lymphatic spread must be invoked in those cases of distant metastasis. Carcinomas of the breast, lung, prostate, and gastrointestinal system, as well as melanomas, are all known to metastasize widely to uveal tissue, and, from there, scleral extension is possible.[125] At this time, a local corneal metastasis has not been reported. Metastasis of sarcoma is rare overall and vanishingly rare in cornea, sclera, or conjunctiva.

The sclera, the major structural tissue of the eye, is prone to extension of tumor from the underlying uveal tract, a frequent site of malignancy, as well as from above, namely, the conjunctiva.[126]

REFERENCES

1. Dice P. Cornea. In: Gelatt KN, ed. *Veterinary Ophthalmology,* 1st ed. Philadelphia: Lea and Febiger, 370:1981.
2. Bernays M, Fleming D, Peiffer RL. Primary corneal papilloma and squamous cell carcinoma associated with pigmentary keratitis in four dogs. *J Am Vet Med Assoc* 214:215, 1999.
3. Russel WO, Wynne ES, Loquvan GS. Studies on ocular squamous cell carcinoma ("cancer eye"): I. Pathological anatomy and historical review. *Cancer* 91:52, 1956.
4. Runnells RA, Benbrook EA. Epithelial tumors of horses. *Am J Vet Res* 7:176, 1942.
5. Lavach JD, Severin GA. Neoplasia of the equine eye, adnexa, and orbit: a review of 68 cases. *J Am Vet Med Assoc* 170:202, 1977.
6. Gelatt KN, Myers VS Jr, Perman V, Jessen C. Conjunctival squamous cell carcinoma in the horse. *J Am Vet Med Assoc* 165:617, 1974.
7. Dugan SJ, Roberts SM, Curtis CR, Severin GA. Prognostic factors and survival of horses with ocular/adnexal squamous cell carcinoma: 147 cases (1978–1980). *J Am Vet Med Assoc* 198:298, 1991.
8. Schwink K. Factors influencing morbidity and outcome of equine squamous cell carcinoma. *Equine Vet J* 14:198, 1987.
9. Gelatt KN. Corneolimbal squamous cell carcinoma in a horse. *Vet Med* 70:53, 1975.
10. Koch SA, Cowles RR. Surgical removal of a squamous cell carcinoma of the equine eye. *Vet Med* 66:327, 1971.
11. Rebhun WC. Treatment of advanced squamous cell carcinoma involving the equine corneal. *Vet Surg* 19:297, 1990.
12. Grier RL, Brewer WG Jr, Paul SR, et al. Treatment of bovine and equine ocular squamous cell carcinoma by radiofrequency hyperthermia. *J Am Vet Med Assoc* 177:155, 1980.
13. Latimer KS, Kaswan RL, Sundberg JP. Corneal squamous cell carcinoma in a dog. *J Am Vet Med Assoc* 11:1430, 1987.
14. Caligiuri R, Carrier M, Jacobson ER, Buergelt CD. Corneal squamous cell carcinoma in a cheetah (*Acinonyx jubatus*). *J Zoo Anim Med* 19:219, 1988.
15. Monlux AW, Anderson WA, Davis CL. The diagnosis of squamous cell carcinoma of the eye ("cancer eye") in cattle. *Am J Vet Res* 18:5, 1957.
16. Kircher CH, Garner FM, Robinson FR. Tumors of the eye and adnexa. *Bull WHO* 50:135, 1974.
17. Miller TR, Gelatt KN. Food animal ophthalmology. In: Gelatt KN, ed. *Veterinary Ophthalmology,* 2d ed. Philadelphia: Lea and Febiger, 628:1991.
18. Martin CL. Canine epibulbar melanomas and their management. *J Am Anim Hosp Assoc* 17:83, 1981.
19. Cotchin E. Melanotic tumors of dogs. *J Comp Pathol Ther* 65:115, 1955.
20. Saunders LZ, Barron CN. Primary pigmented intra-ocular tumors in animals. *Cancer Res* 18:234, 1958.
21. Harling DE, Peiffer RL, Cook CS. Feline limbal melanoma: four cases. *J Am Anim Hosp Assoc* 22:795, 1986.
22. Dublezig RR. Ocular neoplasia in small animals. *Vet Clin North Am Small Anim Pract* 20:837, 1990.
23. Wilcock BP, Peiffer RL. Morphology and behavior of primary ocular melanomas in 91 dogs. *Vet Pathol* 23:418, 1986.
24. Bussanich NM, Dolman PJ, Rootman J, Dolman CL. Canine uveal melanomas: series and literature review. *J Am Anim Hosp Assoc* 23:415, 1987.
25. Collinson PN, Peiffer RL. Clinical presentation, morphology, and behavior of primary choroidal melanomas in eight dogs. *Prog Vet Comp Ophthalmol* 3:158, 1993.
26. Blogg JR, Dutton AG, Stanley RG. Use of third eyelid grafts to repair full thickness defects in the cornea and sclera. *J Am Anim Hosp Assoc* 25:505, 1989.
27. Nasisse MP, Davidson MG, Oliver DK, Brinkman M, Nelms S. Neodymium:YAG laser treatment of primary canine intraocular tumors. *Prog Vet Comp Ophthalmol* 3:152, 1993.
28. Whitley RD. Canine cornea. In: Gelatt KN, ed. *Veterinary Ophthalmology,* 2d ed. Philadelphia: Lea and Febiger, 321:1991.
29. Peiffer RL, Monticello T, Bouldin TW. Primary ocular sarcomas in the cat. *J Small Anim Pract* 29:105, 1988.
30. Dubielzig RR. Ocular sarcoma following trauma in three cats. *JAMA* 184:578, 1984.
31. Grady HG, Blum MF, Kirby-Smith JS. Types of tumor induced by ultraviolet radiation and factors influencing their relative incidence. *J Natl Cancer Inst* 3:371, 1943.
32. Freeman RG, Knox JM. Ultraviolet-induced corneal tumors in different strains of animals. *J Invest Dermatol* 43:431, 1964.
33. Lippincott SW, Blum HF. Neoplasms and other lesions of the eye induced by ultraviolet radiation in strain A mice. *J Natl Cancer Inst* 3:545, 1943.
34. Sabourin CL, Kusewitt OF, Fry RJ, et al. Ultraviolet radiation-induced corneal tumors in the South American opossum, *Monodelphis domestica. J Comp Pathol* 108:343, 1993.
35. Ley RD, Applegate LA, Fry RJ, Sanchez AB. Photoreactivation of ultraviolet radiation-induced skin and eye tumors of the marsupial, *Monodelphis domestica. Cancer Res* 51:6539, 1991.
36. Gilger BC, Whitley RD, McLaughlin SA. Bovine ocular squamous cell carcinoma: a review. In: *Veterinary Annual.* Oxford, UK: Blackwell Scientific, 73:991.

37. Dugan SJ, Curtis CR, Roberts SM, Severin GA. Epidemiologic study of ocular/adnexal squamous cell carcinoma in horses. *J Am Anim Hosp Assoc* 198:251, 1991.

38. Naghshineh R, Sohrabi Hagdoost I, Mokhber-Dezfuli MR. A retrospective study of the incidence of bovine neoplasms in Iran. *J Comp Pathol* 105:235, 1991.

39. Anderson DE, Skinner PE. Studies on bovine ocular squamous carcinoma ("cancer eye"): XI. Effects of sunlight. *J Anim Sci* 20:474, 1961.

40. Kopecky KE, Pugh GW Jr, Hughes DE, Booth GD, Cheville NF. Biological effects of ultraviolet radiation on cattle: bovine ocular squamous cell carcinoma. *Am J Vet Res* 40:1783, 1979.

41. Bailey CM, Hanks DR, Hanks MA. Circumocular pigmentation and incidence of ocular squamous cell tumors in *Bos taurus* and *Bos indicus taurus* cattle. *J Am Anim Hosp Assoc* 196:1605, 1990.

42. French GT. A clinical and genetic study of eye cancer in Hereford cattle. *Aust Vet J* 35:474, 1959.

43. Dugan SJ. Ocular neoplasia. *Vet Clin North Am Equine Pract* 8:609, 1992.

44. Strafuss AC. Squamous cell carcinoma in horses. *J Am Anim Hosp Assoc* 168:61, 1976.

45. Bolton JR, Lees MJ, Robinson WF, Thomas JB, Klein KT. Ocular neoplasms of vascular origin in the horse. *Equine Vet J Suppl* 10:773, 1990.

46. Crawley GR, Bryan GM, Gogolewski RP. Ocular hemangioma in a horse. *Equine Pract* 9:11, 1987.

47. Martin CL, Leipold HW. Mastocytoma of the globe in a horse. *J Am Anim Health Assoc* 8:32, 1972.

48. Hum S, Bowers JR. Ocular mastocytoma in a horse. *Aust Vet J* 66:32, 1989.

49. Hirst LW, Jobi DA, Staskopt M. Benign epibulbar melanocytoma in a horse. *J Am Anim Hosp Assoc* 183:333, 1983.

50. Hacker DV, Moore PF, Buyukmihai NL. Ocular angiosarcoma in four horses. *J Am Anim Hosp Assoc* 189:200, 1986.

51. Fischer CA. Inflammatory disease of the sclera and episclera. In: Peiffer RL, ed. *Comparative Ophthalmic Pathology.* Springfield, IL: Charles C Thomas, chap 11:1983.

52. Paulsen ME, Lavach JD, Snyder SP, Severin GA, Eichenbaum JD. Nodular episclerokeratitis in dogs: 19 cases (1973–1985). *J Am Anim Hosp Assoc* 190:1581, 1987.

53. Williams DL, Barnett KD. Unpublished data, 1994.

54. Smith JS, Bistner S, Riis R. Infiltrative cornea lesions resembling fibrous histiocytoma: clinical and pathologic features in six dogs and one cat. *J Am Anim Hosp Assoc* 169:772, 1976.

55. Mainka SA, Christmas R. Ocular nodular fasciitis in an Asiatic black bear (*Selanantos thibetanus*). *J Zoo Anim Med* 187:1268, 1985.

56. Fischer CA. Sclerouveitis in dogs. *Proc Am Coll Vet Ophthalmol* 3:33, 1972.

57. Fischer CA. A clinicopathologic classification of episcleritis and scleritis in the dog. *Proc Am Coll Vet Ophthalmol* 13:1, 1982.

58. Cook C. *Inflammatory Disease of the Canine Sclera and Episclera: Clinical Classroom 1.* Princeton Junction: Schering Plough, 1984.

59. Crispin SM. Clinical differentiation of canine episcleritis and scleritis. *Vet Annu* 31:132, 1991.

60. Williams DL, Crispin SM. Sclera, episclera and limbus. In: Crispin SM, Peterson-Jones S, eds. *British Small Animal Veterinary Association Manual Of Ophthalmology.* Cheltenham, UK: British Small Animal Veterinary Association, 1993.

61. Lattimer CA, Wyman M, Syzmanski C. Azothiaprine in the management of fibrous histiocytoma in two dogs. *J Am Anim Hosp Assoc* 19:155, 1983.

62. Bellhorn RW, Henkind P. Ocular nodular fasciitis in a dog. *J Am Anim Hosp Assoc* 150:212, 1967.

63. Lavignette AM, Carlton WW. A case of ocular nodular fasciitis in a dog. *J Am Anim Hosp Assoc* 10:503, 1974.

64. Gwin RM, Gelatt KN, Peiffer RL Jr. Ophthalmic nodular fasciitis in the dog. *J Am Anim Hosp Assoc* 176:611, 1979.

65. Blogg RJ. Proliferative keratoconjunctivitis in the collie. *Proc Am Coll Vet Ophthalmol* 8:89, 1977.

66. Mansour AM, Barber JC, Reinecke RD, Wang FM. Ocular choristomas. *Surv Ophthalmol* 93:339, 1989.

67. Hayasaka S, Sekimoto M, Setogawa T. Epibulbar complex choristoma involving the bulbar conjunctiva and cornea. *J Pediatr Ophthalmol Strabismus* 26:251, 1989.

68. Young TL, Buchi ER, Kaufman LM, Sugar J, Tso MO. Respiratory epithelium in a cystic choristoma of the limbus. *Arch Ophthalmol* 108:1736, 1990.

69. Schermer A, Galvin S, Sun T. Differentiation-related expression of a major 64K corneal keratin in vivo and in cell culture suggests limbal location of corneal epithelial stem cells. *J Cell Biol* 103:46, 1986.

70. Gold DH, Weingeist TA. *The Eye in Systemic Disease.* Philadelphia: JB Lippincott, 1990.

71. Wilkes SR, Campbell RJ, Waller RR. Ocular malformation in association with ipsilateral facial nevus of Jadassohn. *Am J Ophthalmol* 92:344, 1981.

72. Feuerstein RC, Mims LC. Linear nevus sebaceous with convulsions and mental retardation. *Am J Dis Child* 104:675, 1962.

73. Panton RW, Sugar J. Excision of limbal dermoids. *Ophthalmol Surg* 22:85, 1991.

74. Pokorny KS, Hyman BM, Jakobiec FA, Perry HD, Caputo AR, Iwamoto T. Epibulbar choristomas containing lacrimal tissue: clinical distinction from dermoids and histologic evidence of an origin from the palpebral lobe. *Ophthalmology* 94:1249, 1987.

75. Ferry AP, Hein HF. Epibulbar osseous choristoma within an epibulbar dermoid. *Am J Ophthalmol* 70:764, 1970.

76. Spencer WH. *Ophthalmic Pathology: An Atlas and Textbook,* 3d ed. Philadelphia: WB Saunders, 1985.

77. Fulton AB, Howard RO, Albert DM, et al. Ocular findings in triploidy. *Am J Ophthalmol* 84:859, 1977.
78. McDonnell JM, Mayr AJ, Martin WJ. DNA of human papillomavirus type 16 in dysplastic and malignant lesions of the conjunctiva and cornea. *N Engl J Med* 320:1442, 1989.
79. Lass JH, Grave AS, Papale JJ, et al. Detection of human papillomavirus DNA sequences in conjunctival papillomas. *Am J Ophthalmol* 96:670, 1983.
80. Lauer SA, Malter JS, Meier JR. Human papillomavirus type 18 in conjunctival intraepithelial neoplasia. *Am J Ophthalmol* 110:23, 1990.
81. Streiten BW, Carillo R, Jamison R, et al. Inverted papilloma of the conjunctiva. *Am J Ophthalmol* 88:1062, 1979.
82. Von Sallman L, Panton D. Hereditary benign intraepithelial dyskeratosis, ocular manifestations. *Arch Ophthalmol* 63:421, 1960.
83. Duke-Elder S. *System of Ophthalmology.* St Louis: CV Mosby, 1965.
84. Lee GA, Hirst LW. Incidence of ocular surface epithelial dysplasia in metropolitan Brisbane. *Arch Ophthalmol* 110:525, 1992.
85. Daxecker F, Philipp W, Mikuz G. Keratoplastik bei unbekanntem Hornhautkarzinom-fallberich. *Fortschr Ophthalmol* 86:189, 1989.
86. Waring GO, Roth AM, Ekins MB. Clinical and pathologic description of 17 cases of corneal intraepithelial neoplasia. *Am J Ophthalmol* 97:547, 1984.
87. Steinhorst U, Von Domarus D. Carcinoma in situ of the cornea. *Ophthalmology* 200:107, 1990.
88. Brown HH, Glasgow BJ, Holland GN, Foos RY. Keratinizing corneal intraepithelial neoplasia. *Cornea* 8:220, 1989.
89. Prezyna AP, Monte JF, Satchindanand SK. Unilateral corneal intraepithelial neoplasia: management of a recurrent lesion. *Ann Ophthalmol* 22:103, 1990.
90. Morsman CD. Spontaneous regression of a conjunctival intraepithelial neoplastic tumor. *Arch Ophthalmol* 107:1490, 1989.
91. Cameron JA, Hidayat AA. Squamous cell carcinoma. *Am J Ophthalmol* 111:571, 1991.
92. Copeland RA, Char DH. Limbal autograft reconstruction after conjunctival squamous cell carcinoma. *Am J Ophthalmol* 110:412, 1990.
93. Ni C, Guo BK. Histological types of spindle cell carcinoma of the cornea and conjunctive: a clinicopathologic report of 8 patients with ultrastructural and immunohistochemical findings in three tumors. *Chin Med J [Engl]* 103:915, 1990.
94. Wolter JR, Bromley WC. Intraepithelial sebaceous epithelioma of lids, conjunctiva, and cornea treated with minimal orbital exenteration. *Ophthalmic Surg* 22:340, 1991.
95. Naumann GH, Apple DA. *Pathology of the Eye.* New York: Springer-Verlag, 1986.
96. Folberg R, McLean IW, Zimmerman LE. Conjunctival melanosis and melanoma. *Ophthalmology* 91:673, 1984.
97. Whitcup SM, Albert DM. A benign nevus of cornea and corneoscleral limbus. *Am J Ophthalmol* 107:304, 1989.
98. Paredaens AD, Kirkness CM, Garner A, Hungerford JL. Recurrent malignant melanoma of the corneal stroma: a case of 'black cornea.' *Br J Ophthalmol* 76:444, 1992.
99. Callender GR. Malignant melanotic tumors of the eye: study of histologic types in 111 cases. *Trans Am Acad Ophthalmol Otolaryngol* 36:131, 1931.
100. McLean IW, Foster WD, Zimmerman LE, Gamel JW. Modifications of Callender's classification of uveal melanoma at the Armed Forces Institute of Pathology. *Am J Ophthalmol* 96:502, 1983.
101. Lee JS, Smith RE, Minkler DS. Scleral melanocytoma. *Ophthalmology* 89:178, 1982.
102. Burki E. Uber Hornhautveranderungen bei einem Fall von multiplem Myelom (Plasmacytom). *Ophthalmology* 135:565, 1958.
103. Beebe WE, Webster RG, Spencer WB. Atypical corneal manifestations of multiple myeloma: a clinical, histopathologic and immunohistochemical report. *Cornea* 8:274, 1989.
104. Hill JC, Mulligan GP. Subepithelial corneal deposits in IgG lambda myeloma. *Br J Ophthalmol* 73:552, 1989.
105. Schellini SA, Bacchi CE. Fibrous histiocytoma of limbus. *Acta Ophthalmol* 67:601, 1989.
106. Lahoud S, Brownstein S, Laflamme MY. Fibrous histiocytoma of the corneoscleral limbus and conjunctiva. *Am J Ophthalmol* 106:579, 1988.
107. Von Heydenreich A. Fibrosarkom der Sklera. *Ophthalmology* 148:416, 1964.
108. Lo GG, Biswas J, Rao NA, Font RL. Corneal myxoma. *Cornea* 9:174, 1990.
109. Odom RB, James WD, Berger TC. *Andrew's Diseases of the Skin,* 9th ed. Philadelphia: WB Saunders, 2000.
110. Cadera W, Silver MM, Burt L. Juvenile xanthogranuloma. *Can J Ophthalmol* 18:169, 1983.
111. Cooper PH, Frierson HF, Kayne AL, et al. Association of juvenile xanthogranuloma with juvenile myeloid leukemia. *Arch Dermatol* 120:371, 1984.
112. Lichtenstein L. Histiocytosis X: integration of eosinophilic granuloma of bone—Letterer-Siwe and Schuller-Christian disease as related manifestations of a single nosologic entity. *Arch Pathol* 56:84, 1953.
113. Dugel PU, Gill PS, Frangieh GT, Rao NA. Ocular adnexal Kaposi's sarcoma in acquired immunodeficiency syndrome, *Am J Ophthalmol* 110:500, 1990.
114. Newsome DA. Noninfectious ocular complications of AIDS. *Int Ophthalmol Clin* 29:95 1989.
115. Dugel PU, Gill PS, Frangieh GT. Treatment of ocular adnexal Kaposi's sarcoma in acquired immune deficiency syndrome. *Ophthalmology* 99:1,127, 1992.
116. Szabo G, Cseh E. Sklera-Neurinom in der Nahe des Limbus. *Ophthalmologica* 106:14, 1943.
117. Quintana M, Lee WR. Intrascleral schwannoma. *Ophthalmologica* 173:64, 1976.

118. Robbins SL, Cotran RS, Kumar V. *Robbins Pathologic Basis of Disease,* 4th ed. Philadelphia: WB Saunders, 1989.

119. Wynagaarden JB, Smith LH, Cecil RL. Textbook *of Medicine,* 17th ed. Philadelphia: WB Saunders, 1985.

120. Singh G, Wilson MR, Foster CS. Long-term follow-up study of mitomycin eye drops as adjunctive treatment of pterygia and its comparison with conjunctival autograft transplantation. *Cornea* 9:331, 1990.

121. Ewing-Chow DA, Romanchuk KG, Gilmour GR, et al. Corneal melting after pterygium removal followed by topical mitomycin C therapy. *Can J Ophthalmol* 27:197, 1992.

122. Cibis GW, Tripathi RC, Tripathi BJ, Harris DJ. Corneal keloid in Lowe's syndrome. *Arch Ophthalmol* 100:1795, 1982.

123. Schwab C, Faschinger C, Ehgartner EM, et al. Ultrastrukturelle befunde der Hornhaut bei Xeroderman pigmentosum. *Fortschr Ophthalmol* 86:181, 1989.

124. Liu S, Christmas TJ, Kirby RS. Combined scleroidal and choroidal metastasis from prostatic carcinoma. *Br J Urol* 70:689, 1992.

125. Shields CL, Shields JA. Metastatic tumors to the uvea. *Int Ophthalmol Clin* 33:3, 1993.

126. Watson PG. Diseases of the sclera and episclera. In: Duane TD, ed. *Clinical Ophthalmology,* vol 4. New York: Harper and Row, 1978.

6

IRIDOCILIARY EPITHELIAL TUMORS

Robert L. Peiffer, Jr., Ronald C. Riis, and Bernard Clerc

The neuroepithelium that lines the posterior surface of the iris and the inner ciliary body and differentiates into retinal pigment epithelium has minimal tendencies toward neoplasia; iris and ciliary body epithelial tumors are extremely uncommon in humans and are occasionally encountered in cats, but are relatively common in dogs. Neoplasia arising from the retinal pigment epithelium is rare in any species. In contrast, these tissues have remarkable tendencies for reactive changes of hypertrophy, hyperplasia, and metaplasia.

ANIMALS

Historical Perspective. A bovine globe was diagnosed as having an "epithelioma of the nonpigmented cells of the ciliary body" in 1929.[1] Cotchin described a ciliary body carcinoma in a 7-year-old male cat.[2] Reports of cases in canine eyes are numerous. A "pigmented sarcoma" described by Leone in 1926, two cases reported by Ball and Zaessinger mentioned by Morgan,[3] and two cases alluded to by Saunders and Barron[4]—a "neuroepithelioma" reported by Nordmann and Hoerner in 1946 and a "tumor arising from the pars ciliaris retinae" described by Veenedall in 1954—were most likely adenomas or adenocarcinomas of the ciliary body. Of additional reported cases, one of Cotchin's cases[5] is of uncertain diagnosis, and a case reported by Saunders and Barron involved the iridal rather than ciliary body pigmented epithelium.[4] Peiffer[6] published the first large series of canine and feline cases in 1983, which was expanded upon by Dubielzig[7] in 1998; additional case reports or small series are found in the contemporary literature.[8–15] To the best of our knowledge, age-related hyperplasia (Fuch's adenoma) has not been described in animals.

Epidemiology. Ciliary body epithelial tumors are the second most common primary intraocular tumor in dogs, occurring about half as frequently as uveal melanomas.[6] They are probably rare tumors in other species. In dogs, adenomas and adenocarcinomas occur at roughly equal frequency. They are unilateral tumors of middle-aged or older animals without apparent breed or sex predisposition.

Clinical Appearance. Ciliary body adenomas and adenocarcinomas may present as either pigmented or nonpigmented cellular proliferations, presumably related to their origin from either the inner nonpigmented or outer pigmented layers, although one might theorize that tumors arising from the pigmented layer might undergo anaplastic changes with loss of melanogenic capability. Nonpigmented tumors appear pink, frequently with prominent surface vascularization, and are more common than pigmented proliferations, which range from gray to dark brown. These tumors usually appear solid (although they may be cystic) and may grow into the retroiridal and/or retrolental spaces and manifest as smooth-surfaced, lobulated space-occupying lesions behind the pupil, or extend through the base of the iris to present as an anterior chamber mass. Extension into the choroid may occur in an occasional case, but this is the exception rather than the rule. Adenomas tend to demonstrate an endophytic growth pattern, primarily involving the ciliary processes, whereas adenocarcinomas are more likely to invade adjacent tissues and present as anterior chamber or, less commonly, episcleral masses. Uveitis, glaucoma, and hemorrhage are not uncommon complications that may occur in either benign or malignant tumors. Uveitis, if it does occur, is postulated to result from soluble products of necrotic tumor tissue. Glaucoma may result when proliferating or invading tumor cells invade the iridocorneal angle, obliterating the ciliary cleft and obstructing the trabecular meshwork and trabecular veins. Involvement must be extensive, however, for increase in intraocular pressure to occur; 50% (180°) of the iridocorneal angle may be able to maintain normal pressure. Glaucoma more commonly occurs secondary to rubeosis irides; preiridal fibrovascular membrane formation is frequently associated with both adenomas and adenocarcinomas. Clinical differentials include other primary anterior uveal tumors, including melanomas, metastatic neoplasms, and benign cystic lesions of the iridal or ciliary epithelium (Figure 6.1).

Gross Features. These tumors vary in pigmentation from gray to dark brown; in general, they appear to lie between the glistening white appearance of medulloepitheliomas and the jet black that may characterize melanocytomas. They tend to have a somewhat irregular lobulated surface with variable vascularization. Adenocarcinomas may extend into iris root and the anterior chamber, posteriorly into the choroid, or intrasclerally and transsclerally. Adenomas tend to remain nodular proliferations of the inner ciliary body. Vitreous hemorrhage and asteroid hyalosis are not uncommon associates. Secondary changes may include those associated with glaucoma or exudative retinal detachment (Figure 6.2).

Histopathologic Features. The morphology of ciliary body epithelial tumors demonstrates a continuous spectrum from well-differentiated monomorphic epithelial cell populations to anaplastic adenocarcinomas with marked atypia and frequent mitoses. Ciliary body adenomas tend to be characterized by sheets and cords of well-differentiated epithelial cells with a distinct tendency to form adenoidal structures with eosinophilic secretory material. Cells are cuboidal or columnar. Melanin granules may be seen within tumor cells, and occasional cases contain areas of tumor necrosis. Although benign tumors may expand into the ciliary body, ciliary cleft, and iris base, extension into corneoscleral tissue is not observed, the majority of cases being confined to the ciliary processes and inner ciliary body stroma (Figure 6.2).

Iridocorneal angle changes include focal closure due to peripheral anterior synechiae related to anterior displacement of the iris leaf by the tumor mass, and/or rubeosis irides. A mild chronic nongranulomatous anterior uveitis may be present. Anterior chamber and/or vitreous hemorrhage may be seen. Asteroid hyalosis is seen in about 30% of cases; exudative retinal detachments are rarely seen.

Adenocarcinomas demonstrate less tendency to form adenoidal structures and tend to be arranged in solid sheets and cords of cells with less eosinophilic secretory material. These neoplasms are variable both in pleomorphism and mitotic index. Melanin granules are less likely to be a feature of adenocarcinomas. Areas of necrosis may be seen. The invasive nature of these tumors is characteristic with extension into choroid and corneoscleral tissues as well as iris and episcleral and orbital tissues. Related ocular pathology is variable, with secondary glaucoma commonly related to rubeosis irides and/or to direct invasion of the ciliary cleft and trabecular meshwork. Choroidal involvement may lead to exudative retinal detachment (Figure 6.3). Although no consistent distinguishing histochemical features between benign and malignant ciliary body epithelial tumors are observed, adenomas are more likely to produce periodic acid-Schiff (PAS)-positive basement membrane material that separates lobules of tumor cells. Both benign and malignant tumors of the ciliary epithelium may produce hyaluronic acid, perhaps related to their embryologic role in synthesis of vitreous.[16] PAS, Alcian blue, and colloidal iron stains reveal both intracellular and extracellular material that is neuraminidase resistant and hyaluronidase sensitive; this material is found inconsistently in both adenomas and adenocarcinomas. This feature may be of value in the histopathologic distinction between primary ciliary body adenocarcinoma and carcinomas elsewhere with metastasis to the eye. These neoplasms are not characterized by collagenous or reticular stroma, nor by mucin production.

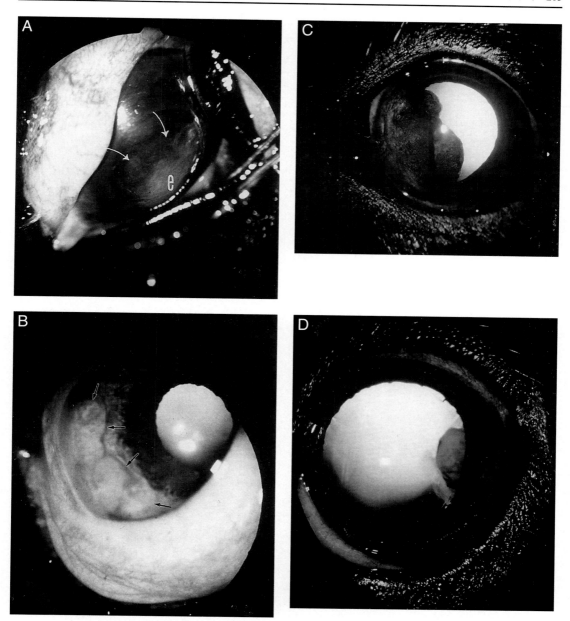

FIG. 6.1—Clinical appearance of ciliary body adenomas or adenocarcinomas. **A:** A pigmented adenoma in a 6-year-old Great Dane was suspected clinically to be an anterior uveal melanoma. The tumor presented as a lobulated dark brown retroiridal mass (arrows) with adjacent corneal edema (e). **B:** A ciliary body adenocarcinoma invaded the iris root in this 9-year-old English springer spaniel to present as a fleshy pink lesion involving the iris base from 7 to 10 o'clock (arrows). **C:** A retroiridal multilobulated lesion is seen in this 10-year-old German shepherd. The diagnosis was that of a low-grade adenocarcinoma. **D:** A ciliary body adenocarcinoma is seen as a pink vascularized retroiridal mass in this male mixed-breed dog. Note that the iris root is also involved. (Photograph D courtesy of Dr. K. Ketring.)

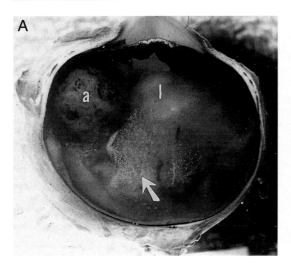

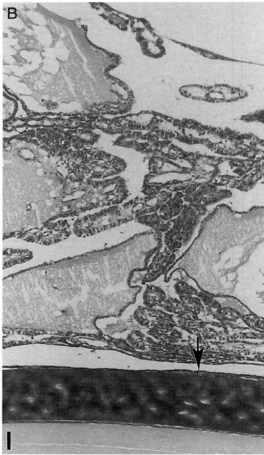

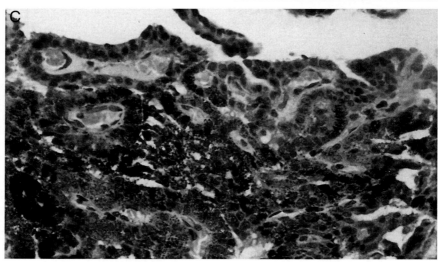

FIG. 6.2—Morphologic features of canine ciliary body adenomas. **A:** Ciliary body adenoma (a) is associated with asteroid hyalosis (arrow) in this 10-year-old beagle cross (l, lens). **B:** An adenoma in the eye of a 9-year-old female German shorthair pointer is characterized by cords of cuboidal cells with organization into adenoidal structures and pools of secretory material. A pseudomembrane of tumor cells line the anterior lens capsule (arrow) (l, lens). PAS, original magnification ×160. **C:** Pigment granules suggest origin from the outer pigmented epithelial layer. This clinical case is depicted in Figure 6.1A. Hematoxylin-eosin, original magnification ×500. (continued)

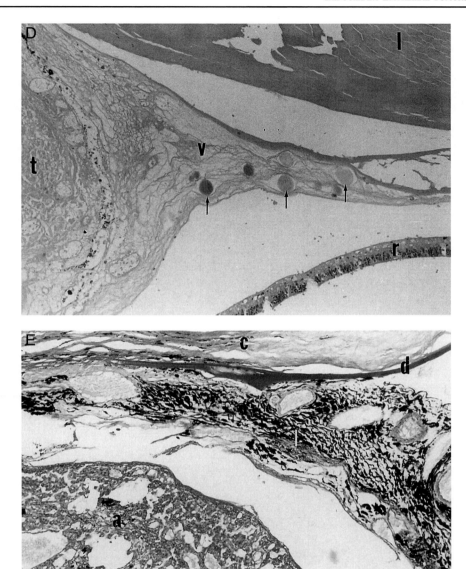

FIG. 6.2 (continued)—**D:** Hyphema and glaucoma complicated a necrotic adenoma (t) in this 8-year-old mixed-breed male. Note the associated retinal detachment (r). The vitreous (v) is characterized by asteroid hyalosis (arrows) (l, lens). Hematoxylin-eosin, ×125. **E:** A ciliary body adenoma (a) in this 7-year-old male Afghan hound resulted in anterior displacement of the iris leaflet with associated collapse of the ciliary cleft and closure of the angle (c, cornea; d, Descemet's membrane; i, iris). PAS, original magnification ×125.

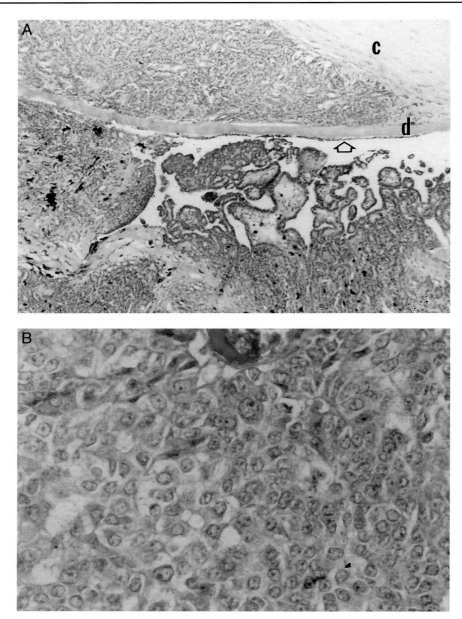

FIG. 6.3—Morphologic features of ciliary body adenocarcinomas. **A:** This neoplasm from a 7-year-old golden retriever was characterized by invasion of the peripheral cornea (c), with tumor cells dissecting along the outer aspect of Descemet's membrane (d). Tumor cells are also forming a neoplastic retrocorneal membrane (arrow). **B:** In this 6-year-old Irish setter, the ciliary body adenocarcinoma was characterized by large nuclei and moderate anisokaryosis. Hematoxylin-eosin, original magnification ×250. (continued)

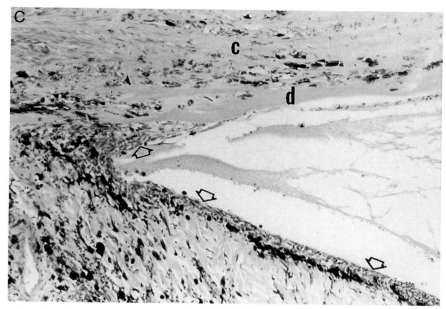

FIG. 6.3 (continued)—**C:** Secondary glaucoma occurred in this 9-year-old Maltese terrier due to preiridal fibrovascular membrane formation, which spans the angle (arrows) (c, cornea; d, Descemet's membrane). Hematoxylin-eosin, original magnification ×200.

A number of cases will lie between the bland morphology of benignity and the characteristic features of aggressive malignancy. It may be of clinical value to distinguish between those of "low grade" malignancy from markedly anaplastic tumors in terms of prognostication for potential metastatic disease.

Immunohistochemistry and Ultrastructure. A small number of cases studied have tended to be vimentin positive and desmin, cytokeratin, S-100 protein, and glial fibrillary acidic protein (GFAP) negative; because of the inconsistency and nonspecificity among cases, immunohistochemistry would appear to be of minimal value in distinguishing benign from malignant and primary from metastatic lesions. S-100 protein may be useful in distinguishing pigmented epithelial tumors from melanomas. Ultrastructural features of these tumors in animals have not been described.

Treatment and Prognosis. Presented with the case of a proliferative intraocular lesion for which routine examination techniques have failed to reveal a specific etiology, clinicians have four

alternatives: (1) to temporize and observe with frequent periodic rechecks to ascertain changes in size and thus indirectly biologic behavior, (2) to perform intraocular aspiration biopsy, (3) to perform excisional biopsy in an attempt to salvage the globe and vision, or (4) to enucleate the globe.

A prudent decision will be preceded by thorough physical and ocular examination, including thoracic radiographics and organ function tests to eliminate the possibility of preexisting metastases. It would appear that, similar to their human counterpart, ciliary body adenocarcinoma metastasis is uncommon. If metastatic disease is present, surgical intervention is generally not indicated, and the logical choice is to provide supportive therapy as necessary as long as the animal is comfortable or consider referral to an oncologist.

If metastatic workup is negative, attempts to define the extent of the tumor should be made, including gonioscopy, ultrasonography, and imaging techniques. Tumors that can be localized to the anterior uvea for less than 90° of circumference should be considered candidates for a partial cyclectomy or iridocyclectomy. The pedunculated nature of ciliary body adenomas

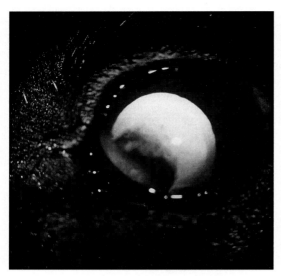

FIG. 6.4—The German shepherd depicted in Figure 6.1 after iridocyclectomy. A focal hemorrhage is present in the anterior vitreous.

may make them amenable to excision[11] simply by cautery-assisted resection of the ciliary processes involved (Figure 6.4). For malignant tumors that have invaded iris root, iridocyclectomy or iridocyclosclerectomy may be considered.

Localized or not, tumors complicated by inflammation, hemorrhage, and/or glaucoma may be either benign or malignant. It has been hypothesized, but not demonstrated, that secondary glaucoma may enhance metastasis of tumor cells; hemorrhage and uveitis may themselves cause secondary glaucoma, and any of these complications is likely to be difficult to control conservatively. It is of interest to note in the literature that the two confirmed cases of distant metastases of ciliary body adenocarcinomas both had glaucoma, and one had undergone intraocular surgery.[12,13] Prudent recommendations would include excision of pedunculated lesions and enucleation of globes harboring poorly defined invasive lesions, or eyes with uveitis or glaucoma. External or endo laser ablation may provide therapeutic options in the future.

Data are lacking to state definitively the advantages and disadvantages of needle aspiration of ocular fluids or intraocular tumors as diagnostic tools. Cytology of aqueous or vitreous aspirates is likely to be of value if cells can be observed during ophthalmic examination, and, if properly performed, the technique demonstrates low incidence of serious complications. However, these tumors tend to be cohesive. Direct biopsy of intraocular tumor masses, though potentially a source of diagnostic cytology, may cause intraocular hemorrhage, seed tumor cells, and enhance metastasis. Clinical distinction between certain intraocular tumors, and between benign and malignant ciliary body epithelial tumors, may be difficult, and needle aspiration may be of value if determination of tumor type (ciliary body epithelial tumor versus melanoma versus metastatic lesion) and biologic behavior (benign versus malignant) will provide information unobtainable by other means that will assist in the management of the particular case.

Medulloepitheliomas. Medulloepitheliomas in animals are rare primitive tumors of the neural epithelium. In humans, they are recognized in the brain, mostly the cerebral hemisphere, and in the eye. Medulloepitheliomas in domestic animals have been reported only in the eye.

Historically, Verhoeff in 1904 first described a "teratoneuroma" as a human intraocular tumor arising from the nonpigmented ciliary epithelium.[17] Because of the tumor's netlike appearance under low-power light microscopy, Fuchs referred to them as "diktyomas," which means netlike.[18] These terms did not gain wide acceptance, and in 1931 the tumor was named *medulloepithelioma,* which now seems to have withstood the test of time.[19]

Medulloepitheliomas in humans are unilateral congenital neoplasms that display no evidence of genetic transmission[20] and appear to be similar in animals. Zimmerman suggested that symptoms and signs leading to the recognition of medulloepitheliomas may not be evident until long after birth.[21]

Clinical diagnosis of these intraocular tumors is based on presenting clinical symptoms and a high index of suspicion. When confronted with an animal with an ocular complaint of poor vision, hyphema, glaucoma, and/or cataract with a mass in the ciliary body, a tumor type should include medulloepithelioma (Figures 6.5 and 6.6). Medulloepitheliomas are embryonal masses arising from the primitive medullary epithelium.[17] The ocular

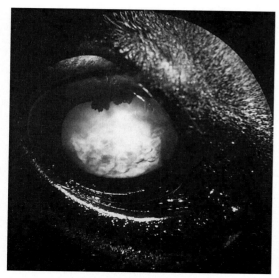

FIG. 6.5—Medulloepithelioma in the eye of a 3-year-old horse. The complaint was hemorrhage in the eye. The vascular network is on the surface of the mass, magnified by the lens. The mass was grossly pink.

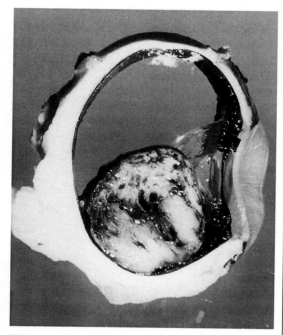

FIG. 6.6—The central calotte of the eye in Figure 6.1 shows the ventral location of the medulloepithelioma arising from the ciliary area.

and cerebral medulloepithelioma has as its hallmark an architectural pattern reminiscent of primitive medullary epithelium and, therefore, a capacity for multiple divergent differentiation. Irrespective of the differentiating capabilities of the fetal medullary epithelium, numerous observations in situ and in vitro, corroborated by electron-microscopic and immunohistochemical studies, have collectively shown that the central medulloblastoma is capable of differentiation along neuronal[16–26] and glial[22,26–33] lines, with sometimes divergent differentiation to both.[26,34,35]

The bipotential differentiating capacity of central medulloblastomas, probably best demonstrated in tissue culture, suggests that it may arise from a primitive neuroepithelial cell capable of two-directional differentiation.[34,35] The medulloblastoma and retinoblastoma are by far the most common of the embryonal tumors of the central nervous system (CNS) in humans,[36] but not in animals. Medulloepitheliomas of the eye in animals, as in humans, are classified into either *nonteratoid* or *teratoid,* and further divided into *benign* or *malignant.* Teratoid medulloepitheliomas contain one or more heterotopic tissues (i.e., nonneural), such as hyaline cartilage, rhabdomyoblasts, undifferentiated mesenchymal cells, and neuroglial cells. Nonteratoid medulloepithelioma contains tissue that resembles medullary epithelium, but may contain tissue derived from secondary optic vesicle, such as retinal pigment epithelium, ciliary epithelium, vitreous, and neuroglia.

By light microscopy, retinoblastomas are characterized by either neuroblastic rosettes (Homer Wright) or rosettes and fleurettes (Flexner-Wintersteiner) that mimic the cytologic and architectural features of rods and cones. Most in vitro studies have failed to demonstrate neuroglial differentiation of retinoblastomas.

Microscopically, medulloepitheliomas in the eye consist mainly of multilayered ribbons of poorly differentiated neuroepithelial cells that resemble the embryonal retina and ciliary epithelium. These sheets of medullary epithelium can fold back upon themselves to form multilayered complex structures (Figures 6.3 and 6.4). Elongated tubules and cystic structures typically contain hyaluronidase-sensitive mucopolysaccharide resembling primitive vitreous (Figure 6.5). Rosettes, larger than those seen in human retinoblastomas, are usually present in medulloepitheliomas.

ELECTRON MICROSCOPY. In defining CNS ependymomas and medulloepitheliomas, some significance has been given to the surface differentiations of the epithelium, particularly the cilia and/or blepharoplasts that constitute evidence in defining the origin.[37] Ocular medulloepithelioma is also papillary, its fine structure resembling ependymoma with definite cilia.[38]

Electron microscopically, cell structures arranged around lumina may have cilia and microvilli projecting into the lumen (Figure 6.6). A band of desmosome-like connections (zonula adherens) form intercellular adhesions near the lumen (Figure 6.7). If the cilia can be examined in cross section, they will show nine pairs of peripheral doublets without a central doublet.[38] These lumina are referred to as *rosettes* and *fleurettes,* both found in medulloepitheliomas and retinoblastomas. The lumen of the rosettes may have numerous elongated microvilli. A thin basement membrane on the basilar surface of the tubules can be enhanced by polarized light. Dense terminal bar complexes can be seen at the intercellular borders near the lumen of the rosette. The cytoplasm of the tumor cells contains scattered mitochondria, short profiles of rough-surfaced endoplasmic reticulum, free polyribosomes, Golgi lamellae, small vesicles, and a few lysosomes. Occasionally, pigment granules may also be present. Human retinoblastoma rosettes and fleurettes have distinctive ultrastructural markers, such as triple membranes around the nucleus and dense cytoplasmic core granules, which medulloepitheliomas lack.[38]

MEDULLOEPITHELIOMA BEHAVIOR. Criteria for malignancy in medulloepitheliomas of humans includes local invasion of other ocular structures and many poorly differentiated neuroepithelial cells with a high mitotic number.[38–41] Some authors believe that the malignant potential is greater in the teratoid variant of medulloepithelioma.[42–45] One report of one cow and four dog ocular teratoid medulloepitheliomas did not speculate on the probability of metastasis, but did classify all as malignant.[43]

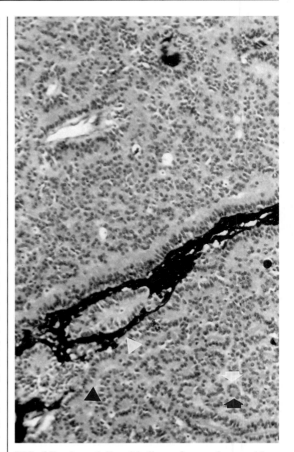

FIG. 6.7—A medulloepithelioma from a 6-year-old German shepherd with a long history of an ocular complaint. Note the cords (triangle) and circular pattern of cells forming lumens or rosette-like structures (arrow). Hematoxylin-eosin, ×10.

The histopathologic criteria for malignancy of both teratoid and nonteratoid medulloepitheliomas are (1) poorly differentiated neuroblastic cells that may resemble retinoblastomas, (2) marked pleomorphism and/or mitoses, (3) sarcomatous characteristics, and (4) invasion of other ocular structures with or without extraocular extension.[46]

Broughton and Zimmerman recommend local excision when the tumor is small and well circumscribed. In most cases, the location of the tumor in the ciliary body enables it to develop into a large size before it produces symptoms and signs. Keep in mind also that these tumors have a tendency to grow circumferentially with only mild thickening of the ciliary body, making ultrasound detection difficult. Enucleation is generally the required treatment for most of these tumors because of the possible extraocular spread and intraocular complications. It appears that these neoplasms generally cause death after extrascleral extension occurs by invasion through the orbit into the CNS. If the tumor is localized within the globe and has benign characteristics, the prognosis is good. An adult animal with an anterior medulloepithelioma has a better prognosis than if it were posteriorly located.[47–49] Metastasis to cervical and retropharyngeal lymph nodes was reported in one horse,[50] with extension from the globe into the orbit.[51] Ocular medulloepitheliomas metastasizing into skeletal muscle and optic nerve of cockatiels has been reported.[52] A large mass protruding from the optic nerve head into the vitreous cavity and posteriorly into the nerve of a horse was diagnosed as malignant medulloepithelioma.[52]

A group of authors reporting on a malignant teratoid medulloepithelioma in a dog retrospectively proposed that a feline chondrosarcoma of the ciliary body and a canine leiomyoma of the ciliary body may indeed be teratoid tumors of the ciliary body.[42,53]

Experiments with oncogenic alkylating[54] and viral[55] agents have shown that glial precursor cells in the embryo, glial precursor cells persisting in adult life, and differentiated glial cells in the adult brain may be involved equally in neoplastic transformation. The susceptibility of the opossum eye to ethylnitrosourea 100 mg/kg in a single or incremental dose at 1–4 weeks of postnatal life induced intraocular teratoid medulloepitheliomas.[54] Intracranial inoculation of rats, mice, and hamsters with human adenovirus type 12 induced neuroectodermal tumors.[55]

A transitional picture between human medulloepithelioma and diffuse anaplastic cerebellar astrocytoma (a rare but well-recognized event) is found mostly in older age groups, an observation that perhaps favors the view that medulloepithelioma is the result of anaplasia rather than an expression of embryonal tumor. The diagnosis of an embryonal tumor should, therefore, rest on its histologic features, not on an age-related presumption.[56]

HISTOCHEMICAL MARKERS. Tumors sectioned for light-microscopic evaluation should be histo-

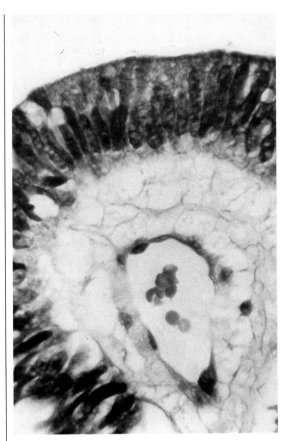

FIG. 6.8—Medulloepithelioma in a horse eye showing the columnar neuroepithelial characteristic morphology. Hematoxylin-eosin, ×40.

chemically stained with (1) hematoxylin-eosin, (2) Weigert's iron hematoxylin-picrofuchsin of van Gieson, (3) silver impregnations for reticulin fibers (Gordon-Sweet's method), (4) Mallory's phosphotungstic acid hematoxylin for muscle fibers, and (5) GFAP. The neuroepithelial tumor cells should also be stained for (1) neuron-specific enolase, (2) vimentin, (3) S-100 protein, and (4) synaptophysin.

In the CNS, GFAP is a marker for astroglial-committed cells. Cells committed to glial differentiation could be the target of oncogenesis at a considerably earlier age of fetal life than has been inferred from transplacental induction of neural tumors with alkylating agents.

Immunocytochemical studies of the glial fibrillary acidic protein in human neoplasms of the

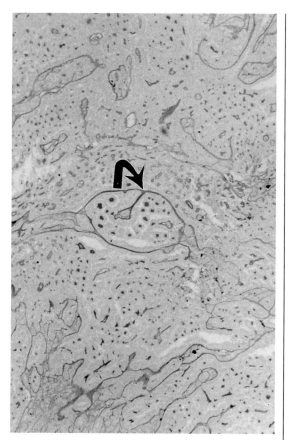

FIG. 6.9—Medulloepithelioma section from Figure 6.3 stained with PAS, ×10. Note the positive areas stained within the lumens (bent arrow).

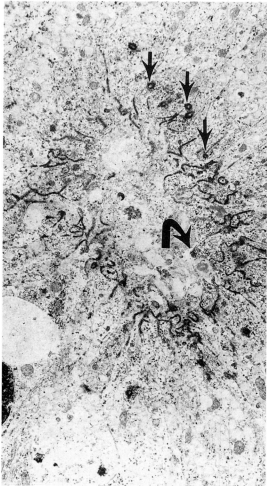

FIG. 6.10—Electron-microscopic view of a horse medulloepithelioma rosette lumina. Note the microvilli projecting into the lumen (bent arrow) and the cross sections of basal bodies or blepharoplasts (three small arrows). ×6000.

CNS found it useful in the diagnosis of astrocytic neoplasms and of mixed gliomas but negative in medulloepitheliomas.[57,58] None of the seven animal ocular medulloepitheliomas in our files are positive for GFAP. Two human ocular cases are reported[59] in which the adenoid patterns were associated with the development of conspicuous papillary formations composed of columnar cells resting on a basement membrane, mimicking the structures of a medulloepithelioma. The adenoid patterns (trabecular and pseudoglandular cell clusters) were interpreted as being anaplastic astrocytes partly because transitions to more mature, typical astrocytomatous areas were demonstrable and partly because some of these cells were immunopositive for GFAP.

An alternative interpretation of a malignant glioma with the presence of papillary structures representing a form of aberrant neoplastic differentiation rather than an expression of a neuroepithelial tumor of embryonal origin is made by Mork et al.,[59] who also state that (1) papillary formations of medulloepitheliomas are never GFAP positive, (2) increased anaplasia in an astrocytic glioma is typically associated with a loss of immunopositivity for GFAP, and (3) therefore only positive GFAP results are significant in the differential diagnosis.

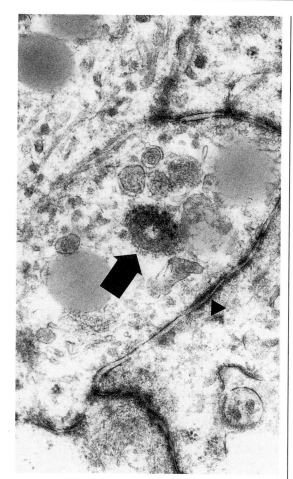

FIG. 6.11—Electron-microscopic appearance of a zonula adherens (triangle) adjacent to the lumen of a horse medulloepithelioma rosette. Also note that the cross section of a cilia (arrow), when perfectly cross-sectioned, should show nine pair of peripheral doublets without a central doublet. ×44,395.

Human CNS medulloepithelioma immunohistochemically stained for the presence of growth factors (basic fibroblast and insulin-like factor 1) were strongly immunoreactive within the neuroepithelial cell population of the tumor.[60] These growth factors may stimulate proliferation and differentiation of tumor cells by autocrine molecular mechanisms. There are no reports of growth factor staining in animal medulloepitheliomas.

The medulloepitheliomas in animals and humans bear a close resemblance, but because this tumor is rare, the number reported is low.

Medulloepitheliomas have been reported in birds,[61] cats,[42,54] cows,[43] dogs,[42,43,53] fish,[44] hamsters,[56] horses,[47–52] mice,[55] opossums,[54] and rats.[55]

HUMANS

Nomenclature. The ciliary body epithelium is derived from the anterior neuroectoderm of the optic cup; the outer layer differentiates into a pigmented monolayer that lies apex to apex with the nonpigmented inner layer. Its functions are to maintain the integrity of the blood ocular barrier in the region of the ciliary body and the secretion of the aqueous humor.

Tumors may arise from either layer and from primitive medulloepithelium (which is nonpigmented regardless of origin) or differentiated ciliary epithelium. The former are referred to as glioneuromas or medulloepitheliomas; the latter may contain heteroplastic elements, which, when present, add the description of *teratoid,* as all three germ layers are not present. The medullary epithelium may play a role in the evolution of true ocular teratomas, an extremely rare neoplasm with ectodermal, mesodermal, and endodermal derivatives. Medulloepitheliomas may be benign or malignant. Neoplasms arising from differentiated ciliary epithelium are labeled as either adenomas or adenocarcinomas.

Historical Perspective. In 1904, Verhoeff suggested the name "teratoneuroma" for a teratoid medulloepithelioma because he observed structures of neural origin in it.[62] Four years later, Fuchs observed that medulloepitheliomas frequently consisted of cells arranged in interlacing cords and coined the term "diktyoma," from the Greek *diktyos* meaning "net."[63] Grinker in 1931 noted that these tumors arise from the medullary epithelium.[64] Spencer and Jesberg formally recognized glioneuromas as choristomatous malformations of these tissues.[65] Studies by Zimmerman and colleagues[66–68] and by Broughton and Zimmerman[69] have been instrumental in the evolution of contemporary nomenclature.

Epidemiology. Glioneuromas are extremely rare, with only a few cases reported in the literature.

Most cases are recognized at birth or shortly thereafter.[66]

Medulloepithelioma is likewise a rare neoplasm, occurring much less commonly than retinoblastoma, which has an incidence of 1:15000. Like retinoblastoma, it is a disease of childhood. Although signs and symptoms most commonly develop between 2 and 4 years, age of initial diagnosis has been reported from 6 months to 41 years. There is no race, gender, or laterality predisposition.[69]

No data are available regarding the occurrence of ciliary body epithelial tumors; suffice to say that they are quite uncommon.

Age-related hyperplasia is rarely seen in the eyes of patients younger than age 50, and thereafter increases in frequency with age from about 10% at age 50–59 to 70% at age 80 and older.[70,71]

Clinical Features. Glioneuromas appear as white fleshy anterior chamber masses, usually located inferonasally or inferotemporally. They may be associated with colobomas of the ciliary body, commonly invading the iris root, and may extend transsclerally.[65,72–74]

Medulloepitheliomas may present with the following signs and symptoms in decreasing frequency: visual impairment; pain; a white-to-pink iris or ciliary body mass that may or may not be cystic (Figure 6.12); leukokoria due to tumor and/or retinal detachment; exophthalmos; glaucoma with megaloglobus; strabismus; dyscoria; epiphora; acquired heterochromia; and intraocular hemorrhage. Rubeosis irides is commonly present. These neoplasms may be associated with lens coloboma cataract and with persistent hyperplastic primary vitreous. Growth is commonly nodular, but may take the form of proliferative vascularized sheets across supporting surfaces, including anterior hyaloid, lens, and iris; iris seeding may occur.[69,75–94] Although usually of ciliary body origin, medulloepitheliomas may arise from the retina or optic nerve.[95–98]

Adenomas and adenocarcinomas of the ciliary epithelium appear as solid ciliary masses; adenomas tend to expand axially into the posterior chamber and anterior vitreous, whereas adenocarcinomas are more likely to invade the iris root and extend extrasclerally. Subluxated lenses, cataract, and glaucoma may occur secondarily. Clinical

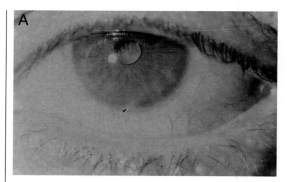

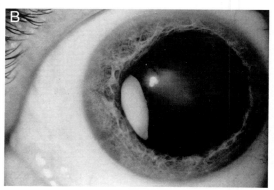

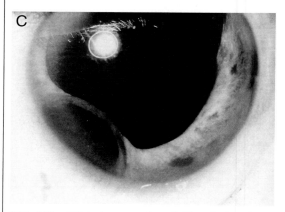

FIG. 6.12—Clinical presentation of ciliary body epithelial tumors. **A:** A 57-year old white man evaluated for cataract was noted to have a small pink tumor at the iris base at 6 o'clock (arrow) that proved to be a medulloepithelioma upon iridocyclectomy. (Courtesy of Joe Wachtel, MD, Georgiana Dvorak Theobald Meeting, 1977.) **B:** The presentation of a medulloepithelioma in this 58-year-old woman was as a white glistening mass lesion of the temporal ora serrata. (Courtesy of J.D. Cameron, MD, Georgianna Dvorak Theobald Meeting, 1988.) **C:** A pigmented adenocarcinoma inferiorly and medially extends through the iris root into the angle structures in this 56-year-old man. Clinically, the tumor was felt to be a melanoma. (Courtesy of N. Zakov, MD, Georgiana Dvorak Theobald Society Meeting, 1978.)

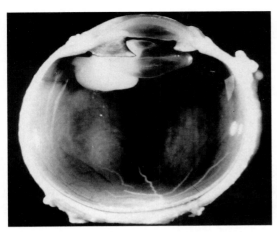

FIG. 6.13—Gross photograph of a malignant teratoid of medulloepithelioma in a 5-year-old girl. (Courtesy of Helmut Buchner, MD, Georgiana Dvorak Theobald Meeting, 1988.)

differentials would include melanomas and metastatic cancer to the ciliary body.[99–105] Age-related hyperplasia is seldom seen clinically except in rare cases where anterior extension into the iris occurs.[105,106]

Gross Pathology. Grossly, glioneuromas and medulloepitheliomas are irregular white or gray masses arising from the ciliary region, extending anteriorly into the iris root, posteriorly into the choroid, and internally into the posterior chamber or vitreous cavity (Figure 6.13).

Adenomas and adenocarcinomas appear as smooth, rounded lesions, of variable pigmentation.

Age-related hyperplasia may be unilateral or bilateral, solitary or multiple, and appears as white-to-gray opaque elongated lesions 0.5–2.0 mm, confined to a ciliary process. Extension into the iris root has been observed, but is rare.[70,71,105,106]

Histopathologic Features. Glioneuromas consist of well-differentiated neural tissue similar to brain, with an eosinophilic fibrillary background and neurons with coarse Nissl substance; neuroblastic rosettes may be encountered.[65,66,72–74]

Medulloepitheliomas have several characteristic histopathologic features that make diagnosis straightforward.[69,107,108] The tumor consists of two elements: rows of undifferentiated neuroepithelial tubules within a fibrillar mucoid matrix. Epithelial cells are arranged in convoluted multilayered patterns of elongated interlacing cords such that they may mimic embryonic retina. The epithelial cells may form rosette structures around a central lumen. Although both Homer Wright and Flexner-Wintersteiner rosettes may be seen, the typical rosettes of medulloepithelioma are larger than those in retinoblastoma. Tubular lumens contain fibrils and hyaluronic acid analogous to vitreous. The matrix consists of loose stroma composed of delicate fibrils with abundant ground substance that likewise resembles primitive vitreous (Figure 6.14A).

Teratoid medulloepitheliomas may contain, in addition, cartilage, neural tissues, and rhabdomyoblastic elements; the latter may mimic ganglion cells by light microscopy, but are differentiated by ultrastructure (Figure 6.14B).[109,110]

Broughton and Zimmerman used the following criteria for malignancy: (1) degree for differentiation of neuroblastic cells, (2) pleomorphism and mitotic activity of these cells, (3) sarcomatous features of heteroplastic tissue in teratoid medulloepitheliomas, and (4) invasion of adjacent tissues with or without extraocular extension. Of their 56 reported cases, 68% were histologically malignant.[69]

Adenomas are composed of cuboidal or columnar epithelial cells arranged in cords or tubules. Adenocarcinomas display loss of adenoidal organization and appear as sheets of cells with typical malignant features. Both benign and malignant tumors can be distinguished from metastatic lesions by their unique characteristic of hyaluronic acid production, evidenced by staining with Alcian blue and treatment with hyaluronidase.[66]

Age-related hyperplasia is characterized by irregular cords of nonpigmented ciliary epithelium separated by often abundant PAS-positive basement membrane-like material (Figure 6.14D and E).

Ultrastructure. Several ocular medulloepitheliomas have been described in the literature.[107,111,112] The tumor cells are arranged around lumina, into which slender microvilli and cilia without central doublets project. Terminal bar complexes and zonula adherens and zonula occludens are present. Invaginating gap junctions are characteristic. Cytoplasm contains sparse

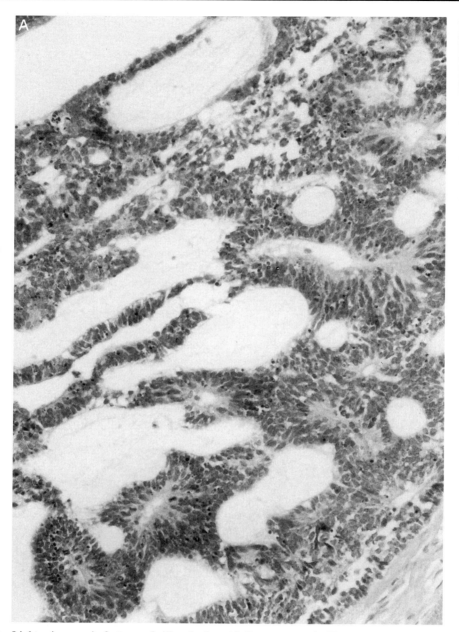

FIG. 6.14—Light-microscopic features of ciliary body epithelium tumors. **A:** The tumor depicted in Figure 6.1B was composed of cords of undifferentiated small cells encircling fibrillar tissue, and characteristic of a small non-teratoid medulloepithelioma. Hematoxylin-eosin, original magnification ×200. (continued)

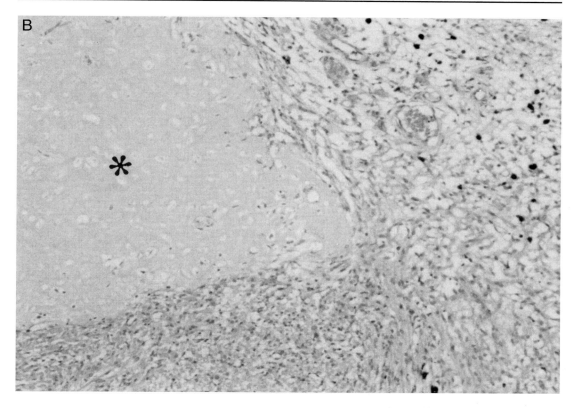

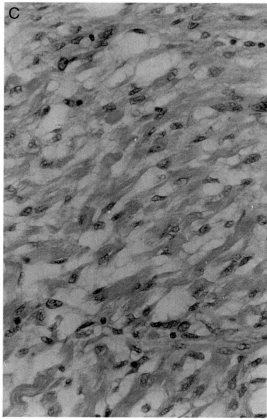

FIG. 6.14 (continued)—**B and C:** A malignant teratoid medulloepithelioma destroyed the globe in this 15-year-old Arabian male. Both cartilaginous differentiation (*) **(B)** and rhabdomyosarcomatous **(C)** differentiation were present. Hematoxylin-eosin, ×100 **(B)** and ×400 **(C).** (Courtesy of H.C. Mansor, MD, Georgiana Dvorak Theobald Meeting, 1980.) (continued)

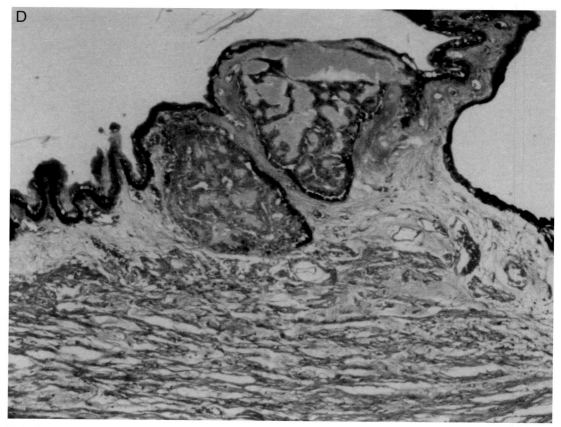

FIG. 6.14 (continued)—**D and E:** Fuch's adenoma (benign hyperplasia) is usually confined to the ciliary processes and anterior ciliary body **(D)**. (continued)

microfilaments, a well-developed Golgi apparatus, and mitochondria. Rough-surfaced endoplasmic reticulum, neurotubules, and polyribosomes are conspicuous toward the lateral aspect of the cells, and melanin granules, lipofucsin, and compound granules are variably present.

Ultrastructural features of a hamartomatous adenoma of the nonpigmented epithelium arising in an anterior uveal coloboma were characterized by cells with convoluted nuclei and complex cell membrane interdigitations; gap junctions and desmosomes are present, with basement membrane production at the basal surface.[113]

Immunohistochemistry. Immunohistochemistry of medulloepitheliomas of the ciliary body[114,115] has shown that neuroepithelial tumor cells are positive for neuron-specific enolase,

vimentin, and often for S-100 protein. Neuroblastic tumor cells are positive for neuron-specific enolase and synaptophysin. Glial-like tumor cells are positive for vimentin, glial fibrillary acidic protein, and S-100 protein.

Treatment and Prognosis. Most ciliary body epithelial tumors are benign or only locally invasive, and thus the prognosis is generally good. Glioneuromas, as choristomatous lesions, are benign, but focally destructive. About two-thirds of medulloepitheliomas have histologic evidence of malignancy, but the mortality rate is only about 10%, though most patients eventually lose the involved eye.[69] In regard to medulloepitheliomas, the most important prognostic feature is extraocular extension. As radiation and chemotherapy are of unestablished benefit, optimal therapy involves

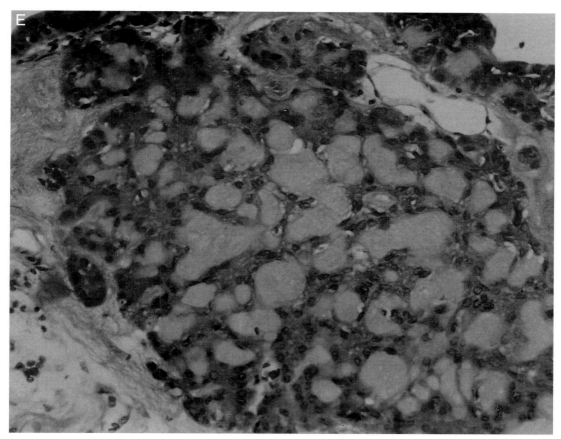

FIG. 6.14 (continued)—Histologically, the lesion is composed of cords of proliferative epithelial cells surrounding PAS-positive material **(E)**. Hematoxylin-eosin, original magnification ×12.5 **(D)** and ×310 **(E)**.

early recognition and surgical intervention, which can take the form of local excision of small circumscribed tumors by iridocyclectomy or block excision; enucleation, if a large extensive tumor is confined to the globe; or exenteration, if orbital extension is present.

The association between pineoblastoma and retinoblastoma is well established. A single case of pineoblastoma associated with a medulloepithelioma has been reported,[104] and the potential for the dual occurrence of these tumors should be appreciated.

Data regarding the biologic behavior of ciliary body epithelial tumors are limited; an adenoma expands slowly and creates morbidity by virtue of being a space-occupying posterior chamber lesion with compression of the lens. Tumor-associated uveitis, glaucoma, and intraocular hemorrhage are more likely to be associated with adenocarcinoma. It would seem that even tumors with malignant features metastasize rarely. Reasonable management would include observation of small suspected adenomas, with iridocyclectomy or enucleation of rapidly growing lesions.

REFERENCES

1. Ball V, Zaessinger J. Cancer des proces ciliares. *Bull Soc Sci Vet Lyon* 32:220, 1929.
2. Cotchin E. Neoplasms in the cat. *Vet Rec* 69:425, 1957.
3. Morgan A. Ocular tumors in animals. *Trans Ophthalmol Soc UK* 89:335, 1960.
4. Saunders LZ, Barron CN. Primary pigmented intraocular tumors in animals. *Can Res* 18:234, 1958.
5. Cotchin E. Further observations on neoplasms in dogs, with particular reference to site of origin and malignancy. *Br Vet J* 110:274, 1959.

6. Peiffer RL Jr. Ciliary body epithelial tumors in the dog and cat: a report of thirteen cases. *J Small Anim Pract* 24:347, 1983.

7. Dubielzig RR. Iridociliary epithelial tumors in 100 dogs and 17 cats: a morphological study. *Vet Ophthalmol* 1:223, 1998.

8. Verwer MAJ, Ten Thije PA. Tumor of the epithelioma of the ciliary body in a dog. *J Small Anim Pract* 8:627, 1967.

9. Bellhorn RW, Henkind P. Adenocarcinoma of the ciliary body. *Pathol Vet* 5:133, 1967.

10. Gelatt KN, Henry JD, Strafuss AC. Excision of an adenocarcinoma of the iris and ciliary body in a dog. *J Am Anim Hosp Assoc* 6:59, 1970.

11. Bellhorn RW, Vainisi SJ. Successful removal of ciliary body adenoma. *Mod Vet Pract* 50:47, 1964.

12. Bellhorn RW. Ciliary body adenocarcinoma in the dog. *J Am Vet Med Assoc* 159:1124, 1971.

13. Glickstein JQ. Malignant ciliary body adenocarcinoma in a dog. *J Am Vet Med Assoc* 165:455, 1974.

14. Peiffer RL Jr, Gwin R, Gelatt KN, Jacobson WE, Williams LW, Hill CW. Ciliary body epithelial tumors in four dogs. *J Am Vet Med Assoc* 172:570, 1978.

15. Schaffer EH, Thyssen C. Adenoma and adenocarcinoma of the iris and ciliary body epithelium in the dog. *Tierarztl Prax* 15:73, 1987.

16. Zimmerman LE, Fine BS. Production of hyaluronic acid by cysts and tumors of the ciliary body. *Arch Ophthalmol* 72:365, 1969.

17. Verhoeff FH. A rare tumor arising from the pars ciliaris retinae (terato-neuroma) of a nature hitherto unrecognized, and its relation to the so-called glioma retinae. *Trans Am Ophthalmol Soc* 10:351, 1904.

18. Fuchs E. Wucherungen und Geschwülste des Ciliarepithels. *Graefes Arch Ophthalmol* 68:534, 1908.

19. Grinker RR. Gliomas of the retina including the results of studies with silver impregnations. *Arch Ophthalmol* 5:920, 1931.

20. Anderson SR. Medulloepithelioma of the retina. *Int Ophthalmol Clin* 2:483, 1962.

21. Zimmerman LE. Verhoeff's "terato-neuroma": a critical reappraisal in light of new observations and current concepts of embryonic tumors. *Am J Ophthalmol* 72:1039, 1971.

22. Camins MB, Cravioto HM, Epstein F, Ransohoff J. Medulloblastoma: an ultrastructural study—evidence of astrocytic and neuronal differentiation. *Neurosurgery* 6:398, 1980.

23. Erwel AE, Brucher JM. Arguments ultrastructurax enforeurde l'appartenance du medulloblastome à la lignée neuronale. *Acta Neurol Belg* 74:208, 1974.

24. Liss L. Glial and parenchymal neoplasms in tissue culture. In: Scharenberg K, Liss L, eds. *Neuroectodermal Tumors of the Central and Peripheral Nervous System.* Baltimore: Williams and Wilkins, 1969:183.

25. Moss TH. Evidence for differentiation in medulloblastomas appearing primitive on light microscopy: an ultrastructural study. *Histopathology* 7:919, 1983.

26. Roessmann U, Velasco ME, Gambetti P, Autilio-Gambetti L. Neuronal and astrocytic differentiation in human neuroepithelial neoplasms: an immunohistochemical study. *J Neuropathol Exp Neurol* 42:113, 1983.

27. Barnard RO, Pambakian H. Astrocytic differentiation in medulloblastoma. *J Neurol Neurosurg Psychiatry* 43:1041, 1980.

28. Deck JHN, Eng LF, Bigbee J, et al. The role of glial fibrillary acidic protein in the diagnosis of central nervous system tumors. *Acta Neuropathol (Berl)* 42:183, 1978.

29. Eng LF, Rubinstein LS. Contribution of immunohistochemistry to diagnostic problems of human cerebral tumors. *J Histochem Cytochem* 26:513, 1978.

30. Mannoji H, Takeshita I, Fukui M, Ohta M, Kitamura K. Glial fibrillary acidic protein in medulloblastoma. *Acta Neuropathol (Berl)* 55:63, 1981.

31. Moss TH. Evidence for differentiation in medulloblastomas appearing primitive on light microscopy: an ultrastructural study. *Histopathology* 7:919, 1983.

32. Palmer JO, Kasselberg AG, Netsky MG. Differentiation of medulloblastoma: studies including immunohistochemical localization of glial fibrillary acidic protein. *J Neurosurg* 55:161, 1981.

33. Velasco ME, Dahl D, Roessmann U, Gambetti P. Immunohistochemical localization of glial fibrillary acidic protein in human glial neoplasms. *Cancer* 45:484, 1980.

34. Herman MM, Rubinstein LJ. Divergent glial and neuronal differentiation in a cerebellar medulloblastoma in an organ culture system: in vitro occurrences of synaptic ribbons. *Acta Neuropathol (Berl)* 65:10, 1984.

35. Markesbery WR, Walsh JW, Frye MD. Ultrastructural study of the medulloblastoma in tissue culture. *J Neuropathol Exp Neurol* 39:30, 1980.

36. Becker LE, Hinton D. Primitive neuroectodermal tumors of the central nervous system. *Hum Pathol* 14:538, 1983.

37. Rubinstein LJ. Embryonal central neuroepithelial tumors and their differentiating potential. *J Neurosurg* 62:795, 1985.

38. Jakobiec FA, Howard GM, Ellsworth RM, Rosen M. Electron microscopic diagnosis of medulloepithelioma. *Am J Ophthalmol* 79:321, 1975.

39. Zimmerman LE. The remarkable polymorphism of tumors of the ciliary epithelium. *Trans Aust Coll Ophthalmol* 2:114, 1970.

40. Zimmerman LE, Font RL, Anderson SR. Rhabdomyosarcomatous differentiation in malignant intraocular medulloepitheliomas. *Cancer* 30:817, 1972.

41. Harry J, Morgan G. Pathology of a unique type of teratoid medulloepithelioma. *Br J Ophthalmol* 63:132, 1979.

42. Barron CN, Saunders LZ. Intraocular tumors in animals: II. Primary nonpigmented intraocular tumors. *Cancer Res* 19:1171, 1959.

43. Langloss JM, Zimmerman LE, Krehribiel JD. Malignant intraocular teratoid medulloepithelioma in three dogs. *Vet Pathol* 13:343, 1976.

44. Lahav M, Albert DM. Medulloepithelioma of the ciliary body in the goldfish (*Carassius auratus*). *Vet Pathol* 15:208, 1978.

45. Saunders LZ, Barron CN. Primary pigmented intraocular tumors in animals. *Cancer Res* 18:234, 1958.

46. Broughton WL, Zimmerman LE. A clinicopathologic study of 56 cases of intraocular medulloepitheliomas. *Am J Ophthalmol* 85:407, 1978.

47. Bistner SI. Medulloepithelioma of the iris and ciliary body in a horse. *Cornell Vet* 64:588, 1974.

48. Szymanski CM. Malignant teratoid medulloepithelioma in a horse. *J Am Vet Med Assoc* 190:301, 1987.

49. Riis RC, Scherlie PH, Rebhun WC. Intraocular medulloepithelioma in a horse. *Equine Vet J* 10:66, 1990.

50. Folger AF. To Tifaelde of Retinaglism Hos Hesten, Aarsskrift, Den Kongelige Veterinaer-og Landbohøjskole, 1919:257-282.

51. Blodi RC, Ramsey FK. Ocular tumors in domestic animals. *Am J Ophthalmol* 64:627, 1967.

52. Eagle RC, Font RL, Swerczek TW. Malignant medulloepithelioma of the optic nerve in a horse. *Vet Pathol* 15:488, 1978.

53. Lahav M, Albert DM, Kircher CH, Percy DH. Malignant teratoid medulloepithelioma in a dog. *Vet Pathol* 13:11, 1976.

54. Jurejelski W Jr, Hudson P, Falk HL. Tissue differentiation and susceptibility to embryonal tumor induction by ethylnitrosourea in the opossum. *Natl Cancer Inst Monogr* 51:123, 1979.

55. Ogawa K. Embryonal neuroepithelial tumors induced by human adenovirus type 12 in rodents. *Acta Neuropathol (Berl)* 78:232, 1989.

56. Rubinstein LJ, Herman MM, Hanberry JW. The relationship between differentiating medulloblastoma and differentiating diffuse cerebellar astrocytoma: light, electron microscopic tissue and organ culture observations. *Cancer* 33:675, 1974.

57. Choi BH, Kim RC. Expression of glial fibrillary acidic protein in immature oligodendroglia. *Science* 223:407, 1984.

58. Tascos NA, Parr J, Gonatos NK. Immunocytochemical study of the GFAP in human neoplasms of the CNS. *Hum Pathol* 13:454, 1982.

59. Mork SJ, Rubinstein LJ, Kepes JJ. Patterns of epithelial metaplasia in malignant gliomas: I. Papillary formations mimicking medulloepitheliomas. *J Neuropathol Exp Neurol* 47:93, 1988.

60. Shiurba RA, Buffinger NS, Spencer EM, Urich H. Basic fibroblast growth factor and somatomedin C in human medulloepithelioma. *Cancer* 68:798, 1991.

61. Schmidt RE, Becker LL, McElroy JM. Malignant intraocular medulloepithelioma in two cockatiels. *J Am Vet Med Assoc* 189:1105, 1986.

62. Verhoeff FH. A rare tumor arising from the pars ciliaris retinae (terato-neuroma) of a nature hitherto unrecognized and its relation to the so-called glioma retinae. *Trans Am Ophthalmol Soc* 10:351, 1904.

63. Fuchs E. Wucherangen and Seshwulste de Ziliarepithels. *Graefes Arch Ophthalmol* 68:534, 1908.

64. Grinker RR. Gliomas of the retina including results of studies with silver impregnation. *Arch Ophthalmol* 5:920,1931.

65. Spencer WH, Jesberg DO. Glioneuroma (choristomatous malformation of the optic cup margin). *Arch Ophthalmol* 89:387, 1973.

66. Zimmerman LE. The remarkable polymorphism of tumors of the ciliary epithelium: Part 1. the Norman McAlister Gregg Lecture. *Trans Aust Coll Ophthalmol* 2:114, 1990.

67. Zimmerman LE. Verhoeff's "terato-neuroma": a clinical reappraisal in light of new observations and current concepts of embryonic tumors—the Fourth F.H. Verhoeff Lecture. *Trans Am Ophthalmol Soc* 69:210, 1971.

68. Zimmerman LE, Sobin LH. Histological typing of tumors of the eye and its adnexae. In: *International Histological Classification of Tumors,* vol 20. Geneva: World Health Organization, 1978.

69. Broughton WI, Zimmerman LE. A clinicopathologic study of 56 cases of intraocular medulloepitheliomas. *Am J Ophthalmol* 85:407, 1978.

70. Iliff WJ, Green WR. The incidence and location of Fuch's adenoma. *Arch Ophthalmol* 88:249, 1972.

71. Bronwyn Bateman J, Foos RY. Coronal adenomas. *Arch Ophthalmol* 97:2379, 1979.

72. Kuhlenbeck H, Haymaker W. Neuroectodermal tumors containing neoplastic neuronal elements: ganglioneuroma, spongioneuroblastoma and glioneuroma. *Milit Surg* 99:273, 1946.

73. Addison DJ, Font RL. Glioneuroma of iris and ciliary body. *Arch Ophthalmol* 102:419, 1984.

74. Manz HJ, Rosen DA, Macklin RD, et al. Neuroectodermal tumors of the anterior lip of the optic cup. *Arch Ophthalmol* 89:382, 1973.

75. Fralick FB, Wilder HC. Intraocular diktyoma and glioneuroma. *Trans Am Ophthalmol Soc* 47:317, 1949.

76. Malone RGS. Dictyoma. *Br J Ophthalmol* 39:429, 1955.

77. DeBuen S, Gonzales-Angulo A. Dictyoma (embryonal medulloepithelioma). *Am J Ophthalmol* 49:606, 1960.

78. Gifford H. A cystic diktyoma. *Surv Ophthalmol* 11:557, 1966.

79. Shields JA, Shields CL, Schwartz RL. Malignant teratoid medulloepithelioma of the ciliary body simulating persistent hyperplastic primary vitreous. *Am J Ophthalmol* 107:296, 1989.

80. Shivde AV, Kher A, Junnarkar RV. Diktyoma. *Br J Ophthalmol* 53:352, 1969.

81. Apt L, Heller MD, Moskovitz M, et al. Dictyoma (embryonal medulloepithelioma): recent review and case report. *J Pediatr Ophthalmol* 10:30, 1973.

82. Green WR, Iliff WJ, Trotter RR. Malignant teratoid medulloepithelioma of the optic nerve. *Arch Ophthalmol* 91:451, 1974.

83. Morris AT, Garner A. Medulloepithelioma involving the iris. *Br J Ophthalmol* 59:276, 1975.

84. Virji MA. Medulloepithelioma presenting as a perforated, infected eye. *Br J Ophthalmol* 61:229, 1977.

85. Yanko L, Behar A. Teratoid intraocular medulloepithelioma. *Am J Ophthalmol* 85:850, 1978.

86. Floyd BB, Minckler DS, Valentin L. Intraocular medulloepithelioma in a 79 year old man. *Ophthalmology* 89:1088, 1982.

87. Brownstein S, Barsoum-Homsy M, Conway VH, et al. Non-teratoid medulloepithelioma of the ciliary body. *Ophthalmology* 91:1118, 1984.

88. Pe'er J, Hidayat AH. Malignant teratoid medulloepithelioma manifesting as a black epibulbar mass with expulsive hemorrhage. *Arch Ophthalmol* 102:1523, 1984.

89. Litricin O, Latkaovic Z. Malignant teratoid medulloepithelioma in an adult. *Ophthalmologica* 191:17, 1985.

90. Canning CR, McCartney ACE, Hungerford J. Medulloepithelioma (diktyoma). *Br J Ophthalmol* 72:764, 1988.

91. Carrillo R, Streeten BW. Malignant teratoid medulloepithelioma in an adult. *Arch Ophthalmol* 97:695, 1979.

92. Hennis H, Saunders R, Shields JA. Malignant teratoid medulloepithelioma of the ciliary body. *J Clin Neuro Ophthalmol* 10:291, 1990.

93. Hausmann N, Stefani FH. Medulloepithelioma of the ciliary body. *Acta Ophthalmol* 69:398, 1991.

94. Mamalis N, Font RL, Anderson CW, Manson MC, Williams AT. Concurrent benign teratoid medulloepithelioma and pineoblastoma. *Ophthalmic Surg* 23:403, 1992.

95. Reese AB. Medulloepithelioma (dictyoma) of the optic nerve. *Am J Ophthalmol* 44:4, 1957.

96. Anderson SR. Medulloepithelioma of the retina. *Int Ophthalmol Clin* 2:483, 1962.

97. Mullaney J. Primary malignant medulloepithelioma of the retinal stalk. *Am J Ophthalmol* 77:499, 1974.

98. Wadsworth JAC. Epithelial tumors of the ciliary body. *Am J Ophthalmol* 32:1487, 1949.

99. Harris JL, Gumucio CC, Ophanion MB. Adenocarcinoma of the ciliary epithelium. *Arch Ophthalmol* 80:217, 1968.

100. Dryja TP, Albert DM, Horns D. Adenocarcinoma arising from the epithelium of the ciliary body. *Ophthalmology* 88:1290, 1981.

101. Shields JA, Augsburger JJ, Wallar PH, et al. Adenoma of the nonpigmented epithelium of the ciliary body. *Ophthalmology* 90:1528, 1983.

102. Jain IS, Gupta A, Ram J. Adenocarcinoma of ciliary epithelium in a young boy. *Ann Ophthalmol* 19:236, 1987.

103. Takagi T, Tsuda N, Watanabe F, et al. An epithelioma of the ciliary body. *Ophthalmologica* 195:13, 1987.

104. Rodrigues M, Hidayat A, Karesh J. Pleomorphic adenocarcinoma of ciliary epithelium simulating an epibulbar tumor. *Am J Ophthalmol* 106:595, 1988.

105. Keyes JEL, Moore PG. Adenomatous hyperplasia of the epithelium of the ciliary body. *Arch Ophthalmol* 19:39, 1938.

106. Zaidman GW, Johnson BL, Salamon SM, et al. Fuchs' adenoma affecting the peripheral iris. *Arch Ophthalmol* 101:771, 1983.

107. Iwamoto T, Witmer R, Landolt E. Diktyoma: a clinical, histological, and electron microscopic observation. *Graefes Arch Klin Exp Ophthalmol* 172:293, 1967.

108. Arora R, Sachdev MS, Mohan M. Intraocular medulloepithelioma: pitfalls in the cytological diagnosis. *Orbit* 6:275, 1987.

109. Zimmerman LE, Font RL, Anderson SY. Rhabdomyosarcomatous differentiation in malignant intraocular medulloepitheliomas. *Cancer* 30:817, 1972.

110. Harry J, Morgan G. Pathology of a unique type of teratoid medulloepithelioma. *Br J Ophthalmol* 63:132, 1979.

111. Jakobiec FA, Howard GM, Ellsworth RM, et al. Electron microscopic diagnosis of medulloepithelioma. *Am J Ophthalmol* 79:321, 1975.

112. Orellana J, Moura RA, Font RL, et al. Medulloepithelioma diagnosed by ultrasound and vitreous aspirate. *Ophthalmology* 90:1531, 1983.

113. Patrinely JR, Font RL, Campbell RJ, et al. Hamartomatous adenoma of the nonpigmented ciliary epithelium arising in iris ciliary body coloboma: light and electron microscopic observations. *Ophthalmology* 90:1540, 1983.

114. Kivela T, Tarkkanhen A. Recurrent medulloepithelioma of the ciliary body: immunohistochemical characteristics. *Ophthalmology* 95:1565, 1988.

115. Desai V, Lieb WE, Donoso LA, et al. Photoreceptor cell differentiation in intraocular medulloepithelioma: an immunohistopathologic study. *Arch Ophthalmol* 108:481, 1990.

7

UVEAL MELANOCYTIC TUMORS

John R.B. Mould, Simon M. Petersen-Jones, Claudio Peruccio, Alessandra Ratto, Joseph W. Sassani, and J. William Harbour

A study of uveal melanomas of dogs, cats, and humans will reveal fascinating similarities and contrasts. In all three species, melanocytic neoplasia is the most common primary intraocular neoplasm. In dogs, the majority arise from the anterior segment and are benign with marked similarities to human melanocytomas. In cats, the most common variant is a diffuse process that arises on the anterior surface of the iris in what can be a prolonged premalignant phase, with malignant transformation frequently accompanied by secondary glaucoma and the tendency for long periods of latency before the clinical manifestations of metastatic disease, which occurs in approximately 30%–50% of patients. In humans, uveal melanomas most commonly arise from the choroid and demonstrate morphologic variants that allow reasonable predictability of biologic behavior; as with cats, the mortality rate is about 50%, and years may pass before metastatic disease may manifest.

Knowledge of uveal melanomas in other species is limited to isolated case reports or small series.

DOGS

Anterior Uveal Melanoma

HISTORICAL PERSPECTIVES. The study of intraocular melanomas in dogs is a generation behind that of comparable lesions in humans. The Callender classification[1] in 1931 was a landmark in understanding the biology of human choroidal melanomas, but it was 50 years before the publication of several series of well-documented cases established the differences between the disease in the two species.

The first series was published in 1958 by Saunders and Barron,[2] who also summarized previous reports of pigmented intraocular tumors of all types and in all species. They described 15 new cases of pigmented tumors in the dog, of which 11 were melanomas. From the high incidence of local recurrence and distant metastases, they concluded that the biologic behavior was similar to that of melanomas in humans, a conclusion that has not been sustained by series published later. Magrane summarized six further cases in 1965,[3] but it was not until the 1980s that larger series established reliable data on which present knowledge is based.[4–9] Wilcock and Peiffer recognized that canine melanomas were distinct from their human counterparts, could not be readily compartmentalized using Callendar's classification scheme, and noted the similarity of many of these canine neoplasms to human melanocytoma.[9]

EPIDEMIOLOGY. Anterior uveal melanoma is regarded as the most common intraocular tumor in dogs,[10–15] as evidenced by the published series and the relative numbers of tumors submitted for pathologic examination. It comprises only a small proportion of all ophthalmic diagnoses and of all neoplasms in dogs. Most recorded cases are in middle-aged or older dogs, with an average age of at least 7 years at the time of diagnosis. There is evidence of a smaller but significant number of cases occurring among younger dogs. Three dogs under 2 years of age were described with benign iris lesions.[16] Other reports have found a bimodal age distribution and described benign spindle cell lesions in young dogs.[4,5] These cases are uncommon, and whether they represent a separate category is not clear. There appears to be no sex predilection for anterior uveal melanomas; suspicion of an autosomal recessively inherited neoplasm has been noted in Labrador retrievers, and published series suggest overrepresentation of German shepherds. Etiologic factors are unknown in

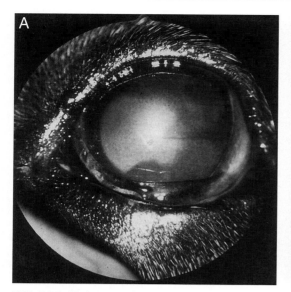
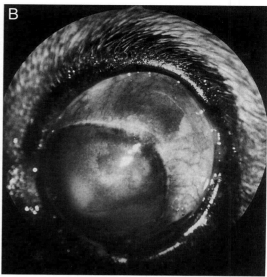

FIG. 7.1—Clinical examination often fails to enable an accurate assessment of the size and distribution of an intraocular tumor. **A:** There is glaucoma with secondary corneal edema, and a pigmented mass can be discerned with difficulty within the eye. **B:** There is an area of scleral and episcleral pigmentation strongly suggesting transscleral extension of a uveal melanoma. Figure 7.4 illustrates the full extent of this tumor.

spontaneous cases, but radiation was shown to induce a high incidence of ciliary-body melanomas in experimental beagles.[17] Anterior uveal melanoma is, therefore, typically a sporadic and uncommon tumor found in older dogs with no other relevant epidemiologic factors.

CLINICAL FEATURES. The clinical features of anterior uveal melanoma relate to the tumor itself and to its secondary effects. Simple intraocular examination often reveals a pigmented mass, but the full extent of tumors arising in the ciliary body and extending around the lens and into the vitreous cavity may not be appreciable clinically as a result of opacity of the cornea and media (Figure 7.1A). Extension into and through the anterior sclera along the emmisaria with the formation of visible subconjunctival pigmented plaques may be more obvious than the primary mass in such cases (Figure 7.1B). In some cases, the tumor weakens the fibrous coat with a resultant neoplastic intercalary staphyloma. Extraocular extension may mimic a uveal prolapse caused by trauma (Figure 7.2). In these cases there will usually be a history of long-standing abnormal appearance to the eye, and a genuine problem in

differential diagnosis is unlikely. Neoplastic cells may also track along the deep corneal surface forming a retrocorneal pigmented plaque (Figure 7.3). In iris ring melanomas, there is circumferential iris darkening and thickening, but the greatest dimension of the tumor in any direction is small. Although the changes are apparent on sectioning the globe, they are much less striking when viewed directly from in front during clinical examination (Figure 7.3). An uncomplicated anterior uveitis may be erroneously diagnosed on the basis of iris thickening, an irregular pupil, and posterior synechiae.

The most common secondary complication of melanomas is glaucoma, and a high proportion of eyes containing melanomas are glaucomatous at the time of enucleation. It might be expected that an apparently focal tumor would leave sufficient functional drainage angle for glaucoma to be a late event, but this is not the case for two reasons. Firstly, even where the tumor has its greatest dimension in one quadrant, tumor cells readily grow around the anterior uvea in an encircling fashion and occlude the entire drainage angle (Figure 7.4). Secondly, tumors may induce ischemia with the release of angiogenic factors

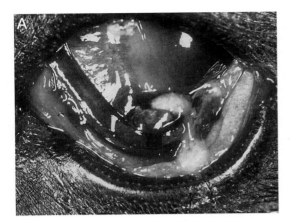

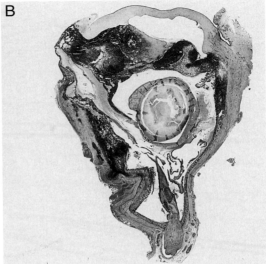

FIG. 7.2—Melanomas occasionally break through the fibrous coats of the eye and clinically resemble traumatic perforation with uveal prolapse. **A:** An irregularly pigmented mass is protruding through the limbus beneath the third eyelid, which is displaced anteriorly. **B:** A diffuse melanoma is present in the iris, ciliary body, and anterior choroid, with the section passing through the staphyloma.

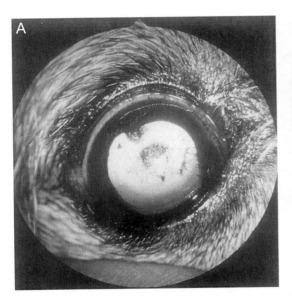

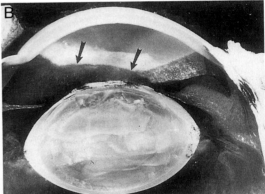

FIG. 7.3—Iris ring melanoma that was mistakenly treated for anterior uveitis for several months. **A:** There is pigment on the anterior lens capsule, focal posterior synechiae, irregular iris thickening, and diffuse darkening of the iris, all of which may be features of iritis. The eye was enucleated 2 months later when glaucoma and scleral pigmentation developed. **B:** On cut surface, the ring-shaped thickening, occlusion of the drainage angle, and scleral invasion are all apparent. To the *left* is invasion of the deep surface of the peripheral cornea by a layer of tumor cells (arrow) obscuring the usual broken appearance of the peripheral corneal pigment still present to the *right*.

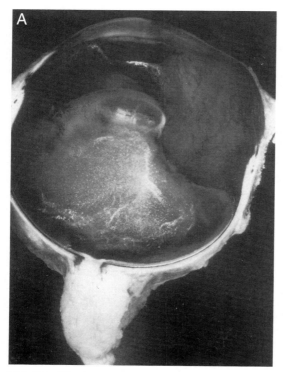
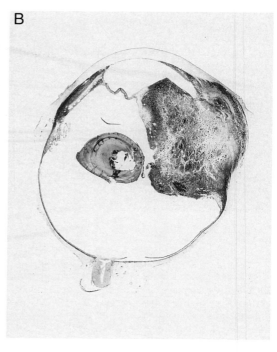

FIG. 7.4—The same eye as in Figure 7.1A. **A:** The lens is subluxated by expansion of the tumor. The vitreous contains asteroid hyalosis. **B:** The section demonstrates the extensive scleral and peripheral corneal invasion over the tumor and the circumferential spread with invasion of the drainage angle opposite the main mass. In **A,** the tumor appears largely uniform, but the section shows variability in appearance as a result of large areas of necrosis.

resulting in neovascular glaucoma (Figure 7.5).[18] Whether the angiogenic factors are released by the tumor itself or by other ocular tissues secondarily affected, such as detached retina, is not known. Globe enlargement may follow glaucoma, and the eye may be distorted further by a focal mass. Hyphema and uveitis may also be present, but, in the authors' experience, clinical signs of uveitis are not as common as is often suggested.

DIAGNOSIS. Among general clinicians, the index of suspicion for intraocular tumors is generally low, with a high proportion of false-negative and false-positive diagnoses among enucleated eyes submitted for pathologic examination.[19] In an older dog, where one eye is steadily deteriorating in general clinical appearance or opacity while the other remains normal, neoplasia should be considered in the differential diagnosis. Ultrasonography is valuable in defining the extent of intraocular masses especially in eyes with severe anterior changes (Figure 7.6). The potential value of imaging techniques has yet to be exploited. General clinical examination should pay particular attention to the possibility of primary tumors elsewhere, including melanomas, which may have metastasized to the eye.

Where clinical and ultrasonographic examinations have indicated a diagnosis of intraocular neoplasia, a tissue diagnosis may be achieved by fine-needle aspiration (FNA) biopsy. The method and results have been described for humans, but there are no reports regarding dogs.[20,21] Needle aspiration biopsy is often objected to on the grounds of the risk of extraocular seeding of tumor cells. Although this is well documented in the case of retinoblastoma,[22] it has not been described in

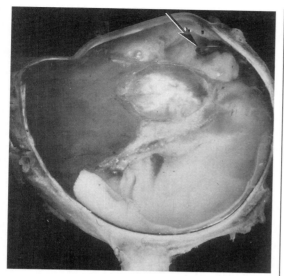

FIG. 7.5—Ciliary-body melanoma resembling that in Figure 7.4. This eye is also glaucomatous but not as a result of circumferential tumor spread. The iris opposite the tumor has a foreshortened appearance (arrow) as a result of neovascularization pulling the iris against the peripheral cornea. The aqueous and vitreous contain excess protein as a result of leakage from the new blood vessels. There is retinal detachment with subretinal fluid adjacent to the posterior limit of the tumor.

reports on the method in other tumor types. The indications have been given as diagnostic uncertainty, patient insistence on confirmation of diagnosis prior to enucleation, and uncertainty as to whether a suspected intraocular tumor is primary or metastatic. Diagnostic uncertainty may occur in dogs for a number of reasons. The uvea in most dogs is heavily pigmented so that other primary and secondary tumors may contain resident melanocytes, giving a deceptive pigmented appearance.[23] Melanomas metastatic to the eye from the oral mucosa have also been described.[7,24] Conversely, amelanotic melanomas may resemble other nonpigmented primary or secondary intraocular tumors (Figure 7.7). The indications for FNA may all apply in dogs but in practice rarely do so. Where a clinical and ultrasonographic diagnosis of neoplasia has been made, and the results of other investigations are normal, most veterinary clinicians would not consider a specific tissue diagnosis essential before deciding on management. Since tumors frequently give rise to intractable glaucoma and a "blind, painful eye," the decision to enucleate is justified regardless of the primary pathology. Application of other treatment modalities that spare the globe, such as laser ablation, should

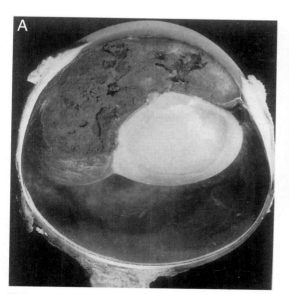

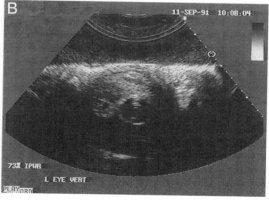

FIG. 7.6—**A:** This heavily pigmented iris tumor fills the anterior chamber. Canine tumors often grow large before definitive diagnosis. **B:** Ultrasonography is effective in demonstrating the full extent of intraocular tumors where clinical examination is limited. Spaces visible within the tumor on cut surface and on scan were filled with blood and large, round, pigment-laden cells but were not lined with endothelium. The lens is subluxated by tumor expansion.

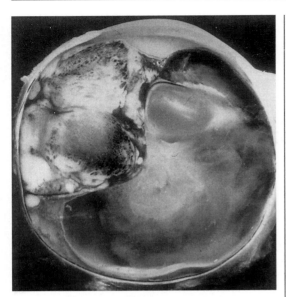

FIG. 7.7—Amelanotic melanoma with a gross morphology similar to those in Figures 7.4 and 7.5. The variation in appearance on cut surface is due to infarction and hemorrhage.

ideally be accompanied by a specific diagnosis that FNA might provide. The possibility remains of a secondary tumor occurring in an eye without evidence of tumor at other sites, but this would be rare.

DIFFERENTIAL DIAGNOSIS. The main differential diagnoses for anterior uveal melanocytic proliferations are other causes of pigmented ocular lesions.[25] These most commonly include pigmented iris cysts; pigmented iris or ciliary-body adenomas; or melanosis secondary to chronic inflammation.

EPIBULBAR MELANOMAS. Epibulbar or limbal melanomas are heavily pigmented tumors arising from cells in the peripheral corneosclera. The tumors may be large and locally invasive into the cornea and sclera. Because of the tendency of uveal melanomas to invade the anterior sclera and form episcleral pigmented plaques, there may be difficulty in distinguishing these tumors from limbal melanomas on superficial examination. An accurate diagnosis is important, since management of limbal melanoma rarely requires enucle-ation. Gonioscopy and ultrasonography should be performed in all cases. Gonioscopy will distinguish limbal melanomas, which are unlikely to invade the drainage angle from anterior uveal melanoma, which readily does so. Only with very long-standing limbal melanoma is there a possibility of intraocular invasion beyond the fibrous coat into the anterior uvea when the primary site may then be in doubt (Figure 7.8).

FRECKLES AND NEVI. Freckles are benign focal accumulations of normal melanocytes, and nevi are proliferations of benign, not fully differentiated, melanocytes, but, in contrast to human pathology, the terms are not often used in the veterinary literature. Heavily pigmented zones may sometimes be encountered in the canine iris, but, where they are plaquelike and constant in size or enlarging only slowly, the management should consist of observation only, supplemented by gonioscopy and ultrasonography, as required (Figure 7.9).

IRIS AND CILIARY BODY CYSTS. Iris and ciliary body (or anterior uveal) cysts are benign pigmented or nonpigmented cysts often seen in larger breeds but especially in mature Labrador and golden retrievers.[26] The cysts arise spontaneously from the posterior iris or ciliary body and consist of a thin shell of pigmented or nonpigmented epithelial cells.[27] They are more likely to be seen clinically after they have detached. They may then float free in the anterior chamber or become fixed between the cornea and iris or attach to the posterior cornea where they may collapse, forming an irregular pigmented shape on the posterior cornea.[28] They are single or multiple and may continue to enlarge once free. Iris cysts are totally benign and usually asymptomatic and may be distinguished from the anterior uveal melanoma by their spherical shape, their transillumination (Figure 7.10), the fact that they can be seen not to be part of or arising from the iris stroma, and the lack of secondary change in the eye. Iris cysts are often quoted as the main differential diagnosis for anterior uveal melanomas, but experienced ophthalmologists are unlikely to have difficulty in distinguishing the two lesions. Ciliary body cysts may present as attached lesions

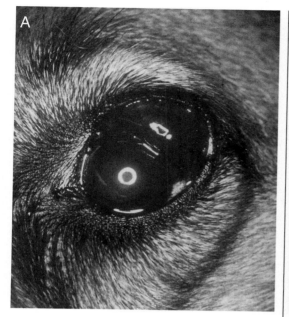

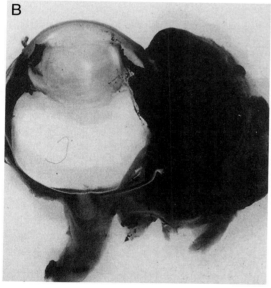

FIG. 7.8—Difficulty in distinguishing a limbal melanoma from a uveal tumor with extraocular extension is unusual. **A:** A large subconjunctival mass has been reportedly present for several months at least. The circular ringflash mark lies directly over the pupil, with the tumor lying dorsolateral to the globe. **B:** The sectioned eye shows the relative size of the intraocular and extraocular components. It is not possible to be certain, but this is probably a limbal melanoma, sufficiently long-standing to have invaded beyond the anterior sclerocornea.

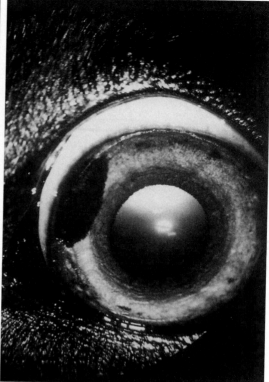

FIG. 7.9—A heavily pigmented zone is present in the medial iris of a young Labrador retriever but is not elevated above the iris surface. There was no change over a 4-year observation period.

of the posterior chamber. Though also benign, an association with glaucoma has be speculated.

MELANOCYTOSIS. Melanocytosis (also described as pigmentary glaucoma in reference to its almost certain sequelae) is seen predominantly in elderly cairn terriers and sporadically in other breeds, including German shepherds and boxers.[29,30] Initially, bilateral hyperpigmentation and thickening of the iris occurs and, with biomicroscopy, pigmented cells can be seen floating free in the aqueous. Invasion of the sclera posterior to the limbus results in prominent patches of subconjunctival pigment (Figure 7.11). The cells become deposited initially inferiorly in the ciliary cleft, and eventually occlusion of the outflow pathway leads to glaucoma. The combination of glaucoma and the

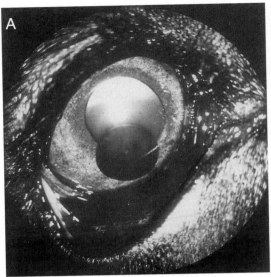

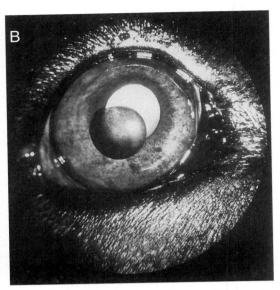

FIG. 7.10—The typical appearance of an iris cyst. **A:** A smooth spherical pigmented mass is present in the anterior chamber but is not part of the iris. **B:** The mass transilluminates.

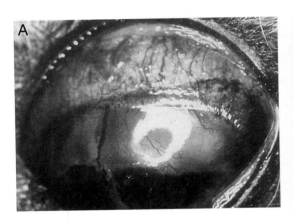

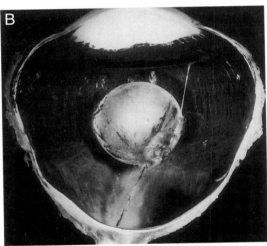

FIG. 7.11—Pigmentary glaucoma in a cairn terrier. **A:** A grossly enlarged glaucomatous globe with extensive pigment invasion of the anterior sclera. **B:** On cut surface, the enlargement is not symmetrical but is greatest in the anterior sclera where there is pigmentary invasion. There is iris and ciliary-body atrophy, and the lens is luxated. Large three-dimensional masses are not present, contrary to what might be expected by the clinical appearance. This could be contrasted with uveal tumors showing scleral invasion as in Figures 7.4 and 7.5.

weakening of the sclera by pigment invasion results in massive enlargement of the anterior globe. Pigmentary glaucoma may be confused with anterior uveal melanoma on the grounds of iris darkening, scleral pigment invasion, and glaucoma. The bilaterality and the breed assist in the diagnosis. Bilateral uveal melanomas have been described in dogs but are very rare.[31,32] In pigmentary glaucoma, the cells invade widely in the eye but do not tend to form three-dimensional masses despite the impression created by the scleral convexities seen clinically. The proliferating cells are large heavily pigmented melanocytes resembling melanocytoma cells, and the lesion likely will ultimately be classified as a form of neoplasia. Investigations into the pathology of the condition are continuing.[33]

MORPHOLOGY

MACROSCOPIC PATHOLOGY. Canine anterior uveal melanomas can be divided into three groups based on pattern of growth of growth, with some individual variation and overlap between categories. Ciliary-body tumors form the largest group, where the greatest tumor diameter is in the ciliary body with invasion anteriorly into the iris, posteriorly into the choroid, and outward into the sclera (Figures 7.4, 7.5, and 7.7). The second group are those tumors arising in the iris and expanding mainly anteriorly into the anterior chamber (Figures 7.7 and 7.12). The third group are iris tumors growing circumferentially in a more or less symmetrical manner and hence termed *ring melanoma* (Figures 7.3 and 7.13). Numerically, this type is the least common but clinically presents the greatest difficulty in diagnosis. On cut surface, the iris is darkened or at least has a dense homogeneous appearance rather than a spongy texture. In all three patterns of growth, there may be scleral invasion, circumferential growth with pigmentation and invasion of the ciliary cleft, invasion of the corneal stroma, and extension along the deep surface of the cornea (Figure 7.14).

Secondary changes may also be present and may be more apparent on sectioning the globe than they were clinically, where they might be obscured by opacity of the cornea and media. Blunt expansion of the tumor, especially arising from the ciliary body, readily displaces the lens, causing subluxation. Tumors extending posteriorly may release fluid into the subretinal space, causing retinal detachment. Asteroid hyalosis is found commonly in canine eyes containing tumors where there is no evidence of it in the fellow eye but the pathogenesis is unclear. Excessive protein content in the aqueous and vitreous (Figure 7.5) may arise from breakdown of the blood-ocular barriers as a result of glaucoma, uveitis, or leakage from new blood vessels with incompetent walls.

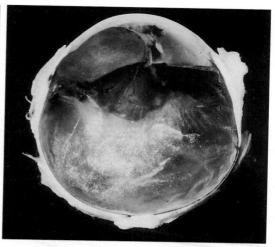

FIG. 7.12—An iris melanoma with anterior extension only (the lens has been removed). There is extensive asteroid hyalosis. There is circumferential spread of the tumor, with tumor cells in the iris and drainage angle opposite the main mass, but this is not visible grossly.

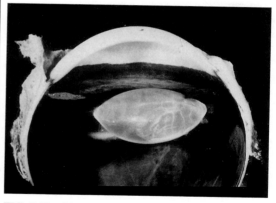

FIG. 7.13—Iris ring melanoma erroneously diagnosed as uncomplicated closed-angle glaucoma. The iris to the *left* is slightly thickened, with a homogeneous appearance and a solid rather than spongy texture. The normal pigment zone in the peripheral cornea has been obscured by a dense sheet of tumor cells (compare Figure 7.3).

MICROSCOPIC PATHOLOGY. Canine anterior uveal melanomas consist of combinations of variably pigmented, spindle or ovoid cells and heavily pigmented, large, round or polyhedral cells.

Spindle cells are fusiform cells with small round or elongated nuclei and indistinct cell

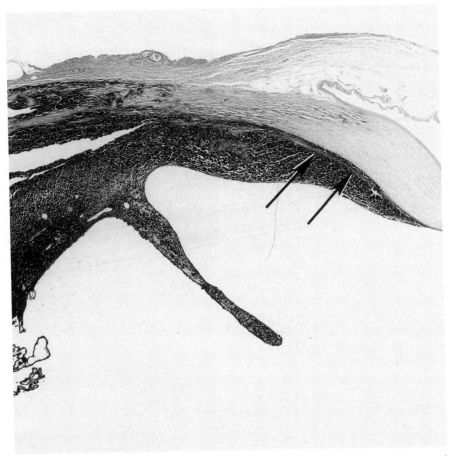

FIG. 7.14—Even the most histologically benign anterior uveal melanomas show considerable potential for local invasion of ocular tissues. This group 1 tumor or melanocytoma (see Table 7.1) shows benign cytologic features but has invaded the sclera posterior to the limbus and the cornea both anterior and posterior to Descemet's membrane (indicated by arrows). Periodic acid—Schiff.

boundaries. Nucleoli are uncommon, and mitotic figures are rare. The cells are often aligned in sheets or bundles forming a swirling pattern. The degree of pigmentation is very variable (Figure 7.15).

Ovoid cells are round or oval and are larger and more pleomorphic than spindle cells, with a higher nucleus-to-cytoplasm ratio. The nuclei are larger, with sparse marginated chromatin and a prominent nucleolus. Cells may be tightly or loosely packed, and cell borders variably distinct. Mitoses are most common in this group but vary with the individual case (Figures 7.15 and 7.16).

Large, round pigment-laden cells or plump cells are much larger, round or polyhedral, with clearly defined borders. Nuclei are relatively small with dense chromatin and rarely nucleoli. Multinucleate cells also occur. Nuclei may be paracentral but most appear to migrate to the cell border as the cells enlarge. The cytoplasm is tightly packed with fine pigment granules. Mitoses are never seen in these cells. Wilcock and Peiffer[9] have suggested that the stem cell of canine melanomas is a poorly pigmented spindle-shaped melanocyte that can mature into the plump pigmented cell which is then incapable of further division. These round cells enlarge, often

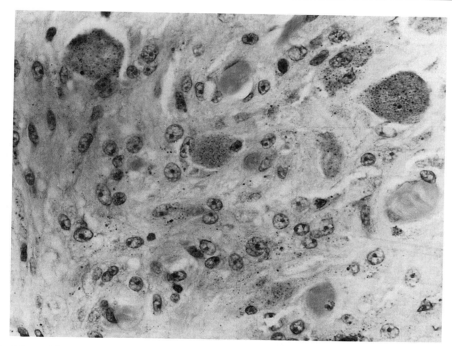

FIG. 7.15—Most of the cells are elongated and ovoid spindle cells with indistinct borders, but there are also a few large, round, pigment-laden cells. Hematoxylin–eosin, bleached.

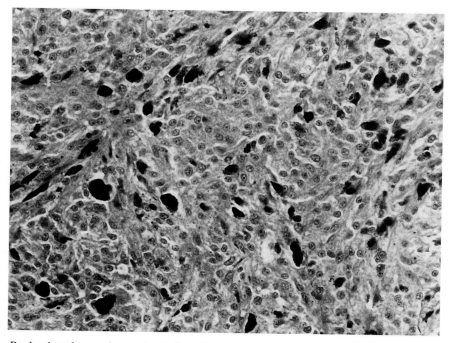

FIG. 7.16—Predominantly round or oval spindle cell melanoma. The cells are cohesive and regular with round or oval nuclei with nucleoli and indistinct cell margins. Larger, heavily pigmented, round or polyhedral cells are distributed randomly through the tumor mass. Hematoxylin–eosin.

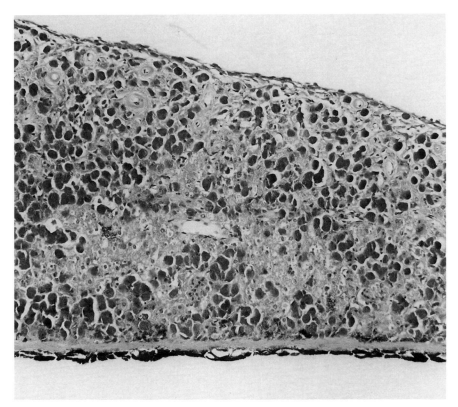

FIG. 7.17—The same dog as in Figure 7.13. This is a group 1 tumor or melanocytoma (see Table 7.1) in which the iris has been invaded by numerous large, round, pigmented-laden cells throughout its circumference. Despite the benign cytology, the eye has been lost as a result of glaucoma. Hematoxylin–eosin, bleached.

to a considerable size, and as they do so the nucleus becomes pyknotic, the cell undergoes lysis, and the original cell border becomes less distinct (Figures 7.17 and 7.18). This process may result in large zones of totally acellular pigment in larger tumors. Although they may be present in large numbers, or even comprise the bulk of the tumor, these plump cells are essentially benign.

It might be suspected that the heavily pigmented plump cells are melanomacrophages and independent of the tumor process on the basis of the different morphology from the spindle cells and the extreme accumulation of pigment. Electron microscopy of these cells, however, has demonstrated only melanosomes and premelanosomes and not phagosomes, indicating that they are true melanocytes and not phagocytes (Figure 7.19).[4,8,9]

The three cell types may be intermixed randomly within the tumor mass, or there may be local aggregations of one cell type to such a degree that there is distinct zoning, with areas of spindle/ovoid cells and areas of large, round pigment-laden cells forming well-defined borders with each other (Figures 7.20–7.22). Bleaching is often essential in evaluating cell types in pigmented canine melanomas, and specific stains for melanin are useful in evaluating nonpigmented tumors (Figure 7.23).

Two classification schemes that have been devised based on the relative proportions of the three cell types are summarized in Table 7.1. There is considerable agreement between the schemes, bearing in mind that there is an arbitrary element in any such classification. These schemes must be used because the metastatic rate is low even in the most malignant of the three tumor categories proposed.

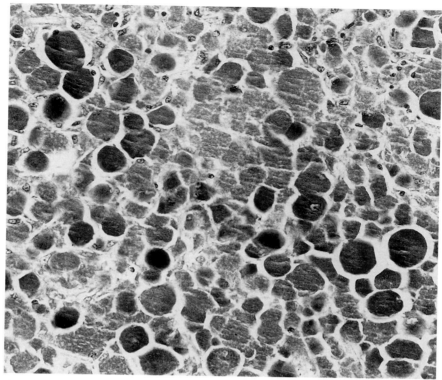

FIG. 7.18—Large, round, pigment-laden cells. The field shows viable large, round cells with small, often peripheral, nuclei and clearly defined cell margins. Lysed cells have indistinct borders. This process may result in large masses of totally acellular pigment within tumors. Hematoxylin–eosin, bleached.

Comparing canine tumor types with the Callender classification for choroidal melanomas is inappropriate for a number of reasons. The human spindle-A cell, with an elongated folded nucleus, is not found in dogs nor is the epithelioid cell with a large nucleus, eosinophilic cytoplasm, and well-defined cell border. The round or oval spindle cells of dogs could be compared with the spindle-B cell of humans but generally are smaller and often less pleomorphic. In addition, the large, round pigment-laden cell, which is such a prominent feature of many canine tumors, is not found in human choroidal melanomas and does not feature in the Callender classification but would be better compared with the cells of anterior and posterior melanocytomas in humans.[34,35] An occasional canine uveal melanoma will demonstrate epithelioid features but lack the nuclear features that characterize human epithelioid melanomas.

IMMUNOHISTOCHEMISTRY. Positive staining of canine anterior uveal melanoma with S-100 has been reported previously.[36] S-100 is effective in identification of melanoma cells in nonpigmented tumors both in formalin-fixed and in glutaraldehyde-fixed tissues (Figure 7.24), although not all cells stain equally. Positive staining with HMB-45 was not demonstrated in glutaraldehyde-fixed specimens.

TREATMENT. The frequent development of glaucoma in eyes containing anterior uveal melanoma means that many such eyes fall into the category of the "blind painful eye" by the time of diagnosis and treatment. Enucleation is the most logical and reliable method of relieving the clinical signs. A tumor that is diagnosed at an earlier stage in an eye that is still pain free and visual may present a difficult choice between

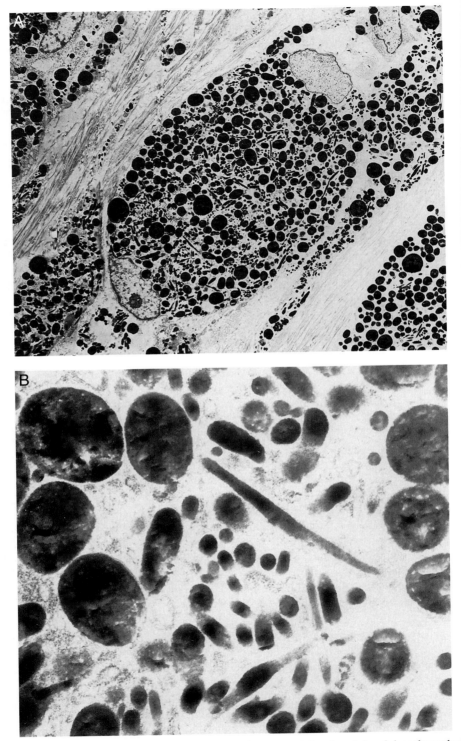

FIG. 7.19—**A:** This large, round, pigment-laden cell contains two peripheral nuclei and densely packed pigment granules. **B:** The pigment consists of non-membrane-bound melanosomes, indicating that it is not a melanomacrophage.

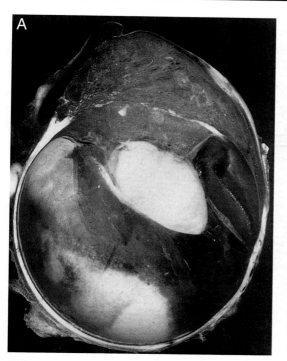

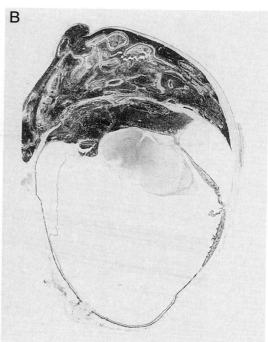

FIG. 7.20—**A:** An exceptional degree of corneal invasion by an anterior uveal melanoma. **B:** The section shows the tumor to have a "marbled" appearance as a result of well-defined zoning of the cell types.

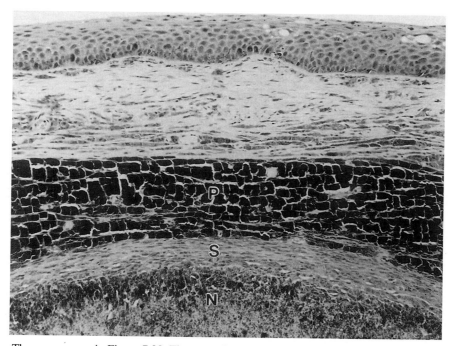

FIG. 7.21—The same eye as in Figure 7.20. The corneal epithelium shows secondary thickening and pigmentation, and the anterior stroma contains lightly pigmented cells. Deep to that is a layer of heavily pigmented, round or polyhedral cells (P) over a layer of lightly pigmented spindle cells (S). The spindle cells then border a large area of necrosis (N). This arrangement was repeated throughout the cornea, giving the appearance seen in Figure 7.20. The necrosis in this case resulted from ischemia rather than individual cell lysis as in Figure 7.18.

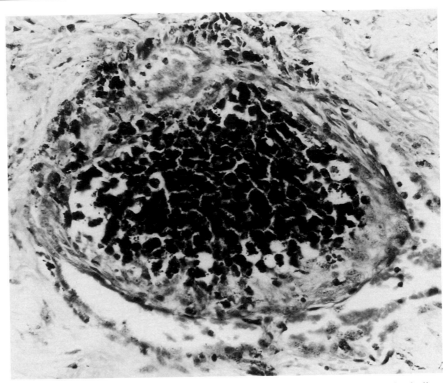

FIG. 7.22—A tumor nodule is present in the sclera and consists of a shell of nonpigmented spindle cells forming a sharp boundary with a central mass of large, round, pigment-laden cells. Hematoxylin–eosin.

temporization and observation, on the one hand, and surgical intervention in the form of enucleation or local resection, on the other. Most anterior uveal melanomas have no metastatic potential, and local complications such as extraocular extension and glaucoma that may develop during observation are not risk factors for metastasis. Since the efficacy of enucleation in preventing metastases is unproven, it has been suggested that enucleation of eyes without secondary changes is difficult to justify.[9]

Local resection can be performed with small circumscribed anterior tumors but remains a technically difficult procedure in dogs, with a high incidence of operative and postoperative complications, especially where scleral flaps are required for access to posterior tumors in the ciliary body. Because of the heavy pigmentation of the canine anterior uvea and the tendency of tumors to grow circumferentially, it can be very difficult clinically to define the limits of a

melanoma. The practical result is that few canine cases meet the criteria for local resection, and it is not often performed. In humans, earlier recognition, more closely confined tumors, and better surgical success rates combine to make iridectomy relatively common.[37]

Transscleral tumor ablation with the Nd-YAG has been reported in 16 dogs.[38] Diode laser treatment likewise offers promise of being efficacious in selected neoplasms. The method does not enable a histologic diagnosis but is justified on the grounds that few intraocular tumors have metastatic potential and enucleation has no proven benefit for the few that do. Laser treatment has therefore been attempted as a means of tumor ablation without the need for enucleation. The effects of the treatment on tumor remission or ablation have been very variable for undetermined reasons, but side effects of the treatment have been few and mild. Whether laser treatment influences metastatic potential is not yet clear.

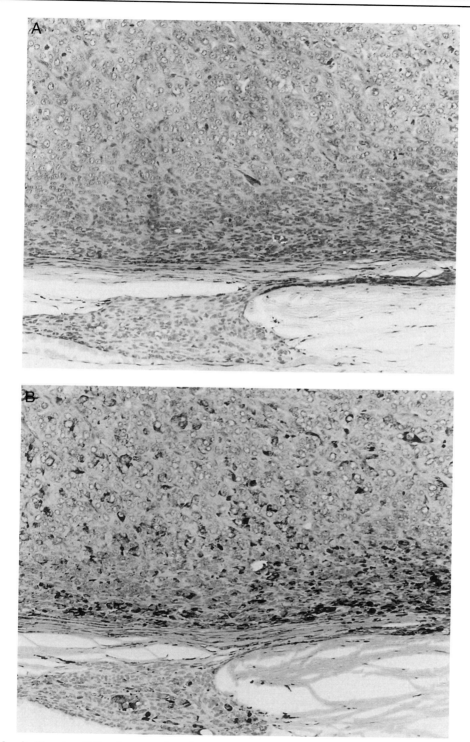

FIG. 7.23—**A:** "Amelanotic" melanoma of predominantly round/oval cells with an island of tumor within the sclera. Hematoxylin–eosin. **B:** The same field stained for melanin demonstrates the presence of considerable amounts of pigment. Fontana-Masson.

TABLE 7.1—Proposed classification schemes for canine anterior uveal melanoma

	Bussanich et al.[8]		Wilcock and Peiffer[9]
Tumor class	Characteristics	Tumor class	Characteristics
Group 1	Over two-thirds plump cells Remainder spindle cells with a few ovoid cells Densely pigmented No mitotic figures Minimal intrascleral spread Small average size	Melanocytoma	Predominance of plump cells Variable number of benign spindle cells Mitotic figures rare
Group 2	Mixture of three cell types Average mitotic index* of 1 Moderately pigmented Larger average size	Benign spindle cell melanoma	Largely benign spindle cells Moderate number of plump cells Mitotic figures rare
Group 3	Over two-thirds ovoid cells Poorly pigmented Average mitotic index* of 23 Largest tumor size	Potentially malignant spindle cell melanoma	More pleomorphic spindle cells Mitotic index* at least 4 (most higher) Pigmentation variable with few darkly pigmented Plump cells rare

*Mitotic index = total mitoses per 10 high-power fields

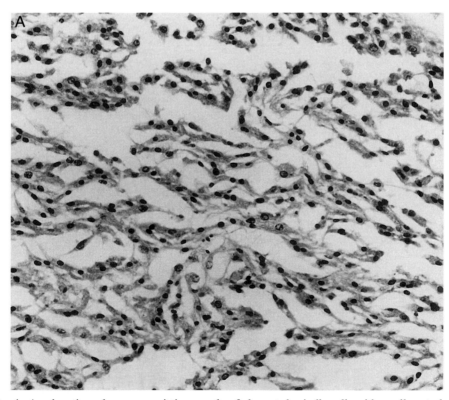

FIG. 7.24—**A:** Amelanotic melanoma consisting mostly of elongated spindle cells with small central nuclei. The cell borders are well defined and the cells lack cohesion. Hematoxylin–eosin. (continued)

PROGNOSIS AND BIOLOGIC BEHAVIOR. Obtaining long-term follow-up data on dogs with cancer is notoriously difficult where cases are seen at referral centers and particularly with pathologic specimens submitted to laboratories. A true assessment of the metastatic potential of canine anterior uveal melanomas appeared only with the publication in the 1980s of larger series with adequate follow-up periods.[4-9] Table 7.2 shows that metastatic deaths from canine anterior uveal melanomas are uncommon. Deaths occurred at rates of 0%–8.7%, with an overall rate of 4.7%. The total number of published cases in the literature is only 14 (with some further cases suspected), and single cases are still worthy of publication.[36,39,40] Metastatic deaths follow a consistent pattern within a few months, with tumor deposits in multiple sites, some of them unusual (Table 7.3).

Various histologic features have been assessed as possible prognostic indicators. Necrosis, inflammation, degree of pigmentation, and presence of tumor cells in cornea, ciliary cleft, or episclera were not useful predictors of biologic behavior. Mitotic index was found to be the single most reliable criterion, with tumors of proven malignant behavior having indices of at least 4 per 10 high-power fields.[9] The mitotic index was also high in two single cases reported.[36,40] It has been suggested that simply finding mitoses is suspicious of malignancy.[14] In documented cases of metastatic spread, the primary tumors have showed conventional features of malignancy such as anaplasia and cellular and nuclear pleomorphism.

Difficulties in classification of canine anterior uveal melanomas stem from the use of the term *malignant*.[5,42,43] On criteria such as invasion or

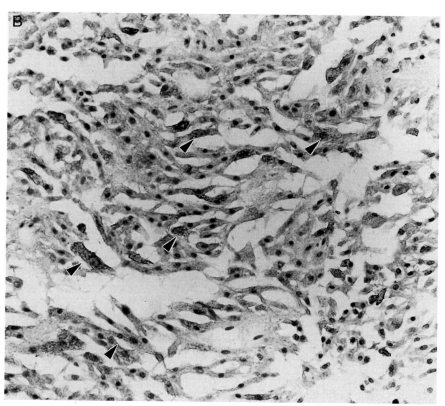

FIG. 7.24 (continued)—**B:** All cells are positive for S-100 to some degree, with some strongly positive (arrowheads). S-100, DAB method.

TABLE 7.2—Published incidence of confirmed metastatic deaths from canine anterior uveal melanoma

References	Total cases	Cases with follow-up	Follow-up period	Cases with confirmed metastases	Metastatic death rate (%)
Diters et al.[4]	23	15	5 mos to 5 yrs (most >2 yrs)	0 (One dog died with a "hepatic mass.")	0
Ryan and Diters[5]	31	23	3 mos to >4 yrs (most >2 yrs)	2	8.7
Trucksa et al.[7]	29	29	2 to >3 yrs	0 (One dog died of disseminated melanoma interpreted as arising from a primary oral tumor.)	0
Bussanich et al.[8]	14	14	4 mos to >4 yrs (most >3 yrs)	1	7.1
Wilcock and Peiffer[9]	72	48	1 to 5 yrs	3 (One further dog died with cachexia and liver failure.)	6.3
Total		129		6	4.7

TABLE 7.3—Summary of confirmed metastatic deaths from canine anterior uveal melanoma

References	Cases with confirmed metastases	Survival time following diagnosis	Metastatic sites
Michael[41]	1	5 months	Ovaries, kidneys, and spleen
Saunders and Barron[2]	2	Case 1: 6 months	Parietal pleura, pericardium, bronchial lymph nodes, lungs, liver, pituitary plus local invasion of the brain
		Case 2: Euthanasia at time of diagnosis	Lung (solitary tiny lesion)
Magrane[3]	1	8 months	Nasal cavity, upper gum, lungs, stomach, and adrenal gland
Ryan and Diters[5]	2	Case 1: 2 months	Kidney, adrenal glands, lung, bronchial lymph nodes, atrium, ventricular myocardium plus local extension to optic chiasm
		Case 2: Euthanasia (ocular melanoma not noted prior to euthanasia)	Liver, spleen, kidney, and lungs
Schäffer and Funke[6]	1	Euthanasia at time of diagnosis	Lungs and kidneys (one further case with orbital recurrence and suspected thoracic metastases)
Dietz et al.[39]	1	1 month	Lungs, heart, liver, spleen, and kidneys
Bussanich et al.[8]	1	4 months	Liver, lungs, and kidneys
Wilcock and Peiffer[9]	3	Maximum, 3 months	Visceral metastases (one further case suspected)
Friedman et al.[40]	1	Euthanasia at time of diagnosis	Lung, right atrium
Minami and Patnaik[36]	1	3 months	Lung, left ventricular wall, and kidneys

destruction of adjacent tissues, many canine tumors should be classified as malignant. The eye is susceptible to functional loss and pain as a result of tumor expansion and invasion, and most eyes containing melanomas are ultimately non-functional and lost. Even tumors in the most benign group 1 or melanocytoma category (see Table 7.1) have considerable potential for local invasion and functional loss, especially where the drainage angle is occluded (Figure 7.14). It has been pointed out, however, that in many other sites in the body the same lesion would be regarded with much less alarm.[9] Regardless of the effects on the globe, most dogs will survive. Since the term malignant implies life threatening, its use in the context of canine anterior uveal melanoma is best restricted to metastatic potential alone.[40]

Choroidal Melanoma

HISTORICAL PERSPECTIVES. In 1958, Saunders and Barron[2] summarized 18 previously reported cases of canine pigmented intraocular tumors, including those of epithelial origin. It is interesting, however, that of these 18 cases six were choroidal melanomas and only three were anterior uveal melanomas (a further four cases had inadequate details of site of origin), giving the impression of a much higher incidence of choroidal melanomas than is currently accepted. Their own series of 15 new cases included nine anterior uveal melanomas and only one choroidal melanoma (with one further tumor of uncertain site of origin) and is, therefore, more consistent with later reports. As with anterior uveal tumors, only in the last two decades have further published reports documented this tumor more fully.[44–51]

EPIDEMIOLOGY. Canine choroidal melanoma is much less common than anterior uveal melanoma and is estimated at only 5% of total intraocular melanomas in this species.[51] Most reported cases have occurred in mature or older dogs, with an average age of 6.5 years in the largest published series.[51] No breed predisposition is apparent in cases from the pet population, but three cases have been described in young experimental beagles.[44,46,47] This may represent a breed susceptibility but is more likely the result of regular screening revealing covert lesions that would have been unnoticed in a pet dog, at least at the same age.

CLINICAL FEATURES. Most published cases provide little detail of clinical features because the reports concern enucleated globes submitted for pathologic analysis. In some cases a pigmented fundic mass was identified either at routine examination or for reasons not given, but in many cases the presentation related to secondary effects of the tumor, such as chronic uveitis, glaucoma, blindness, or intraocular hemorrhage.

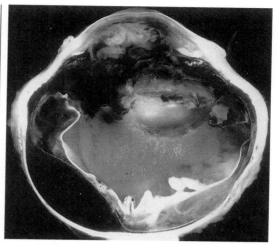

FIG. 7.25—A dark choroidal mass with overlying retinal detachment, intraocular hemorrhage, and glaucoma. The mass was an organized hematoma. The cause of the hemorrhage was not identified.

DIAGNOSIS AND DIFFERENTIAL DIAGNOSIS. Insufficient information is available on the clinical appearance of choroidal tumors and on supportive diagnostic tests such as fluorescein angiography and ultrasonography to give clear diagnostic criteria. Differential diagnoses include other causes of a subretinal mass, such as metastatic choroidal tumor, granuloma, or hematoma (Figure 7.25); other causes of pigmentary proliferation, such as postinflammatory pigmentation or choroidal nevi; and other causes of retinal detachment, glaucoma, and uveitis. Ultrasound-guided FNA was used in one case, and the resultant cytology was suggestive of choroidal melanoma.[50]

MORPHOLOGY

MACROSCOPIC PATHOLOGY. The primary site of uveal melanomas involving the ciliary body and choroid may be arguable but have been conventionally regarded in the modern literature as anterior uveal melanomas with posterior extension. Melanomas are only described as choroidal where the entire tumor is within the choroid. Published cases of canine choroidal melanomas show a very similar gross appearance consisting of a heavily pigmented subretinal mass with a smooth profile and tapering edges and a clearly delineated margin. In some larger tumors, however, the mass was virtually filling the posterior globe.

Many cases arise adjacent to the optic nerve (Figure 7.26). Retinal detachment is a common finding and varies from local detachments associated with the mass to total stalk detachment. In the largest series, the majority of dogs had total detachments, with subretinal hemorrhage and proteinaceous exudate.[51]

MICROSCOPIC PATHOLOGY. Reports of the microscopic features of choroidal melanomas in dogs have described a combination of variably pigmented spindle or oval cells and large, heavily pigmented round or polyhedral cells in various proportions. The most detailed scheme for classification of the cell types has been proposed by Collinson and Peiffer.[51] Type 1 cells are large, plump, pigmented cells with eccentric pyknotic nuclei similar to those seen in anterior uveal melanomas (Figure 7.27).

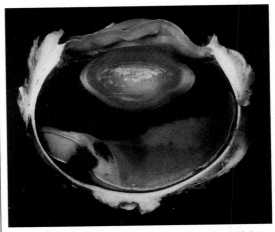

FIG. 7.26—Horizontal section through a choroidal melanoma lateral to the optic disk and invading the overlying retina.

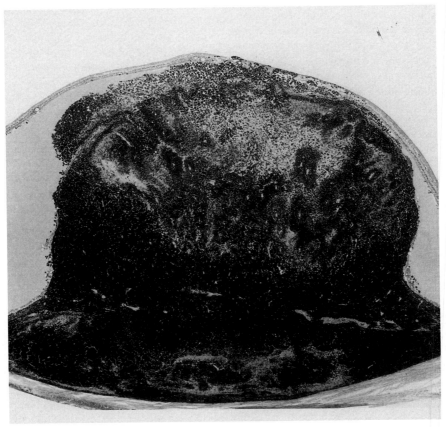

FIG. 7.27—Low power section of the tumor in Figure 7.26. The paler areas in the optical half of the tumor are areas of necrosis containing darker islands with pale centers where tumor cells are surviving around blood vessels. There is a secondary retinal detachment and proteinaceous subretinal fluid.

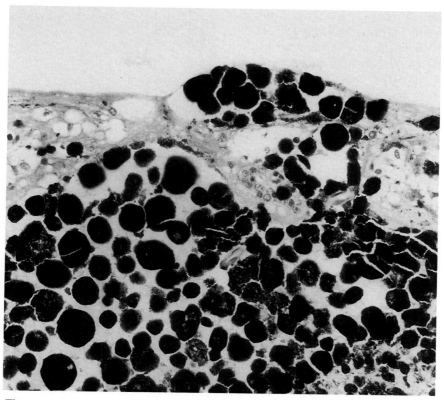

FIG. 7.28—The tumor consists entirely of Type I cells, which are large, heavily pigmented, and roughly circular with a small nucleus. Tumor cells are invading the disorganized and atrophic retina.

Type 2 cells are plump spindle cells with oval nuclei and single nucleoli. Type 3 cells are thin spindle cells with elongated nuclei and occasional spindle cells. Type 4 cells are of small epithelioid type with nuclear pleomorphism, a high nucleus-to-cytoplasm ratio, and a high mitotic index (Figure 7.28). Type 1 cells are always heavily pigmented, but pigmentation is variable in the other cell types. In most of the reported cases, the mitotic index is low or zero, and tumors with significant mitotic indices are uncommon.

Some cases show invasion into, and in some cases through, the sclera and into the optic nerve. Other histopathologic changes have included invasion through Bruch's membrane, detachment and atrophy of overlying retina, neovascular glaucoma, necrosis, anterior and posterior uveitis, and minor cataract formation.

The impression is left that although choroidal melanomas occur with less frequency than their anterior uveal counterparts, there are no distinguishing morphologic differences between the two groups.

TREATMENT. All of the reported cases have resulted in enucleation, and no other treatment modalities have been described. In view of the low metastatic potential of canine choroidal melanomas, it seems reasonable to manage small pigmented posterior-segment masses, not causing pain or blindness, by periodic observation and ultrasonography, provided that other diagnoses have been excluded as far as possible.

PROGNOSIS. Canine choroidal melanomas appear to have a very low potential for metastatic disease or fatal local extension. There are older reports of deaths,[52,53] but full details were not provided and there are no reports in the modern literature. This low metastatic potential is consistent with the benign cytology and the low mitotic indices reported. One tumor consisted predominantly of type 4 cells with a high mitotic index and transscleral and optic nerve invasion, but the case was lost to follow-up.[51] Most of the cases described could be categorized as melanocytomas resembling more the choroidal nevi of humans and without the spectrum of malignant potential of human choroidal melanomas. Canine cases resembling human choroidal melanomas in cytologic features and metastatic potential are of comparative interest but rare (Figures 7.29 and 7.30).

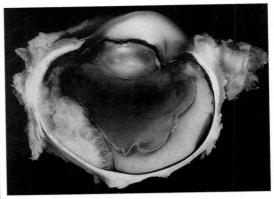

FIG. 7.29—Amelanotic choroidal melanoma with secondary retinal detachment. Amelanotic choroidal melanomas are rare in dogs, and a metastatic tumor might be suspected on the gross appearance.

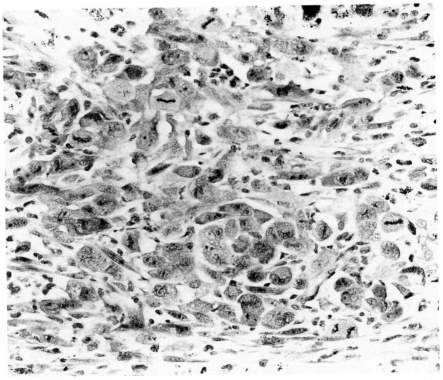

FIG. 7.30—The same eye as in Figure 7.29. The tumor is a poorly differentiated melanoma consisting mainly of epithelioid cells with large nuclei and nucleoli and clearly defined cell borders. Some spindle cells are also present. Several mitotic figures can be seen. It is rare for the cell types in a canine choroidal melanoma to correlate so well with the Callender classification and to demonstrate such malignant cytologic features. Hematoxylin–eosin.

CATS

Historical Perspectives. Saunders and Barron described 15 cases of intraocular tumors in dogs and, in passing, mentioned cases reported by other authors that involved different species, including horses, cats, rabbits, and fish.[2] In 1967, Whitehead[54] listed four cases of malignant melanoma among the tumors seen in 165 cats in a 5-year period. In 1969, Engle and Brodey,[55] in a retrospective study of 395 neoplasms from 372 cats, histologically diagnosed at the University of Pennsylvania Veterinary Hospital, found three primary intraocular malignant melanomas.

In 1970, Bellhorn and Henkind[56] described eight cases of intraocular malignant melanoma in domestic cats. Patnaik and colleagues[57] found a single ocular tumor in a cat, a melanoma having diffuse visceral metastasis, in a series of 289 non-hematopoietic neoplasms from 264 cats. In 1977, Cardy[58] published a case report on a primary intraocular malignant melanoma in a Siamese cat; the same year, Peiffer et al.[59] described a nodular malignant melanoma of the iris and the ciliary body in a Siamese cat, and, in 1978, Souri[60] observed a case of a diffuse anterior uveal melanoma in a domestic cat, with scleral involvement as well.

Acland et al.[61] published descriptions of four cases of diffuse iris melanoma in cats. These tumors were unusual because they were associated with slowly progressive diffuse heterochromia and glaucoma. In 1981, three articles concerning feline uveal melanomas appeared in literature: Chaudieu and Fonk[62] coauthored the report on a case of diffuse malignant melanoma involving the iris, the ciliary body, and the sclera, and infiltrating the choroid; Albert et al.[63] made

the cat the first animal model of a virally induced uveal melanoma; and Shadduck et al.,[64] in a second related work, discussed this potential model of the human counterpart.

In 1982, Niederkorn et al.[65] studied the relationship between enucleation and the appearance of second primary tumors in cats bearing virally induced intraocular tumors (primarily melanomas). In 1985, Schäffer and Funke[6] classified histologically five primary intraocular malignant melanomas in cats.

In the same year, Peiffer[66] presented a report on 17 feline globes with primary uveal melanomas and three feline limbal melanomas. In 1986, Dubielzig et al.[67] summarized information gathered in the study of 39 cases of primary ocular melanoma, and Harling et al.[68] described the clinical features and biologic behavior of limbal melanoma arising from the dendritic melanocytic cells of the corneoscleral junction in four cats.

In 1988, another three articles concerning feline uveal melanomas were published: Bertoy et al.[69] considered a case of intraocular melanoma with multiple metastasis in a cat; Schwink and Betts[70] diagnosed a malignant melanoma of the iris in a cat; and Patnaik and Mooney[71] reported on 16 feline intraocular uveal melanomas. In 1990, Wilcock et al.[72] described 38 diffuse iris melanomas in a series of 131 enucleated glaucomatous feline eyes. In 1991, Duncan and Peiffer[73] considered the structural features and behavior of 38 feline primary anterior uveal melanomas. The histogenesis of the lesion was postulated and mitotic index, full-thickness iris involvement, and the presence of tumor cells in the scleral venous plexus shown to be ominous prognosticators, and the tendency for many cases

TABLE 7.4—Features of patients described in case reports.

Authors	Year	Sex	Age	Breed	Eye
Cardy[58]	1977	M	14	Siamese	?
Peiffer et al.[59]	1977	F	12	Siamese	Left
Souri[60]	1978	M	3, 5	DSH	Left
Acland et al.[61]	1980	F	7	DSH	Right
		M	11	Persian	Left
		M	7	Persian	Left
		M	13	DSH	Left
Chaudieu and Fonk[62]	1981	M	12	Siamese	Left
Bertoy et al.[69]	1988	M	11	DSH	Right
Schwink [70]	1988	M	8	Persian	Left

to have long latencies between enucleation and metastatic death noted.

Feline uveal melanomas have also been considered in several review papers, in textbooks, and in publications.[74–85]

Epidemiology. Approximately 1.5% of all cats in a clinical practice may be expected to have tumors, and less than 2% of all these feline neoplasms affect the eye.[75,86] The most common primary intraocular neoplasm in cats is malignant melanoma of the anterior uvea and is usually unilateral.[75] In a study that considered 38 cats with uveal melanomas, male and female were represented approximately equally (19 to 14), as were left and right globes (17 to 15). Breed information on 23 cats including domestic shorthair, domestic longhair, and Siamese cats indicated no breed predisposition. Affected cats were 4–20 years old, with a mean age of 10.5 years.[75] Among the seven case reports found in literature concerning 10 cats (Table 7.1), three were Siamese, four DSH, three Persian (eight males and two females); affected cats were 3.5–14.0 years old, with an average age of 9.8 years.

Clinical Features

CLINICAL SIGNS. Malignant melanomas usually originate in the iris and ciliary body, but extension to the peripheral choroid and transscleral extension occurs.

Benign limbal melanomas (Figure 7.31) have been observed in cats.[19,66,68]

The iris involvement is characterized by the presence of one or more golden to dark brown pigmented foci that slowly (over months to years) coalesce to form larger pigmented areas and eventually involve most of the iris as it becomes diffusely hyperpigmented (Figure 7.32), thicker, and less mobile.[76] Amelanotic variants have been described.[75,87] Thickening and distortion of the iris due to the infiltrative neoplastic melanocytes may become so pronounced as to cause obstruction of the filtration angle and secondary glaucoma (Figure 7.33). In many cases, slit-lamp examination enables the identification of clumps of pigmented cells in the aqueous humor, with occasional cases with pigmented cells on the anterior lens capsule.

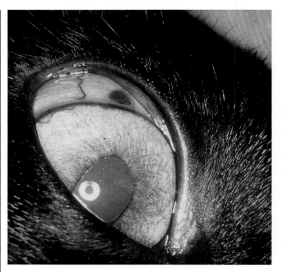

FIG. 7.31—Benign limbal melanoma in a 5-year-old Siamese male cat.

Although iris hyperpigmentation and the signs associated with secondary glaucoma are the most common presenting complaints, the disease may be accompanied by iris atrophy, hyphema, or pseudouveitic syndromes.

DIAGNOSTIC TECHNIQUES. A thorough clinical examination allows a strong presumptive clinical diagnosis as well as localization and determination of the extent of the tumor. Biomicroscopy is most useful in identifying pigmented cells in the anterior chamber and the thickening and smoothing of the iris surface that accompanies the hyperpigmentation; gonioscopy is necessary to identify involvement of the drainage angle. In early disease, the pectinate fibers are hyperpigmented; with progression, the neoplastic cells obliterate the ciliary cleft. Oblique observation of the dilated eye may allow the direct examination of the ciliary body that is better visualized in anesthetized cats by indirect ophthalmoscopy and associated scleral depression. Transillumination can help differentiate uveal melanomas from uveal cysts. Iris transillumination may be useful in determining extent of the neoplasm. Ultrasonography is most useful in eyes where associated alterations in the media hinder direct obser-

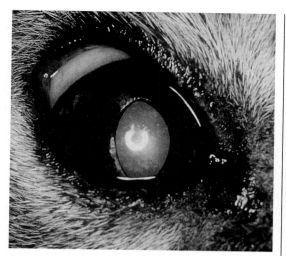

FIG. 7.32—Diffuse pigmentation of the iris in a case of malignant melanoma in a 15-year-old DSH male cat.

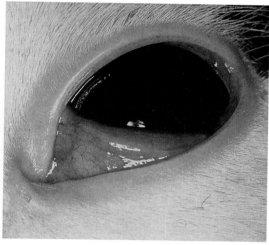

FIG. 7.33—Diffuse malignant melanoma involving the anterior uveal tract and secondary glaucoma in a 5-year-old DSH male cat.

vation and in further determining ciliary-body and posterior-segment involvement. High-frequency ultrasonography may be of value in determining anterior uveal thickness as an indicator of extent of involvement.

The most significant challenge is the differentiation of iris melanoma from benign processes and, in the case of amelanotic melanomas, other proliferative disease, including lymphoma and granulomatous inflammation. Iris hyperpigmentation may occur due to melanocytic hyperplasia induced by chronic inflammation, and benign melanocytic proliferations undoubtedly occur.

Iridal biopsy has been considered useful for differentiating melanoma from benign pigmentary changes.[83] The histogenesis of the disease includes a premalignant phase, however, and either FNA or incisional biopsy at this stage may not be a reliable predictor of future behavior. Paracentesis and cytologic examination of aqueous humor have the same limitations compounded by minimal cellularity. These invasive procedures have been correlated with an increased incidence of metastasis in humans and have potential for serious complications, including intraocular hemorrhage and seeding.[70,75]

Radiographic studies of the thorax and abdomen, thorough clinical examination and screening organ function tests, are indicated to determine the presence or absence of metastatic disease. Other modalities including fluorescein angiography, fluorophotometry, and the uptake of radioactive labels have diagnostic potential but have not been explored.

DIFFERENTIAL DIAGNOSIS. As alluded to in the previous section, melanoma must be clinically differentiated from nonneoplastic tumors, including pigmented cysts, freckles, or nevi (Figure 7.34); discoloration consequent to granulomatous and nongranulomatous inflammation (Figure 7.35); and other intraocular tumors (ciliary-body adenoma or adenocarcinoma, lymphosarcoma, and metastatic tumors).

Common distinguishing features of malignant melanoma include an increase in extent on repeated examinations (although progression may be quite slow in the premalignant phase), prominent vascular supply (not always evident), presence of satellite lesions, extension into the iridocorneal angle as detected by gonioscopy, and the presence of complicating factors, including glaucoma.

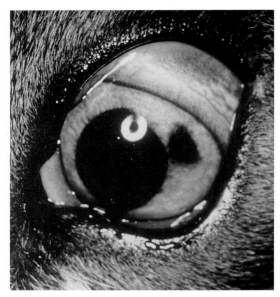

FIG. 7.34—Stationary pigmentation of the iris in a 4-year-old DSH female cat.

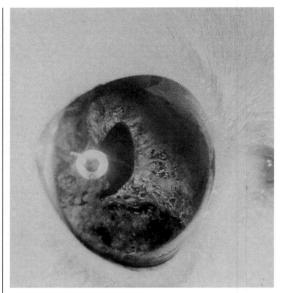

FIG. 7.35—Discoloration and pigmentation of the iris due to anterior uveitis in a 7-year-old Persian male cat.

Tumors of the pigmented ciliary-body epithelium may also provide a difficult clinical distinction from nodular anterior uveal melanomas. This distinction may be made only upon histopathologic examination following enucleation.

Of key importance in the differential diagnosis is that between intraocular malignant melanoma with extraocular extension versus benign limbal melanomas, which, while uncommon compared with dogs, are seen in cats (Figure 7.31).[19,66,68]

BIOLOGIC BEHAVIOR. Diffuse iris melanomas should be regarded as potentially aggressive malignant neoplasms with a potential for metastatic disease that can have long latency periods.[73] They may extend through the sclera into the orbit or extend to the cranial cavity via the optic nerve and may spread to distant organs.[19,58,61,75] The tendency of feline uveal melanomas is to metastasize first to regional lymph nodes and later to all visceral organs and to the skeletal system. Metastasis to the lungs, pleura, heart, pericardium, mediastinum, hilar lymph nodes, diaphragm, omentum, liver, spleen, bone, and brain has been docu-

mented.[56,69,70] In one study of feline ocular melanomas, 10 of 16 uveal melanomas had metastasis prior to enucleation.[71] Some authors distinguish diffuse melanoma of the iris from nodular melanomas, the former representing a biologically different type of melanoma that is locally infiltrative, invades the intertrabecular spaces, plugs the drainage mechanism, and causes glaucoma, but is not as likely to produce distant metastasis.[61,93]

Metastasis can be detected up to several years following clinical diagnosis and/or enucleation. The metastatic rate in one study was 63%.[71]

In one study, cases with proven or suspicious metastatic disease had a significantly greater tumor mass in the enucleated eye than did cases in which follow-up evaluation failed to show evidence of metastatic disease. This suggests that there is an advantage to early diagnosis and enucleation.[16]

Malignant melanomas metastatic to the eyes have been reported in animals but rarely.[53] Melanomas in the eye should be interpreted as primary until proven otherwise.[58]

The number of cases with long-term follow-up is limited, and hard data regarding survival rates are somewhat elusive. However, we believe that adequate data are available to encourage clinicians to consider these neoplasms as a potentially malignant, life-threatening condition that is best managed by enucleation if confined to the globe or, if orbital extension has occurred, by exenteration. Controversy exists as to whether all cases of diffuse primary hyperpigmentation will progress to malignancy, but we believe that this is the case. The neoplastic cells can gain egress from the globe via the aqueous outflow pathways, and shedding of cells may occur early in the course of the disease. Thus, the earlier the enucleation, the better is the prognosis. Surgery should be preceded by a thorough physical examination, including chest radiographs to rule out preexisting metastatic disease or the possibility of a primary site of a melanoma elsewhere in the body with metastasis in the globe.[19]

As regards the comparative aspects, in a study of 3,432 cases of uveal melanoma in human patients, no metastasis to the regional lymph nodes was observed. It has been stated that uveal melanomas in humans do not metastasize to the regional lymph nodes, in contrast to the melanomas of other sites, because of the absence of lymphatic vessels in the uveal tract.[89–91]

Cancer cells in cats might enter the lymphatic vessels from the periocular lymphatics following transscleral extension.[71]

ETIOLOGY. Uveal melanomas have been experimentally produced in cats by injection of the Gardner strain of feline sarcoma virus (GFeSV).[63–65,92] The feline leukemia virus (FeLV) status of clinical cases has received little attention,[70] and the relationship between FeLV (feline retrovirus) and intraocular malignant melanoma is unclear.[70] In one study, the findings in all 14 cats among 16 with ocular melanoma were tested for FeLV were normal.[71] A relationship between trauma and uveal melanomas in cats has been proposed but never proven.[77]

TREATMENT. Enucleation is indicated for an affected globe following clinical diagnosis and workup for the presence of metastatic disease. We recommend early enucleation recognizing that there are no data that define the efficacy of surgery in altering the natural course of the disease, regardless of when performed. Intraocular melanomas in cats have a greater tendency to metastasize and are more malignant than dermal melanomas, with higher rates of death and metastasis.[71]

Nodular tumors of limited extent could potentially be managed by sector iridectomy or iridocyclectomy, and nodular iris melanoma would theoretically be amenable to laser ablation. No data are available regarding the application of these techniques to nodular or diffuse iris melanoma. In the latter, the multifocal nature of the disease process, the documented early dissemination of neoplastic cells via the aqueous humor with entrapment within the trabecular meshwork, and the involvement of the iris root and pectinate ligament would seem to contraindicate laser therapy as an effective management tool.

Histopathologic Features. Feline ocular melanomas are commonly reported as heavily pigmented masses, although they may rarely be poorly pigmented or nonpigmented (amelanotic) growths. Most commonly, they arise from diffusely transformed cells on the anterior iris surface (diffuse iris melanoma) and infiltrate the stroma in an anterior-posterior direction (Figures 7.36 and 7.37),[14,56,58,61,73] or originate in the ciliary body and infiltrate the same and the sclera (Figure 7.38).[59,60,71] The tumor mass can be contiguous to the lens and may obliterate the drainage angle and displace the iris, the ciliary processes, and the lens (Figure 7.39), infiltrating the anterior chamber. The cornea may be invaded by neoplastic tissue, and its rupture is possible.[58,60,69,72] Rarely, the neoplasm can replace the whole globe.[71]

A clear-cut case of primary choroidal melanoma in cats has not been reported. This contrasts sharply with humans, where the incidence of anterior uveal tract melanoma is no higher than 20%.[56,79]

TERMINOLOGY. In human uveal melanomas, morphologic classifications have evolved that correlate well with clinical behavior.[1] They are based

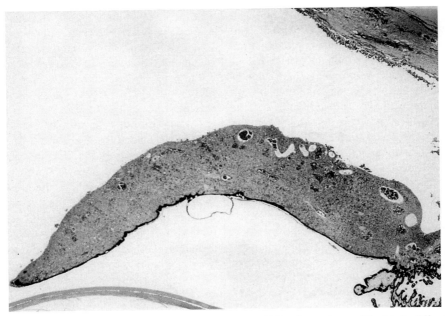

FIG. 7.36—Anterior uveal malignant melanoma in an 11-year-old Persian male cat. The iris is diffusely infiltrated by neoplastic melanocytes with variable amount of pigment. Note the cystic degeneration of the iris epithelium. Hematoxylin–eosin, ×22.5.

on cell type, from narrow spindle cell to large polygonal cell, and on the amount of reticulin present. Spindle cell areas with abundant reticulin are the least malignant, whereas polyhedral cell areas with no reticulin are the most malignant. In Callender's classification, human ocular melanomas are schematically divided by cell type as spindle A, spindle B, fascicular, necrotic, mixed, and epithelioid, in order of increasing malignancy. Although similar histologic characteristics and cell types occur in animals, correlation with biologic behavior has not been demonstrated and attempting to apply this scheme to cat melanomas is inapproprate.[56,58,60,61,71]

In fact, the use of identical terminology implies similarities that may or may not exist, and only serves to confuse the issue from a comparative perspective.[73]

Kircher's classification and nomenclature, included in the International Histologic Classification of Tumors in Domestic Animals,[78] was based on the study of approximately 300 cases of ocular tumors in domestic animals, on file at the Armed Forces Institute of Pathology, Washington, DC.

The primitive melanogenic ocular tumors were divided as follows:

A. Neoplasms of the eyelid and conjunctiva
  1. Benign melanoma
  2. Malignant melanoma
B. Neoplasms of the uveal tract
  1. Benign melanoma
  2. Malignant melanoma
    (a) Spindle cell type
    (b) Epithelioid cell type
    (c) Mixed-cell type

This classification suggested that benign and malignant melanomas of the eyelids and conjunctiva did not differ morphologically from those of the skin.

In this collection, melanomas of the conjunctiva were found only in dogs and horses, and malignant melanomas were the most important intraocular neoplasms in dogs and cats. Benign melanomas of the uveal tract that had not been found in animals were classified as mixed-cell type, the most common variant in animals. Kircher's classification established no correlation between cell type and prognosis for intraocular malignant melanomas in animals.

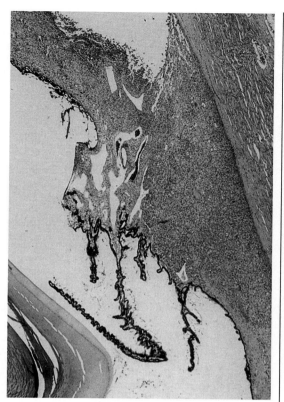

FIG. 7.37—Nonpigmented anterior uveal melanoma in the left eye of a 6-year-old male DSH cat. The tumor infiltrated the iris and the ciliary body with an anterior-posterior progression. Hematoxylin–eosin, ×3.3.

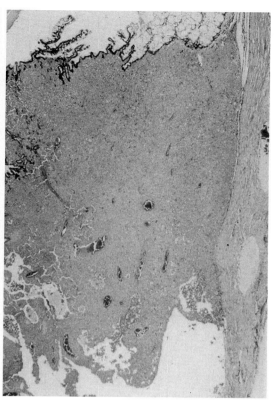

FIG. 7.39—Anterior uveal malignant melanoma in an 11-year-old male cat. Tumor cells invaded the ciliary cleft and trabecular meshwork and obliterated the drainage angle. Hematoxylin–eosin, ×22.5.

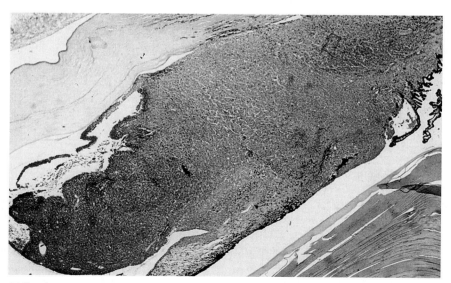

FIG. 7.38—Feline intraocular melanoma originated in the ciliary body and infiltrated the same and part of the anterior chamber. Hematoxylin–eosin, ×22.5.

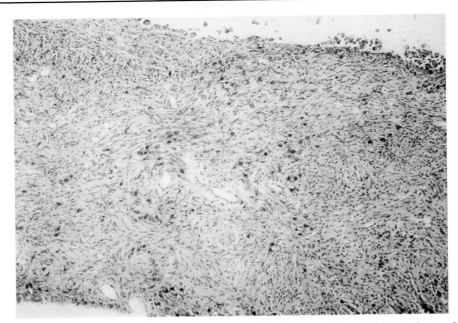

FIG. 7.40—Diffuse spindle-cell-type iris melanoma in a cat. The tissue was characterized by sheets of elongated melanocytes with ovoid nuclei. Mononuclear densely pigmented cells were visible among spindle cells. Hematoxylin–eosin, ×125.

The difficulties encountered in attempting to apply this classification to canine melanomas has been discussed earlier: Bellhorn and Henkind[56] described four major cell types encountered in their series of feline ocular melanomas—epithelioid cells, spindle cells, cells with indistinct borders and pleomorphic nuclei, and plump cells. This scheme has been modified over the years,[54,56] and a simplified terminology has been proposed for feline ocular melanomas: in most cases, one cellular form predominates and is the basis for the categorization of the neoplasms in one of three groups—spindle, plump spindle, or pleomorphic cell.[73]

MORPHOLOGY. Spindle cell neoplasms are characterized more commonly by sheets of streaming elongated cells, but sometimes they may take whorled or interwoven patterns (Figure 7.40).[81] Cell boundaries are indistinct, but sometimes it is possible to see small, clear clefts between cells (Figure 7.41). The cytoplasm is lacy and palely stained with eosin, or compact and eosinophilic. Groups of cells can have abundant cytoplasm with only a fine dusting of pigment granules. Between spindle cells, scattered mononuclear, densely pig-

mented cells can be seen in variable numbers, with larger, coarse, melanin granules. Spindle cells have flattened ovoid nuclei, 7.5 μm long and 1.5 μm wide, with vesicular or finely stippled chromatin patterns. Frequently, small prominent nucleoli are present, but multiple nucleoli are rarely seen.[73] These tumors were previously classified as "type B spindle cell melanomas."[71,78] In a group of 38 intraocular feline malignant melanomas, they represented only 8%.[73]

Plump spindle cell neoplasms are the most common group of pigmented intraocular melanomas in cats.[73] These neoplasms are composed of elongated to polygonal cells with oval to round vesicular nuclei. Nuclear length in elongated cells is similar to spindle cells, but the width is greater, with an average of 5 μm. Round nuclei are 5–7 μm in diameter.[73] Cell boundaries are frequently indistinct, except in areas with polygonal cells. These cells can be cohesive or noncohesive, darkly pigmented, and have round nuclei with single small nucleoli (Figure 7.42). The number of mitoses is extremely variable from 1 to 15 per high-power dry field.[58,60,69] These tumors were previously classified as "mixed-cell type melanomas."[56,60,71,78]

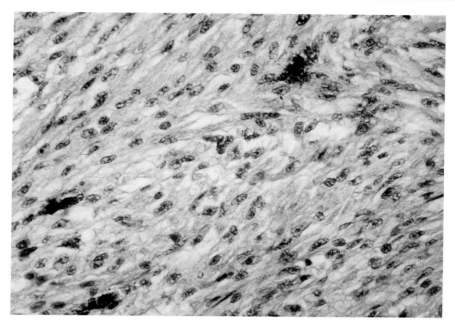

FIG. 7.41—Spindle cell anterior uveal melanoma in a cat: the cytoplasm are lacy, and the nuclei are ovoid with small nucleoli. There are many clear clefts between cells. Hematoxylin–eosin, ×425.

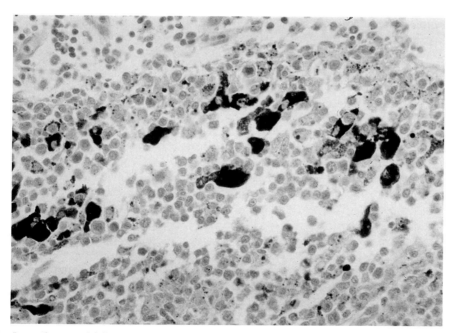

FIG. 7.42—Low-pigmented feline uveal melanoma plump spindle type. In this area, there is a predominance of noncohesive polygonal melanocytes with round nuclei. Hematoxylin–eosin, ×425.

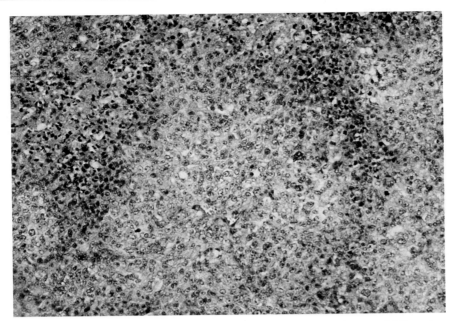

FIG. 7.43—Round, densely packed melanocytes with vesicular nuclei in a nonpigmented feline pleomorphic uveal malignant melanoma. Hematoxylin–eosin, ×225.

Pleomorphic cell neoplasms are characterized by a predominance of polygonal or round melanocytes with variable melanin content, arranged in dense sheets and infiltrated between stromal fibers (Figure 7.43).[61] Polygonal melanocytes have rounded hyperbasophilic, sometimes vesicular nuclei and prominent large nucleoli, about one-third of the size of the nucleus. The cytoplasm can be foamy and abundant, homogeneous and eosinophilic (Figure 7.44). In polygonal cells with large basophilic nuclei, nucleoli can be difficult to distinguish.[73] Hyperbasophilic cells occasionally contain eosinophilic intranucleolar inclusions that are interpreted as cytoplasmic invaginations.[61,73] Their nuclei can also be multiple and/or large and bizarre (multilobed) with large and prominent nucleoli (Figure 7.45).

Balloon cells also are seen in pleomorphic melanomas.[15,61,73] They are large melanocytes with central, round nuclei with finely stippled chromatin and abundant vacuolated cytoplasm containing a fine dusting of pigment granules. Cell boundaries are particularly prominent in these cells.[61,73]

Macrophages also containing melanin (melanophages) can be seen throughout the neoplastic tissue (Figure 7.46).[61] These neoplasms were previously classified as "epithelioid"[56,59,71,78] or "plump-epithelioid cell tumors."[58] In one study, seven cases of pleomorphic feline uveal melanoma were described among 38 collected cases.[73]

Occasionally, neoplasms are encountered with features such that compartmentalization into one of the aforementioned subgroups is difficult; these include neoplasms with features similar to melanocytomas as described for dogs and humans. Nuclear morphology is less uniform, however.

In intraocular feline melanomas, the amount of pigmentation, hemorrhage, and necrosis varies from tumor to tumor, and within the same tumor.[71,81] They are commonly highly vascular neoplasms, and some of their blood channels are without apparent endothelial lining. Necrosis, although not common, is both a cause and result of hemorrhage. Proteolytic products of necrotic tumor cells can induce intraocular lymphocytic and plasmacytic infiltrates, neovascularization of the iris (rubeosis iridis), and secondary cataract. Extension commonly follows vascular channels.[75] Polymorphonuclear leukocyte response is possible when the tumor produces corneal rupture.[58] Retinal detachment can occur, usually associated with extension to the choroid.[59] Loss of ganglion cells, axonal loss

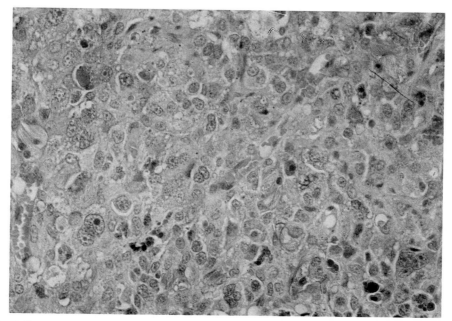

FIG. 7.44—Feline uveal malignant melanoma pleomorphic cell type. Polygonal neoplastic melanocytes with vesicular nuclei and prominent nucleoli are present. Hematoxylin–eosin, ×425.

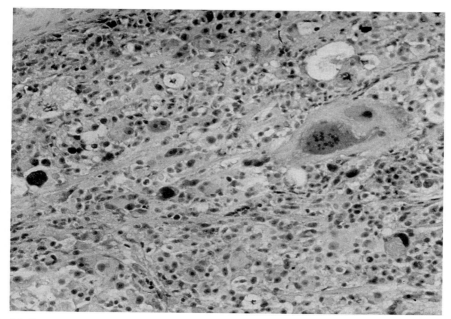

FIG. 7.45—Malignant cells with large and bizarre nuclei and multiple nucleoli in a pleomorphic nonpigmented feline uveal melanoma. Hematoxylin–eosin, ×233.

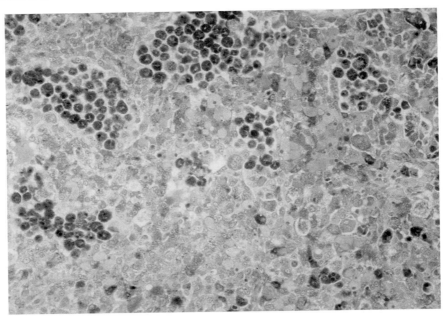

FIG. 7.46—In this case, cells are predominantly "epithelioid" with moderate to marked nuclear pleomorphism. Balloon cells and macrophages with abundant intracytoplasmic melanin are present. Hematoxylin–eosin, ×225.

and gliosis in the nerve fiber layer and optic nerve head (revealed by Bodian silver staining), changes indicative of chronic glaucoma, may be seen.[61]

HISTOCHEMISTRY. Feline ocular melanomas are in general morphologically distinct; on occasion, however, differentiation between hypopigmented/amelanotic melanoma and poorly differentiated ciliary-body tumor, or between intraocular fibrosarcoma and spindle cell malignant melanoma, can be challenging. Tumors of the pigmented ciliary-body epithelium may also be difficult to distinguish from plump spindle type ciliary-body melanoma. By staining the tissue for S-100 protein, one encounters a lack of detectable antigen in ciliary-body adenoma/adenocarcinoma and in posttraumatic sarcoma, and a positive result in melanoma.[14,77] By staining the tissue with anticytokeratin antibody, the result should be negative in melanoma and sarcoma, and positive in ciliary-body epithelial tumors.

Only rarely is it necessary to bleach the tissues with potassium permanganate, prior to staining with hematoxylin–eosin or other methods, in order to appreciate nuclear morphology.

ELECTRON MICROSCOPY. There are few studies about ultrastructural examination of intraocular feline melanomas. In a review of 38 primary anterior uveal melanomas, structural features of two were characterized by selective scanning and transmission electron microscopy. Ultrastructurally, the tumor cells demonstrated round or linear intracytoplasmic melanosomes that appeared as individualized blebs or buds off the anterior surface of the iris.[73] Shadduck et al.[64] examined by electron microscopy fragments of early and advanced melanomas induced by intraocular injection of G-strain feline fibrosarcoma virus, and portions of cell cultures derived from these tumors. The presence of mixed populations of cells and the major histologic features were confirmed. Melanosomes in various stages of development were identified in "spindle shaped" and "epithelioid" tumor cells. Albert et al.[63] described the ultrastructural appearance of induced feline melanomas: transformed melanocytes were basically similar to melanoma cells described in human eyes.

Prognosis. With slight equivocation, clinical and morphologic features of ocular melanomas in cats provide imprecise guidelines for prognostication. Rapidly growing neoplasms are more likely to metastasize than are slowly growing neoplasms. Larger melanomas likely have a poorer prognosis than do smaller ones. Extraocular extension

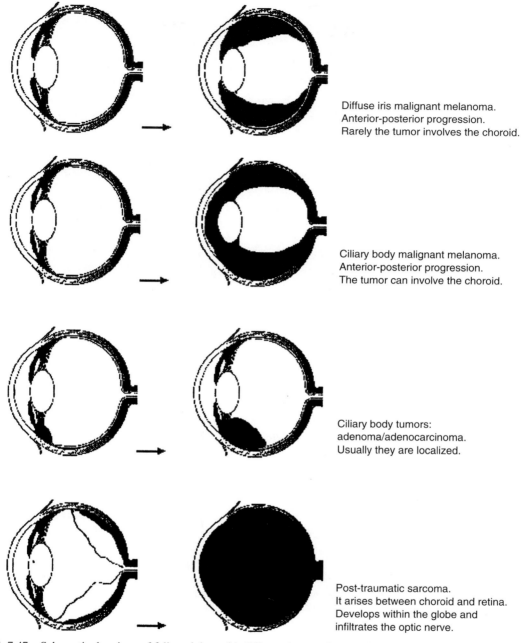

Diffuse iris malignant melanoma.
Anterior-posterior progression.
Rarely the tumor involves the choroid.

Ciliary body malignant melanoma.
Anterior-posterior progression.
The tumor can involve the choroid.

Ciliary body tumors:
adenoma/adenocarcinoma.
Usually they are localized.

Post-traumatic sarcoma.
It arises between choroid and retina.
Develops within the globe and
infiltrates the optic nerve.

FIG. 7.47—Schematic drawings of feline globes with different intraocular neoplasms at different stages of development.

increases the likelihood of both local recurrence and metastatic disease. Cellular type, reticulin content, and necrosis have been studied and found not to be reliable predictors of biologic behavior.

Duncan and Peiffer[73] used a grading scheme to note the degree of pigmentation and nuclear vari-

ability. Tumor location and extent also were catalogued (Figure 7.47). Mitotic index, nuclear-cytoplasmic (N/C) ratio, and number of nucleoli were compared between fatal and nonfatal groups of tumors. The number of mitotic figures was significantly greater in the fatal group; no significant

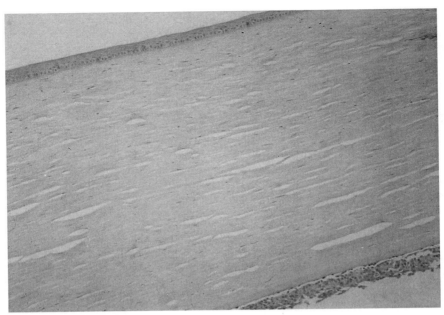

FIG. 7.48—A Siamese male cat. Malignant melanocytes on the posterior corneal surface. This eye was affected by a poorly pigmented diffuse iris melanoma, plump spindle type.

differences were found between two groups in N/C ratio and in number of nucleoli or in the degree of pigmentation. All fatal cases demonstrated tumor within the lumens of scleral veins.

Nests of neoplastic cells may be seen in the vitreous and on the corneal endothelium (Figure 7.48), or appear floating into the anterior chamber and invading the drainage pathway.[60,61,73] These cells can invade and proliferate within the ciliary cleft and trabecular meshwork, with access to the scleral veins; the presence of malignant cells within these vessels represents a negative prognostic factor.[56,69,73] The globe and orbit are devoid of lymphatics; unless the neoplasm gains access to the conjunctival lymphatics by transscleral extension, metastasis occurs by hematogenous routes via the uveal vasculature or the scleral veins.

HUMANS

Overview

HISTORICAL AND EMBRYOLOGIC CONSIDERATIONS. Neural crest cells are derived from ectoderm located at the margin of the neural plate.[94] They can be divided into upper cranial and lower truncal components. The cranial segment is important in the embryology of the head.[95] The cells of the cranial neural crest migrate into *primary mesenchyme,* which is composed of mesoderm, and the composite tissue is termed *secondary mesenchyme.*[96] It had been believed that much of the structures of the head and neck, including many ocular tissues, were derived from the mesodermal component of this tissue, but many of these structures have been demonstrated to arise from the neural crest cells of this secondary mesenchyme.[97,98] The neural crest-derived ocular and periocular tissues include the corneal stroma and endothelium, anterior-chamber angle, iris stroma, and melanocytes of the eyelids, conjunctiva, and uvea. Hu and colleagues[99] have suggested that, during embryogenesis, iris melanocytes migrate and mature to become choroidal melanocytes. Retinal pigment epithelium also produces melanin; however, it is of neuroepithelial origin.

Adult melanocytes are characterized by the presence of melanin pigment and the enzyme tyrosinase.[99] Boissy and associates[100] have noted that cutaneous melanocytes have been postulated to protect the dividing epithelial cells from mutations caused by ultraviolet light, and to scavenge free radicals generated in epithelial cells. They contrast these functions with the proposed function of uveal melanocytes, absorbing scattered light within the eye to prevent background "light noise," which might degrade the retinal function. They postulate that epidermal and uveal melanocytes represent two distinct populations with the ability to differentiate in culture independent of their respective normal environments.

Cramer[101] has suggested that during histogenesis, contrary to traditional beliefs, melanocytes do not "drop off" the epidermis to populate the dermis. Rather, melanocytes migrate up from the dermis into the epidermis in normal histogenesis and in normal tissue maintenance. Furthermore, he asserts that the precursor of cutaneous melanocytes is a pluripotential cell and not a melanoblast, which is a cell committed to melanocyte differentiation. Similarly, Huley and associates[102] have proposed that, contrary to previous reports, melanization initially is primarily dermal, and there also is minimal, if any, migration of premelanocytes from epidermis to dermis.

TERMINOLOGY AND CLASSIFICATION. Ocular melanocytic lesions can be divided logically into (1) eyelid skin and conjunctival lesions and (2) uveal lesions. It is appropriate to create these two broad divisions because descriptive terminology, and histologic and prognostic classification systems, are shared within each of these two groups but differ between them. As an example, *junctional* is used to describe melanocytes located between the epithelium and the underlying connective tissue of skin and conjunctiva. For conjunctiva, melanocytes in the substantia propria are termed *subepithelial* and correspond to dermal melanocytes, which are similarly located in the skin. There is no similar descriptive terminology used for uveal lesions. Conversely, uveal melanomas are classified on a cytologic basis using a modification the Callender system, which classified tumors based on cell type into spindle A, spindle B, fascicular, mixed, epithelioid, and necrotic.[1,103] The Callender system or its modifications are not used in classifying skin or conjunctival lesions, although melanoma cells in these areas may be described clinically as being of a "spindle or epithelioid" cell type. The subsequent discussion dwells on uveal lesions, with readers referred to other sections to explore melanocytic lesions of the human skin and conjunctiva.

Nevus and Malignant Melanoma

EPIDEMIOLOGIC OVERVIEW. During a 10-year period ending December 1976, ocular melanomas comprised 16% of all melanomas and 70% of ocular malignant disease in Alberta, Canada.[104] Similarly, Mahoney and associates[105] noted that melanomas comprised 70.4% of ocular cancers in New York between 1975 and 1986. In the Third National Cancer Survey, 1968 to 1971, there were 432 patients with noncutaneous melanomas; 79% of these tumors were ocular melanomas.[106]

Mahoney and colleagues[105] found an average age-adjusted annual incidence of ocular melanomas in New York State of 4.9 per 1,000,000 among men and 3.7 per 1,000,000 among women. Osterlind[107] noted an age-standardized incidence of ocular melanoma of 0.75 per 100,000 in males and 0.60 per 100,000 in females in Denmark from 1943 to 1982. The relative incidence of uveal melanomas can be garnered from the latter study in which 80% of the melanomas were in the choroid, 10% in the ciliary body and iris, 5% in the conjunctiva, and 5% in "multiple regions." The relative frequencies of the various Callender cell types were 12% epithelioid, 36% spindle cell, and 51% mixed. It also is of interest to note that the incidence of cutaneous melanoma increased by five- to sixfold during the period of that study although the incidence of ocular melanoma remained stable. The findings of Osterlind are similar to those of Hayton and associates,[108] who studied ocular melanomas in Alberta, Canada, and noted that 82% of ocular melanomas arose from the choroid. The melanomas were classified as spindle cell in 53% of cases, mixed-cell type in 23%, epithelioid in 8%, and fascicular in 1%.

Uveal melanomas rarely can occur in children,[109,110] and even congenital cases have been reported.[111] Pediatric uveal melanomas do not differ significantly from the adult counterpart.[109,110] Multifocal lesions[112,113] or bilateral tumors[114,115] are extremely uncommon presentations of uveal melanoma.

Gallagher and colleagues[116] have suggested that increased risk of ocular melanoma is associated with light eye and hair color and with indoor occupation. Holly and associates[117] found an increased risk of uveal melanoma associated with increasing numbers of large nevi, light eye color, a tendency to sunburn, and exposure to ultraviolet or black lights. Seddon and colleagues[118] have postulated a subset of patients whose ocular melanomas are hormonally responsive. Nevertheless, receptor studies and case-control studies have failed to confirm a strong association with hormonal or reproductive history.[118–120] A rare example of a suspected occupational association with uveal melanoma was a cluster of choroidal melanomas that occurred among chemical workers in West Virginia.[121]

Although familial occurrence of uveal melanocytic tumors has been reported, it is extremely rare to find a family history of ocular or skin melanoma among uveal melanoma patients.[122,123]

Iris Melanoma

CLINICAL FEATURES. Iris melanomas most often are asymptomatic lesions that may be noted by the patient to be enlarging, especially if old photographs are examined for comparison.[124] Slight growth of iris melanocytic lesions during puberty does not necessarily signify malignant change, and these lesions may remain dormant for many years before substantial growth is detected. Occasional patients will complain of pain or decreased vision from elevated intraocular pressure. On average, patients with iris melanomas are 10–20 years younger than those harboring choroidal melanomas. Approximately 80% of iris melanomas and suspicious nevi are located in the inferior one-half of the iris (Figure 7.49).[124,125] Although melanocytic iris lesions most often involve lightly pigmented irides, it is not known whether this finding represents an actual predilection for an increased occurrence in such individuals or merely represents increased ease of detection because of contrast with a light-background iris color.[126]

The clinical distinction between iris nevi and melanomas can be difficult. Jakobiec and Sil-

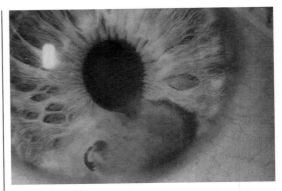

FIG. 7.49—Clinical photograph of iris melanoma located in the inferior quadrant of the iris.

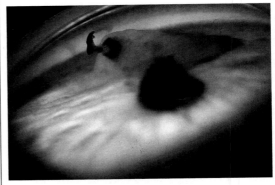

FIG. 7.50—Goniophotograph of the same iris melanoma as the lesion in Figure 7.22 demonstrates that the mass also involves the anterior-chamber angle. Lesions in this location may represent anterior extension of a ciliary-body tumor.

bert[124] made the distinction between lesions originating from the iris versus primary ciliary-body tumors that secondarily involve the iris (Figure 7.50). In their histopathologic review of 189 iris lesions originally diagnosed a melanomas, many of the lesions were reclassified as nevi. Interestingly, clinical features such as lesion color, location, ocular symptoms, pigment dust in the angle, pupil distortion, glaucoma, tapioca appearance, sector cataract, episcleral vessel dilation, anterior-chamber angle involvement, and ectropion uveae did not help in distinguishing between benign and malignant lesions. However, in a more recent study, larger size, pigment dispersion, prominent tumor vascularity, elevated intraocular

TABLE 7.5—Iris melanocytic lesions: histopathologic diagnostic categories

Lesion group	Definition	Iris lesions	Iris and ciliary body lesions	Total (%)	
1	Melanocytosis	1	3	4	(2)
2	Melanocytoma	5	5	10	(5)
3	Epithelioid cell nevus	5	0	5	(3)
4	Intrastromal spindle cell nevus	17	25	42	(23)
5	Spindle cell nevus with surface plaque	58	16	74	(38)
6	Borderline spindle cell nevus	11	19	30	(16)
7	Spindle cell melanoma	1	11	12	(7)
8	Mixed spindle cell and epithelioid cell melanoma	3	5	8	(4)
9	Epithelioid cell melanoma	2	2	4	(2)
Total		103	86	189 (100)	

Modified from Jakobiec and Silbert.[124]

pressure, and ocular symptoms were found to be significantly associated with histologic malignancy among resected tumors.[127] In this same study, larger size was the only predictive feature for growth of iris melanocytic lesions that were not initially treated. Ciliary-body extension and ring formation have been shown to be statistically associated with malignancy.[124] Iris angiography has been used for diagnostic purposes, but its usefulness is now questioned.[128–131] More recently, high-frequency anterior-segment ultrasound has been used to evaluate the size, location, and internal acoustic characteristics of these lesions, although the capability of this modality to aid in distinguishing benign from malignant melanocytic lesions has not been established.[132] In some cases, FNA biopsy may be required to determine the diagnosis and initiate proper treatment.[133]

Documentation of substantial growth over a relatively short time is the most important criterion in distinguishing iris nevi from melanomas.[124,134] Among all iris melanocytic lesions, only a small minority are melanomas. Territo and associates[135] reviewed 288 lesions consistent with iris nevus or melanoma. Of these patients, 43 (14.9%) were managed initially by surgical excision of the iris lesion, whereas 235 (81.6%) were thought to have a low-grade lesion and were managed by observation. Only 8 (4.6%) of 175 lesions observed eventually were documented to grow and require treatment. Other iris lesions can also mimic iris melanoma, including primary iris cysts, essential iris atrophy, iris foreign body, peripheral anterior synechia, and iris metastases.[134]

MORPHOLOGY. Jakobiec and Silbert[124] divided melanocytic iris lesions into nine histologic categories (Table 7.5; for illustrations of specific Callender cell types mentioned, see examples in the section *Ciliary Body and Choroid Melanoma*). Their first six groups refer to morphologic varieties of nevi and include lesions that previously would have been classified as spindle-A melanomas. Nevertheless, the authors state that all of these lesions are cytologically benign and clinically behave accordingly. Group 7 includes spindle cell melanomas that cytologically are equivalent to spindle-B melanomas of the choroid. Group 8 contains a combination of spindle and epithelioid cells. Group 9 includes tumors that are composed almost entirely of epithelioid cells. As can be seen from Table 7.5, the majority of melanocytic iris lesions that were clinically worrisome were nevertheless benign histologically following excisional biopsy.

Marcus and associates[136] have reported that silver staining of nucleolar organizer region-associated proteins is an objective means that can be used to differentiate iris nevi from melanomas. In their study, all iris nevi demonstrated counts lower than 1.9, and all iris melanomas had counts greater than 2.8.

TREATMENT. Because of the difficulty in distinguishing benign from malignant iris melanocytic tumors, and in light of the low metastatic rate of these tumors in general, the management of these tumors continues to be challenging and controversial. In a study by Harbour et al.[127] of 285 iris melanocytic tumors, 32 of which were histologically diagnosed as melanoma, only two of the patients developed metastasis, and both had been treated promptly. Thus, iris melanoma has a relatively low metastatic rate, and it is unclear whether prompt treatment alters the ultimate outcome. Thus, most ocular oncologists are relatively conservative in recommending treatment, and the indications for treatment that most experts would agree on include large size, increased intraocular pressure, ocular symptoms, and documented growth.[125,134,137] Treatment options include local resection (iridectomy or iridocyclectomy), plaque brachytherapy, and enucleation. Local resection is performed when the tumor is localized without dispersion and is less than about 4 clock hours in basal dimensions. Plaque radiotherapy is gaining popularity in unresectable tumors in which the vision in the affected eye is critical (e.g., poor vision in the fellow eye).[138] Enucleation is usually reserved for large or multifocal lesions that cannot be resected, or in cases with extensive involvement of the trabecular meshwork and secondary glaucoma that cannot be managed clinically. FNA biopsy is rarely needed but may occasionally be useful to rule out a simulating lesion, such as a metastatic iris lesion. The role of observation for those lesions that involve the anterior face of the ciliary body is more controversial, and some authors recommend earlier excision for such lesions.[137]

PROGNOSIS. Patients with iris melanoma have been reported to have an excellent prognosis. Perhaps, some of this reputation can be attributed to the fact that many lesions previously labeled "melanomas" actually should be reclassified as nevi.[124] However, most recent reports have suggested a low metastatic rate even for confirmed iris melanomas. Shields et al.[139] found that only 5% of their patients with histologically proven iris melanoma developed metastasis.

When Geisse and Robertson[131] reviewed published reports of iris melanomas and those on record at the Mayo Clinic, they found 1043 reported cases of iris melanomas, of which 31 (3%) had metastasized. There were no reports of metastasis from spindle-A lesions, thereby supporting the previous reclassification of these neoplasms as nevi by Jakobiec and Silbert.[124] The metastatic rates for spindle-B and epithelioid lesions were 10.5% and 6.9%, respectively. Information on the initial surgical treatment was available on 21 of the 31 lesions that metastasized. Of note is that 13 (62%) of the 21 metastasizing lesions were either incompletely excised or were transected at the initial surgery. These and other reports documenting the incidence of metastasis from iris melanomas still may overestimate the metastatic rate for true iris lesions, because the reports may include some lesions predominantly arising in the ciliary body.[124] Davidorf[140] has postulated that iris melanomas are not inherently different from other ocular melanomas, but that their extremely small average volume at the time of diagnosis (55 mm^3) is the major feature contributing to their excellent prognosis compared with other uveal melanomas. Ultrasound biomicroscopy may prove useful clinically in documenting the extent of ciliary-body involvement in anterior-segment melanocytic lesions.[141]

Ciliary Body and Choroid Melanoma

CLINICAL FEATURES. Servodidio and Abramson[142] reviewed the presenting signs and symptoms of 193 uveal melanoma patients. Table 7.6 summarizes their findings. Most of the patients presented with visual disturbance, but 41% were asymptomatic. Anteriorly located melanomas involving the ciliary body may present with episcleral sentinel vessels, tilting of the lens, or cataract. Any unilateral alteration of intraocular pressure, either elevation or depression, may be associated with anterior uveal melanomas.[143] Shields and associates[144] noted elevated intraocular pressure in 17% of eyes harboring ciliary-body melanomas. Such findings should alert clinicians to the need for a thorough dilated fundus examination, including examination of the ciliary body.

On ophthalmoscopic examination, choroidal melanocytic lesions represent a continuum from small, flat, discrete nevi (Figure 7.51) to suspicious lesions (Figure 7.52) and, finally, to frank melanomas (Figures 7.53 and 7.54). Choroidal melanomas vary in color from amelanotic to green-black. They seldom are jet black; however, retinal pigment epithelial hyperplasia often is a dark black lesion. Melanomas may have overly-

TABLE 7.6—Presenting signs and symptoms in choroidal melanomas

Patients included (*n*=193)

Eye	Sex	Age
OD, 94	Female, 94	<60 years old, 30
OS, 99	Male, 99	>60 years old, 127
Tumor size		Tumor location (*n*=193)
Small (<3.0 mm long), 30		Posterior to the equator, 111
Medium (3.1–8.0 mm long), 111		Anterior to the equator, 54
Large (8.1 mm or longer), 52		Ciliary body, 28
Presence of tumor or retinal detachment in macula		
Yes, 32		
No, 161		

Presenting signs and symptoms	Patients treated (*n*=168)
Routine eye examination, 65	Radioactive plaque, 112
Problem in fellow eye, 15	Iodine 125, 49
Visual acuity/field defect, 77	Cobalt 60, 63
Flashes/floaters, 30	Enucleation, 44
Pain, 5	Local surgery, 8
Metastatic disease, 1	Noninvasive therapy, 4

Modified from Servodidio and Abramson.[142]

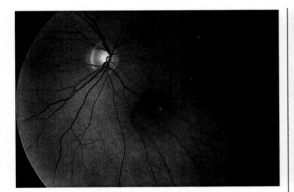

FIG. 7.51—Fundus photograph of a small, flat, discrete, typical choroidal nevus.

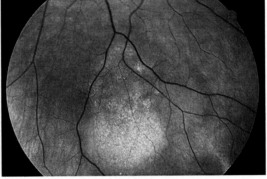

FIG. 7.52—Fundus photograph of a suspicious nevus with mild elevation and shallow, localized retinal detachment.

ing orange lipofuscin pigment and subretinal fluid, which are predictive of future growth.[145]

Melanomas usually begin as a relatively flat or placoid lesion (Figure 7.55). They are slow growing and gradually become more dome shaped before breaking through Bruch's membrane to assume a characteristic "mushroom" configuration when large (Figure 7.56). Diffuse melanomas are less typical lesions that grow in an infiltrative pattern so that their radial dimensions exceed their thickness. The uniform appearance of these latter lesions makes them more difficult to detect than the more typical lesion, thereby often leading to a delay in diagnosis and the possibility of orbital extension (Figure 7.57).[146,147] They are very uncommon and were reported to comprise 4.5% of 400 melanomas from the files of the Armed Forces Institute of Pathology.[146]

The accuracy in diagnosing choroidal melanoma has risen dramatically in the past half-century, largely due to equipment such as the indirect ophthalmoscope and ophthalmic ultrasound, as well as increased awareness of the clinical features of this

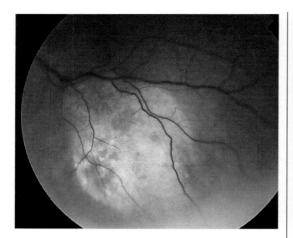

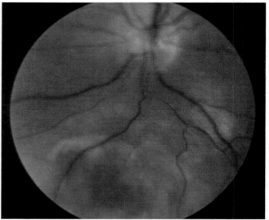

FIG. 7.53—Fundus photograph of a localized, elevated choroidal melanoma with typical green-black pigmentation.

FIG. 7.54—Fundus photograph of a large choroidal melanoma adjacent to the optic disc.

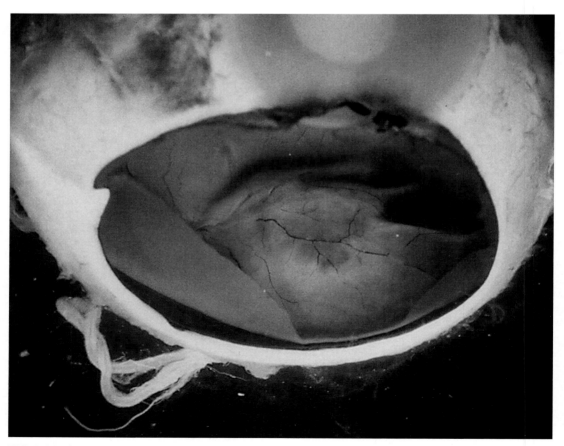

FIG. 7.55—**A:** Gross pathologic specimen demonstrating relatively placoid choroidal melanoma adjacent to the macula. (continued)

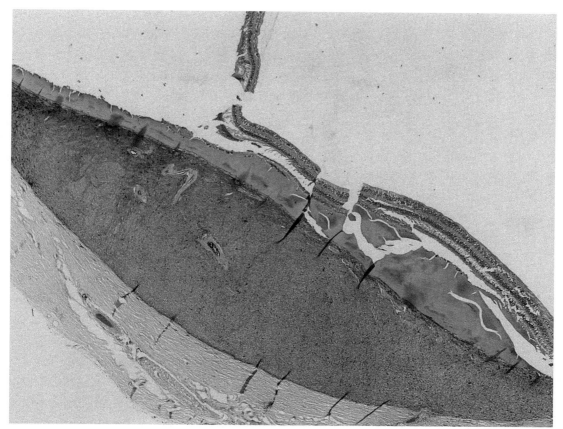

FIG. 7.55 (continued)—**B:** Low-power photomicrograph of placoid choroidal melanoma. Hematoxylin–eosin, ×4.

disorder. Earlier reports indicated a false-positive diagnostic rate of 1.4%–20%.[148–155] However, a recent report from the Collaborative Ocular Melanoma Study (COMS)[156] found that 99.5% of tumors diagnosed as uveal melanomas and enucleated in the study were in fact melanomas by histopathologic verification.

The cornerstone of diagnosis in uveal melanoma is careful ophthalmoscopy by an experienced observer.[157–159] The most important ancillary study is ultrasonography with both A scan and B scan.[159] The low internal reflectivity seen with A scan is highly characteristic of melanoma and distinguishes it from other choroidal lesions such as metastasis and hemangioma. Fluorescein angiography and magnetic resonance imaging are occasionally helpful, but the P-32 test is no longer felt to be of significant utility. Ultrasonography is particularly useful in the presence of opaque media.[154,160] Approximately 7%–10% of enucleated eyes in the past contained unsuspected uveal melanomas, particularly in glaucomatous eyes with opaque media.[154,155,161–163]

MORPHOLOGY AND PROGNOSIS. The Callender classification for melanomas of the ciliary body and choroid, originally published in 1931,[1] attempted to combine morphologic and prognostic features. According to this classification, spindle cell type was one of the major categories, characterized by the presence of sheets, whorls, and irregular arrangements of cells resembling fibroblasts. Spindle cells were subdivided into two spindle cell subtypes: subtype A (Figure 7.58), with a delicate reticular nucleus and no nucleolus, and subtype B (Figure 7.59), with a sharply defined,

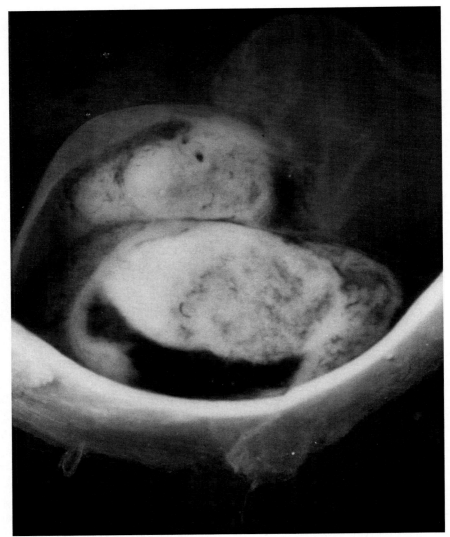

FIG. 7.56—**A:** Gross pathologic specimen demonstrating the "mushroom" or "collar button" configuration of a choroidal melanoma that has broken through Bruch's membrane. (continued)

small, round nucleolus and a coarse nuclear network. The second major category was epithelioid cell type (Figure 7.60), comprised of polygonal, large cells with large, round to oval nuclei possessing one or two small, round, discrete nucleoli. Mixed-cell type (Figure 7.60), the most common variety, was composed of a mixture of spindle (either A or B) and epithelioid cells. Callender also recognized a fascicular cell type in which the cells are arranged in a palisade pattern, but this pattern was subsequently reclassified as a variant of the spindle-B cell type. The final category

according to the original Callender classification was the necrotic cell type, characterized by degenerated cells that could not be placed in another category. Since Callender's original classification system was reported, it has been modified by Callender by himself and others.[72] For example, most tumors originally classified as spindle-A melanomas are now thought to represent nevi, based on their bland cytologic characteristics and their low frequency of metastasis.[165] A new variety of epithelioid cell also has been described that is characterized by less cytoplasm and a smaller

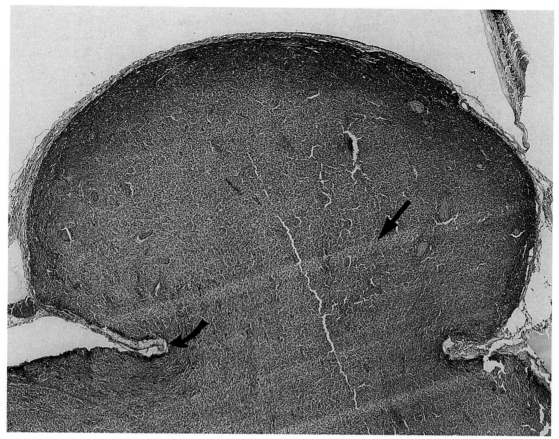

FIG. 7.56 (continued)—**B:** Photomicrograph of a lesion similar to that in **A.** Indentation is caused by the constricting band of Bruch's membrane (curved arrow). Note the "chatter mark" artifact from a microtome knife (straight arrow), and the retina draped over the "dome" of the mass. Hematoxylin–eosin, ×10.

nucleus marked by a large eosinophilic nucleolus in contrast to the epithelioid cell originally described by Callender.[166]

Callender associated histologic characteristics with survival prognosis for uveal melanomas, and numerous studies have validated his findings.[108,167–173] Packard[172] reported that the 5-year survival rate for individuals with spindle cell tumors, mixed tumors, and epithelioid tumors was 85%, 58%, and 57%, respectively. McLean and colleagues[173] examined small melanomas of the choroid and ciliary body and found the following survival rates: spindle A, 90%; spindle B, 84%; mixed, 40%; and epithelioid, 0%. Of note, however, is that survival for patients with uveal melanoma does not parallel that of age-matched controls for up to 15 years after tumor diagnosis (Table 7.7). Thus, in their study of ocular

melanoma in Alberta, Canada, Hayton and associates[108] found that 15% of their patients died of metastasis more than 10 years after diagnosis. Therefore, studies discussing prognosis in uveal melanoma must follow cases for at least 15 years in order to produce meaningful results.[171]

One of the difficulties with the Callender system is the common disagreement among experienced ophthalmic pathologists regarding the proper histologic classification of a given tumor.[165,171,174,175] The source of this disagreement has been based, in part, on the lack of objective criteria for each category.[165] In addition, the criteria for diagnosing various cell types have shifted over time.[165] In reality, histologic types probably represent arbitrary stages along a continuum of malignant transformation from the benign nevus to the highly malignant tumor containing epithelioid cells.[175]

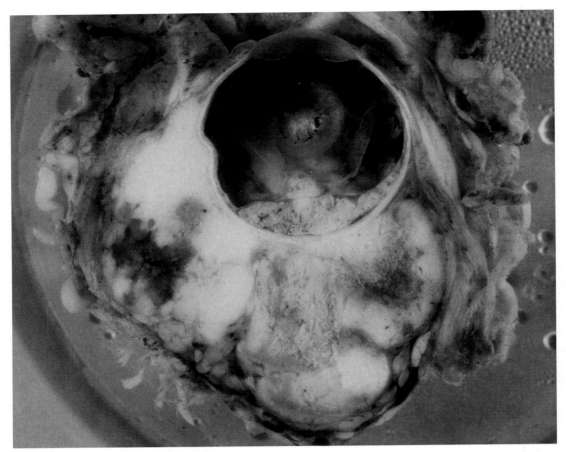

FIG. 7.57—**A:** Gross orbital exenteration pathologic specimen of diffuse choroidal melanoma that has exited the eye and filled the orbit. (continued)

Other histologic features have also been found to correlate with prognosis. Gamel and McLean, studying nuclear features (chromatin clumping, minimum nuclear diameter, nucleolar diameter, chromatin margination, maximum nuclear diameter, and abundant cytoplasm), found that these correlated well with cell type.[175] The standard deviation of the nucleolar area (SDNA) and the inverse of the SDNA (ISDNA) reflect nuclear pleomorphism and correlate with survival in uveal melanoma.[176] Seddon and associates[177] have shown that the ISDNA and the number of epithelioid cells per high-power field each correlates with tumor survival. Gamel and colleagues[178] have suggested that another nucleolar measurement, the mean of the largest nucleoli (MLN), is more easily measured than the SDNA and corre-lates well with largest tumor dimension, SDNA, and cell type as a predictor of tumor mortality. Furthermore, increased predictive power is achieved when largest tumor dimension is used as a covariant with SDNA, cell type, or MLN. Although these morphometric features of the nucleolus represent objective predictors of tumor mortality and may more accurately reflect the full spectrum of malignancy than the arbitrary stages found in the Callender system,[179] they require equipment not normally found in a histopathology laboratory. Folberg and associates[180] have identified nine vascular patterns and networks (at least three back-to-back closed vascular loops) that were found to be most strongly associated with metastatic death. Similarly, melanomas possessing vascular patterns typical of nevi are less

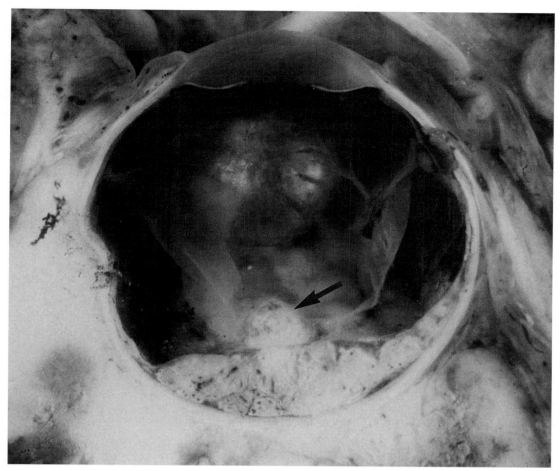

FIG. 7.57 (continued)—**B:** Higher magnification of **A** showing diffuse choroidal melanoma with a small "mushroom" component (arrow).

lethal than are melanomas with vascular networks.[181] Clinical features have also been associated with prognosis, with larger tumor size and anterior tumor location predictive of poorer prognosis.[108,169,171,172] These clinical features approximate the accuracy of histologic cell type in predicting patient survival.[171]

TREATMENT AND PROGNOSIS. The treatment of ciliary-body and choroidal melanoma has evolved dramatically over the past half-century and continues to be the object of controversy. Historically, enucleation was performed for an eye containing a lesion suspected of being a melanoma. However, Zimmerman and colleagues[173,182–184] proposed in the 1970s that enucleation may actually hasten the

systemic dissemination of melanoma cells. This hypothesis was based on a major assumption that the mortality rate from the tumor was probably about 1% per year. In addition, Wagoner and Albert[185] found that 2.4% of 1214 melanomas had evidence of metastasis at the time of diagnosis. This number was significantly larger than previously had been estimated. Seigel and associates[186] failed to find a significant difference in the pattern of patients who died of uveal melanomas compared with patients who died of other cancers. Manschot and van Peperzeel[187] questioned whether the growth rate of uveal melanomas was consistent with tumor fatalities within 2 years of enucleation secondary to tumor cells disseminated at the time of enucleation.

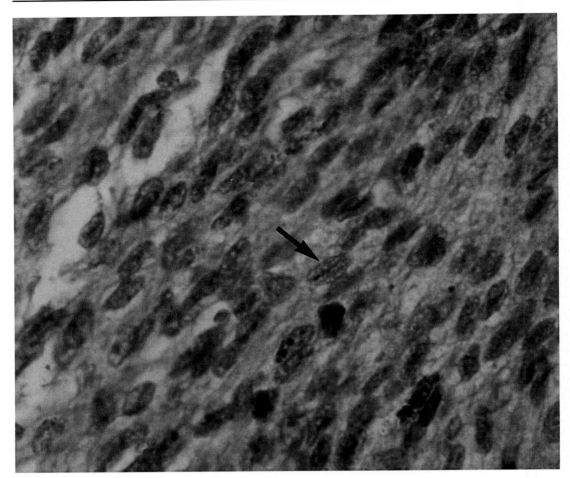

FIG. 7.58—Photomicrograph of spindle cell uveal melanoma. Note the spindle-A cell (arrow) characterized by a nuclear chromatin "stripe." Hematoxylin–eosin, ×200.

Gass[188] evaluated the growth rate of choroidal and ciliary-body melanomas prior to enucleation and concluded that, contrary to the conclusions of Zimmerman and associates, melanomas do not have a uniform slow growth rate prior to enucleation. Rather, Gass found that mitotic index, tumor cytology, tumor size, and tumor-related mortality all correlated with growth rate, which tended to be uniform for a particular tumor but which varied considerably between tumors. Additionally, Gass[158] demonstrated that mortality was not significantly increased if small suspected melanomas were observed for documented growth prior to enucleation. After the observations by Gass, most ocular oncologists began to follow small, indeterminate melanocytic tumors for documented growth prior to enucleation. Although the validity of the "Zimmerman hypothesis" is now questioned on several grounds, this hypothesis had the important effect of inspiring the development of alternative treatment modalities, such as plaque radiotherapy and local resection.[159]

The COMS has provided insights into many treatment questions regarding uveal melanoma. For many years, there was controversy over whether patients should undergo prophylactic external beam irradiation prior to enucleation to reduce the chance of metastatic disease. However, a well-designed, prospective trial has clearly shown no survival benefit to this prophylactic

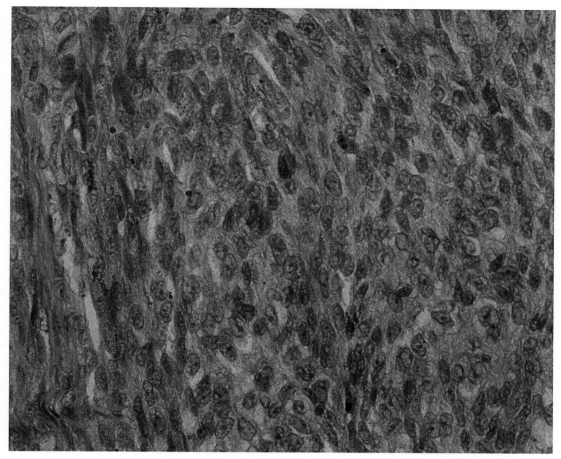

FIG. 7.59—Photomicrograph of spindle-B cell uveal melanoma characterized by the presence of a distinct nucleolus but limited amount of cytoplasm and lack of distinct cell borders. Hematoxylin–eosin, ×100.

radiotherapy in patients with large choroidal melanomas.[189] In another arm of the COMS, the survival following enucleation versus plaque radiotherapy is being compared for medium-sized tumors. The results of this trial should settle the important issue of whether these two therapies are indeed equivalent with regard to survival. Other eye-sparing therapies have been developed, such as local tumor resection,[190] charged-particle radiotherapy,[191] stereotactic radiosurgery,[192] and transpupillary thermotherapy.[193] None of these have been compared with enucleation in a prospective, controlled trial, so the appropriate indications for each form of therapy will remain controversial into the foreseeable future.

The prognosis for patients with uveal melanoma depends on many clinical and histologic factors, as already mentioned. In 1992, however, Diener-West and colleagues[194] performed a meta-analysis of the literature in order to reach some conclusions about prognosis based on size. They reported 5-year mortality rates of 16% for small tumors, 32% for medium tumors, and 53% for large tumors. This remains the best estimate in the literature of prognosis for all tumor sizes. In a recent report from the COMS, the metastatic death rate was studied among patients with large tumors.[195] Of 1003 patients entering the study, 46% had died (similar to the 53% in the Diener-West study), with a median

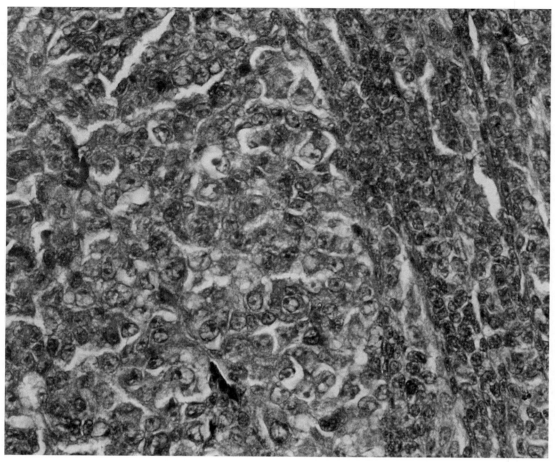

FIG. 7.60—Photomicrograph of mixed-cell uveal melanoma. Compare the epithelioid cell population on the *left* two-thirds of the photomicrograph, characterized by marked variation in nuclear size, distinct cell borders, and abundant cytoplasm, to the spindle cell population on the *right.* Hematoxylin–eosin, ×100.

TABLE 7.7—Survival of patients with uveal melanoma grouped on the basis of cell type and size

	Number of cases	Survival (%)		
		5 Years	10 Years	15 Years
Spindle type				
Small	405	97.8	89.6	87.3
Medium	476	88.0	73.8	69.0
Large	183	76.8	60.3	45.9
Mixed type				
Small	266	77.7	67.1	61.3
Medium	512	59.0	46.4	40.1
Large	527	43.2	30.2	25.5

From McLean et al.[173]

survival time of 7.4 years. Of the patients who died, 62% had confirmed melanoma metastasis, and metastasis was suspected in 21%. The most common sites of metastasis were liver (93%), lung (24%), and bone (16%).

ACKNOWLEDGMENTS

J.R.B.M. and S.P.-J. are grateful to Prof. W.R. Lee, University of Glasgow, for access to laboratory and photographic facilities; to Prof. J.S. Boyd, University of Glasgow Veterinary School, for ultrasonography facilities; and to Dr. I.A.P. MacCandlish, University of Glasgow Veterinary School, for immunocytochemistry.

REFERENCES

1. Callender GR. Malignant melanotic tumors of the eye: a study of histologic types in 111 cases. *Trans Am Acad Ophthalmol Otolaryngol* 36:131, 1931.
2. Saunders LZ, Barron CN. Primary pigmented intraocular tumors in animals. *Cancer Res* 18:234, 1958.
3. Magrane WG. Tumors of the eye and orbit in the dog. *J Small Anim Pract* 6:165, 1965.
4. Diters RW, Dubielzig RR, Aguirre GD, Acland GM. Primary ocular melanoma in dogs. *Vet Pathol* 20:379, 1983.
5. Ryan AM, Diters RW. Clinical and pathological features of canine ocular melanomas. *J Am Vet Med Assoc* 184:60, 1984.
6. Schäffer EH, Funke K. Das primär-intraokulare maligne Melanom bei Hund und Katze. *Tierarztl Prax* 13:343, 1985
7. Trucksa RC, McLean IW, Quinn AJ. Intraocular canine melanocytic neoplasms. *J Am Anim Hosp Assoc* 21:85, 1985.
8. Bussanich NM, Dolman PJ, Rootman J, Dolman CL. Canine uveal melanomas: series and literature review. *J Am Anim Hosp Assoc* 23:415, 1986.
9. Wilcock BP, Peiffer RL. Morphology and behaviour of primary ocular melanomas in 91 dogs. *Vet Pathol* 23:418, 1986.
10. Peiffer RL. Primary intraocular tumors in the dog. *Mod Vet Pract* 60:383, 1979.
11. Trucksa RC. Canine ocular melanocytic neoplasms. In: Peiffer RL, ed. *Comparative Ophthalmic Pathology.* Springfield, IL: Charles C Thomas, 1983:170.
12. Buyukmihci NC. Tumors of the eye. In: Theilen GH, Madewell BR, eds. *Veterinary Cancer Medicine,* 2d ed. Philadelphia: Lea and Febiger, 1987:chap 23.
13. Swanson JF, Dubielzig RR. Ocular tumors. In: Withrow SJ, MacEwen EG, eds. *Clinical Veterinary Oncology.* Philadelphia: JB Lippincott, 1989:chap 28.
14. Dubielzig RR. Ocular neoplasia in small animals. *Vet Clin North Am* 20:837, 1990.
15. Wilcock BP. The eye and ear. In: Jubb KVF, Kennedy PC, Palmer N, eds. *Pathology of Domestic Animals,* vol 1, 4th ed. San Diego: Academic, 1993:chap 4.
16. Gelatt KN, Johnson KA, Peiffer RL. Primary iridal pigmented masses in three dogs. *J Am Anim Hosp Assoc* 15:339, 1979.
17. Taylor GN, Dougherty TF, Mays CW, Lloyd RD, Atherton DR, Jee WSS. Radium-induced eye melanomas in dogs. *Radiat Res* 51:361, 1972.
18. Peiffer RL, Wilcock BP, Yin H. The pathogenesis and significance of pre-iridal fibrovascular membrane in domestic animals. *Vet Pathol* 27:41, 1990.
19. Peiffer RL. The differential diagnosis of pigmented ocular lesions in the dog and cat. *Calif Vet* 5:14, 1981.
20. Augsburger JJ, Shields JA. Fine needle aspiration biopsy of solid intraocular tumors: indications, instrumentation and techniques. *Ophthalmic Surg* 15:34, 1984.
21. Augsburger JJ, Shields JA, Folberg R, Lang W, O'Hara BJ, Claricci JD. Fine needle aspiration biopsy in the diagnosis of intraocular cancer. *Ophthalmology* 92:39, 1985.
22. Stevenson KE, Hungerford J, Garner A. Local extraocular extension of retinoblastoma following intraocular surgery. *Br J Ophthalmol* 73:739, 1989.
23. Bloom F. Melanocarcinoma of the iris in a dog. *J Am Vet Med Assoc* 100:439, 1942.
24. Barron CN, Saunders LZ, Jubb KV. Intraocular tumors in animals: III. Secondary intraocular tumours. *Am J Vet Res* 24:835, 1963.
25. Peiffer RL. Differential diagnosis and therapy of canine intraocular tumors. *Mod Vet Pract* 60:539, 1979.
26. Corcoran KA, Koch SA. Uveal cysts in dogs: 28 cases (1989–1991). *J Am Vet Med Assoc* 203:545, 1993.
27. Carter JD, Mausolf F. Clinical and histologic features of pigmented ocular cysts. *J Am Anim Hosp Assoc* 6:194, 1970.
28. Bedford PGC. The anterior uveal cyst as an unusual cause of corneal pigmentation in the dog. *J Small Anim Pract* 21:97, 1980.
29. Covitz D, Barthold S, Diters R, Riis R. Pigmentary glaucoma in the cairn terrier. *Trans Am Coll Vet Ophthalmol* 15:246, 1984.
30. Petersen-Jones SM. Abnormal ocular pigment deposition associated with glaucoma in the cairn terrier. *J Small Anim Pract* 32:19, 1991.
31. Buckler GK. An uncommon condition in a dog. *Vet Rec* 13:1361, 1933.
32. Roperto F, Restucci B, Crovace A. Bilateral ciliary body melanomas in a dog. *Prog Vet Comp Ophthalmol* 3:149, 1993.
33. Petersen-Jones SM, Mould JRB. Ocular pigment deposition resulting in secondary glaucoma in cairn terriers. *Invest Ophthalmol Vis Sci* 33(suppl):2354, 1992.
34. Reidy JJ, Apple DJ, Steinmetz RL, Craythorn JM, Lotfield K, Gieser SC, Brady SE. Melanocytoma: nomenclature, pathogenesis, natural history and treatment. *Surv Ophthalmol* 29:319, 1985.
35. Frangieh GT, Elbaba F, Traboulsi EI, Green WR. Melanocytoma of the ciliary body: presentation of four cases and review of nineteen reports. *Surv Ophthalmol* 29:328, 1985.
36. Minami T, Patnaik AK. Malignant anterior uveal melanoma with diffuse metastasis in a dog. *J Am Vet Med Assoc* 12:1894, 1992.
37. Foulds WS. The diagnosis and management of tumours of the iris and ciliary body. In: Oosterhuis JJ, ed. *Ophthalmic Tumours.* Dodrecht, The Netherlands: Dr W Junk, 1985:173.
38. Nasisse MP, Davidson MG, Olivero DK, Brinkmann M, Nelms S. Neodymium:YAG laser treatment of primary canine intraocular tumors. *Prog Vet Comp Ophthalmol* 3:152, 1993.

39. Dietz HH, Jensen OA, Berg Jørgensen J. Malignant melanoma of the uvea in the dog. *Nord Vet Med* 38:68, 1986.

40. Friedman DS, Miller L, Dubielzig RR. Malignant canine anterior uveal melanoma. *Vet Pathol* 26:523, 1989.

41. Michael SJ. Melanosarcoma of the eye with metastasis to the kidneys and ovaries. *J Am Vet Med Assoc* 113:253, 1948.

42. Trucksa RC. Benign vs malignant [letter to the editor]. *J Am Vet Med Assoc* 184:904, 1984.

43. Ryan AM, Diters RW. Benign vs malignant [letter to the editor]. *J Am Vet Med Assoc* 184:905, 1984.

44. Weisse I, Stötzer H. Intraokuläres Melanom bei einem jungen Beagle. *Berl Munch Tierarztl Wochenschr* 17:328, 1971.

45. O'Toole D, Murphy J. Spindle B cell melanoma in the choroid of a dog. *J Small Anim Pract* 24:561, 1983.

46. Aguirre GD, Brown G, Shields JA, Dubielzig RR. Melanoma of the choroid in a dog. *J Am Anim Hosp Assoc* 20:471, 1984.

47. Dubielzig RR, Aguirre GD, Gross SL, Diters RW. Choroidal melanomas in dogs. *Vet Pathol* 22:582, 1985.

48. Weisse I, Frese K, Meyer D. Benign melanoma of the choroid in a beagle: ophthalmological, light, and electron microscopic investigations. *Vet Pathol* 22:586, 1985.

49. Schoster JV, Dubielzig RR, Sullivan L. Choroidal melanoma in a dog. *J Am Vet Med Assoc* 203:89, 1993.

50. Morgan RV, Patton CS. Choroidal melanoma in a dog. *Cornell Vet* 83:211, 1993.

51. Collinson PN, Peiffer RL. Clinical presentation, morphology and behavior of primary choroidal melanomas in eight dogs. *Prog Vet Comp Ophthalmol* 3:158, 1993.

52. Hopper HD. Some dog neoplasms. *Cornell Vet* 35:137, 1945.

53. Smythe RH. *Veterinary Ophthalmology.* London: Baillière, Tindall, Cox, 1956:321.

54. Whitehead JE. Neoplasia in the cat. *Vet Med Small Anim Clin* 62:357, 1967.

55. Engle GC, Brodey RS. A retrospective study of 395 feline neoplasms. *J Am Anim Hosp Assoc* 5:21, 1969.

56. Bellhorn RW, Henkind P. Intraocular malignant melanoma in domestic cats. *J Small Anim Pract* 10:631, 1970.

57. Patnaik AK, Liu SK, McClelland AJ. Nonhematopoietic neoplasms in cats. *J Natl Cancer Inst* 54:855, 1975.

58. Cardy RH. Primary intraocular malignant melanoma in a Siamese cat. *Vet Pathol* 14:648, 1977.

59. Peiffer RL Jr, Seymour WG, Williams LW. Malignant melanoma of the iris and ciliary body in a cat. *Mod Vet Pract* 58:853, 1977.

60. Souri E. Intraocular melanoma in a cat. *Feline Pract* 8:43, 1978.

61. Acland GM, McLean IW, Aguirre GD, Trucksa R. Diffuse iris melanoma in cats. *J Am Vet Med Assoc* 176:52, 1980.

62. Chaudieu G, Fonk Y. Cas clinique: melanome malin primaire uveal epitheloide unilateral chez un chat. *Point Vet* 13:37, 1981.

63. Albert DM, Shadduck JA, Craft JL, Niederkorn JY. Feline uveal melanoma model induced with feline sarcoma virus. *Invest Ophthalmol Vis Sci* 20:606, 1981.

64. Shadduck JA, Albert DM, Niederkorn JY. Feline uveal melanomas induced with feline sarcoma virus: potential model of the human counterpart. *J Natl Cancer Inst* 67:619, 1981.

65. Niederkorn JY, Shadduck JA, Albert DM. Enucleation and the appearance of second primary tumors in cats bearing virally induced intraocular tumors. *Invest Ophthalmol Vis Sci* 23:719, 1982.

66. Peiffer RL Jr. Spontaneous ocular melanomas in the dog and cat: a comparative morphologic study. *Invest Ophthalmol Vis Sci* 26(suppl):21, 1985.

67. Dubielzig RR, Everitt J, Shadduck JA, Albert DM. Feline ocular melanoma and posttraumatic sarcoma. *Proc Am Coll Vet Ophthalmol* 17:436, 1986.

68. Harling DE, Peiffer RL Jr, Cook CS, Belkin PV. Feline limbal melanoma: four cases. *J Am Anim Hosp Assoc* 22:795, 1986.

69. Bertoy RW, Brightman AH, Regan K. Intraocular melanoma with multiple metastasis in a cat. *J Am Vet Med Assoc* 192:87, 1988.

70. Schwink K, Betts DM. Malignant melanoma of the iris in a cat. *Vet Med* 2:35, 1988.

71. Patnaik AK, Mooney S. Feline melanoma: a comparative study of ocular, oral, and dermal neoplasms. *Vet Pathol* 25:105, 1988.

72. Wilcock BP, Peiffer RL Jr, Davidson MG. The causes of glaucoma in cats. *Vet Pathol* 27:35, 1990.

73. Duncan DE, Peiffer RL. Morphology and prognostic indicators of anterior uveal melanomas in cats. *Prog Vet Comp Ophthalmol* 1:25, 1991.

74. Albert DM, Shadduck JA, Liu HS, Sunderman FW, Wagoner MD, Dohlman HG, Papale JJ. Animal models for the study of uveal melanoma. *Int Ophthalmol Clin* 20:143, 1980.

75. Williams LW, Gelatt KN, Gwin RM. Ophthalmic neoplasms in the cat. *J Am Anim Hosp Assoc* 17:999, 1981.

76. Martin CL. Feline ophthalmologic diseases: the globe and ocular neoplasia. *Mod Vet Pract* 63:449, 1982.

77. Buracco P, Peruccio C, Cornaglia E, Capurro C, Ratto A, Bocchini V, Morrison WB. Neoplasie oculari melanocitiche del cane e del gatto ed aspetti comparativi. *Veterinaria* 3:49, 1989.

78. Kircher CH, Garner FM, Robinson FR. X: Tumours of the eye and adnexa. *Bull WHO* 50:135, 1974.

79. Saunders LZ, Rubin LF. *Ophthalmic Pathology of Animals.* Basel: S Karger, 1975:218.

80. Peiffer RL Jr. Il tratto uveale. In: Peruccio C, Monti F, Solarino A, eds. *Atlante di Oftalmologia Veterinaria*. Turin: Edizioni Medico Scientifiche, 1985:227.

81. Cordy DR. Tumors of the nervous system and eye. In: Moulton JE, ed. *Tumors in Domestic Animals*, 3d ed. Berkeley: University of the California Press, 1990:chap 14.

82. Jones TC, Hunt RD. *Patologia Veterinaria*, vol 2. Padua: Piccin, 1987:chap 28.

83. Walde I, Schaffer EH, Kostlin RG. *Atlas of Ophthalmology in Dogs and Cats*. Philadelphia: BC Decker, 1990:chap 18.

84. Slatter D. *Fundamentals of Veterinary Ophthalmology*, 2d ed. Philadelphia: WB Saunders, 1990:322.

85. Nasisse MP. Feline ophthalmology. In: Gelatt KN, ed. *Veterinary Ophthalmology*, 2d ed. Philadelphia: Lea and Febiger, 1991:552 (chap 14).

86. Priester WA, McKay FW. The occurrence of tumors in domestic animals. *Natl Cancer Inst Monogr* 54:42, 1980.

87. Bjerkas E, Aresan F, Peiffer RL. Diffuse amelanotic iris melanoma in a cat. *Vet Comp Ophthalmol* 7:150, 1997.

88. Thrall DE. Radiographic diagnosis of metastatic pulmonary neoplasia. *Comp Continuing Educ* 1:131, 1979.

89. McCullough B, Schaller J, Shadduck JA, Yohn DS. Induction of malignant melanomas associated with fibrosarcoma in gnotobiotic cats inoculated with Gardner-feline fibrosarcoma virus. *J Natl Cancer Inst* 48:1893, 1972.

90. Pack GT, Gerber DM, Scharnagel IM. End results in the treatment of malignant melanoma: a report of 1,190 cases. *Ann Surg* 136:905, 1952.

91. Rapini RP, Golitz LE, Greer RO Jr, Krekorian EA, Poulson T. Primary malignant melanoma of the oral cavity: a review of 117 cases. *Cancer* 55:1543, 1985.

92. Lubin JR, Albert DM, Essex M, De Noronha F, Riis R. Experimental anterior uveitis after subcutaneous injection of feline sarcoma virus. *Invest Ophthalmol Vis Sci* 24:1055, 1983.

93. Rones B, Zimmerman LE. The production of heterochromia and glaucoma by diffuse malignant melanoma of the iris. *Trans Am Acad Ophthalmol Otolaryngol* 61:447, 1957.

94. Brazel SM, Sullivan TJ, Thorner PS, Clarke MP, Hunter WS, Morin JD. Iris sector heterochromia as a marker for neural crest disease. *Arch Ophthalmol* 110:233, 1992.

95. Kirby ML, Bockman DE. Neural crest and normal development: a new perspective. *Anat Rec* 209:1, 1984.

96. Bahn CF, Falls HF, Varley GA, Meyer RF, Edelhauser HF, Bourne WM. Classification of corneal disorders based on neural crest origin. *Ophthalmology* 91:558, 1984.

97. Johnston MC, Noden DM, Hazelton RD, Coulombre JL, Coulombre AJ. Origins of avian ocular and periocular tissues. *Exp Eye Res* 29:27, 1979.

98. Jakobiec FA, Tannenbaum M. In: Duane TD, ed. *Clinical Ophthalmology*. Hagerstown, MD: Harper and Row, 1980.

99. Hu F, Teramura DJ, Mah K. Normal uveal melanocytes in culture. *Pigment Cell Res* 1:94, 1987.

100. Boissy RE, Trinkle LS, Nordlund JJ. Neural-tube-derived melanocyte subsets undergo commitment to their distinct lineages in culture. *Cell Differ Dev* 30:129, 1990.

101. Cramer SF. The origin of epidermal melanocytes: implications for the histogenesis of nevi and melanomas. *Arch Pathol Lab Med* 115:115, 1991.

102. Hulley PA, Stander CS, Kidson SH. Terminal migration and early differentiation of melanocytes in embryonic chick skin. *Dev Biol* 145:182, 1991.

103. Callender GR, Wilder HC, Ash JE. Five hundred melanomas of the choroid and the ciliary body followed for five years or longer. *Am J Ophthalmol* 25:962, 1942.

104. Birdsell JM, Gunther BK, Boyd TA, Grace M, Jerry LM. Ocular melanoma: a population-based study. *Can J Ophthalmol* 15:9, 1980.

105. Mahoney MC, Burnett WS, Majerovics A, Tanenbaum H. The epidemiology of ophthalmic malignancies in New York State. *Ophthalmology* 97:1143, 1990.

106. Scotto J, Fraumeni JJ, Lee JA. Melanomas of the eye and other noncutaneous sites: epidemiologic aspects. *J Natl Cancer Inst* 56:489, 1976.

107. Osterlind A. Trends in incidence of ocular malignant melanoma in Denmark 1943–1982. *Int J Cancer* 40:161, 1987.

108. Hayton S, Lafreniere R, Jerry LM, Temple WJ, Ashley P. Ocular melanoma in Alberta: a 38 year review pointing to the importance of tumor size and tumor histology as predictors of survival. *J Surg Oncol* 42:215, 1989.

109. Leonard BC, Shields JA, McDonald PR. Malignant melanomas of the uveal tract in children and young adults. *Can J Ophthalmol* 10:441, 1975.

110. Barr CC, McLean IW, Zimmerman LE. Uveal melanoma in children and adolescents. *Arch Ophthalmol* 99:2133, 1981.

111. Broadway D, Lang S, Harper J, Madamat F, Pritchard J, Tarawenh M, Taylor D. Congenital malignant melanoma of the eye [review]. Cancer 67:2642, 1991.

112. Volcker H, Naumann G. Multicentric primary malignant melanomas of the choroid: two separate malignant melanomas of the choroid and two uveal naevi in one eye. *Br J Ophthalmol* 62:408, 1978.

113. Pe'er J, Bernstein-Lifshitz L. Case report: anterior and posterior uveal melanomas in one eye. *Arch Ophthalmol* 106:22, 1988.

114. Shammas HF, Watzke RC. Bilateral choroidal melanomas: case report and incidence. *Arch Ophthalmol* 95:617, 1977.

115. Eide N. Simultaneous bilateral primary choroidal melanoma. *Acta Ophthalmol (Copenh)* 67:216, 1989.

116. Gallagher RP, Elwood JM, Rootman J, Spinelli JJ, Hill GB, Threfall WJ, Birdsell JM. Risk factors for ocular melanoma: Western Canada Melanoma Study. *J Natl Cancer Inst* 74:775, 1985.

117. Holly EA, Aston DA, Char DH, Kristiansen JJ, Ahn DK. Uveal melanoma in relation to ultraviolet light exposure and host factors. *Cancer Res* 50:5773, 1990.

118. Seddon JM, MacLaughlin DT, Albert DM, Gragouda ES, Ference MD. Uveal melanomas presenting during pregnancy and the investigation of oestrogen receptors in melanomas. *Br J Ophthalmol* 66:695, 1982.

119. Hartage P, Tucker MA, Shields JA, Augsburger J, Hoover RN, Fraumeni JF Jr. Case-control study of female hormones and eye melanoma. *Cancer Res* 49:4622, 1989.

120. Holly EA, Aston DA, Ahn DK, Kristiansen JJ, Char DH. Uveal melanoma, hormonal and reproductive factors in women. *Cancer Res* 51:1370, 1991.

121. Albert DM, Puliafito CA, Fulton AB, Robinson NL, Zakov ZN, Dryja DP, Smith AB, Eagan E, Leffingweil SS. Increased incidence of choroidal malignant melanoma occurring in a single population of chemical workers. *Am J Ophthalmol* 89:323, 1980.

122. Paridaens D, Lyons CJ, McCartney A, Hungerford JL. Familial aggressive nevi of the iris in childhood. *Arch Ophthalmol* 109:1552, 1991.

123. Singh AD, Wang MX, Donoso LA, Shields CL, De Potter P, Shields JA. Genetic aspects of uveal melanoma: a brief review. *Semin Oncol* 23:768, 1996.

124. Jakobiec F, Silbert G. Are most iris 'melanomas' really nevi? A clinicopathologic study of 189 lesions. *Arch Ophthalmol* 99:2117, 1981.

125. Van Klink F, De Keizer R, Jager M, Kakebeeke-Kemme H. Iris nevi and melanomas: a clinical follow-up study. *Doc Ophthalmol* 82:49, 1992.

126. Kliman GH, Augsburger JJ, Shields JA. Association between iris color and iris melanocytic lesions. *Am J Ophthalmol* 100:547, 1985.

127. Harbour JW, Augsburger JJ, Eagle RC Jr. Initial management and follow-up of melanocytic iris tumors. *Ophthalmology* 102:1987, 1995.

128. Demeler U, Von DD. The clinical picture, fluorescence angiography and histology of a ring melanoma of the iris [author's translation] [in German]. *Klin Monatsbl Augenheilkd* 168:387, 1976.

129. Demeler U. Iris angiograms in malignant melanoma of the uvea [in German]. *Ophthalmologica* 177:70, 1978.

130. Jakobiec F, Depot M, Henkind P, Spencer W. Fluorescein angiographic patterns of iris melanocytic lesions. *Arch Ophthalmol* 100:1288, 1982.

131. Geisse LJ, Robertson DM. Iris melanomas. *Am J Ophthalmol* 99:638, 1985.

132. Pavlin CJ, McWhae JA, McGowan HD, Foster FS. Ultrasound biomicroscopy of anterior segment tumors. *Ophthalmology* 99:1220, 1992.

133. Grossniklaus HE. Fine-needle aspiration biopsy of the iris. *Arch Ophthalmol* 110:969, 1992.

134. Shields JA, Sanborn GE, Augsburger JJ. The differential diagnosis of malignant melanoma of the iris: a clinical study of 200 patients. *Ophthalmology* 90:716, 1983.

135. Territo C, Shields CL, Shields JA, Augsburger JJ, Schroeder RP. Natural course of melanocytic tumors of the iris. *Ophthalmology* 95:1251, 1988.

136. Marcus D, Mawn L, Egan K, Albert D. Nucleolar organizer regions in iris nevi and melanomas. *Am J Ophthalmol* 114:202, 1992.

137. McGalliard JN, Johnston PB. A study of iris melanoma in Northern Ireland. *Br J Ophthalmol* 73:591, 1989.

138. Shields CL, Shields JA, De Potter P, Singh AD, Hernandez C, Brady LW. Treatment of non-resectable malignant iris tumours with custom designed plaque radiotherapy. *Br J Ophthalmol* 79:306, 1995.

139. Shields CL, Shields JA, Materin M, Gershenbaum E, Singh AD, Smith A. Iris melanoma: risk factors for metastasis in 169 consecutive patients. *Ophthalmology* 108:172, 2001.

140. Davidorf FH. The melanoma controversy: a comparison of choroidal, cutaneous, and iris melanomas. *Surv Ophthalmol* 25:373, 1981.

141. Pavlin CJ, Harasiewicz K, Sherar MD, Foster FS. Clinical use of ultrasound biomicroscopy. *Ophthalmology* 98:287, 1991.

142. Servodidio CA, Abramson DH. Presenting signs and symptoms of choroidal melanoma: what do they mean? *Ann Ophthalmol* 24:190, 1992.

143. Shields M, Klintworth G. Anterior uveal melanomas and intraocular pressure. *Ophthalmology* 87:503, 1980.

144. Shields CL, Shields JA, Shields MB, Augsburger JJ. Prevalence and mechanisms of secondary intraocular pressure elevation in eyes with intraocular tumors. *Ophthalmology* 94:839, 1987.

145. Collaborative Ocular Melanoma Study Group. Factors predictive of growth and treatment of small choroidal melanoma: COMS report no. 5. *Arch Ophthalmol* 115:1537, 1997.

146. Font RL, Spaulding AG, Zimmerman LE. Diffuse malignant melanoma of the uveal tract: a clinicopathologic report of 54 cases. *Trans Am Acad Ophthalmol Otolaryngol* 72:877, 1968.

147. Shammas HF, Blodi FC. Orbital extension of choroidal and ciliary body melanomas. *Arch Ophthalmol* 95:2002, 1977.

148. Shields JA. Lesions simulating malignant melanoma of the posterior uvea. *Arch Ophthalmol* 89:466, 1973.

149. Ferry AP. Lesions mistaken for malignant melanoma of the posterior uvea: a clinicopathologic analysis of 100 cases with ophthalmoscopically visible lesions. *Arch Ophthalmol* 72:463, 1964.

150. Chang M, Zimmerman LE, McLean I. The persisting pseudomelanoma problem. *Arch Ophthalmol* 102:726, 1984.

151. Blodi FC, Roy PE. The misdiagnosed choroidal melanoma. *Can J Ophthalmol* 2:209, 1967.

152. Howard GM. Erroneous clinical diagnoses of retinoblastoma and uveal melanoma. *Trans Am Acad Ophthalmol Otolaryngol* 73:199, 1969.

153. Shields JA, McDonald PR. Improvements in the diagnosis of posterior uveal melanomas. *Arch Ophthalmol* 91:259, 1974.

154. Robertson DM, Campbell RJ. Errors in the diagnosis of malignant melanoma of the choroid. *Am J Ophthalmol* 87:269, 1979.

155. Davidorf FH, Letson AD, Weiss ET, Levine E. Incidence of misdiagnosed and unsuspected choroidal melanomas: a 50-year experience. *Arch Ophthalmol* 101:410, 1983.

156. Anonymous. Accuracy of diagnosis of choroidal melanomas in the Collaborative Ocular Melanoma Study: COMS report no. 1. *Arch Ophthalmol* 108:1268, 1990 [erratum in *Arch Ophthalmol* 108:1708, 1990].

157. Zimmerman LE. Problems in the diagnosis of malignant melanomas of the choroid and ciliary body: the 1972 Arthur J. Bedell Lecture [review]. *Am J Ophthalmol* 75:917, 1973.

158. Gass JD. Observation of suspected choroidal and ciliary body melanomas for evidence of growth prior to enucleation. *Ophthalmology* 87:523, 1980.

159. Shields JA, Shields CL, Donoso LA. Management of posterior uveal melanoma [review]. *Surv Ophthalmol* 36:161, 1991.

160. Shields JA, Augsburger JJ. Cataract surgery and intraocular lenses in patients with unsuspected malignant melanoma of the ciliary body and choroid. *Ophthalmology* 92:823, 1985.

161. Kirk HQ, Petty RW. Malignant melanoma of the choroid: a correlation of clinical and histological findings. *Arch Ophthalmol* 56:843, 1956.

162. Makley TA, Teed RW. Unsuspected intraocular malignant melanomas. *Arch Ophthalmol* 60:475, 1958.

163. Litricin O. Unsuspected uveal melanomas. *Am J Ophthalmol* 76:734, 1973.

164. Yanoff M. Glaucoma mechanisms in ocular malignant melanomas. *Am J Ophthalmol* 70:898, 1970.

165. McLean IW, Zimmerman LE, Evans RM. Reappraisal of Callender's spindle: a type of malignant melanoma of choroid and ciliary body. *Am J Ophthalmol* 86:557, 1978.

166. McLean IW, Foster WD, Zimmerman LE, Gamel JW. Modifications of Callender's classification of uveal melanoma at the Armed Forces Institute of Pathology. *Am J Ophthalmol* 96:502, 1983.

167. Wilder HC, Callender GR. Malignant melanoma of the choroid: further studies on prognosis by histologic type and fiber content. *Am J Ophthalmol* 22:851, 1939.

168. Wilder HC, Paul EV. Malignant melanoma of the choroid and ciliary body: a study of 2535 cases. *Milit Surg* 109:370, 1951.

169. Flocks M, Gerende JH, Zimmerman LE. The size and shape of malignant melanomas of the choroid and ciliary body in relation to prognosis and histologic characteristics: a statistical study of 210 tumors. *Trans Am Acad Ophthalmol Otolaryngol* 59:740, 1955.

170. Paul EV, Parnell BL, Fraker M. Prognosis of malignant melanomas of the choroid and ciliary body. *Int Ophthalmol Clin* 2:387, 1962.

171. McLean MJ, Foster WD, Zimmerman LE. Prognostic factors in small malignant melanomas of choroid and ciliary body. *Arch Ophthalmol* 95:48, 1977.

172. Packard RBS. Pattern of mortality in choroidal malignant melanoma. *Br J Ophthalmol* 64:565, 1980.

173. McLean IW, Foster WD, Zimmerman LE. Uveal melanoma: location, size, cell type, and enucleation as risk factors in metastasis. *Hum Pathol* 13:123, 1982.

174. Gass JD. Problems in the differential diagnosis of choroidal nevi and malignant melanoma: 33d Edward Jackson Memorial Lecture. *Trans Am Acad Ophthalmol Otolaryngol* 83:19, 1977.

175. Gamel JW, McLean IW. Quantitative analysis of the Callender classification of uveal melanoma cells. *Arch Ophthalmol* 95:686, 1977.

176. Gamel JW, McLean IW, Greenberg RA, Zimmerman LE, Lichtenstein SJ. Computerized histologic assessment of malignant potential: a method for determining the prognosis of uveal melanomas. *Hum Pathol* 13:893, 1982.

177. Seddon JM, Polivogianis L, Hsieh LL, Albert DM, Gamel JW, Gragoudas ES. Death from uveal melanoma: number of epithelioid cells and inverse SD of nucleolar area as prognostic factors. *Arch Ophthalmol* 105:801, 1987.

178. Gamel JW, McCurdy JB, McLean IW. A comparison of prognostic covariates for uveal melanoma. *Invest Ophthalmol Vis Sci* 33:1919, 1992.

179. Donoso LA, Augsburger JJ, Shields JA, Greenberg RA, Gamel J. Metastatic uveal melanoma: correlation between survival time and cytomorphometry of primary tumors. *Arch Ophthalmol* 104:76, 1986.

180. Folberg R, Rummelt V, Parys-Van Grinderderen R, Hwang T, Woolson RF, Pe'er J, Gruman LM. The prognostic value of tumor blood vessel morphology in primary uveal melanoma. *Ophthalmology* 100:1389, 1993.

181. Rummelt V, Folberg R, Rummelt C, Gruman LM, Hwang T, Woolson RF, Yi H, Naumam GO. Microcirculation architecture of melanocytic nevi and malignant melanomas of the ciliary body and choroid: a comparative histopathologic and ultrastructural study. *Ophthalmology* 101:718, 1994.

182. Zimmerman LE, McLean IW, Foster WD. Does enucleation of the eye containing a malignant melanoma prevent or accelerate the dissemination of tumour cells? [review]. *Br J Ophthalmol* 62:420, 1978.

183. Zimmerman LE, McLean IW. An evaluation of enucleation in the management of uveal melanomas [review]. *Am J Ophthalmol* 87:741, 1979.

184. Zimmerman LE, McLean IW, Foster WD. Statistical analysis of follow-up data concerning uveal melanomas, and the influence of enucleation. *Ophthalmology* 87:557, 1980.

185. Wagoner MD, Albert DM. The incidence of metastases from untreated ciliary body and choroidal melanoma. *Arch Ophthalmol* 100:939, 1982.

186. Seigel D, Myers M, Ferris F, Steinhorn SC. Survival rates after enucleation of eyes with malignant melanoma. *Am J Ophthalmol* 87:761, 1979.

187. Manschot WA, Van Peperzeel HA. Choroidal melanoma: enucleation or observation? A new approach. *Arch Ophthalmol* 98:71, 1980.

188. Gass JD. Comparison of uveal melanoma growth rates with mitotic index and mortality. *Arch Ophthalmol* 103:924, 1985.

189. Anonymous. Collaborative Ocular Melanoma Study (COMS) randomized trial of pre-enucleation radiation of large choroidal melanoma: II. Initial mortality findings—COMS report no. 10. *Am J Ophthalmol* 125:779, 1998.

190. Foulds WS, Damato BE, Burton RL. Local resection versus enucleation in the management of choroidal melanoma. *Eye* 1:676, 1987.

191. Char DH, Kroll SM, Castro J. Long-term follow-up after uveal melanoma charged particle therapy. *Trans Am Ophthalmol Soc* 95:171, 1997.

192. Mueller AJ, Talies S, Schaller UC, Horstmann G, Wowra B, Kampik A. Stereotactic radiosurgery of large uveal melanomas with the gamma-knife. *Ophthalmology* 107:1381, 2000.

193. Oosterhuis JA, Journee-de Korver HG, Keunen JE. Transpupillary thermotherapy: results in 50 patients with choroidal melanoma. *Arch Ophthalmol* 116:157, 1998.

194. Diener-West M, Hawkins BS, Markowitz JA, Schachat AP. A review of mortality from choroidal melanoma: II. A meta-analysis of 5-year mortality rates following enucleation, 1966 through 1988. *Arch Ophthalmol* 110:245, 1992.

195. Anonymous. Assessment of metastatic disease status at death in 435 patients with large choroidal melanoma in the Collaborative Ocular Melanoma Study (COMS): COMS report no. 15. *Arch Ophthalmol* 119:670, 2001.

8

FELINE OCULAR SARCOMAS

Richard R. Dubielzig

Few of the neoplasms discussed in this chapter are species specific or at least lack a similar counterpart. From this perspective, as well as others, feline ocular sarcomas represent one of the most interesting processes discussed in this text. Recognized only within the past two decades, it has fascinated ocular pathologists with a spectrum of morphology, from fibrous and osseous to epithelioid and round cell proliferations. The common association with prior trauma, sometimes occurring years prior to encogenesis, and the frequent finding of ruptured lenses has generated queries in regard to cell of origin. Unfortunately for affected cats, the neoplasm is very aggressive and few survive its ravages.

HISTORICAL PERSPECTIVES

Feline ocular sarcomas are the second most commonly occurring primary ocular neoplasm in cats, diffuse iris melanoma being the most common. Ocular sarcomas are important because of their malignant potential and unique association with long-standing prior ocular disease. Woog et al.[1] reported a single case of osteosarcoma occurring in a phthisical feline eye in 1983. The affected eye had been traumatized 8 years before removal of the tumor. Association between trauma and the occurrence of ocular sarcomas was made in 1984 by Dubielzig,[2] who reported on three cases of ocular sarcomas following trauma in cats. These tumors occurred several years following the traumatic event. Characteristic features included histologic evidence of long-standing lens rupture and circumferential distribution of the sarcoma within the globe. Invasion of the optic nerve leading to blindness and neurologic complications was also reported. Peiffer et al.[3] reported on 13 cats with ocular sarcomas in 1988. Only five of the cats had histories of previous trauma. Six other cats had

histories of chronic uveitis of undetermined cause. Four cats had tumors that were localized in the globe, and all of these cats had intact lenses. Nine cats had tumors that lined the inner aspect of the globe, and all of these eyes had long-standing lens rupture. Seven of the 13 cats died of complications caused by tumor regrowth or metastasis. Dubielzig et al.[4] reported on 13 cases (including the three cases described previously) in 1990. Tumor types included spindle cell, anaplastic sarcoma, and osteosarcoma. All 11 cats where a history was available had prior ocular disease. In six, trauma was established to be the cause of the initial ocular problem. Dubielzig et al.[5] reported on the morphology of 10 additional cases, including ultrastructural and immunohistochemistry. Cassotis et al.[6] reported on an immunohistochemical survey of 38 cases showing convincing evidence of a lens epithelial cell origin for all but the round cell variant tumors.

TERMINOLOGY

The establishment of a nomenclature scheme that most correctly identifies ocular sarcomas in cats is complicated because tumors show varied differentiation. The term *posttraumatic sarcoma* has been used to highlight that many of these globes have the unique historical feature of previous trauma. The term has lost favor with individuals who feel that uveitis without trauma may also be a risk factor in ocular sarcoma. The term *primary ocular sarcoma* of cats avoids the controversy of whether uveitis is a risk factor but does not separate out localized sarcomas that may not be related to previous ocular damage in any way. Although sarcomas that occur in traumatized cat globes are in fact primary to the eye, they can also be thought of as being secondary to trauma. Using primary ocular sarcoma as a generic term for tumors that develop secondary to trauma seems unnecessarily confusing. I suggest the general term *feline ocular sarcoma.*

Dubielzig et al.[5] showed morphologic evidence that approximately half of these tumors possibly arise from lens epithelial cells. Wong et al.[7] presented in vitro ocular epithelial proliferation and ultrastructural data suggesting that the ciliary body epithelium is a possible progenitor. A purest might argue that a tumor that is derived from an epithelial cell should not be called a sarcoma. Nonetheless, these tumors are morphologically mesenchymal in their appearance. Other types of differentiation include fibrosarcoma, anaplastic sarcoma, giant cell sarcoma, Schwann cell tumor, osteosarcoma, and normal cell sarcoma. The nomenclature scheme that I suggest would be to use the generic term *feline ocular sarcoma* to name the phenomenon of carcinogenesis in previously damaged feline globes. Individual cases can be named in accordance with the differentiation of the tumor cells.

EPIDEMIOLOGY

Feline ocular sarcomas most often occur in globes previously damaged. The time between the original disease and the development of the tumor can be as short as several months and as long as 10 years. There is controversy regarding whether previous trauma is the only risk factor to the development of feline ocular sarcoma. An actual history of trauma is recorded in only about half of the cases published. Interestingly, long-standing lens rupture is a morphologic feature of all the cases published except four of the 13 cases reported by Peiffer et al.[3] Those same four cases are also the only cases of localized ocular sarcoma reported. One might certainly wonder whether localized ocular sarcoma is a different disease. Dubielzig et al.[8] studied the proliferative tissue reactions in dog and cat globes at differing times after spontaneous trauma and found that tissues of several cell lines proliferate, including lens epithelial cells. No differences were found in the proliferative reaction in dogs or cats, and one might wonder why cats have the risk of ocular sarcoma following traumas and not dogs. Hendrick et al.[9] discovered that cats are at risk of developing sarcomatous lesions at the site of vac-cination. One might speculate that cats are at risk of developing malignant tumors associated with the proliferative phase of wound healing or chronic inflammation; however, six cases screened using immunohistochemistry and polymerase chain reaction for feline sarcoma virus and feline leukemia virus failed to demonstrate viral presence.[10]

CLINICAL FEATURES

Most feline ocular sarcomas occur in globes that were previously injured and are presented for examination when the appearance of the damaged eye changes. This usually is a process of swelling or a change in color. Often the damaged globe undergoes a color change by which it becomes opaquely white or pink, which is an indication of tumor infiltration into the cornea or proliferation within the anterior chamber. Interestingly, there is seldom a history of pain caused by these tumors in the early stages. Recently, because of the heightened awareness of the risk factors associated with previously traumatized eyes, owners are instructed to observe the traumatized eyes carefully for changes, and globes with sarcomas are removed at earlier stages.

These tumors are malignant and can spread by direct invasion of the optic nerve, leading to blindness and neurologic disease or direct extension into the orbit, leading to reoccurrence locally. Lymph node and hematogenous metastasis have also been reported with feline ocular sarcoma.

MORPHOLOGY

Gross Appearance. The most characteristic gross appearance of feline ocular sarcomas is that of a globe filled internally by a solid tan neoplasm (Figure 8.1). In later stages of the disease, transscleral infiltration or optic nerve penetration are common features (Figure 8.2).

Light-Microscopic Features. Histologically, feline ocular sarcomas are highly variable. Dubielzig et al.[5] reported that approximately half of the tumors show morphologic features of lens epithelial cell differentiation. By light microscopy, these consist of plump spindle cells surrounded by a thick smooth PAS (periodic acid-Schiff)-positive basement membrane (Figure 8.3). Other tumors include spindle cells with no basement membrane, round anaplastic cells forming solid sheets (Figure 8.4), giant cells, osteosarcomas, and schwannoma. The morphologic features of these different patterns are not different from the same tumors seen elsewhere in the body.

Electron Microscopy. Feline ocular sarcomas showing a pattern of differentiation suggesting an epithelial origin have thick basement membrane structures between individual cells (Figure 8.5). Where tumor cells contact each other, there are desmosomal attachment structures, and where tumors attach to basement membranes, there are hemidesmosomes[5] (Figure 8.6). Dense bundled rodlets have been described within the cytoplasm that were identical to those seen in nonpigmented nonciliary epithelium.[7]

Immunohistochemistry. Dubielzig et al.[5] and Cassotis et al.[6] reported that feline ocular sarcomas that have differentiation suggesting lens epithelial cell origin stain positively with vimentin, muscle-specific actin, TGF-B (transforming growth factor β), and bFGF (basic fibroblast growth factor). Lens epithelial cells show a similar staining pattern when they proliferate in traumatized globes within an intact lens capsule.[8] The immunohistochemical staining patterns of feline ocular sarcomas, made up exclusively of round cells, have failed to provide helpful clues as to the tissue of origin.

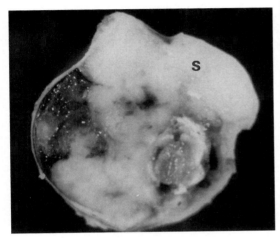

FIG. 8.1—Gross appearance of advanced feline ocular sarcoma. The globe is sectioned in the vertical plane. The figure shows scleral infiltration (S).

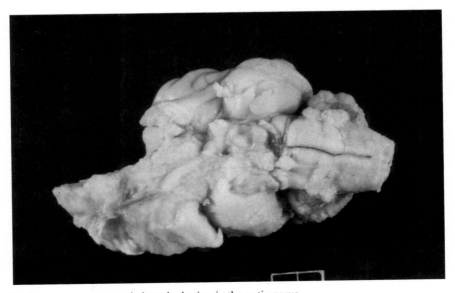

FIG. 8.2—Ocular sarcoma metastasis into the brain via the optic nerve.

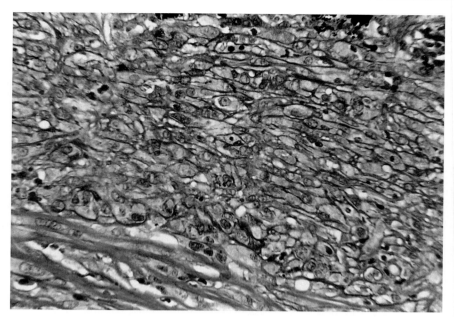

FIG. 8.3—Photomicrograph of feline ocular sarcoma showing plump spindle cells surrounded by a thick, smooth PAS (periodic acid—Schiff)-positive membrane. These tumors are thought to be of lens epithelial origin. PAS, ×250.

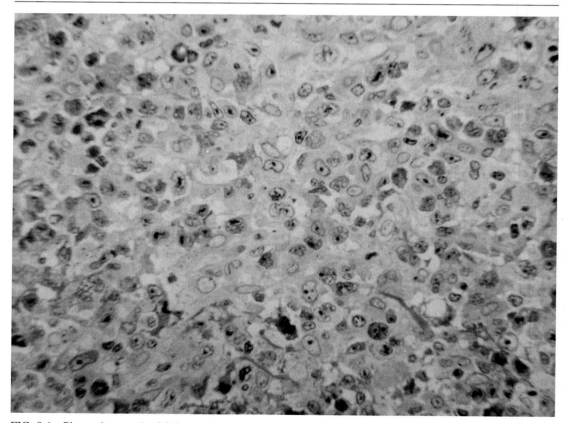

FIG. 8.4—Photomicrograph of feline ocular sarcoma showing anaplastic round cells. Hematoxylin-eosin, ×500.

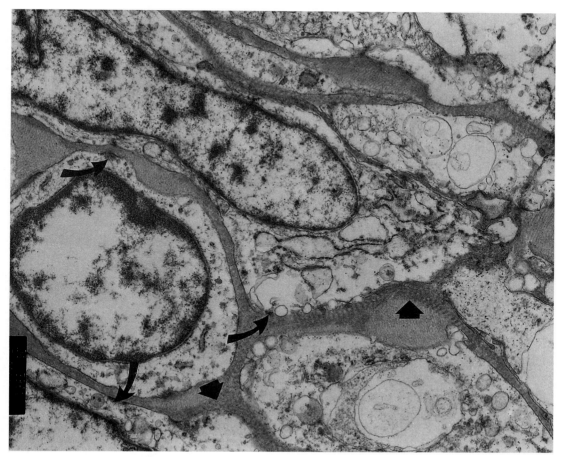

FIG. 8.5—Electron micrograph of feline ocular sarcoma. Thick basement membranes separate individual cells. Hemidesmosomes attach cells to basement membranes (curved arrows). Within basement membranes are areas of long-spacing collagen with characteristic 100-nm banding (arrowheads). ×14,000.

TREATMENT

Little is known about the effectiveness of specific treatment modalities for feline ocular sarcoma. The most helpful approach to treatment would be to educate owners about the increased risk of malignancy in cat eyes that have been previously traumatized and recommend that blind traumatized globes be enucleated. Likewise, globe-sparing cosmetic procedures for chronic glaucomas such as pharmacologic ablation of the ciliary body and evisceration with intraocular prosthesis should both be avoided in cats. Any change in the appearance of a quiet, previously damaged globe should lead to evaluation for possible enucleation. It is not known whether early removal reduces the risk of metastasis, but that conclusion is reasonable. A surgeon should be mindful of the tendency

for feline ocular sarcoma to infiltrate the optic nerve. The nerve should be removed as close to the foramen as possible, and the proximal-most segment of nerve should be specifically examined histologically to identify tumor infiltration.

PROGNOSIS

The majority of cases of feline ocular sarcomas reported have been malignant. In more than half of the reported cases, the cats have died from tumor-related causes within months of the original surgery. Causes of death have included invasion of the brain through the optic nerve, local recurrence in the orbit, and distant metastasis. Early identification and removal offer the best chance of enhancing long-term survival of cats

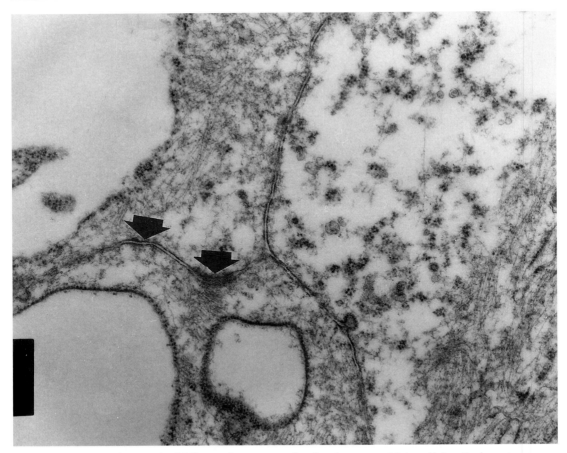

FIG. 8.6—Electron micrograph of feline ocular sarcoma showing desmosomal intercellular attachments (arrows). ×35,000.

with ocular sarcoma. Little is known about specific treatment modalities, including radiation, chemotherapy, or immunotherapy, as adjuncts to surgery in treating feline ocular sarcomas.

REFERENCES

1. Woog J, Albert DM, Gondor JR, Carpenter JJ. Osteosarcoma in a phthisical feline eye. *Vet Pathol* 20:209, 1983.
2. Dubielzig RR. Ocular sarcoma following trauma in three cats. *J Am Vet Med Assoc* 184:578, 1984.
3. Peiffer RL, Monticello T, Bouldin TW. Primary ocular sarcomas in the cat. *J Small Anim Pract* 29:105, 1988.
4. Dubielzig RR, Everitt J, Shadduck JA, Albert DM. Clinical and morphologic features of post-traumatic ocular sarcomas in cats. *Vet Pathol* 27:62, 1990.
5. Dubielzig RR, Hawkins KL, Toy KA, Rosebury WS, Mazur M, Jasper TG. Morphologic features of feline ocular sarcomas in 10 cats: light microscopy, ultrastructure, and immunohisto-chemistry. *Vet Comp Ophthalmol* 4:7, 1994.
6. Cassotis NJ, Dubielzig RR, Davidson MG. Immunohistochemical analysis of primary ocular sarcomas in cats: 38 cases. *Proc Am Coll Vet Ophthalmol* 30:72, 1999.
7. Wong CJ, Peiffer RL, Oglesbee S, Orborne C. Feline ocular epithelial response to growth factors. *Am J Vet Res* 57:1748, 1996.
8. Dubielzig RR, Hawkins KL, Buyukmihci NC, Corea ME. Cellular proliferation within the globe after trauma in enucleated cat and dog eyes. *Invest Ophthalmol Vis Sci* 34:970, 1993.
9. Hendrick MJ, Goldschmidt MH, Shofer FS, Wang Y, Somlyo AP. Postvaccinal sarcomas in the cat: epidemiology and electron probe microanalytical identification of aluminum. *Cancer Rec* 52:5391, 1992.
10. Cullen CL, Haines DM, Jackson ML, Peiffer RL, Grahn BM. The use of immunohistochemistry and the polymerase chain reaction for detection of feline leukemia virus and feline sarcoma virus in six cases of feline ocular sarcoma. *Vet Ophthalmol* 1:189, 1998.

9 OPTIC NERVE NEOPLASIA

Nedim C. Buyukmihci, Karen E. Chancellor, and Thomas W. Bouldin

ANIMALS

Primary neoplasia of the optic nerve is uncommon especially when compared with the prevalence of neoplasms arising from other parts of the eye. Secondary involvement through invasion from surrounding structures occurs more frequently, but these are no more specific to the optic nerve than they are to other tissue within the orbit. These neoplasms of the orbit are relatively rare in themselves and are covered in a different chapter. Metastatic involvement of the optic nerve from hematogenous spread is extremely rare.

Currently, little is known about the biologic behavior of most optic nerve neoplasms, particularly in species other than dogs. No clinical features reliably distinguish one type of neoplasm from another. Because these tumors occur infrequently, few data are available to provide guidelines for the treatment and prognosis of specific types when a diagnosis is made. Much of the literature is anecdotal, describing single or a few cases, although much can be gained by reviewing this information. It can be seen, for example, that these neoplasms usually are aggressive and result in death.

Early diagnosis of an optic nerve neoplasm presents a challenge to a veterinarian. Veterinary patients do not communicate to us whether they are having visual field loss, something that may indicate an early compressive or invasive lesion of the optic nerve. Instead, the human guardian must observe signs of disease—signs that usually are not appreciated until advanced disease unless the person is an astute observer.

If an animal is fortunate and brought to a veterinarian during the earliest stages of disease, the nature of the eye may allow for early diagnosis. The clear ocular media provide the opportunity to visualize abnormalities before they become serious in terms of the life of the animal. The intraocular portion of the optic nerve—the optic disc—can be observed with ophthalmoscopy. Even if a neoplasm involves the extraocular portion of the nerve and cannot be directly visualized, indirect signs, however subtle, may be of great help. There may be displacement of the globe within the orbit and neuro-ophthalmic signs of disease. As with orbital disease, contemporary imaging techniques have dramatically enhanced diagnostics.

In most situations, there will be diminution or loss of both the direct and consensual pupillary response to light in the affected eye due to damage to the afferent branch of the pupillomotor pathway. The direct and consensual pupillary responses of the opposite eye, however, will be intact in cases of unilateral disease, assuming no coincidental disease is present to confound the situation. Subtle anisocoria may be present because of the unequal distribution of pupillomotor fibers, which tend to provide greater stimulation of the ipsilateral iris sphincter muscle. Because the eye with the neoplasm would be contributing less pupillomotor input, the net effect would be to have a slightly more dilated pupil on the side of the tumor.

Vision would be decreased or lost in the affected eye. The guardian may notice this when the animal bumps objects on the same side as the tumor. Patching the eye in question in the examination room may have little to no effect on the animal's ability to navigate the room. When the patch is placed over the unaffected eye, however, the animal might be reluctant to move, become preoccupied with removing the patch, or not be able to navigate the room. Subtle decrease in visual capabilities is unlikely to be demonstrable.

Ophthalmoscopic examination, preferably by the indirect technique initially, may reveal an enlarged optic disc protruding into the vitreous cavity (Figure 9.1). The margins of the optic disk

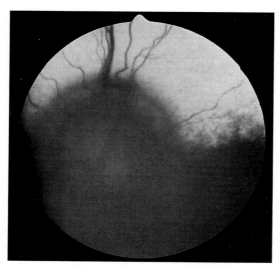

FIG. 9.1—Optic nerve meningioma in an 8-year-old spayed female boxer dog, right eye. The optic disc is enlarged and out of focus due to edema and neoplastic infiltration.

may appear blurred, and there may be hemorrhage on the surface. Whereas direct ophthalmoscopy can be used, taking advantage of the stereopsis provided by indirect ophthalmoscopy can provide a more striking and convincing view of an enlarged and protruding optic disc.

In many cases, there may be no involvement of the optic disc. Instead, the portion of the optic nerve posterior to the lamina cribrosa, invisible to the examiner, may be involved. In these situations, the loss of vision and pupillary responses to light would be a major clue to the presence of an optic nerve problem.

Exophthalmos or other deviation of the globe may be present if the tumor is of significant size. The degree and direction of displacement of the globe would depend on the size and location of the tumor. Initially, there would be rostral displacement due to the location of the lesion at the orbital apex. This is best visualized by observing the animal from above. As the tumor grows larger, the globe would be displaced to the side opposite the tumor as well as rostrally. Protrusion of the third eyelid is a frequent occurrence with large tumors as is reduction or prevention of ocular motility. With or without obvious bulbar deviation, attempts at retropulsing the globe

would be met with resistance compared with the unaffected side. Careful attempts at retropulsion generally can demonstrate this resistance and localize the mass. Ophthalmoscopic examination may reveal indentation of the posterior aspect of the globe as manifested by folding or gray discoloration of the retina or tapetum. Retropulsion simultaneous with ophthalmoscopy may make this more pronounced.

One of the most common systematic errors seen in cases of a space-occupying lesion of the orbit is the misinterpretation of the signs for those of glaucoma. The prominent eye can be misleading. When an eye enlarges due to glaucoma, however, the cornea does so as well. In addition to measuring intraocular pressure, comparison of corneal diameters in animals having one normal eye should be helpful in this regard. More importantly, globes that are prominent due to glaucoma usually can be retropulsed to some degree into the orbit and demonstrate other signs associated with the elevated intraocular pressure, including episcleral injection, corneal edema and striae, lens dislocations, and characteristic fundus changes.

Although pain is not a feature of optic nerve neoplasia itself, secondary, painful changes such as exposure keratitis or orbital inflammation may be present.

If the tumor has grown into the globe, it may have extended into the adjacent choroid or between the sensory retina and retinal epithelium. This almost always would lead to separation of the sensory retina from the retinal epithelium or detachment of the entire retina from the choroid, either situation easily recognizable ophthalmoscopically.

If the ocular media are opaque, preventing examination of the eye's interior, one must rely on other diagnostic procedures. Such eyes generally are not salvageable, and it may be difficult to establish that they do not contain a neoplasm by using noninvasive techniques. Ultrasound may provide the necessary evidence for the presence of an intraocular mass. Even if this cannot be accomplished, if the eye is painful and is considered permanently blind, enucleation and orbital exploration followed by histologic examination can clarify the cause as well as provide relief.

Skull radiography, venography, contrast orbitography, or ultrasonography may be of help.[1,2] None of these methods, however, is likely to lead to an unequivocal diagnosis of optic nerve neoplasia. The techniques listed help localize the lesion or provide information about its extent within the orbit. Computed tomography or magnetic resonance imaging (MRI) have been helpful in determining not only nerve involvement, but whether there has been intracranial extension, which would be strongly suggestive of neoplasia.[3,4]

Occasionally, abnormal tissue will be adequately accessible to enable incisional or needle biopsies.[5,6] If the lesion is known to be small and well circumscribed, lateral orbitotomy can theoretically provide a method for removing the tumor completely and also for saving the globe (although vision may be lost, and the vasculature to the globe must be preserved).[5,6] This rarely is the case and, at the very least, excision of the affected orbital portion of the optic nerve is necessary. Practically, this also entails enucleation of the globe even though it may be normal, but this is justified to ensure total removal. Fortunately, primary neoplasms usually are unilateral, allowing for a considerable degree of visual function to be retained through the remaining normal eye.

Unfortunately, in most cases, these neoplasms are extensive before the animal is brought to a clinician for consultation. The tumor may have invaded the orbital tissue or wall. Thus, even with procedures such as exenteration, neoplastic tissue often remains, and recurrence is frequent. Metastatic disease or intracranial extension frequently follows and results in death. Exenteration followed by radiation therapy may extend the animal's life in some of these cases.

At least three conditions may mimic optic nerve neoplasia. Normal, but exuberant, myelination of the optic disk may be mistaken by a novice for neoplastic infiltration of the optic disc. In these cases, there will be no evidence of optic nerve dysfunction.

Inflammation of the optic nerve may result in a swollen, protruding optic disc due to edema and infiltration by inflammatory cells. Animals with space-occupying intracranial disease also may have protrusion of the optic disk due to edema or blockage of axoplasmic flow. These conditions may have associated loss of optic nerve function. Optic neuritis often appears to be sudden in onset, and there may be hemorrhage within the superfi-

cial layers of the optic disk. Lesions involving the brain and causing swelling of the optic disc usually would be expected to have other neurologic signs associated with them. Nevertheless, differentiation of these two conditions from optic nerve neoplasia may be difficult. A positive response to a short course of systemic corticosteroid therapy may be of some use. Practitioners must be aware, however, that these drugs may ameliorate the inflammatory component present with neoplasms, as well, making a positive response to therapy unreliable as a means of diagnosis.

Meningioma. This is the most common primary neoplasm of the optic nerve, at least in dogs.[7–16] It has been reported in rats.[17] Meningiomas arise from arachnoidal epithelial cells of the orbital portion of the optic nerve sheath (Figure 9.2). Although the cells may differ in shape, size, and other characteristics, they all are comprised of the same cell ultrastructurally, and subdivision is of minimal value.[18] Bone and cartilage (Figure 9.2B) are produced in some tumors as are psammoma bodies. In dogs, affected individual animals have been reported usually to be over 6 years of age.[8,19] No breed predilection is apparent.[19]

Clinical signs generally are typical for a mass destroying the optic nerve or a space-occupying lesion of the posterior region of the orbit (Figure 9.1). Occasionally, the neoplasm may extend into the globe, resulting in retinal detachment or separation, uveitis, or glaucoma. When there is ossification, this may make it easier to distinguish radiographically. The most important sign, however, is diminution of optic nerve function. Unilateral blindness and loss of pupillary responses to light are frequent findings.

Although well-circumscribed optic nerve meningiomas might be excised successfully, enucleation usually is necessary. Whereas meningiomas rarely metastasize, they can invade the cranium via the optic nerve and cause more serious central nervous system (CNS) damage.[11–13]

Sarcoma. There have been several reports of sarcomas occurring in traumatized cat eyes.[20–22] Most of these tumors have been fibrosarcomas, but some have been osteosarcomas and others were anaplastic sarcomas. Although the type of trauma was unknown, in each case the alleged

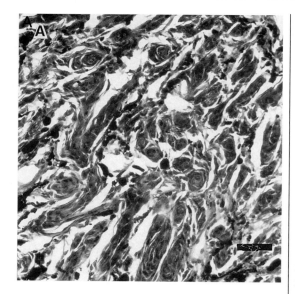

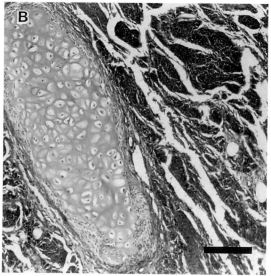

FIG. 9.2—Optic nerve meningioma in a 7-year-old female Scottish terrier, right eye. **A:** Notice the compact whorls of meningothelial cells. Bar = 100 μm, hematoxylin-eosin. **B:** There is prominent cartilage formation. Bar = 150 μm, hematoxylin-eosin.

occurrence was several years prior to the discovery of neoplasia. Most of the eyes were phthisical and had lens rupture. Although not primary to the optic nerve, these tumors are mentioned here because of their propensity for growth into and along the optic nerve, often into the brain, resulting in death.

The pathogenesis in these cases is unclear. Perhaps chronic inflammation allowed for transduction of normal cellular oncogenes into feline leukemia virus (FeLV) sequences. In only one case was the FeLV status of these cats known, and it was negative.[20] The pluripotential lens epithelium and retinal epithelium are possibilities as sources of tissue that transformed independently of whether FeLV was present.

Although neoplasia of this sort appears to be extremely rare, the reported cases point to the need for being circumspect in dealing with phthisical eyes, particularly in cats. Such eyes are of no use to an affected animal regardless of the question of neoplasia. If there is a change in character, such as chronic inflammation or enlargement, enucleation with radical optic neurectomy is indicated. When doing this, however, care needs to be taken to avoid putting strong traction on the optic nerve, as there have been several anecdotal accounts of animals that became blind due to optic nerve dysfunction in their normal eye after an otherwise routine enucleation.[23] A working hypothesis for this unfortunate outcome is traction-related damage to the contralateral optic nerve at the level of the optic chiasm.

Medulloepithelioma. Because medulloepitheliomas primarily are tumors of the ciliary epithelium, their major points are discussed in Chapter 6. The tissue of origin, however, is neuroepithelium. Because neuroepithelium is present all along the optic pathways during development, this type of tumor can occur in the optic nerve.

There have been at least three cases of medulloepithelioma involving the optic nerve, apparently as primary lesions.[24–26] As is typical for these tumors, the animals generally were young: an 18-month-old female standardbred horse[25] and a 4-month-old male thoroughbred.[26] The history and clinical findings in both suggested that the tumor arose from the intraocular portion of the optic nerve. Although the former animal's case was not followed after exenteration of the orbit, neoplastic tissue along the surgical margin of the optic nerve suggested the likelihood of recurrence. In the latter case, the colt was euthanatized.

In the remaining case, the animal was a 9-year-old paint horse that had exophthalmos and a mass in the right vitreous cavity.[24] A dilated pupil and loss of pupillary responses to light indicated optic nerve involvement. Although enucleation was done, there was regrowth with spread into the brain, prompting euthanasia 2 months later. The tumor was diagnosed as a primary optic nerve tumor of neuroepithelial origin. Although the authors avoided calling this tumor a medulloepithelioma, partly because of location, the clinical and microscopic findings appeared strikingly similar to the previous case.

Glioma. These are tumors arising from the neuroglia of nervous tissue. Because these appear rarely to involve the optic nerve, a classification scheme based on clinical or microscopic features is premature. It is presumed that the classification scheme used for similar neoplasms arising in CNS tissue would be applicable.[27]

The two reported cases of glioma involving the optic nerve involved black Labrador retrievers.[28,29] In the first case, the tumor appeared to involve only the optic nerve and had caused retinal separation. There was no recurrence up to 18 months after enucleation.

In the second case, the tumor had caused a painful exophthalmos and had grown into the globe. Necropsy following euthanasia revealed tumor in the ventral part of the brain as well as in the eye and orbit. It was not clear, however, from the description in the report whether the tumor was primary to the optic nerve. The account could not refute the possibility that the mass arose in the brain and had grown down the optic nerve to the eye.

Miscellaneous. Cavernous hemangioma of the optic nerve has been diagnosed in an adult captive rhesus monkey.[30] This extended as a racemose hemangioma involving the retina, providing a striking funduscopic picture of greatly enlarged and tortuous retinal vessels. The diagnosis was made during a routine examination of the eye, and no clinical signs were referable to the tumor. A necropsy failed to demonstrate abnormalities of the brain. The vessels of the tumor were thin walled and did not contain muscularis. Although they did not connect with the central retinal artery, they were connected with the central retinal vein. Abnormal vessels occu-

pied the entire thickness of retina, which was attenuated and cystic. The pathologic changes did not extend to the macula.

Astrocytoma arising from the optic disc has been reported in a 12-year-old castrated male golden retriever.[31] Although neoplastic cells extended along the optic nerve, the dog was free of neurologic signs or evidence of neoplastic regrowth for at least 6 months after enucleation.

Summary. As more primary optic nerve neoplasms are studied, methods of diagnosis and treatment and our view of prognoses may have to be altered. In this regard, all veterinarians who establish a diagnosis of optic nerve neoplasia should carefully document it. History, clinical findings, and long-term follow-up are essential if progress is to be made in the establishment of accurate prognoses and the administration of appropriate treatment. Histologic confirmation of all removed tissues is necessary to provide crucial background information.

HUMANS

A variety of primary and metastatic tumors have been reported in the optic nerve of humans.[32] The vast majority of these neoplasms are astrocytomas or meningiomas, with metastases and other types of primary tumors being rare. The following discussion focuses on the two common neoplasms of the retrobulbar optic nerve and its sheath.

Optic Nerve Gliomas

HISTORICAL PERSPECTIVES. Optic nerve gliomas were first described in the 1800s, and Verhoeff[33] recorded a notable systematic histologic study of 11 cases in 1922. Numerous accounts of patients with optic nerve glioma have been reported since. The histopathology of this neoplasm is now well defined, but its etiology and treatment remain topics of current research and debate.

TERMINOLOGY AND BACKGROUND. Neoplasms of the CNS are currently classified by their putative cell of origin, which in turn is based on the phenotypic expression of the constituent neoplastic cells. The term *glioma* is imprecise, because it refers to any neoplasm composed of glial cells (i.e., all forms of astrocytoma, oligodendroglioma, and ependymoma). When used in the context of *optic nerve glioma,* however, the term *glioma* has become synonymous with *astrocytoma.*

Astrocytomas, which are the most common type of primary brain tumor, arise in all parts of the brain and spinal cord, but are most frequent in the cerebrum. Cytologically, astrocytomas form a spectrum ranging from tumors composed of very well differentiated astrocytes with minimal cytologic atypia (astrocytoma, grade 1 or 2) to those composed of less well differentiated astrocytes with cytologic atypia and mitotic activity (astrocytoma, grade 3; anaplastic astrocytoma) to those composed of poorly differentiated astrocytes with severe cytologic atypia, mitotic activity, and areas of necrosis (astrocytoma, grade 4; glioblastoma multiforme).

Patient survival is closely associated with the histologic grade of the astrocytoma.[34] Grade 1 astrocytomas are typically slowly growing neoplasms with a median survival period measured in decades. Grade 2 and grade 3 astrocytomas have intermediate growth rates, with median survival periods of approximately 4 years and 2 years, respectively. Grade 4 astrocytomas (glioblastomas) are rapidly growing neoplasms with a median survival period of approximately 1 year, even if treated aggressively.

Aside from histologic grade, astrocytomas may also be subclassified morphologically into subtypes based on the cytologic features of the neoplastic cells.[35] This histologic subtyping of astrocytomas is important clinically, because prognosis is closely related to the subtype of astrocytoma. Most astrocytomas are of the *diffuse* subtype. Diffuse astrocytomas (also referred to as *fibrillary* astrocytomas) most commonly occur in the cerebral hemispheres of adults, but may be found in all age groups and in all parts of the CNS, including the optic nerve. These astrocytomas are so named because the neoplastic astrocytes, regardless of degree of differentiation, diffusely infiltrate surrounding brain. Diffuse astrocytomas also have a proclivity for developing increasing anaplastic changes over time (*malignant degeneration*). Because of their

invasiveness, rapid growth, and tendency for malignant degeneration, patients with diffuse astrocytomas have a poor prognosis. Fortunately, diffuse astrocytomas occur only rarely in the anterior visual pathways.[36]

Another important, but less common, subtype of astrocytoma is the *pilocytic* variety. Pilocytic astrocytomas arise most commonly in the cerebellum, region of the hypothalamus, and anterior visual pathways of children, but may occur in all parts of the CNS and in both children and adults. The tumor is so named because it is composed in part of greatly elongated (piloid, hairlike) astrocytes. In contrast to diffuse astrocytomas, pilocytic astrocytomas are almost always well differentiated (grade 1–2), are generally less infiltrative, and rarely undergo malignant degeneration. Their circumscribed nature and slow growth rate give patients with pilocytic astrocytomas a good prognosis.

Astrocytomas, regardless of grade or histologic subtype, rarely metastasize outside the CNS. Despite this lack of extracranial metastasis, all astrocytomas are potentially lethal due to their mass effect causing raised intracranial pressure and brain herniation. These neoplasms also destroy brain tissue locally so that focal neurologic deficits are common. Seizures and hydrocephalus are additional potential complications.

Astrocytomas of the anterior visual pathways (optic nerve, optic chiasm, and optic tract) are often referred to as *optic nerve gliomas,* even though the vast majority of these tumors are more specifically pilocytic astrocytomas and often appear to arise in the optic chiasm or optic tract. Because tumors located in the optic nerve are much more amenable to complete surgical resection (and therefore have a much better prognosis) than those located more posteriorly in the chiasmal region, some authors subdivide gliomas of the anterior visual pathways into optic nerve gliomas and chiasmal gliomas.[37] Although this subdivision has merit, many authors use the term *optic nerve glioma* for pilocytic astrocytomas arising anywhere along the anterior visual pathways. The much less common diffuse astrocytoma arising in the anterior visual pathways is often referred to as a *malignant optic glioma,* since this neoplasm invariably shows histologic features of anaplasia and a correspondingly poor prognosis.[36]

EPIDEMIOLOGY. Optic nerve gliomas (those with intraorbital involvement) are generally considered rare tumors, accounting for only about 1% of CNS astrocytomas.[38] They were the fifth most common orbital tumor (2.5%) in Henderson's series of 1376 consecutive orbital tumors seen at the Mayo Clinic between 1948 and 1987 (see Henderson,[39] 43–52). Reflecting their predominant occurrence in childhood, optic nerve gliomas were the second most common orbital tumor (14% of 212 cases) when Henderson's series was restricted to patients of age 15 years or less.

There is wide agreement that optic nerve gliomas (pilocytic astrocytomas of the anterior visual pathways) occur primarily in children. Alvord and Lofton[40] reported that of 623 optic nerve gliomas recorded in the literature, 59% were in the first decade, 22% in the second decade, 6% in the third decade, and the remaining 13% in older patients. Rush et al.[41] found in their series of 85 histologically verified optic nerve gliomas that patients ranged from less than 1 year to 46 years of age, with a median age of 6½ years for tumors arising in the optic nerve and 11 years for those arising in the chiasm. Most series show females being more frequently affected than males; in the 85 cases of Rush et al.,[41] 58% were females.

Numerous studies have confirmed the association of neurofibromatosis type 1 (NF-1) with optic nerve glioma. Rush et al.[41] found in their series of 85 cases that 15% of the 33 cases located in the optic nerve and 23% of the 52 cases located in the optic chiasm were associated with NF-1. Conversely, Lewis et al.[42] observed in a prospective study of 217 patients with NF-1 that 15% had radiologic evidence of an optic nerve or chiasmal glioma, although only 5% of these patients were clinically symptomatic. Of these NF-1 patients with radiologic evidence of optic nerve glioma, 15% had involvement of both optic nerves. Interestingly, NF-1 appears to have a favorable effect on the prognosis of patients with optic nerve glioma.[43]

Malignant (anaplastic) diffuse astrocytomas arising in the anterior visual pathways are tumors of adults. The mean age at presentation was 52 years

in the 30 cases reviewed by Taphoorn et al.[44] Both men and women are affected, although there is a slight male predominance.

CLINICAL FEATURES. Optic nerve gliomas typically present with some degree of visual loss. Proptosis is common in tumors involving the intraorbital optic nerve. Disturbances of ocular motility, pain, and papilledema or disc pallor may also be present. Patients with tumors involving the chiasmal region may develop hypothalamic dysfunction, hydrocephalus, or seizures.

Optic nerve gliomas are typically slowly growing neoplasms with a very good prognosis. In fact, the slow rate of growth of these tumors prompted some authors to consider them hamartomas rather than true neoplasms.[45,46] Most authors, however, regard optic nerve gliomas as true neoplasms (see Henderson,[39] 245). The location of the glioma within the anterior visual pathways is extremely important in determining prognosis. When confined to the optic nerve, these relatively circumscribed tumors can often be totally excised. In this situation, one can expect an excellent prognosis with little chance for recurrence. However, when the astrocytoma involves the chiasm, complete excision is technically impossible, and the likelihood of continued growth and invasion of surrounding brain structures by the tumor should be anticipated (Figure 9.3).

Malignant diffuse astrocytomas of the anterior visual pathways typically present with progressive visual loss in middle-aged adults. The clinical presentation often mimics optic neuritis, with complete visual loss occurring within a few weeks.[36]

MORPHOLOGY. Astrocytomas arising in the optic nerve usually produce a fusiform or globular enlargement of the nerve. If the tumor also involves the intracranial portion of the anterior visual pathways, the tumor may be constricted by the optic foramen so that the neoplasm develops a "dumbbell" shape. The optic foramen may be enlarged by the tumor. The cut surfaces of the tumor are usually firm, although areas of cystic degeneration are common. The leptomeninges are often extensively infiltrated by astrocytoma to

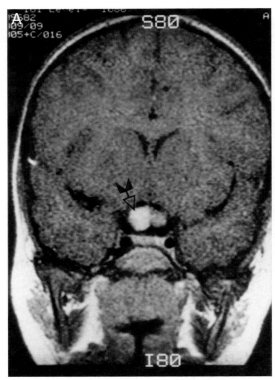

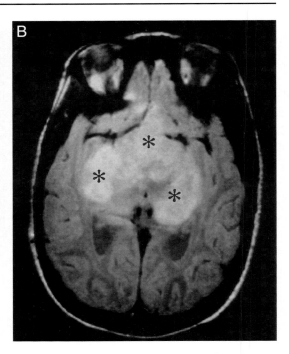

FIG. 9.3—Magnetic resonance imaging of optic nerve gliomas. **A:** T1-weighted coronal image of brain from a child with neurofibromatosis type 1 (NF-1) and an optic nerve glioma. There is an enhancing lesion (arrow) of the right optic chiasm, which is enlarged. The left optic chiasm also shows slight enhancement and enlargement. **B:** Axial proton density image of brain from a child with NF-1 and a glioma of the anterior visual pathways. There is abnormal signal intensity (asterisks) bilaterally from the regions of the optic chiasm and optic tracts. (Scans courtesy of Mauricio Castillo, MD, Chapel Hill, NC.)

form a circumferential ring of tumor around the nerve (Figure 9.4). Despite infiltration of the leptomeninges by tumor, there is rarely infiltration of the dura mater.

Optic gliomas may involve any portion of the anterior visual pathways, with the region of the chiasm being more often involved than the optic nerve. Of the 623 cases collected from the literature by Alvord and Lofton,[40] 75% initially involved the region of the chiasm and 25% initially involved the optic nerve. Of those tumors initially involving the chiasm, half were limited to the optic chiasm, and half involved the chiasm and adjacent structures. Rush et al.[41] found in their series of 85 optic gliomas that 61% involved the chiasm and 39% involved the optic nerve; 20% of their chiasmal gliomas extended to the hypothalamus or optic tract, and 70% of their optic nerve gliomas

extended to the intracanalicular or intracranial optic nerve. Optic nerve gliomas involving both optic nerves are uncommon: only one of the 34 cases reported in the Mayo Clinic series (see Henderson,[39] 245) and only three of the 63 cases reported by Yanoff et al.[47] were bilateral. It has been suggested that bilateral optic nerve gliomas are found only in patients with neurofibromatosis.[41]

Optic nerve glioma is identical histologically to pilocytic astrocytoma arising in the cerebellum (juvenile pilocytic astrocytoma; cystic cerebellar astrocytoma of childhood) and elsewhere in the CNS.[47,48] The neoplasm is moderately cellular and often shows two patterns of cellular growth. In one pattern, the neoplastic astrocytes are elongated to form spindle-shaped cells (piloid astrocytes). These piloid cells often bundle together to form thick perivascular sheaths. In the second pattern,

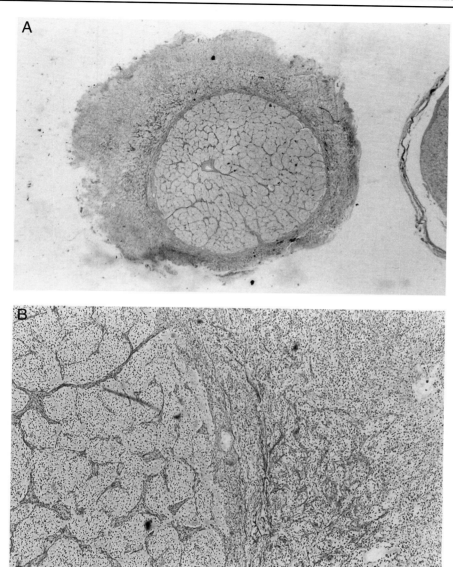

FIG. 9.4—Optic nerve glioma. **A:** Cross section of optic nerve shows diffuse enlargement of nerve by an infiltrating pilocytic astrocytoma. There is also extensive infiltration of the leptomeninges. **B:** At higher magnification, the hypercellularity of the optic nerve (*left*) and leptomeninges (*right*) reflects the diffuse infiltration of these structures by astrocytoma. Note the preservation of connective tissue septa within the nerve.

the cells are more stellate and associated with considerable extracellular matrix and numerous extracellular microcysts (*microcystic degeneration*). Vascular endothelial proliferation and scattered atypical nuclei are common in pilocytic astrocytomas arising in the anterior visual pathways and elsewhere in the CNS and do not indicate a poor prognosis. Definite features of anaplasia, such as mitotic figures and areas of tumor necrosis, are rare in pilocytic astrocytomas of the optic nerve or chiasm. In keeping with pilocytic astrocytomas in other locations in the CNS, those of the anterior visual pathways rarely undergo malignant degeneration over time.

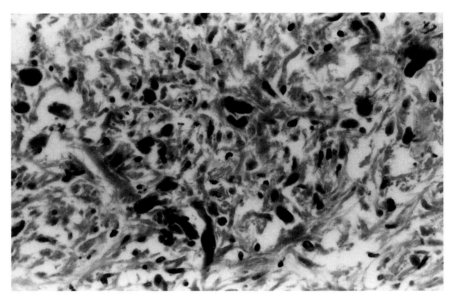

FIG. 9.5—Optic nerve glioma. Multiple darkly staining, oval to elongated Rosenthal fibers are present in this pilocytic astrocytoma of the optic nerve.

A characteristic degenerative change found in many pilocytic astrocytomas, regardless of location in the CNS, is the presence within the neoplastic cells of intensely eosinophilic, intracellular hyaline structures. These oval to rod-shaped structures are termed *Rosenthal fibers* and represent an alteration in intracytoplasmic glial filaments (Figure 9.5). Rosenthal fibers were found in about half of the 63 cases of optic nerve glioma studied by Yanoff et al.[47] These structures are characteristic of pilocytic astrocytomas, but are not pathognomonic, as similar structures may be found in areas of old gliosis within the brain or spinal cord.

Another, less common, degenerative change in pilocytic astrocytomas is the presence of granular, eosinophilic bodies within the cytoplasm of the neoplastic cells.[47] Granular eosinophilic bodies, like Rosenthal fibers, are not restricted to pilocytic astrocytomas.[49]

Optic nerve gliomas frequently infiltrate and expand the leptomeninges. Over 75% of the 63 optic nerve gliomas studied by Yanoff et al.[47] showed leptomeningeal spread. The infiltrating tumor cells evoke proliferation of fibroblasts, which also contributes to the enlargement of the glioma-infiltrated leptomeninges (Figure 9.4).

Hyperplasia of arachnoidal (meningothelial) cells is a common and prominent feature in some optic nerve gliomas. Foci of meningothelial hyperplasia were present in 56% of the cases in one large series[47] and were often distinct from areas of astrocytoma invading the leptomeninges. Microscopically, these foci of meningothelial hyperplasia are indistinguishable from meningioma and may present a diagnostic problem for pathologists when separate from the infiltrating astrocytoma. This is especially true when the biopsy of the enlarged optic nerve is superficial. Zimmerman[50] has emphasized that the proliferating arachnoidal cells in meningeal hyperplasia remain intradural, whereas the neoplastic cells typically invade the dura mater and surrounding orbital tissues.

Ultrastructural and immunocytochemical studies of optic nerve gliomas confirm that the constituent cells have astrocytic differentiation. Electron microscopy reveals abundant intermediate filaments within the tumor cells' cytoplasm, and immunostained sections reveal positive staining of these intermediate filaments for glial fibrillary acidic protein (GFAP) (see Burger and Scheithauer,[51] 77–96). The majority of optic nerve gliomas have proliferation indices (Ki-67) of less than 1%.[52]

As previously noted, the rare malignant optic glioma of adulthood has histologic features of a high-grade diffuse astrocytoma (anaplastic astrocytoma or glioblastoma multiforme). These anaplastic features include high cellularity, marked cellular and nuclear atypia, mitotic activity, vascular endothelial proliferation, and foci of tumor necrosis.[36]

TREATMENT AND PROGNOSIS. The treatment of optic nerve glioma is controversial.[37] The results of any treatment are difficult to evaluate in optic nerve gliomas because of their usually slow progression. For tumors limited to the optic nerve, serial MRI enables the growth characteristics of a tumor to be monitored over time so that surgical excision can be delayed until the neoplasm shows definite extension posteriorly toward the chiasm (see Henderson,[39] 249–252).

When the optic chiasm is involved by tumor, complete excision is not feasible, and radiotherapy is often employed in an attempt to slow the growth of the neoplasm. Unfortunately, radiation can have serious, long-term consequences, especially in children. For this reason, combination chemotherapy has been employed in some cases. The use of chemotherapy with radiotherapy allows the radiotherapy to be delayed, thus possibly avoiding some of the adverse side effects of radiation in children.[53]

The rare malignant optic gliomas arising in adults are usually treated with surgery and radiotherapy. These rapidly growing, poorly differentiated astrocytomas cannot be completely excised and are not responsive to radiotherapy, so nearly all patients succumb within 1 year of clinical presentation.[44]

Optic Nerve Meningiomas

HISTORICAL PERSPECTIVES. Meningiomas were well described in the 1800s, and by 1928 Mayer had collected 40 cases of orbital meningiomas, although his series did not distinguish primary meningioma of the optic nerve sheath from the more common intracranial meningioma with secondary extension into the orbit.[54] One of the first descriptions of an unequivocal primary optic nerve sheath meningioma has been credited to Coston in 1936.[54] Since that time, numerous series have documented the occurrence of primary optic nerve meningiomas. The histopathology of the optic nerve meningioma is now well defined, but its etiology and treatment remain topics of current research.

TERMINOLOGY AND BACKGROUND. Meningiomas are neoplasms that are considered to arise from the meningothelial (arachnoidal) cells of the arachnoid mater. The arachnoid mater is the layer of meninges sandwiched between the inner pia mater and outer dura mater and covers the entire CNS, including the intraorbital portion of the optic nerve. Meningiomas are found in all parts of the CNS, but most commonly arise from the intracranial (intracranial meningioma) or spinal meninges (intraspinal meningioma). Much less frequently, meningiomas arise from the meninges around the optic nerve (optic nerve meningioma) or from meningeal tissue within the stroma of the choroid plexus (intraventricular meningioma). Rarely, these neoplasms are unassociated with meninges, arising ectopically in sites such as cranial bone, paranasal sinus, orbit, lung, and skin (see Burger and Scheithauer,[51] 259–262).

Meningiomas involving the orbit (orbital meningiomas) may be subdivided into *primary* and *secondary* types. Primary orbital meningiomas arise within in the orbit, whereas secondary orbital meningiomas arise elsewhere and extend into the orbit. These secondary tumors originate from a variety of sites adjacent to the orbit, including the sphenoid ridge, basofrontal region, parasellar area, superior orbital fissure, and paranasal sinuses (see Henderson,[39] 377). The term *primary orbital meningioma* is not synonymous with *optic nerve* (optic nerve sheath) *meningioma*, as primary orbital meningiomas include those of optic nerve sheath origin and those arising ectopically in the orbit.[55] Determination of whether an orbital meningioma is primary or secondary can sometimes be difficult and is rather subjective.

Most meningiomas are well differentiated histologically. Those showing anaplastic features are classified as atypical meningiomas or malignant meningiomas, depending on the degree of hypercellularity and atypia, frequency of mitotic figures, and presence of necrosis (see Burger and Scheithauer,[51] 277–283). Meningiomas are also sometimes subclassified microscopically into a large variety of morphologically distinctive variants, such as meningotheliomatous, transitional, fibrous, psammomatous, secretory, microcystic, lymphoplasmacytic, chordoid, papillary, and metaplastic (see Burger and Scheithauer,[51] 262–269). This large number of histologic variants reflects the diverse microscopic appearances of meningiomas. Most intracranial meningiomas are meningotheliomatous, transitional, or fibrous. With the exception of the more aggressive papillary and chordoid variants, the numerous histologic variants of meningioma have a similar biologic activity (see Burger and Scheithauer,[51] 262–269).

EPIDEMIOLOGY. Meningiomas are common tumors of the CNS, but only occasionally involve the orbit. Thus, among 546 surgically verified meningiomas seen at the Mayo Clinic between 1980 and 1987, only 7.5% involved the orbit, and only 1.6% were considered primary orbital meningiomas (see Henderson,[39] 378). Meningiomas accounted for 10.1% of the tumors in Henderson's series of 1376 consecutive orbital tumors, being the fourth most common primary orbital tumor and the third most common secondary orbital tumor (see Henderson,[39] 377).

Secondary orbital meningiomas are much more common than primary orbital meningiomas. Dutton[54] found that 90% of the 5000 patients with orbital meningiomas reported in the literature had secondary meningiomas. Of the remaining 10% with primary orbital meningiomas, 96% had optic nerve sheath meningiomas and 4% had ectopic meningiomas; 92% of the optic sheath tumors arose from the nerve sheath within the orbit, and 8% arose from the nerve sheath within the optic canal.

Optic nerve meningiomas may occur at any age. Like their intracranial and intraspinal counterparts, however, optic nerve meningiomas are most common in adulthood and show a female preponderance. Among 256 patients with optic nerve meningioma reported in the literature, the mean age was 40.8 years (range, 2.5 to 78 years) and 61% were female.[54] Some studies suggest that the primary orbital meningiomas occurring in childhood are more aggressive.[55,56] Right and left optic nerves are approximately equally affected, with 95% of the tumors being unilateral and 5% being bilateral.[54] It is unclear whether the bilateral tumors represent multifocal meningiomas or the intracranial spread of a meningioma to involve both optic nerves.

There is broad agreement that the incidence of neurofibromatosis in patients with optic nerve meningioma is higher than the incidence of neurofibromatosis within the general population. Dutton found that among seven reported series of optic nerve meningiomas in which evidence of neurofibromatosis was specifically sought, 9% of the 142 cases were associated with neurofibromatosis.[54]

CLINICAL FEATURES. Visual loss, proptosis, optic disc atrophy, papilledema, decreased ocular motility, and optociliary shunt vessels are the most common clinical findings in optic nerve meningioma.[54] Visual loss of gradual onset is the most frequent presenting symptom. Papilledema is much more common with primary orbital meningiomas than with secondary orbital meningiomas (see Henderson,[39] 380). Orbital pain, generalized headache, and edema of the eyelid are among the other reported clinical findings.

Optic nerve meningiomas are best visualized radiologically with MRI.[57] A diffuse tubular enlargement of the nerve is most common, although both globular and fusiform shapes are also seen. Calcification may be present within the tumor and is a helpful feature for differentiation from optic nerve glioma. Tram tracking, a radiographic sign in which the radiographically denser, tumor-infiltrated, optic nerve sheath surrounds the more radiolucent optic nerve, is another helpful feature favoring optic nerve meningioma.[58]

MORPHOLOGY. Optic nerve meningiomas grow primarily in the subarachnoid space around the optic nerve (Figure 9.6). The tumor may grow eccentrically or completely encircle the nerve. As the tumor enlarges, it compresses the underlying nerve, leading to optic atrophy. Actual invasion of the optic nerve is uncommon, being found in only two of the 25 cases of optic nerve meningioma studied histologically by Karp

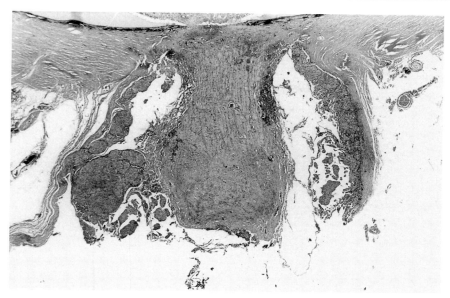

FIG. 9.6—Optic nerve meningioma. The retrobulbar optic nerve is surrounded by a meningioma arising in the optic nerve sheath. (This case was presented by Helmut Buettner, MD, at the annual meeting of the Theobald Society, New Orleans, LA, 1986.)

et al.[55] The tumor is initially encapsulated by the dura mater, but often invades the overlying dura mater and may extend beyond the dura mater into the surrounding orbital tissues. Some meningiomas extend anteriorly within the optic nerve sheath to the globe, but only infrequently do meningiomas invade the sclera (4%), choroid (4%), or optic disc (8%).[55] Meningiomas may also extend posteriorly within the optic nerve sheath to the optic canal or middle cranial fossa. Primary orbital meningiomas that extend intracranially are similar to primary intracranial meningiomas in that they act as mass lesions, but rarely invade brain.

Histologically, primary orbital meningiomas are typically well differentiated and resemble their intracranial counterparts. Most show features of the meningotheliomatous or transitional variant (see Henderson,[39] 384–387; and Karp et al.[55]) The tumors are moderately cellular, with the neoplastic cells having indistinct cell borders, large amounts of eosinophilic cytoplasm, and oval nuclei (Figures 9.7 and 9.8). The oval nuclei and large amounts of cytoplasm give the neoplastic cells an epithelial (meningotheliomatous) appearance. The neoplastic cells may form small nodules, around which spindle-shaped cells whorl (Figure 9.9). Psammoma (oval, lamellated, calcified) bodies are found in some meningiomas. Large, hyperchromatic nuclei that are occasionally present in meningiomas represent a degenerative change rather than evidence of anaplasia. The anaplastic changes that characterize atypical and malignant meningiomas, such as conspicuous mitotic activity and foci of tumor necrosis, are exceptional in optic nerve meningiomas.

TREATMENT AND PROGNOSIS. The therapeutic approach to optic nerve meningiomas is controversial.[59] Optic nerve meningiomas without intracranial extension are rarely fatal, although loss of vision is usual. When the tumor is confined to the orbit, observation may be preferable to surgery, since surgery may only hasten the progression to blindness. When the optic nerve meningioma extends to the intracanalicular or intracranial portions of the optic nerve, treatment decisions become more complex. Radiotherapy has been used in some cases, with improvement in visual acuity following irradiation being reported.[54,60]

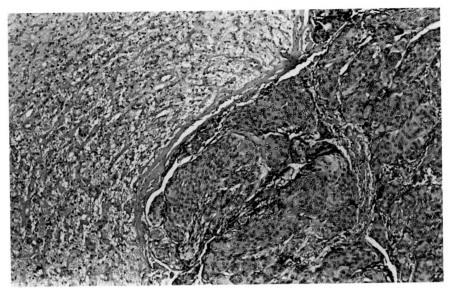

FIG. 9.7—Optic nerve meningioma. The meningioma (*right*) compresses the optic nerve (*left*), which is atrophic and gliotic. The meningioma demonstrates a typical lobular growth pattern.

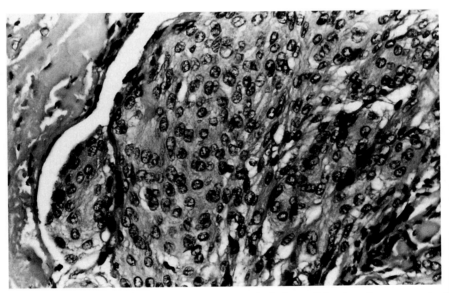

FIG. 9.8—Optic nerve meningioma. The neoplastic cells have indistinct cell borders, large amounts of cytoplasm, and pale, oval nuclei typical of the meningotheliomatous variant of meningioma. Some nuclei show vacuolation, a common finding in meningioma.

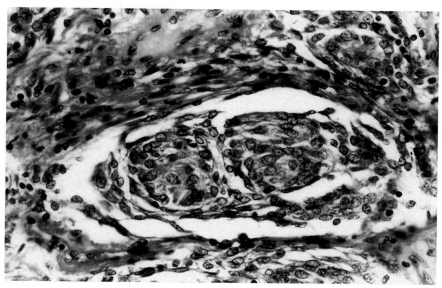

FIG. 9.9—Optic nerve meningioma. The neoplastic meningothelial cells form small discrete lobules. Cells at the periphery of a lobule are often spindle shaped and give the appearance of whorling around the nodule.

REFERENCES

1. Johnston GR, Feeney DA. Radiology in ophthalmic diagnosis. *Vet Clin North Am Small Animal Pract* 10:317, 1980.
2. LeCouteur RA, Scagliotti RH, Beck KA, Holliday TA. Indirect imaging of the canine optic nerve, using metrizamide (optic thecography). *Am J Vet Res* 43:1424, 1982.
3. Fike JR, LeCouteur RA, Cann CE. Anatomy of the canine orbital region: multiplanar imaging by CT. *Vet Radiol* 25:32, 1984.
4. LeCouteur RA, Fike JR, Scagliotti RH, Cann CE. Computed tomography of orbital tumors in the dog. *J Am Vet Med Assoc* 180:910, 1982.
5. Harvey CE. Exploration of the orbit. In: Bistner SI, Aguirre G, Batik G, eds. *Atlas of Veterinary Ophthalmic Surgery.* Philadelphia: WB Saunders, 1977:258.
6. Koch DB, Leitch M, Beech J. Orbital surgery in two horses. *Vet Surg* 9:61, 1980.
7. Abrams K, Toal RL. What is your diagnosis? *J Am Vet Med Assoc* 196:951, 1990.
8. Andrews EJ. Clinicopathologic characteristics of meningiomas in dogs. *J Am Vet Med Assoc* 163:151, 1973.
9. Barnett KC, Kelly DF, Singleton WB. Retrobulbar and chiasmal meningioma in a dog. *J Small Anim Pract* 8:391, 1967.
10. Barron CN, Saunders LZ, Jubb KV. Intraocular tumors in animals: III. Secondary intraocular tumors. *Am J Vet Res* 24:835, 1963.
11. Buyukmihci N. Orbital meningioma with intraocular invasion in a dog: histology and ultrastructure. *Vet Pathol* 14:521, 1977.
12. Dugan SJ, Schwarz PD, Roberts SM, Ching SV. Primary optic nerve meningioma and pulmonary metastasis in a dog. *J Am Anim Hosp Assoc* 29:11, 1993.
13. Geib LW. Ossifying meningioma with extracranial metastasis in a dog. *Pathol Vet* 3:247, 1966.
14. Langham RF, Bennett RR, Zydeck FA. Primary retrobulbar meningioma of the optic nerve of a dog. *J Am Vet Med Assoc* 159:175, 1971.
15. Paulsen ME, Severin GA, LeCouteur RA, Young S. Primary optic nerve meningioma in a dog. *J Am Anim Hosp Assoc* 25:147, 1989.
16. Rubin LF, Jortner B. Clinico-pathologic conference. *J Am Vet Med Assoc* 146:148, 1965.
17. Yoshitomi K, Everitt JI, Boorman GA. Primary optic nerve meningiomas in F344 rats. *Vet Pathol* 28:79, 1991.
18. Cordy DR. Tumors of the nervous system and eye. In: Moulton JE, ed. *Tumors in Domestic Animals,* 3d ed. Berkeley: University of California Press, 1990:640.
19. Braund KG, Ribas JL. Central nervous system meningiomas. *Compend Continuing Educ Pract Vet* 8:241, 1986.
20. Barrett PM, Merideth RE, Alarcon FL. Central amaurosis induced by an intraocular, posttraumatic fibrosarcoma in a cat. *J Am Anim Hosp Assoc* 31:242, 1995.
21. Dubielzig RR. Ocular sarcoma following trauma in three cats. *J Am Vet Med Assoc* 184:578, 1984.
22. Dubielzig RR, Everitt J, Shadduck JA, Albert DM. Clinical and morphologic features of posttraumatic ocular sarcomas in cats. *Vet Pathol* 27:62, 1990.

23. Stiles J, Buyukmihci NC, Hacker DV, Canton DD. Blindness from damage to optic chiasm [letter to editor]. *J Am Vet Med Assoc* 202:1192, 1993.

24. Bistner S, Campbell RJ, Shaw D, Leininger JR, Ghobrial HK. Neuroepithelial tumor of the optic nerve in a horse. *Cornell Vet* 73:30, 1983.

25. Eagle RC, Font RL, Swerczek TW. Malignant medulloepithelioma of the optic nerve in a horse. *Vet Pathol* 15:488, 1978.

26. Ueda Y, Senba H, Nishimura T, Usui T, Tanaka K, Inagaki S. Ocular medulloepithelioma in a thoroughbred. *Equine Vet J* 25:558, 1993.

27. Jones TC, Hunt RD. *Veterinary Pathology,* 5th ed. Philadelphia: Lea and Febiger, 1983.

28. Barnett KC, Grimes TD. Retrobulbar tumour and retinal detachment in a dog. *J Small Anim Pract* 13:315, 1972.

29. Spiess BM, Wilcock BP. Glioma of the optic nerve with intraocular and intracranial involvement in a dog. *J Comp Pathol* 97:79, 1987.

30. Bellhorn RW, Friedman AH, Henkind P. Racemose (cirsoid) hemangioma in rhesus monkey retina. *Am J Ophthalmol* 74:517,1972.

31. Caswell J, Curtis C, Gibbs B. Astrocytoma arising at the optic disc in a dog. *Can Vet J* 40:427, 1999.

32. Rao NA, Spencer WH. Optic nerve. In: Spencer WH, ed. *Ophthalmic Pathology,* 4th ed. Philadelphia: WB Saunders, 1996:518.

33. Verhoeff FH. Primary intraneural tumours (gliomas) of the optic nerve. *Arch Ophthalmol* 51:120 (part 2) and 239 (part 3), 1922.

34. Daumas-Duport C, Scheithauer BW, O'Fallon J, Kelley P. Grading of astrocytomas: a simple and reproducible method. *Cancer* 62:2152, 1988.

35. Kleihues P, Cavenee WK, eds. *Pathology and Genetics of Tumours of the Nervous System.* Lyon, France: IARC, 2000:6.

36. Hoyt WF, Meshel LG, Lessell S, Schatz NJ, Suckling RD. Malignant optic glioma of adulthood. *Brain* 96:121, 1973.

37. Jacobson DM. Gliomas of the anterior visual pathways. *Neurosurg Clin North Am* 10:683, 1999.

38. Russell DS, Rubinstein LJ. *Pathology of Tumours of the Nervous System,* 5th ed. Baltimore: Williams and Wilkins, 1989:370.

39. Henderson JW. *Orbital Tumors,* 3d ed. New York: Raven, 1994.

40. Alvord EC Jr, Lofton S. Gliomas of the optic nerve or chiasm: outcome by patient's age, tumor site, and treatment. *J Neurosurg* 68:85, 1988.

41. Rush JA, Younge BR, Campbell BJ, MacCarty CS. Optic glioma: long-term follow-up of 85 histopathologically verified cases. *Ophthalmology* 89:1213, 1982.

42. Lewis RA, Gerson LP, Axelson KA, Riccardi VM, Whitford RP. Von Recklinghausen neurofibromatosis: II. Incidence of optic gliomata. *Ophthalmology* 91:929, 1984.

43. Deliganis AV, Geyer JR, Berger MS. Prognostic significance of type 1 neurofibromatosis (von Recklinghausen disease) in childhood optic glioma. *Neurosurgery* 38:114, 1996.

44. Taphoorn MJB, De Vries-Knoppert AEJ, Ponssen H, Woblers JG. Malignant optic glioma in adults. *J Neurosurg* 70:277, 1989.

45. Hoyt WF, Baghdassarian SA. Optic glioma of childhood: natural history and rationale for conservative management. *Br J Ophthalmol* 53:793, 1969.

46. Miller NR, Iliff WJ, Green WR. Evaluation and management of gliomas of the anterior visual pathways. *Brain* 97:743, 1974.

47. Yanoff M, Davis RL, Zimmerman LE. Juvenile pilocytic astrocytoma ("glioma") of optic nerve: clinicopathologic study of sixty-three cases. In: Jakobiec FA, ed. *Ocular and Adnexal Tumors.* Birmingham, AL: Aesculapius, 1978:685.

48. Eggers H, Jacobiec FA, Jones IS. Optic nerve gliomas. In: Jones IS, Jacobiec FA, eds. *Diseases of the Orbit.* Hagerstown, MD: Harper and Row, 1979:417.

49. Murayama S, Bouldin TW, Suzuki K. Immunocytochemical and ultrastructural studies of eosinophilic granular bodies in astrocytic tumors. *Acta Neuropathol (Berl)* 83:408, 1992.

50. Zimmerman LE. Arachnoid hyperplasia in optic nerve glioma [correspondence]. *Br J Ophthalmol* 64:638, 1980.

51. Burger PC, Scheithauer BW. Tumors of the central nervous system. In: Rosai J, ed. *Atlas of Tumor Pathology,* 3d ser, fasc 10. Washington, DC: Armed Forces Institute of Pathology, 1994.

52. Cummings TJ, Provenzale JM, Hunter SB, Friedman AH, Klintworth GK, Bigner SH, McLendon RE. Gliomas of the optic nerve: histological, immunohistochemical (MIB-1 and p53), and MRI analysis. *Acta Neuropathol (Berl)* 99:563, 2000.

53. Packer RJ, Sutton LN, Bilaniuk LT, Radcliffe J, Rosenstock JG, Siegal KR, Bunin GR, Savino PJ, Bruce DA, Schut L. Treatment of chiasmatic/hypothalamic gliomas of childhood with chemotherapy: an update. *Ann Neurol* 23:79, 1988.

54. Dutton JJ. Optic nerve sheath meningiomas. *Surv Ophthalmol* 37:167, 1992.

55. Karp LA, Zimmerman LE, Borit A, Spencer W. Primary intraorbital meningiomas. *Arch Ophthalmol* 91:24, 1974.

56. Wright JE, McNab AA, McDonald WI. Primary optic nerve sheath meningioma. *Br J Ophthalmol* 73:960, 1989.

57. Mafee MM, Goodwin J, Dorodi S. Optic nerve sheath meningiomas. *Radiol Clin North Am* 37:37, 1999.

58. Dutton JJ. Optic nerve gliomas and meningiomas. *Neurol Clin* 9:163, 1991.

59. Volpe NJ, Gausas RE. Optic nerve and orbital tumors. *Neurosurg Clin North Am* 10:699, 1999.

60. Kennerdell JS, Maroon JC, Malton M, Warren FA. The management of optic nerve sheath meningiomas. *Am J Ophthalmol* 106:450, 1988.

10

RETINOBLASTOMA IN HUMANS AND ANIMALS

Daniel M. Albert, Jacques Lasudry, and Gia Klauss

In many regards, retinoblastoma (RB) is an intriguing cancer. This tumor represents a prototype for several aspects of the pathogenesis of a broad range of cancers. One of the most intriguing features is that spontaneous cases appear to be almost exclusively limited to humans. Although the RB gene is ubiquitously present in vertebrates, only one convincing case of spontaneous RB in animals other than human has been reported so far.[1]

HISTORICAL PERSPECTIVE

Petrus Pavius of Amsterdam has been credited with providing the first published description in 1597 of a probable RB.[2,3] For the next two centuries, little was written concerning the tumor until James Wardrop, in 1809, recognized RB as a discrete entity. Until then, it had been lumped together with other neoplasms as *fungus haematodes.* The latter term was meant to describe extremely vascular fungating tumors frequently encountered on the limbs and the breasts. Through meticulous dissections, and without the help of the microscope, Wardrop demonstrated that the ocular form of this disease arose from the retina of children and could be distinguished from the more general classification of "soft cancer."[3] In addition to his description, Wardrop strongly advocated early enucleation to save the patient's life and persisted in this belief in spite of the absence of anesthesia at the time and even though he himself never achieved a cure. Wardrop accurately attributed his failures to the advanced stage of the disease at the time of enucleation and to the optic nerve having always been involved.[4] In the 1850s, with the introduction of chloroform as a general anesthetic and the availability of the ophthalmoscope for earlier diagnosis, enucleation became accepted as an appropriate treatment. Consequently, more surgical specimens from survivors became available for histopathologic study, and clinicopathologic correlations were established. Enucleation has been the main factor responsible for improved prognosis, with the survival rate improving from 5% in 1869 to 57% in 1916.

The era of conservative treatment began with the first attempt at radiotherapy in 1903, by H.L. Hilgartner.[2] In 1930, radioactive episcleral plaques were first applied, using radon seeds and, later, cobalt 60. Since the 1950s, cryotherapy, photocoagulation, and chemotherapy have been introduced both as primary and as adjunctive treatments, particularly for small RBs.[5,6]

As increasing numbers of patients survived the disease, the role of heredity in RB gradually became apparent. As early as 1821, multiple cases in the same family were reported, and, in 1868, Albrecht Von Graefe raised the suspicion that RB might be a hereditary disease. During the first half of the 20th century, studies of survivors led to the conclusion that sporadic cases occur either as somatic mutations (in which case, the mutations affect only the somatic cells) or as new germinal mutations (in which case, the patient can transmit the disease to his or her offspring). The somatic mutations were recognized to be the most common.[3]

In 1971, Alfred Knudson, using a statistical distribution analysis, postulated his "two-hit" hypothesis for the causation of RB. In the dominantly inherited form, one mutation is inherited via the parental germinal cells, and the second occurs in somatic cells. In the nonhereditary form, both mutations occur in somatic cells, in the postzygotic stage.[7,8] Soon after, David Comings suggested that the two mutational events occur on both alleles of the retinoblastoma susceptibility gene (RB gene).[9] Other clues indicating a genetic disturbance located on a chromosome of the "D group" (which included the then morphologically similar chromosomes 13, 14, and 15) had been reported in 1962.[2,3] Subsequent intensive molecular genetic research led to localization of the susceptible segment on the subband 14 of the long arm of the chromosome 13 (13q14). The RB gene was isolated in 1986 and sequenced soon after.[10–13] The elucidation of the growth-suppressor gene activity of the RB gene proved to be an important prototype in our understanding of cancer-related suppressor genes.

TERMINOLOGY

The histologic description of RB has long been a controversial issue.[3,4] A report on *glioma of the retina* in 1953 cites 40 different names that had been given to the tumor. It is therefore not surprising that terminology has varied widely over time. Even after James Wardrop described RB as a separate entity, most writers continued to group it with *fungus haematodes* for many years. Wardrop's observation that RB arose from the retina met with controversy until the retinal origin of the tumor was definitely demonstrated in 1836 by histopathologic techniques.[3] In 1864, Rudolf Virchow concluded that RB was a tumor of glial origin and applied the term *glioma of the retina* to it. This remained the most widely used name for the tumor for many years. Independently, Simon Flexner in 1891 and Hugo Wintersteiner in 1897 described the characteristic rosettes that are named after them. To emphasize the resemblance of the tumor cells to photoreceptor cells and the layer bordering the primitive ventricle cavity, they proposed the term *neuroepithelioma.* Eventually, Frederick Verhoeff, referring to the histologic resemblance of the majority of tumor cells to the cells of the embryonic undifferentiated retina, proposed the term *retinoblastoma,* which was adopted by the American Ophthalmological Society in 1926.[4]

In 1970, a rare, but distinct, variant of RB was identified. Clinically, the affected eyes in this entity display small tumors that are often partially calcified but still viable, and that exhibit neither growth nor a threat to vision. Histologically, these tumors appear to be composed entirely of benign well-differentiated cells. To emphasize the benign behavior of these tumors, they have been named in the English literature *retinocytomas* or *retinomas.*[4,14,15]

Finally, the term *trilateral retinoblastoma* has been coined to describe the rare occurrence of an ectopic RB located in the midbrain and presenting as a primary malignant neoplasm in addition to the intraocular tumors.[16,17]

EPIDEMIOLOGY

RB is the most common malignant intraocular tumor of infancy and early childhood, and it is the second most common primary malignant intraocular tumor in any age group.[18,19] Its frequency in the United States and Western Europe has been evaluated to be between 1 in 20,000 and 1 in 15,000 live births, with no sex predilection.[4]

Its frequency has gradually increased since the beginning of the 20th century, with stabilization after the 1960s.[18–20] This is presumed to be the consequence of (1) a predictable increase in the number of patients affected by the heritable type of RB with improved diagnosis and treatment, and (2) more complete registration of the cases. Some evidence has suggested that African-American and American-Indian populations might have a higher occurrence rate.[18,19] A report by Tamboli et al., however, showed no difference in incidence of RB by either sex or race.[20]

Age at Presentation and Distribution. The vast majority of patients with active disease are diagnosed by 3–4 years of age, and the incidence of RB rapidly decreases with age.[4,18,21] Over time, it has become apparent that age at presentation is highly related to the type of RB, i.e., sporadic or familial (hereditary), unilateral or bilateral. The hereditary type usually involves both eyes and occurs earlier.

Several circumstances can affect the presentation and hence influence the time of diagnosis. In developing countries where ophthalmologic care is limited or unavailable, the diagnosis is generally made at an advanced stage, frequently when extraocular extension and metastases are present. In such cases, the prognosis is poor. The cure rate is low, and so is the likelihood for a patient to transmit the genetic predisposing trait. As a result, familial presentation of the disease may be less frequent than in developed countries.[21]

In developed countries, about 40% of RB cases are of the hereditary type, whereas 60% are sporadic.[5] With an overall penetrance of approximately 90%, 10% of the individuals carrying the hereditary mutation will not develop an ocular tumor but will still transmit the trait to 50% of their offspring.[22]

Bilateral involvement, with possible multifocal tumors in each eye, is present at the time of diagnosis in 25%–30% percent of the cases and virtually always indicates the hereditary type. Diagnosis is generally made at approximately 10–15 months. In the hereditary type, early presentation within the first days of life is not uncommon.[5,21]

In the remaining 70%–75% of cases, tumors are unilateral and unifocal, and are generally diagnosed later than the hereditary type. The majority of them are sporadic, with the average age at diagnosis approximately 21–30 months.[21]

The earlier the onset of the disease, the more likely it is to be of the hereditary type. Although hereditary unilateral disease appears to be somewhat delayed in onset when compared with bilateral disease, presentation after age 4 appears to be confined to the nonhereditary unilateral type.[5,21] It is very unlikely that two consecutive mutational events will hit both alleles of the RB gene in more than one retinoblast in a given individual. Therefore, virtually all bilateral cases are of the hereditary type, which implies that the initial mutation affects every cell, somatic and germinal.[22] In most bilateral cases, the initial mutation is not inherited but rather occurs as a new germline mutation.[23] About 12%–15% of the patients without a previous family history have an RB that is indistinguishable clinically from the other 85%, but carry the initial mutation in their germinal cells as well, and thus transmit de novo the susceptibility to their offspring.[22] Of such cases, 90% have the mutation on the allele inherited from the father. Demonstration of the new germline mutation by DNA studies in such patients is important for two reasons: to assess the risk to the patient's offspring, and to assess the risk of the patient developing a second primary malignancy later in life (vide infra).[22]

Risk Factors. The more complete registration and tracking of patients and the better prognosis for hereditary cases appear to be only partial explanations for the increase incidence over the century. The question of environmental or nutritional influences has been raised, but so far, except for a positive familial history, no conclusive risk factor has been identified.[24] Among other issues that must be considered with caution, parental age has been the object of several studies. High paternal age (over 50 years old) and high maternal age (over 35 years old) were associated with sporadic hereditary RB but not with sporadic nonhereditary RB, in a Dutch report.[25] A Japanese study, however, failed to reveal any relation to either paternal and maternal age, or to the month of birth (seasonal variations), for sporadic RB.[26] Similarly, an established statistical association between paternal employment in the military or in the metal industry and sporadic hereditary RB needs further substantiation.[27] The major contribution of the epidemiologic studies concerning risk factors for RB has been to demonstrate that none is obvious.[24] The elucidation of the molecular mechanisms involved in the inactivation of both copies of the RB gene in the tumor cells lead to new directions for research.

MORPHOLOGY

Light Microscopy. Several histologic features are characteristic of RB, so that, in most cases, the clinical diagnosis is readily confirmed by histopathology.

GROWTH PATTERNS. Three macroscopic growth patterns described in RB can be appreciated by clinicians.[18,19,21]

In the *endophytic* type, independently from the layer of origin, the tumor expands in the inner layers of the retina, toward the center of the globe. This leads to the development of tumoral protrusions at the vitreoretinal interface and the gradual loss of visualization of the retinal vessels.[21] Loose clusters of viable tumor cells can then seed into the vitreous and aggregate onto previously uninvolved areas of the retina to start new tumoral foci. Eventually, tumor cells may also pass into the anterior chamber and form a pseudohypopyon.[21] Cells may accumulate into the trabecular meshwork and even follow the aqueous outflow of the eye.[4] This is sometimes misinterpreted as the manifestation of a granulomatous iridocyclitis, or endophthalmitis. Glaucoma and inflammation may occur. The whole sequence, which can mimic an endophthalmitis with vitritis, has been termed a *masquerade syndrome.*[21]

In the *exophytic* type, the tumor expands mainly from the outer layers of the retina, toward the choroid.[18,19] At first, there is an elevation of the retina. As a result of tumor growth, a retinal detachment can occur. Tumor cells may subsequently spread beneath the retina in the subretinal space, deposit onto the retinal pigment epithelium, rupture Bruch's membrane, invade the choroid, and eventually follow the ciliary vessels or nerves, resulting in local extension into the orbit. Choroidal blood vessels may be invaded, resulting in hematogenous spread.[4,21,28]

Both endophytic and exophytic patterns are usually found within the same globe, especially in large tumors.[4] The patterns of growth carry little prognostic significance in themselves.[18,19] Vitreous seeding, however, indicates a poorer prognosis.[21]

A third growth pattern, the *diffuse infiltrating* type, which was described in 1958, occurs in about 1.5% of all RBs.[29] The mean age at presentation is also older than usual, averaging 6.1 years, with a range of 1–11 years. Boys have been affected in 60% of the reported cases. This growth pattern has an atypical and diffuse, rather than discrete, involvement of the retina. The clinical diagnosis is much more difficult than when a discrete mass is seen, and it is consequently often delayed for several months. The most common misdiagnoses of the diffuse infiltrative type are uveitis, traumatic iritis, or *Toxocara canis* infestation.[21,29]

RBs, regardless of the pattern of growth, demonstrate a tendency to invade the optic disc and spread into the substance of the optic nerve or the subarachnoidal space. Direct extension to the orbit and the brain are possible sequelae. Meningeal carcinomatosis may occur following invasion into the subarachnoidal space surrounding the optic nerve.[4]

TISSUE ARCHITECTURE. As the tumor enlarges, the blood supply usually becomes insufficient, resulting in a typical histologic pattern. Dilated capillaries are surrounded by sleeves of viable tumor cells with an approximate thickness of 90–110 μm. Beyond this layer, oxygen diffusion is presumed to be insufficient to support cell survival, resulting in areas of ischemic coagulative necrosis surrounding the islands of viable tumor cells.[4] Among the necrotic cells, the vessels are frequently noted to be occluded by endothelial hyperplasia (Figures 10.1–10.4).[18,19]

A characteristic finding in RB is laminar hematoxylinophilic staining of the vessel walls of the tumor. This may even occur at a distance from the tumor, in such sites as the internal limiting membrane, the iris vessels, or the trabecular meshwork. This staining is due to deposits of DNA released by tumor cell necrosis. Calcification is another common finding and is present mainly in the areas of necrosis.[18,19] The amount of inflammation elicited by the necrosis is variable. Among the necrotic cells, perivascular lymphocytes can be seen.[4,18,19]

Spontaneous regression is a rare but well-documented entity. Its occurrence may be marked by ischemic coagulative necrosis, along with intense inflammatory reaction and calcification, bone formation, reactive proliferation of the retinal pigment epithelium and/or the ciliary epithelial cells, and subsequent phthisis bulbi.[30] Two distinct pathways of tumor cell death have been recognized.[18] At the periphery of the tumor cell cuffs, cells die without involvement of inflammatory cells and follow the pathway of *apoptosis.* A predictable sequence of events occurs. The nuclei and the cytoplasm of tumor cells condense and shrink and then split into pieces that are phagocytosed by neighboring viable cells. *Emperipolesis* also occurs. Here, lymphocytes are seen to be ingested by the targeted cells, and their presence in the cytoplasm causes the lysis of the tumor cells.[18]

Retinocytomas, or *retinomas,* have the most differentiated tissue architecture.[4] These are benign tumors composed of cells exhibiting photoreceptor differentiation with almost no mitoses. Ophthalmoscopically, they usually appear as small lesions covered by unremarkable retinal vessels; the underlying retinal pigment epithelium shows variable degrees of alteration.[14,15,31]

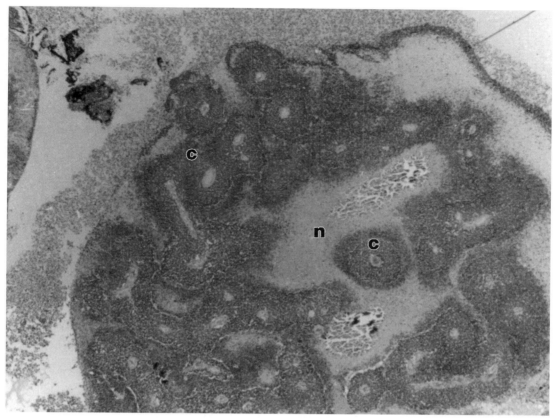

FIG. 10.1—Typical tissue architecture of retinoblastoma shows prominent tumor organization into cuffs (c) of cells about vessel loops, separated by large eosinophilic areas of necrosis (n). The resultant tumor is very friable. As the tumor enlarges, tumor cells seed into the vitreous. Hematoxylin–eosin, ×40.

HISTOLOGIC FEATURES OF PROGNOSTIC SIGNIFICANCE. The *degree of differentiation* of RB is positively correlated with the patient's prognosis. Undifferentiated tumors have a more anaplastic behavior and a greater metastatic potential, and therefore carry a worse prognosis (Figures 10.5–10.6).[4,18,21] However, they are also more radiosensitive than well-differentiated tumors. The *amount of seeding* into the vitreous and the anterior chamber negatively affects the prognosis. Spread through the aqueous outflow pathway or through the conjunctival lymphatics can lead to hematogenous dissemination or to extension to the regional lymph nodes, respectively. In the event of *massive choroidal invasion,* tumor cells gain access to the most vascularized tissue of the body, and the chances of hematogenous spread are greatly increased.[4,18]

The *extent of tumor invasion of the substance of the optic nerve or subarachnoidal space of the nerve* is an extremely important diagnostic criterion. When the tumor does not involve the optic disk, the prognosis is favorable. As soon as the tumor extends beyond the lamina cribrosa, the prognosis worsens drastically, and an 80%–100% mortality rate is reported when tumor is seen at the level of surgical transection (Figure 10.7).[4,19,21,28]

CYTOLOGY. Typically, RB is a tumor composed mainly of undifferentiated cells (Figure 10.8).[4] Differentiated RB composed almost entirely of

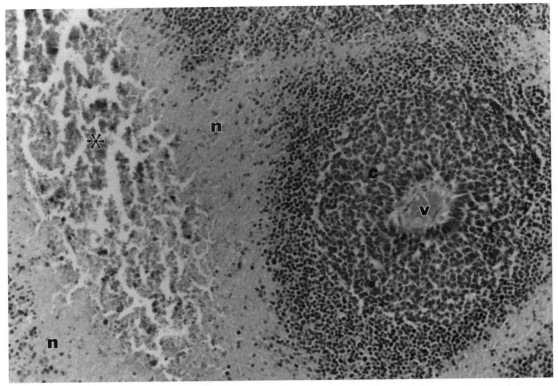

FIG. 10.2—Cuffs of cells (c) survive for approximately 100 μm from central vessel (v) beyond which necrosis ensues. Calcification areas (asterisk) in the middle of the necrotic areas (n) are a highly characteristic feature of retinoblastoma. Hematoxylin–eosin, ×200.

rosettes and fleurettes can present but is extremely uncommon. Most RBs will show foci of differentiated or even highly differentiated tumor among larger poorly differentiated areas.[18,19,28] The degree of differentiation is generally judged by the number of *Flexner-Wintersteiner rosettes* (FWRs), which are composed of a circular arrangement of cuboidal tumor cells joined together at their apex by terminal bars (zonula adherens-like structures) and arranged around a lumen (Figure 10.9). The alignment of these structures resembles the so-called *outer limiting membrane* of the normal retina. The empty lumen, corresponding to the subretinal space, contains hyaluronidase-resistant acid mucopolysaccharides similar to those surrounding the outer segments of the rods and cones, along with abortive portions of inner segments of photoreceptor cells. FWRs are considered

pathognomonic of RB. No other neoplasm displays as many and as differentiated ones, although similar structures can be seen in retinal dysplasia (but without any feature of anaplasia) and in medulloepithelioma.[4]

Less frequent are the *Homer Wright rosettes* (HWRs), in which the cells are arranged around a core of fibrils (Figure 10.10).[4] They can also be found in medulloepithelioma, neuroblastoma, and cerebellar medulloblastoma.

The highest degree of differentiation is seen in the *fleurettes* first described by Ts'o and colleagues, in which the tumor cells display less hyperchromatic nuclei and prominent abortive inner segments, and to a lesser extent outer segments, in an arrangement reminiscent of a fleur-de-lis (Figure 10.11).[4,14,15,31]

As a rule, metastatic tumors are very poorly differentiated, and also show much less necrosis

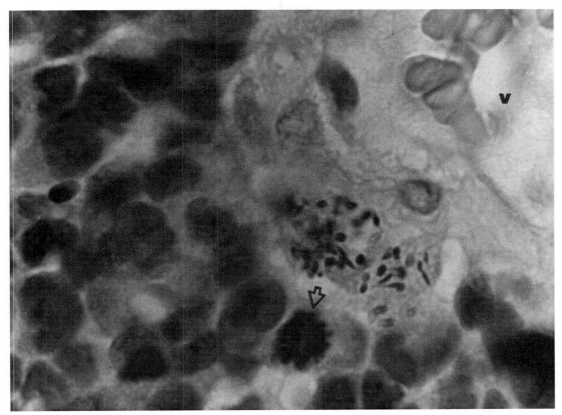

FIG. 10.3—Mitotic activity (arrows) is prominent among the viable tumor cells in the perivascular cuffs (v, blood vessel). Hematoxylin–eosin, ×2000.

than primary intraocular tumors.[4] In trilateral RB, the ectopic midbrain tumor usually demonstrates a high degree of differentiation, exhibiting abundant FWRs and even fleurettes.[4,32]

Electron Microscopy. The cells composing FWRs and fleurettes show ultrastructural features of photoreceptor cell differentiation. Characteristic cilia with a "9+0" pattern, cytomembranes resembling nuclear envelope, annulate lamellae, triple-membrane structures involving the nuclear and cytoplasmic membranes, bristle-coated vesicles, dense-core granules, and zonula adherens-like junctions are all features commonly found in RB.[4,33,34]

Immunohistochemistry. The nature of the putative precursor cell from which RB evolves is

still controversial.[28,35-38] Immunohistochemical studies to date have not enabled investigators to validate either of the main theories of RB cytohistogenesis, i.e., whether the transforming mutational event occurs in a hypothetical sublineage committed to cone differentiation, or whether the cell of origin is a multipotential neural retinoblast. The latter hypothesis takes into account the rare cases of neoplastic transformation toward rods and Müller cells. In the multipotential retinoblast hypothesis, the predominance of the cone phenotype is explained by the "default" hypothesis, according to which rods fail to develop because of the absence of an appropriate extrinsic differentiation signal normally provided by the retinal microenvironment.[35-37] Although true neuronal differentiation has long been accepted, the existence of glial

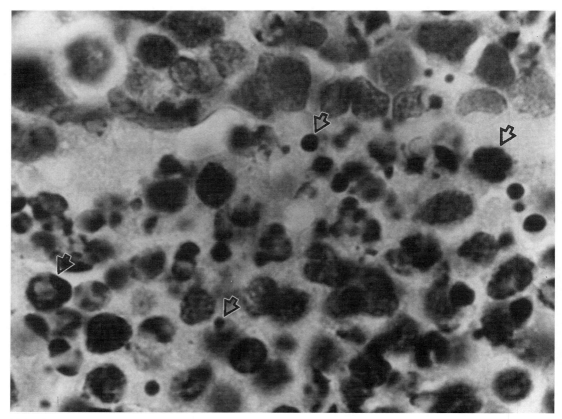

FIG. 10.4—At the periphery of the cuffs, tumor cell necrosis can follow the pathway of apoptosis. In a highly organized sequence, the nuclei and cytoplasm of the tumor cells condense and shrink and then split into pieces that are phagocytosed by neighboring viable cells (arrows). Hematoxylin–eosin, ×2000.

differentiation has been controversial because it has been difficult to distinguish from reactive glial proliferation.[28] In a report of 22 cases of RB, Nork et al. demonstrated that all cells of the tumors were either Müller cells or photoreceptors, and that both rods and cones are elaborated.[38] The Müller cells were shown to be neoplastic in two of the tumors by their lack of immunochemical labeling with anti-p110RB1 antibody.

PATHOGENESIS AND GENETICS OF RETINOBLASTOMA

The RB gene has been demonstrated to be a tumor-suppressor gene prototype. Normally, it encodes for a protein that exerts negative control over cellular proliferation.[11,23,39,40] The encoded protein (pRb) has a molecular weight of approximately 110 kilo-Daltons and interacts inside the nucleus with the transcription of other genes, depending on its degree of phosphorylation. During quiescent G_0 and early G_1 phases of the cell cycle, only underphosphorylated pRb is found. The phosphorylated form is produced by cell cycle-dependent kinases and is associated with DNA synthesis during late G_1 and S phases.[37]

The RB gene is a dominant growth-suppressor gene: a single wild-type allele is enough to ensure proper cell cycle control. In accordance with Knudson's hypothesis as expanded by Coming, malignant growth results from the absence of any normal pRb, when both alleles of the RB gene are affected by a mutational event.[7-9] This can occur in two different ways with regard to the first "hit." The initial mutation may be inherited, and, in this

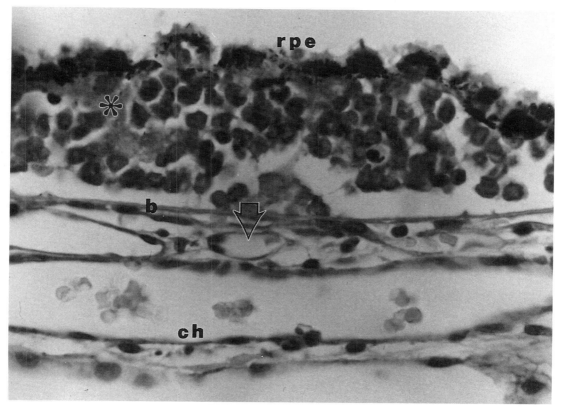

FIG. 10.5—Tumor cells that have seeded into the subretinal space are seen spreading (asterisk) under the retinal pigment epithelium (rpe). After eroding Bruch's membrane (b), they will gain access to the richly vascularized choroid (ch) (arrow). Hematoxylin–eosin, ×800.

case, the paternal allele is the one affected in 90% of the cases.[41] On the other hand, the initial mutation may occur sporadically, affecting alleles of both parental origin equally. In about 15% of the sporadic cases, the mutation occurs soon enough during embryogenesis to be present in the germinal cells as well.[23]

Regarding the second "hit," the remaining chromosome 13 can be affected by an independent mutation or can undergo a recombination with the affected chromosome 13 in such a way that the cell becomes homozygous for the initial RB gene defect. This phenomenon is referred to as *loss of heterozygosity*.[42] It is still uncertain whether the inactivating mutations of both alleles of the RB gene, though proven to be necessary, are also sufficient to lead to uncontrolled neoplastic growth. It has been suggested that

retinoma (or *retinocytoma*) might result from this sequence alone, whereas *retinoblastoma* would require additional chromosomal abnormalities.[23]

CLINICAL FEATURES

Clinical Presentation and Differential Diagnosis. The presenting signs and symptoms depend primarily on the size and progression of the tumor at the time of diagnosis. In Third World countries, extensive extraocular spread is common at the time of presentation and carries a most unfavorable prognosis for life. In developed countries, the most common presenting sign is leukocoria, which is a white pupillary reflex[21] that occurs when the tumor has reached a size large enough to induce noticeable alteration of the reflected light from a retinoscope or from the flash of a camera

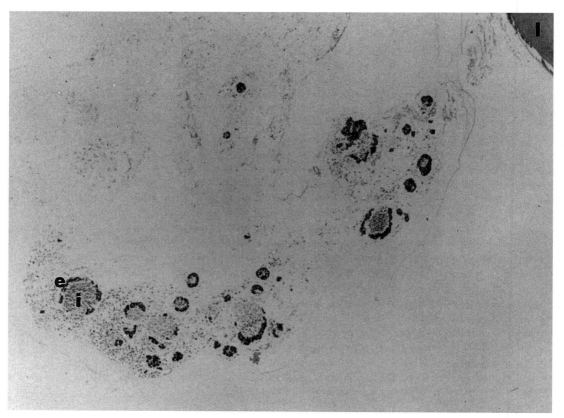

FIG. 10.6—Tumor cells that are seeding into the vitreous organize into islands of cells that show the reverse image of the perivascular cuffing principle: the inner cells (i) are the necrotic ones, being further apart from the nutrient supply than the peripheral, or external, cells (e) (l, lens). Hematoxylin–eosin, ×40.

(Figure 10.12). (Several anecdotal cases have been diagnosed as a result of the parents looking at family pictures and wondering why one eye of their child looked white while the fellow eye looked red.) Acquired strabismus, which is the second most frequent presenting sign of RB, occurs when a lesion, even small, involves the macula.[21] Although it is an uncommon occurrence, it dictates that all infants or young children with strabismus have a careful fundic examination.

Less commonly, an RB can present as a masquerade syndrome. As the tumor enlarges, tumor cells can seed into the vitreous and into the anterior chamber, where they can settle in a manner suggestive of a hypopyon, forming a pseudohypopyon. As previously noted, true inflammatory signs can present as well in the course of the disease.[21] Rubeosis iridis is frequent, causing het-

erochromia; the rubeotic vessels bleed easily. Vitreous hemorrhage can also occur. It is of primary importance that clinicians remember that spontaneous hyphema and refractory inflammation in a child require careful examination to exclude the possibility of an underlying RB.

Secondary glaucoma can result from pseudohypopyon, spontaneous hyphema, extensive peripheral anterior synechiae, or pupillary block. These in turn may be caused by tumor proliferation in the vitreous and exudative retinal detachment. Severe periocular inflammation has been described in association with tumor necrosis simulating endophthalmitis or panophthalmitis.

If left untreated, local extension and distant metastatic spread will occur.[4,21] The tumor can exit the globe anteriorly at the level of the angle, or posteriorly through the scleral emisseria, and

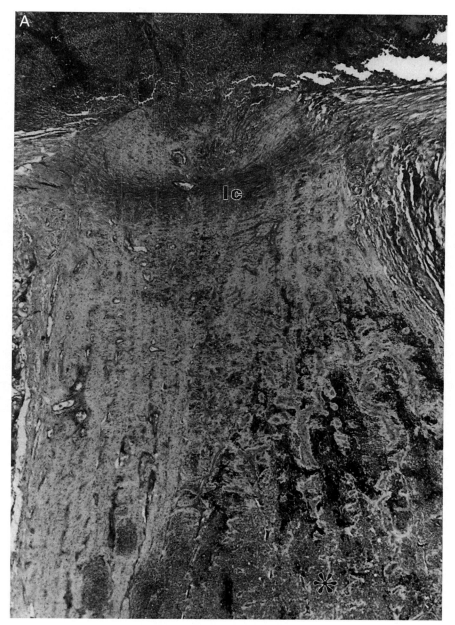

FIG. 10.7—**A:** Massive optic nerve invasion (asterisk) can be seen here beyond the lamina cribrosa (lc). (continued)

spread through the lymphatics to the regional preauricular and cervical lymph nodes.[4,21] Intracranial involvement is usually the result of direct optic nerve invasion, but direct spread into the orbital bones or beyond the orbit through the optic foramen has been described.[4] The most fre-quent sites of distant metastases include the bones and viscera. Metastatic extension is usually wide-spread and occurs most often within the first 2 years of treatment.

Spontaneous regression is a rare but well-established feature of RB. It is said that this

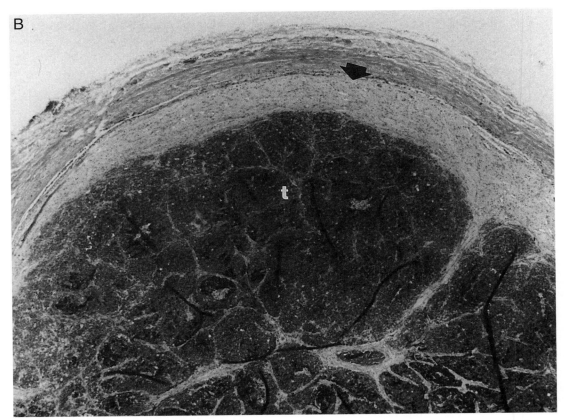

FIG. 10.7 (continued)—**B:** On cross section, massive tumor involvement of the optic nerve (t) is seen leaving only a thin layer of optic nerve tissue at the periphery (arrow). Hematoxylin–eosin, ×40.

occurs more frequently in RB than any other tumor. Eight cases of spontaneous regression were reported in a review of 700 eyes with RB from the Armed Forces Institute of Pathology files.[43] In most cases, this follows tumor necrosis and inflammation, and phthisis bulbi usually ensues. As a rule, any phthisical eye of uncertain cause, even in an adult, should be suspected of regressed RB.[30]

Controversy exists regarding the relationship of retinocytoma (or retinoma) to spontaneous regression.[4,31] These tumors typically do not show progression and do not lead to phthisis bulbi, and thus enable useful vision to be retained. However, a case of malignant transformation of apparent retinocytoma has been reported.[21]

Second primary tumors frequently occur late in life in the survivors of the hereditary type of RB. Statistics regarding occurrence vary among authors.[6,44–47] Although the risk is greatly increased by radiotherapy and chemotherapy, this outcome also prevails for patients who have not received these treatments. Up to about 90% of irradiated patients and about 70% of nonirradiated patients are reported to develop such tumors 32 years after diagnosis. An increased risk of second tumors of the bones and soft tissues of the head has been shown for children receiving external beam radiation before the age of 12 months.[48] The inherited genetic anomaly at the RB locus predisposes most commonly to the development of osteosarcomas both in and outside the irradiation field. An increased risk has been suggested for other malignant neoplasias, like spindle cell sarcoma, chondrosarcoma, rhabdomyosarcoma, neuroblastoma, glioma, leukemia, sebaceous cell carcinoma, squamous cell carcinoma, and malignant melanoma.[6,21] It has been stated that second

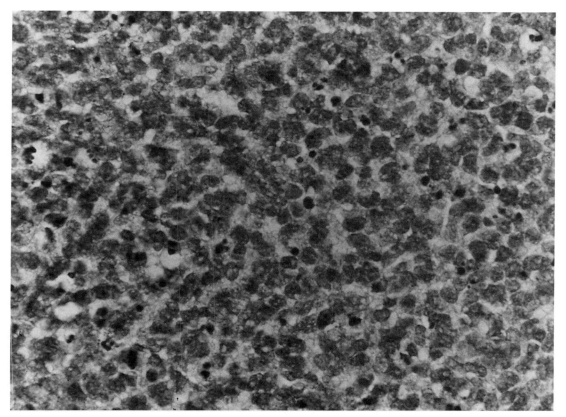

FIG. 10.8—Monomorphic appearance of the basophilic tumor cells in an undifferentiated retinoblastoma. Hematoxylin–eosin, ×500. (Courtesy of Dr. T.M. Nork.)

primary malignancies account for more deaths than do RBs themselves. An approximate 25% cumulative risk of death from second primary tumors 40 years after diagnosis has been reported in a large cohort.[44]

Approximately 2%–5% of the children affected by the hereditary type of RB have a trilateral form. To date, this presentation has been almost uniformly fatal.[4,21,34,49] A recent case report documented successful treatment of a single child with chemotherapy and local therapy, with the child remaining free of recurrence 26 months after initial diagnosis.[50] The primitive neuroectodermal component is a primary tumor that typically arises in the pineal gland or parasellar region, in addition to the intraocular tumors. It differs from a brain metastasis in several aspects. It occurs without evidence of extraocular tumor extension or other metastases and is often diagnosed earlier than metastases. As previously mentioned, it is also better differentiated than most metastases.[4,33,51]

Overall, prognosis for survival for patients with RB is good when prompt and adequate diagnosis and management are available. Long-term survival of more than 85% of patients has been reported. Survival declines when the tumor has extended outside the eye.[21]

Treatment. RB is a life-threatening tumor. Prompt diagnosis and treatment are mandatory to preserve survival and vision. Eyes with a poor prognosis for useful vision are usually enucleated.[21] It is important to obtain as great a length of optic nerve as possible with the globe, to avoid the risk of leaving tumor in the orbit and also to enable good pathologic staging. For tumor DNA analysis, fresh tissue samples should be harvested

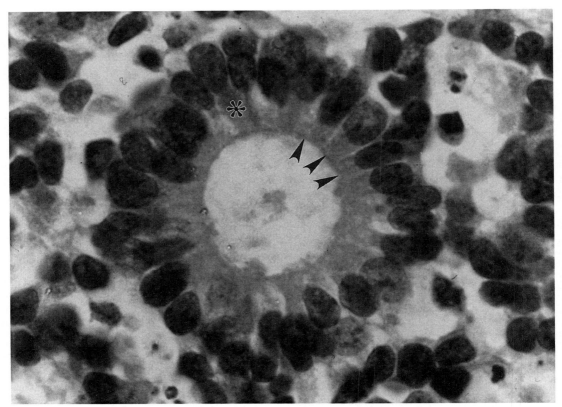

FIG. 10.9—Flexner-Wintersteiner rosettes are highly characteristic of retinoblastoma. Cuboidal tumor cells are organized in rosettes arranged around a lumen containing abortive portions of photoreceptor inner segments (asterisk). The cells are joined by zonula adherens-type structure reminiscent of the outer limiting membrane (arrowheads). Hematoxylin–eosin, ×1250. (Courtesy of Dr. T.M. Nork.)

before fixation. In the past, in unilateral cases, the affected eye was almost routinely enucleated.[5,21]

With the development of effective modern conservative treatments, enucleation of eyes with visual potential can frequently be avoided.[52,53] RB is usually a radiosensitive tumor. Radiation therapy remains the most widely used primary treatment in favorable unilateral and bilateral cases.[5,6] The treatment planning is essentially guided by anatomic considerations. Generally, multiple large tumors are managed by external beam radiation therapy. When dealing with smaller tumors, radioactive episcleral plaques, cryotherapy, or photocoagulation techniques are frequently used.[5,21,53] Iodine 125 is currently the isotope of choice for radioactive episcleral plaque.[6]

When the tumor is small and located posteriorly, photocoagulation therapy is preferred. In this technique, burns are produced by a laser (or infrequently a xenon arc) and are applied around the tumor to obliterate the tumor's retinal feeder vessels. A more anterior location of the tumor allows the use of cryotherapy. Freezing is applied transsclerally in a triple or quadruple freeze-and-thaw cycle. The aim of treatment is to incorporate the whole tumor mass into an ice ball, thus destroying the tumor directly.[5,52]

More recently, experimental treatment modes have been introduced, including the use of local techniques following systemic chemotherapy, photodynamic therapy, or particle radiation treatment. Chemotherapy has been used for unfavorable cases with extraocular extension, generally in conjunction with radiotherapy.[54]

The use of external beam radiation (EBR) has been shown to be associated with an increased

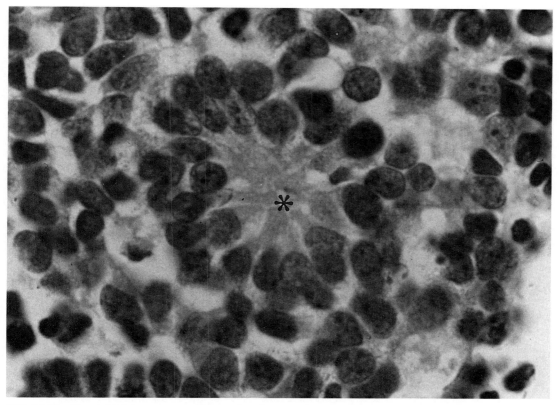

FIG. 10.10—Homer Wright rosettes, which are less frequent than Flexner-Wintersteiner rosettes, are composed of cells arranged around a cobweb-like tangle of fibrils (asterisk). Hematoxylin–eosin, ×1250. (Courtesy of Dr. T.M. Nork.)

risk of second primary tumor development both within and outside of the radiation field, particularly when administered to children younger than 12 months of age.[48] Subsequent disfiguring abnormalities in orbital development may occur with attendant social consequences.[55,56] Emphasis has been placed more recently on the development of new treatment protocols in an effort to avoid EBR and enucleation. Chemoreduction with combinations of carboplatin, vincristine sulfate, and teniposide or etoposide has been successfully employed to reduce tumor size. Subsequent use of local therapy such as applying laser, cryotherapy, thermotherapy, or plaque radiotherapy to the residual tumor has been shown to be an effective alternative, thus sparing the use of EBR or enucleation.[57–61] Cyclosporine has been employed as a multidrug-resistance reversal agent when used with chemotherapeutics.[50,61] Ther-

motherapy for small RBs without vitreal seeds has been reported as an effective therapy, with lasting tumor regression in 86% of tumors in one study.[62]

RETINOBLASTOMA IN ANIMALS.

The naturally occurring animal cases of RB found in the literature have been the object of a critical review.[63] Prior to 1993, a total of 14 individual animals had been reported to have RB in 12 reports in the literature. All tumors were unilateral. Four instances were in fish, three in horses, two in dogs, and one each in a calf, cat, chicken, monkey, and sheep. In addition, two anecdotal cases in horses and two cases in fish were alluded to without description. All of the reported cases in which enough pathologic evidence was presented for independent evaluation proved, under current

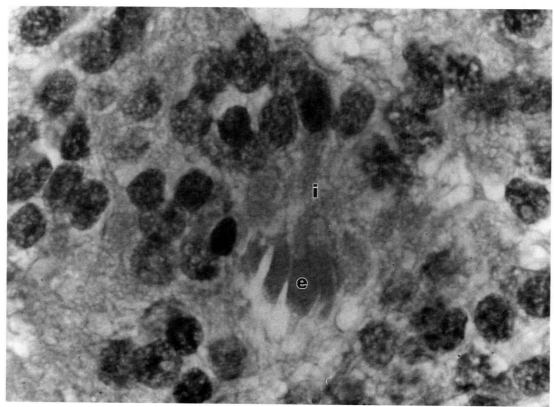

FIG. 10.11—The highest degree of differentiation is achieved by the fleurette, which shows prominent portions of photoreceptor inner segments (i) and, to a lesser degree, outer segments (e). Hematoxylin–eosin, ×1250. (Courtesy of Dr. T.M. Nork.)

morphologic criteria, to be either medulloepithelioma, adenocarcinoma, glioma, gliosis, or dysplasia, rather than RB.

The confusion might have arisen because these entities share some superficial resemblance with RB, such as acini that have a rosette-like configuration, or cause gliosis of the retina. However, these cases did not meet the usual criteria for confirming the diagnosis of RB.

Subsequent to that review, a single case of spontaneous RB in a dog has been reported.[1] Histologically, the intraocular tumor was found to involve the retina and infiltrate the posterior choroid. The tumor was comprised largely of small neuroblastic cells, with large, hyperchromatic nuclei and scanty cytoplasm. There was pseudorosette formation with preservation of cells surrounding blood vessels and necrosis at sites distant from vessels. Hematoxylinophilic staining of blood vessel walls was a feature. Areas of differentiation within the tumor revealed FWRs, with Alcian blue-positive staining within the centers. Immunocytochemical analysis of the tumor revealed strong positive staining for retinal S antigen, which suggests photoreceptor differentiation and is characteristic of human RB cells.[64,65] Glial fibrillary acid protein immunoreactivity was demonstrated in a few cells. Enzyme histochemical analysis of carbonic anhydrase was strongly positive within tumor cells of FWRs, indicating differentiation into red- and green-sensitive cones and Müller cells.[38] Nick end labeling of DNA (TUNEL) to identify apoptosis revealed a pattern similar to that of human RB, and TUNEL-positive labeling of blood vessel basal laminae, corresponding to the hematoxylinophilic staining, suggested accumulation of disintegrated tumor cell DNA.[66,67]

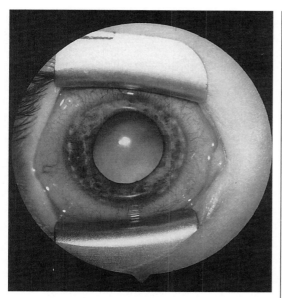

FIG. 10.12—Clinical presentation of a leukocoria, a white pupillary reflex, in a 3-year-old boy without a familial history of retinoblastoma. The child's aunt felt that his right eye had been crossing since he was an infant. He had been treated for the previous 6 months for recurrent inflammation of his right eye. The clinical examination disclosed a large retinoblastoma that had seeded into the vitreous and invaded the optic nerve. Prominent rubeosis iridis, extensive peripheral anterior synechiae, and elevated intraocular pressure close to 40 mmHg accounted for the recurrent inflammatory presentation. (Courtesy of Dr. B.J. Kushner.)

Although no fresh tissue was available to identify mutations in the RB1 gene, the histopathologic and histochemical characteristics of the tumor suggest that this is the first substantiated case of spontaneous RB in a nonhuman species. The RB1 tumor-suppressor gene is conserved among vertebrates.[12,13] Unlike the situation in humans, in which loss of both RB1 alleles apparently results in RB development, this is not sufficient in experimental mouse models. Concomitant loss of p53 function is often necessary for RB tumorigenesis in mice, but mutations in p53 are rarely seen in human RB.[68] The tumor-suppressor protein p53, like pRB, is an important regulator of the cell cycle, causing apoptosis of abnormal cells. Apoptosis of tumor cells in RB is a common histologic feature but becomes rare with malignant transformation (metastasis and extraocular

extension). Certain immortalized cell lines from human RBs have been demonstrated to have nuclear exclusion of p53.[69] Although high levels of wild-type p53 are found within these cells, the abnormal cytoplasmic localization suggests a dysfunctional p53 phenotype, which may account for the lack of apoptosis in these cell lines and in metastatic and extraocular RB. The rarity of naturally occurring RB in animals suggests the presence of additional mechanisms of cell cycle control and tumor suppression in nonhuman species.

EXPERIMENTAL MODELS

There is a strong need for improvement in the treatment of RB. Although enucleation achieves a high cure rate when performed early, alternative treatments designed to preserve vision need to be developed. Local or systemic extraocular spread requires the use of radiotherapy and/or chemotherapy, both of which carry risks of morbidity. It has been difficult to develop experimental methods of therapy because naturally occurring RB is not seen with any frequency in animal species other than humans. Several approaches have been used to produce both in vitro and in vivo experimental models, including various carcinogenic chemicals, oncogenic viruses, cell cultures with graft techniques, and genetic alterations.

Chemical Induction of Retinoblastoma-like Tumors. An in vivo rat model was developed in 1980 to produce intraocular malignant tumors following injection of nickel subsulfide in the vitreous body.[70] Nickel subsulfide, Ni_{3S2}, is the most carcinogenic of numerous nickel compounds that have been tested in rats. Administration of Ni_3S_2 to rats by inhalation, implantation into heterotopic tracheas, or parenteral injections into muscle, testis, or kidney, results in malignant tumors at the site of deposition. In the model described, a suspension of 0.5 mg Ni_3S_2 in 20 ml of NaCl vehicle was administered to albino Fischer-344 strain rats by a single injection into the vitreous body of one eye.

Of the 15 rats, 14 developed malignant tumors in the injected eyes after a latency of approximately 8 months. Five eyes displayed multiple tumors. The 21 tumors that were induced by the nickel subsulfide included 11 melanomas, 4 RB-like tumors,

3 gliomas, and 3 unclassified malignant neoplasms. The RBs were poorly differentiated, with variable occurrence of mitotic figures and neuroepithelial rosettes. When compared with the malignant tumors produced by the other routes of administration of Ni_3S_2, the intravitreal injection showed a higher tumor yield with a shorter latency. This was thought to result from the persistence of a high intravitreal concentration of the carcinogenic chemical due to the absence of blood supply to the vitreous, and its isolation from the systemic vascular supply by the blood-retina barrier and the ciliary epithelium.

Other previous animal models of ocular tumor induction by carcinogenic chemicals did not result in RB. These models included production of tumors in mice by intraocular injection of 20-methylcholanthrene, in rats by intraperitoneal injection of ethionine and N_2-fluorenylacetamide, in dogs by intravenous injection of radium 226 and thorium 228, and in rats by intraocular introduction of platinum foil and cellophane film. The majority of the tumors produced were melanomas.

Viral Induction of Retinoblastoma-like Tumors. Viruses have been demonstrated to produce tumors in animals since the beginning of the century. Increasing evidence has accumulated for their implication in certain human cancers. A select group of viruses have been implicated in human cancers. Among the DNA viruses, these include *papova viruses, herpes viruses,* and the *hepatitis B virus.* Among the RNA viruses, these include the *human T leukemia virus* and the *human immunodeficiency virus.*[71]

In contrast to the situation in humans, many viruses are known to cause cancer in animals, either as a consequence of natural infection or after experimental inoculation. Such viruses cause changes referred to collectively as *transformation* in a variety of mammalian cells grown in vitro. The cytologic appearance, rate of multiplication, colonial morphology, antigenic characteristics, and chromosome pattern are generally altered in the transformed cultures. Following the injection of such transformed cells into an animal of the same species, a malignant tumor develops at the site of inoculation. The changes in the cells are then referred to as *neoplastic transformation.*[72,73]

DNA VIRUS-INDUCED RETINOBLASTOMA-LIKE TUMORS. The first evidence that oncogenic DNA viruses could be used to produce in vitro neoplastic transformation of uveal and retinal tissues was reported in 1968.[74] Explant cultures of adult hamster retina, choroid, and iris were infected with either simian virus 40 (SV40), the LLE 46 strain of human adenovirus type 7 (AdV7), human polyoma virus, or human adenovirus type 12 (AdV12). Most cultures underwent transformation. After several in vitro passages, the transformed cells injected subcutaneously into irradiated adult hamsters produced solid tumors at the site of injection, thus demonstrating their acquired tumorigenicity.

Oncogenic viruses may produce tumors with similar morphology in many different tissues. In some cases, the tumor morphology may be determined by the causative virus. In this hamster model, adenovirus-induced transformation characteristically led to small cell sarcoma. Papova viruses, such as SV40, commonly induced spindle cell tumors regardless of whether the transformed tissue was from the retina or uvea. The tumors produced were poorly differentiated. Some of them showed weak resemblance with RB, but no rosettes or neural elements were identified.[74]

Subsequently, the transforming properties of AdV12 in ocular tissues were investigated closely in rats and mice.[75-79] AdV12 displays a highly carcinogenic potential in rodents, especially for replicating neuroblastic cells in the central nervous system. In these in vivo models, CDF inbred albino rats and C3H/BifB/Ki mice received a single intraocular injection of virus. The tumors produced exhibited both histologic and electron-microscopic features reminiscent of RB. Specifically, incomplete HWRs, along with giant tumor cells, were seen in multicentric foci of tumors arising from transformed cells in the retina and in the optic nerve. Ultrastructural findings such as nuclear triple-membrane structures and cilia with a 9+0 tubule pattern were interpreted to indicate a neuroblastic origin of the tumors.[80]

Cell lines were successfully derived from the AdV12-induced retinal tumors and proved to be transplantable in several graft models using rats and mice. Tumor cells were injected in animals of the same species either subcutaneously or intravitreally. A predictable model of tumor growth in newborn inbred CDF rats and in syngeneic Fischer-344 strain rats was produced with the intravitreal injection technique.[75,81,82] When compared with their tumor of origin, the grafted cells were less differentiated, showing very few of the typical RB features. Some of the recipient rats had been immunosuppressed by whole body irradiation prior the transplantation, but exhibited the same tumor growth and degree of inflammation, suggesting that the tumor cells were not strongly immunogenic.

An RB-like tumor was also produced in two of 21 newborn baboons after intravitreal injection of AdV12. Here, as opposed to rodents, the tumors showed FWRs. This difference was hypothesized to be related to the stage of maturation of the retina at the time of inoculation: mature for the baboon, whereas still actively replicating for the rodent.[83]

Unlike AdV12, the herpes viruses have been implicated as etiologic agents in cancer in both humans and animals. Herpes simplex virus type 2 (HSV2) has been associated with cervical carcinoma. Both HSV1 and HSV2 can clinically infect the cornea, uvea, and retina in humans. The fact that HSV2 is responsible for the majority of neonatal herpes infections suggested the question of whether it might have a role in a childhood tumor like RB and prompted an investigation into its carcinogenic potential for the mammalian retina. An in vitro model of malignant transformation of hamster retina by HSV2 was established and was the first neoplasm of ocular tissue induced experimentally by a herpes virus.[84] Explants of 3-week-old hamster retina were incubated with HSV2. Suspensions of transformed cells were then injected subcutaneously into nude mice to induce tumor growth. Portions of these tumors were injected subcutaneously into corticosteroid immunodepressed 3-week-old hamsters. The resulting malignant cells showed poor differentiation, making positive identification of the precursor cell difficult. The presence of neurosecretory granules and retinoic acid receptors was consistent with the retinal origin of the tumor.

RNA VIRUS-INDUCED RETINOBLASTOMA-LIKE TUMORS. In contrast to DNA viruses, many RNA viruses are oncogenic in their host of origin, while showing less cytopathogenicity. Grouped in the Oncovirinae subfamily, these retroviruses mainly cause naturally occurring tumors of the reticuloendothelial and hematopoietic system (leukemias and lymphomas) or of the connective tissue (sarcomas). An RB-like tumor with structures closely resembling FWRs has been produced in newborn kittens after intravitreal injection of feline leukemia virus. Injection of feline sarcoma virus, on the other hand, has led to ocular melanomas.[85]

Cell Lines and Graft Models. Several successful graft models have been produced with human RB cell lines. These models have proven useful in providing reproducible systems for in vivo treatment trials. Cell lines provide the in vitro counterpart of these experiments.

The first successfully established human RB cell line, Y-79, was fully characterized in 1974. The line was derived from a hereditary RB in a 2½-year-old girl.[86] Despite a tendency for dedifferentiation of cells in tissue culture in general, these cultured cells resembled the cells of the original tumor by light and electron microscopy. In particular, frequent nuclear envelope infoldings and triple-membrane structures, cytoplasmic microtubules, bristle-coated vesicles, stacked annulate lamellae, macula adherens-type junctions, and RNA-directed DNA polymerase activity were all features found in both cultured Y-79 and original tumor cells. Genetically, Y-79 cells are affected by a partial deletion of one allele of the RB gene and an as yet uncharacterized mutation in the other.[87]

Y-79 cells were successfully transplanted subcutaneously or intraocularly into immune-deficient *nude mice* in 1977.[88] The homozygous mouse with the mutation *nude (nu/nu)* is born without a thymus and has a severe defect in cellular immunity and in graft tissue rejection. Freshly removed human RB cells were also successfully transplanted into the anterior chamber of nude mouse eyes. The combination of prior cyclophosphamide-induced immunodepression with the relative immunologic privilege of the anterior chamber as injection site further contributed to immunotolerance of the grafted tumor cells. By 1980, more than 10 human RB cell cultures had been established and grown intraocularly as well as subcutaneously in nude mice, without the need of prior immunodepression.[89] The transplanted cells retained many characteristics of the tumor of origin. In particular, some of the intraocular tumors displayed a high degree of vascularity and a comparable level of differentiation, whereas no major karyotypic changes were detected.

The rabbit anterior chamber was found to be a successful recipient site for the second described human RB cell culture, WERI-Rb1, which was established in 1977 from a 1-year-old girl without a family history of RB. The original tumor was poorly differentiated. In the WERI-Rb1 cell line, the entire RB gene is homozygously deleted.[90]

CONTRIBUTIONS OF THE MODELS. One of the main advantages offered by the anterior or posterior chamber as recipient site for grafted RB cells is that direct visibility of tumor progression makes reproducible grading systems possible. Following the introduction of these models, various treatment modalities were explored, including radiotherapy, chemotherapeutic agents, and photodynamic therapy.

In *photodynamic therapy* (PDT), a photosensitizing drug, such as a hematoporphyrin derivative (HpD), is first injected intravenously. If the tumor blood supply is adequate, the HpD is thought to accumulate preferentially in the tumor cells. Subsequent exposure to a light of appropriate wavelength in the presence of oxygen leads to intracellular production of markedly cytotoxic superoxide ions. This in turn destroys the local tumor while hopefully sparing the surrounding normal tissues.[91] Analysis of the damage induced by PDT in Y-79 cells indicates that the mechanism involved is the production of lipid peroxide under anaerobic conditions, and that the first target organelle is the mitochondria, followed by plasma membrane disruption and pyknosis.[92]

Reports thus far about the success rate of PDT have been variable and demonstrate the necessity of making a clear distinction between in vitro and in vivo results. Whether there is a preferential affinity of the tumor cells for the HpD is still controversial.[93] In cell culture, tumor cells are more likely to be exposed to a much higher concentration of HpD than can be achieved in vivo, where toxicity to the surrounding tissues is a limiting factor.[93]

Partial control of tumor growth was possible in the nude mouse and F344 rat grafts, but has been limited by damage caused to normal surrounding tissues, attenuation of the light penetrating the tumor tissue, and the dependence of HpD cellular uptake on the tumor's vascular supply. Poorly vascularized tumors showed a poor response to PDT, which suggests an alternative hypothesis in which tumor regression would result from primary PDT-induced vascular endothelium damage, with subsequent tumor vessel collapse.[91,93-95]

In *chemotherapy* experiments, cyclophosphamide has been shown the most effective among the various conventional agents tested in nude mice.[96] Equally effective, diaziquone (aziridinylbenzoquinone, AZQ) is a promising new drug under investigation. As a result of AZQ's liposolubility and low ionization, it shows a high affinity for the central nervous system. Furthermore, AZQ does not require metabolic activation in the liver, offering the possibility of high-dosage local administration with reduced systemic toxicity.[97]

Gene therapy has been explored using an adenoviral vector containing the herpes simplex thymidine kinase gene (AdV-TK). When the prodrug gangcyclovir is administered, the transduced viral kinase and existent cellular kinases create a product that inhibits DNA synthesis in dividing cells. In vitro transduction of Y-79 RB cells with AdV-TK and incubation with gancyclovir results in cell death. Using the nude mouse-Y-79 RB vitreal explant model, intratumoral injection of AdV-TK followed by intravitreal gancyclovir administration results in decreased tumor burden in these eyes.[98]

DIFFERENTIATING AGENTS. In Y-79 cell cultures, several factors have been shown to induce morphologic changes, growth inhibition, or specific antigen and protein expression, all of which have been interpreted as cellular differentiation. These include sodium butyrate and dibutyril-cAMP, retinoic acid, serum-free conditions, and RPE-derived growth factors.[99,100]

Vitamin D compounds have been shown to be promising antineoplastic agents. Calcitriol receptors have been found in Y-79 cells, and treated cells exhibited decreased tumor induction as a subcutaneous graft in athymic mice.[101-103]

With the addition of sodium butyrate to Y-79 cells grown in vitro, a marked synergistic effect was achieved as compared with a glucocorticoid alone. However, no effect was obtained when these drugs were used in combination in the nude mouse.[104] Nevertheless, Y-79 cells were successfully grafted into the peripheral retinas of F344 rats after the cells had been exposed to a combination of retinoic acid and butyrate to induce their prior differentiation. The transplanted cells integrated into the host retina without signs of further invasion, displayed FWRs, and developed elaborate synaptic contacts with the surrounding neuropil.[105]

Alterations of Retinoblastoma Gene Function. Conceivably, the complex function of the RB gene can be interrupted at numerous points. Regulation of the expression and translation of the gene, synthesis, and regulatory function of the encoded protein are all specific steps that, if interfered with, will result in partial or total loss of gene function. Several experimental models have been produced that demonstrate the effects of interrupting different aspects of this pathway.

SIMIAN VIRUS 40 LARGE T ANTIGEN TRANSGENIC MOUSE. The first model of heritable RB was a transgenic mouse produced by the genomic integration and expression of a transgene consisting of the luteinizing hormone b subunit (bLH) promoter region from -1.09 Kb to $+9$ bp relative to the transcription initiation site, linked to the SV40 early region, from *Bgl*I to the *Bam*HI.[106,107] The latter restriction fragment lacked the SV40 early promoter region but contained the protein-coding region for the large T antigen (SV40Tag) and the short t antigen (SV40tag), including the translation initiation and transcription termination site. The viral oncogene SV40Tag contains a conserved amino acid sequence with homology to the transforming domain of two other viral oncogenes: adenovirus E1A and human papillomavirus 16 E7. This region is required for transforming function of SV40Tag and also for its specific binding to pRb. The chimeric transgene was injected after purification into fertilized single-cell ovocytes and integrated randomly into the murine genome.

As intended by the investigators, the transgenic F_0 mice produced pituitary adenomas. A single male, fortunately fertile, unexpectedly developed bilateral intraocular tumors. From this mouse, a strain was successfully established. Tumors of this male founder on histopathologic examination were found to be RBs. The derived mouse line represented the first animal model of hereditary RB. All of the transgene-bearing mice develop bilateral multifocal RB, and about a quarter have a primary midbrain intracranial tumor in addition to the ocular tumors, consistent with the presentation of trilateral RB.

All subsequent studies of the tumors in this transgenic mouse confirmed their close identity to human RB. The ocular tumors were multifocal and bilateral, and invaded adjacent structures in an identical fashion. They were composed of small undifferentiated cells with relatively large hyperchromatic nuclei and scanty cytoplasm. Both FWRs and HWRs were seen, as well as perivascular cuffs of viable tumor cells surrounded by areas of necrosis and calcification.

Recognizable ultrastructural findings that also correlated with human RB included microtubules, dense-core neurosecretory granules, cilia without a central tubule (9+0 pattern), nuclear triple-membrane structures, and evidence of photoreceptor differentiation.

The antigenic profile of the murine intraocular tumors further paralleled that of human RB.[108] Along with the constant origin of the murine RB in the inner nuclear layer and the predominance of HWRs, immunohistochemical characterization suggested that the tumor cells were possibly derived from bipolar cells.

As noted, about a quarter of these transgenic mice have a primitive neuroectodermal tumor of the midbrain showing a probable multicentric origin below or adjacent to the ependymal layer of the cerebral aqueduct. In general, the midbrain tumors were less differentiated than the concurrent intraocular tumors. Although incomplete rosettes were observed, true FWRs or HWRs or fleurettes were lacking.[109] Immunohistochemical and ultrastructural findings confirmed the midbrain tumors to be highly undifferentiated. The pineal was not the site of origin in this model. Rather, the tumor was thought to arise from neuroblasts in the subependymal layer, which is hypothesized to retain the capacity to undergo transformation. Accordingly, it can give rise to ectopic RB reminiscent of the undifferentiated midbrain tumors observed in human trilateral RBs, which are occasionally suprasellar or parasellar instead of pineal.

This transgenic mouse model of RB has been used extensively in the development and testing of chemotherapeutic agents and other alternative therapies.

Local chemotherapy delivery systems have been investigated because of side effects associated with systemic administration. Carboplatin has been shown to inhibit tumor development in a dose-dependent fashion when administered via intravitreal injection alone or in combination with external beam radiation.[110,111] However, a dose-dependent retinal toxicity was observed when tested in rabbits.[110] Subconjunctival carboplatin inhibited tumor growth in this mouse model, but the addition of cryotherapy did not effect tumor control.[112]

Vitamin D compounds have been tested and shown to be effective in reducing the size of intraocular tumors.[113] The antineoplastic properties of vitamin D compounds in RB may be related to induction of apoptosis, as has been demonstrated in other tumor cell lines.[114,115] Additionally, vitamin D compounds induce transcriptional activation of p21, a cyclin-dependent kinase inhibitor.[116] Transcription of p21 is induced by p53 in response to DNA damage, and p21 acts to halt the cell cycle to allow DNA repair, thus modulating cellular proliferation and differentiation.[117,118] The vitamin D_3 analog 1,25-(OH)2-16-ene-23-yne vitamin D_3 was demonstrated to be nontoxic at doses that effectively inhibit tumor growth in the bLH-Tag and athymic/Y-79 mouse models.[119,120] A promising new vitamin D analog, 1-α-hydroxyvitamin D_2, is currently being investigated in these mouse models.[121]

Ferromagnetic hyperthermia (FMH), a focal ocular heating system, was shown to have a synergistic effect in tumor control when combined with EBR. Thus, combination with FMH may be a useful method to decrease the dose of radiation necessary for tumor control in children.[122]

NEOPLASTIC INDUCTION TARGETED TO THE RETINA. Many of the known genes for retinal markers have either not been well characterized or are expressed only in fully differentiated photoreceptor cells and not in retinoblasts. In the mouse embryo, both natural murine and transgenic human interstitial retinol binding protein (IRBP) genes are expressed in the photoreceptor cells and, to a lesser extent, in the pinealocytes. IRBP expression takes place by at least around embryonic day 17, earlier than opsin, and when cones and rods are about to enter their respective differentiation pathway.[123]

In an attempt to direct tumorigenesis in a specific manner to cells in the photoreceptor cell lineage, a transgenic mouse was produced by using the transforming capacity of SV40Tag under the control of the *human* IRBP promoter.[123] The resulting transgenic mice developed, at an embryonic or early postnatal stage, intraocular and brain tumors with a variable incidence and severity. This variability is thought to result from the effect of the site of integration on the levels of expression of the transgene. Mice that exhibited retinal tumors consistently developed brain tumors as well. Both intraocular and brain tumors were highly undifferentiated. The eyes of 2-month-old mice harbored tumors that involved mainly the outer retinal layers and seemed to spare the inner plexiform and ganglion cell layers. No FWRs were detected. Instead, HWRs and peculiar rosettes composed of a single layer of cuboidal cells surrounding capillaries were seen. Immunohistochemical study detected labeling for NSE, S-Ag, and Leu-7, as seen in normal retina. There was, however, no evidence of photoreceptor-specific antibodies, such as opsin and phosphodiesterase. The brain tumors, which involved the diencephalon, showed an immunohistochemical profile similar to that of the ocular tumors.[123]

A third transgenic mouse model of hereditary RB was created by using SV40Tag, driven this time by the *murine* IRBP promoter (IRBP-SV40Tag).[124] Southern-blot analysis of the genome of the positive mice revealed patterns consistent with single integration sites of multiple copies of the IRBP-SV40Tag transgene in head-to-tail tandem arrays. The number of copies per founder ranged from five to approximately 50. Noteworthy, the mice with a higher transgene copy number were consistently smaller than their negative littermates. A strain was produced from the founder with the lower copy number. All of the positive mice in his offspring developed intraocular and pineal tumors at a very early age. By 2 weeks of age, the photoreceptor cell layer and the pineal gland were extensively replaced by tumor cells. The intraocular tumors resembled undifferentiated RB with no apparent rosettes.

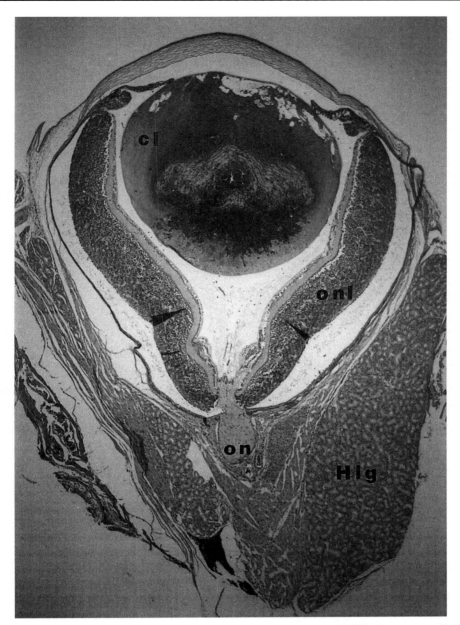

FIG. 10.13—Cross section of a 2-week-old interstitial retinol binding protein (IRBP) simian virus 40 (SV40) T antigen (IRBP-Tag) transgenic mouse eye. The expression of SV40Tag oncogene driven by the mouse IRBP promoter has led to widespread tumorigenesis in the outer nuclear layer (onl) (cl, cataractous lens; Hlg, Harderian lacrimal gland; on, optic nerve). Hematoxylin–eosin, ×40.

The pineal tumors, on the other hand, resembled highly differentiated RB with abundant HWRs. Northern-blot analysis of both ocular and pineal tumors and their corresponding cell cultures revealed that the tumor cells expressed SV40Tag and IRBP but not opsin. This suggested that the tumors arose from precursor cells that expressed IRBP but not opsin. Therefore, the murine IRBP promoter had precisely targeted SV40Tag expression to photoreceptor cells of the developing retina prior to their terminal differentiation (Figures 10.13–10.15).[124]

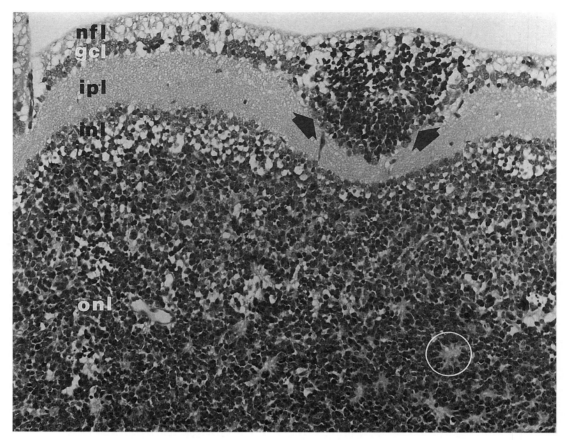

FIG. 10.14—This 2-week-old interstitial retinol binding protein (IRBP) T antigen (Tag) mouse retina shows disturbance of normal embryogenesis. The inner row of the inner nuclear layer (inl) seems to be partially differentiated, but the outer plexiform layer has failed to develop. A small tumoral focus is seen starting in the ganglion cell layer (gcl) (arrows). The whole thickness of the outer nuclear layer (inl) has been replaced by small basophilic tumor cells showing a tendency toward Homer Wright rosette formation (encircled) (nfl, nerve fiber layer; ipl, inner plexiform layer). Hematoxylin–eosin, ×200.

Human papilloma virus (HPV) is associated with the development of cervical and anogenital carcinomas in humans. Two viral oncogenes, HPV E6 and E7, belong to the same class of viral oncoproteins as SV40Tag and are associated with malignant transformation in HPV infection. The HPV E7 gene product has been shown to bind and inactivate pRB in vitro and in vivo.[125,126] E7 does not bind p53, and E6 functionally inactivates p53 while leaving pRB function intact.[127,128] Using the HPV oncoproteins, transgenic mouse models have been created to examine the roles that pRB and p53 play in RB.

Transgenic mice were created with the a-crystallin promoter fused to SV40Tag, in order to direct Tag expression within the lens. These mice develop microphthalmos, cataract, and lenticular tumors, but do not develop retinal tumors.[129] Lines of transgenic mice were produced that expressed HPV E6/E7 under the control of the a-crystallin promoter to direct expression of E6/E7 to the lens.[130,131] A single line of these mice was found to express E6 and E7 in the retina, with concomitant functional loss of p53 and pRB. Tumors resembling RB arose from the bipolar cell layer of the retina and displayed HWRs histologically. Triple-membrane structures and basal bodies were observed by electron microscopy. Tumors occasionally extended to the brain via the optic nerve and metastasized to cervical lymph

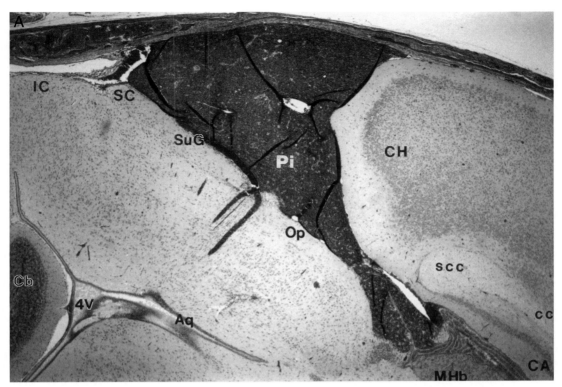

FIG. 10.15—**A:** This 2-week-old interstitial retinol binding protein (IRBP) T antigen (Tag) mouse pineal gland shows complete replacement by small basophilic tumor cells. The tumor, which is still confined to the gland at this time, fills the entire transverse fissure of the cerebrum (3V, third ventricle; 4V, fourth ventricle; Aq, cerebral aqueduct; CA, Ammon's horn; Cb, cerebellum; cc, corpus callosum; CH, cerebral hemisphere; ChP, choroid plexus; hbc, habenular commissure; IC, inferior colliculus; MHb, median habenular nucleus; Op, optic nerve layer of the superior colliculus; pc, posterior commissure; Pi, pineal gland; PiRe, pineal recess of the third ventricle; SC, superior colliculus; scc, splenius corpus callosum; SCO, subcommissural organ; sss, superior sagittal sinus; SuG, superficial gray layer of the superior colliculus). Sagittal section, hematoxylin–eosin, ×40. (continued)

nodes. The incidence and frequency of RB development varied when these mice were mated to other genetic strains, thus indicating that other cellular genes play a role in tumorigenesis.

Alterations of the Murine Retinoblastoma Gene. At the same time that transgenic mice are produced to explore the consequences of the expression of a viral oncoprotein known to bind and probably inactivate p110 Rb and p53, other mice were created in which the normal murine RB gene itself was mutated.[132–134] The murine pRb shows 91% homology with its human counterpart. It is expressed ubiquitously in the mouse embryo at approximately embryonic day 13 (E13), with a maximum level in the liver and the brain.[135] The murine RB gene promoter has been characterized and shares 80% homology with the human sequence.[136] Using a positive-negative selection strategy, mouse embryonic stem cells were specifically mutated for one allele of the RB gene, resulting in an inactive gene. By breeding techniques, both heterozygous and homozygous embryos were obtained.[132–134]

In mice, the homozygous state for the inactivating mutation proved to be incompatible with life, and all of the homozygous embryos died before E16. The homozygous embryos developed in apparent synchrony with their normal littermates up to E11.5. After that, they showed developmental abnormalities to various degrees, the most consistent of which were defective erythropoiesis

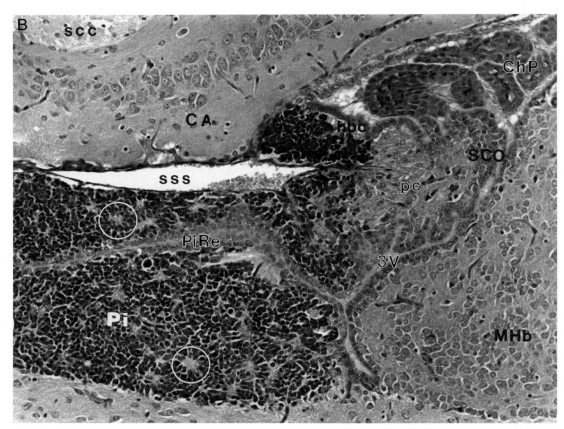

FIG. 10.15 (continued)—**B:** The pineal gland tumor shows a higher degree of differentiation than the corresponding intraocular tumors, showing numerous Homer Wright rosettes (encircled). Sagittal section, hematoxylin–eosin, ×400.

and neurogenesis. Around E12–E15, the liver normally replaces the yolk sac as the source of erythropoiesis, and this is reflected in the peripheral blood formula by a gradual shift from prevalence of nucleated red blood cells to prevalence of mature enucleated red blood cells. The homozygous embryos failed to achieve this shift and showed a persistent predominance of primitive nucleated red blood cells, suggesting either a deregulation of production of more primitive erythrocytes or a defect in end-stage differentiation of the erythroid precursor cells.[132–134]

Concurrently with the defective erythropoiesis, widespread neuronal apoptosis and ectopic mitoses were found predominantly in the hindbrain, the spinal cord, and the dorsal root ganglia. By the time the embryos died, no abnormalities were apparent in the retina. As a possible explanation, it was suggested that the homozygous mice may die before the retina reaches a susceptible stage.[132–134]

Interestingly, the introduction of multiple copies of a wild-type human RB gene-containing transgene, under the human RB promoter, resulted in the rescue of the homozygous-deficient embryos from the lethal phenotype, suggesting that the homozygous RB gene mutation was the sole mechanism involved in the generation of the observed phenotype.[133]

None of the mice heterozygous for the RB gene mutation developed RB despite periods of observation of up to 11 months. A proposed explanation was that the number of susceptible retinal stem cells in the mouse is too small to compensate for the low rate of spontaneous deactivating mutation of the remnant wild allele, which is necessary for a detectable frequency of tumors. Nonetheless, a significant number of heterozygous mice developed brain tumors, including adenocarcinoma of the pituitary, after latency periods of 4–12 weeks. These tumors consistently showed loss of the remaining wild-type RB gene allele.[132–134]

FUTURE PROSPECTS AND SPECULATIONS

Spontaneous RB in animals is exceedingly rare. Experimental production of RB-like tumors proves that the retina in other species can undergo malignant transformation. Knowledge of the experimental methods used to produce RB-like tumors is important when considering the results.

The induction of RB-like tumors by means of diverse carcinogens might deserve to be studied in more detail in light of the more recent molecular biologic data on their pathogenesis and possible implication as risk factors.

The viral induction of RB-like tumors is a complex mechanism that involves the effects of various viral genes, including regulatory genes and oncogenes, as well as host reactions to the viral infections.

Transgenic animals express only restricted portions of the viral genome in a controlled manner. The amount of viral oncoproteins present in the cells can be measured, but also important is the precise determination of the time of onset of their action. The identification of unique promoters in retinal cells that are expressed at specific times during development is needed. By selection of the appropriate promoter, viral oncogenes can be targeted to an exclusive cell type at a specific frame of embryogenesis. This represents a powerful tool for studying sequences of tissue-specific differentiation, as well as the tumor thus derived.

However, even transgenic expression of viral oncogenes is an approximation of the situation in humans. Indeed, it is now clear that pRb is not the only cell cycle regulatory protein targeted in these models by the SV40 T antigen. This antigen is known to interact with the p53 gene product, and its interaction with other growth-suppressor proteins is under investigation. New insights into these complex interaction pathways have been provided by the study of highly selective oncoproteins like HPV16 E6 and E7. HPV16 E7 inhibits pRb while leaving p53 intact. When driven by the IRBP promoter, HPV16 E7 expression does not lead to retinal tumorigenesis but rather to extensive *programmed cell death*—or *apoptosis*—of the photoreceptor cells.[127]

Furthermore, evidence for a role of viruses in human RB is lacking thus far. In this respect, polymerase chain reaction (PCR) assays of 50 human RBs for the presence of five human DNA tumor viruses (AdV12, BK virus, JC virus, HPV16, and HPV18) have been unable to detect any viral gene in the tumor cells.[137]

As biotechnology advances, new treatment strategies will be created. Complete genetic analyses of RB tumor cells will identify the specific mutations responsible for the neoplastic transformation. From this knowledge, new drugs can be designed to directly target the mutated molecule, whether it is a defective enzyme, transcription factor, or receptor.

The issue of potential reversibility of malignant behavior (tumor cell *reconstitution*) upon restoration of the missing RB gene into RB culture cells or homozygous animals has not yet been resolved. Divergent results have been reported by several research teams.[86,138–143] The RB gene seems to be a relatively weak tumor suppressor.[23]

Few reports address the issue of the differences that might exist between *negative cell growth control*, preventing a cell from entering into a neoplastic growth state, and *tumor suppression activity*, which implies a capacity of the neoplastic tumor growth to regress to a controlled state.

CONCLUSIONS

Since its recognition as a specific tumor in 1809, RB has been extensively studied. Clinicians recognized that survival of patients depended on early diagnosis. Pathologists were later able to describe the course of the disease and identify important prognostic features, such as the degree of optic nerve involvement. The introduction of radiotherapy gave rise to successful conservative treatment. Subsequently, it became apparent that, later in life, second primary tumors arose both within and outside the field of irradiation.

Chemotherapy was found to have a useful, albeit limited, role as an adjunct in the treatment of RB. Epidemiologists, statisticians, and geneticists have progressively studied the early clinical observations of the peculiar hereditary transmission of the disease. RB has been demonstrated to be a prototype of a group of cancers caused by a transmittable genetic defect. Molecular biologists cloned the RB gene and demonstrated its tumor-suppressor activity. Together with the development of effective experimental models, exploration of the molecular mechanisms of oncogenesis now raises promising future prospects for treatment. Precise risk-factor determination for the offspring and relatives has become a reality. Genetic therapy represents a major promise for the future.

REFERENCES

1. Syed NA, Nork TM, Poulsen GL, Riis RC, George C, Albert DM. Retinoblastoma in a dog. *Arch Ophthalmol* 115:758, 1997.
2. Duke-Elder S, Dobree JH. Diseases of the retina. In: Duke-Elder S, ed. *System of Ophthalmology.* London: Henry Kimpton, 672:1967.
3. Albert DM. Historic review of retinoblastoma. *Ophthalmology* 94:654, 1987.
4. Zimmerman LE. Retinoblastoma and retinocytoma. In: Spencer WH, ed. *Ophthalmic Pathology.* Philadelphia: WB Saunders, 1292:1985.
5. Petersen RA. Retinoblastoma: diagnosis and nonradiation therapies. In: Albert DM, Jakobiec FA, eds. *Principles and Practice of Ophthalmology.* Philadelphia: WB Saunders, Chap 268:1993.
6. Cassady JR. Radiation therapy for retinoblastoma. In: Albert DM, Jakobiec FA, eds. *Principles and Practice of Ophthalmology.* Philadelphia: WB Saunders, chap 269:1993.
7. Knudson AG Jr. Mutation and cancer: statistical study of retinoblastoma. *Proc Natl Acad Sci USA* 68:820, 1971.
8. Knudson AG Jr. The genetics of childhood cancer. *Cancer* 35:1022, 1975.
9. Comings DE. A general theory of carcinogenesis. *Proc Natl Acad Sci USA* 70:3324, 1973.
10. Yunis JJ, Ramsay N. Retinoblastoma and subband deletion of chromosome 13. *Amer J Dis Child* 132:161, 1978.
11. Dryja TP, Rapaport J, Joyce JM, Petersen R. Molecular detection of deletions involving band q14 of chromosome 13 in retinoblastoma. *Proc Natl Acad Sci USA* 83:7391, 1986.
12. Friend SH, Bernards R, Rogelj S, Weinberg R, Rapaport J, Albert DM, Dryja TP. A human DNA segment with properties of the gene that predisposes to retinoblastoma and osteosarcoma. *Nature* 323:643, 1986.
13. Lee W-H, Bookstein R, Hong F, Young L-J, Shew J-Y, Lee EY-HP. Human retinoblastoma susceptibility gene: cloning, identification, and sequence. *Science* 235:1394, 1987.
14. Ts'o MOM, Zimmerman LE, Fine BS. The nature of retinoblastoma: I. Photoreceptor differentiation—a clinical and histopathologic study. *Am J Ophthalmol* 69:338, 1970.
15. Ts'o MOM, Fine BS, Zimmerman LE. The nature of retinoblastoma: II. Photoreceptor differentiation—an electron microscopic study. *Am J Ophthalmol* 69:350, 1970.
16. Bader JL, Miller RW, Meadows AT, Zimmerman LE, Champion LAA, Voûte PA. Trilateral retinoblastoma. *Lancet* 2:582, 1980.
17. Jakobiec FA, Ts'o MOM, Zimmerman LE, Danis P. Retinoblastoma and intracranial malignancy. *Cancer* 39:2048, 1977.
18. Sang DN, Albert DM. Retinoblastoma: clinical and histopathologic features. *Hum Pathol* 13:133, 1982.
19. Sang DN, Albert DM, Kuo PK. Retinoblastoma: clinical observations and histopathological study. *Int Ophthalmol Clin* 22:73, 1982.
20. Tamboli A, Podgor MJ, Horm JW. The incidence of retinoblastoma in the United States: 1974 through 1985. *Arch Ophthalmol* 108:128, 1990.
21. Shields JA, Shields CL. *Intraocular Tumors: A Text and Atlas.* Philadelphia: WB Saunders, chaps 18-22:1992.
22. Dryja TP. Assessment of risk in hereditary retinoblastoma. In: Albert DM, Jakobiec FA, eds. *Principles and Practice of Ophthalmology.* WB Saunders, Philadelphia, chap 267:1993.
23. Gallie BL, Dunn JM, Hamel PA, Muncaster M, Cohen BL, Phillips RA. How do retinoblastoma tumours form? *Eye* 6:226, 1992.
24. Buckley JD. The aetiology of cancer in the very young, *Br J Cancer* 18(suppl):8, 1992.
25. DerKinderen DJ, Koten JW, Tan KE, Beemer FA, Van Romunde LK. Parental age in sporadic hereditary retinoblastoma. *Am J Ophthalmol* 110:605, 1990.
26. Matsunaga E, Minoda K, Sasaki MS. Parental age and seasonal variation in the births of children with sporadic retinoblastoma: a mutation-epidemiologic study. *J Hum Genet* 84:155, 1990.
27. Bunin GR, Petrakova A, Meadows AT, Emanuel BS, Buckley JD, Woods WG, Hammond GD. Occupation of parents of children with retinoblastoma: a report from the Children's Cancer Study Group. *Cancer Res* 50:7129, 1990.
28. Sahel JA, Albert DM. Pathology of the retina and the vitreous. In: Albert DM, Jakobiec FA, eds. *Principles and Practice of Ophthalmology.* Philadelphia: WB Saunders, 2261:1993.
29. Bhatnagar R, Vine AK. Diffuse infiltrating retinoblastoma. *Ophthalmology* 98:1657, 1991.
30. Khodadoust AA, Roozitalab HM, Smith RE, Green WR. Spontaneous regression of retinoblastoma. *Surv Ophthalmol* 21:467, 1977.

31. Gallie BL, Phillips RA, Ellsworth RM, Abramson DH. Significance of retinoma and phthisis bulbi for retinoblastoma. *Ophthalmology* 89:1393, 1982.

32. Albert DM, Lahav M, Lesser R, Craft J. Recent observations regarding retinoblastoma: 1. Ultrastructure, tissue culture growth, incidence, and animal models. *Trans Ophthalmol Soc UK* 94:909, 1974.

33. Craft JL, Robinson NL, Roth NA, Albert DM. Scanning electron microscopy of retinoblastoma. *Exp Eye Res* 27:519, 1978.

34. Zimmerman LE. Trilateral retinoblastoma. In: Blodi FC, ed. *Retinoblastoma.* New York: Churchill Livingstone, 185:1985.

35. Gonzalez-Fernandez F, Lopes MBS, Garcia-Fernandez J, Foster RG, De Grip WJ, Rosemberg S, Newman SA, VandenBerg SR. Expression of developmentally defined retinal phenotypes in the histogenesis of retinoblastoma. *Am J Pathol* 141:363, 1992.

36. Bogenmann E, Lochrie MA, Simon MI. Cone cell-specific genes expressed in retinoblastoma. *Science* 240:76, 1988.

37. Hurwitz RL, Bogenmann E, Font RL, Holcombe V, Clark D. Expression of the functional cone phototransduction cascade in retinoblastoma. *J Clin Invest* 85:1872, 1990.

38. Nork TM, Schwartz TL, Doshi HM, Millecchia LL. Retinoblastoma: cell of origin. *Arch Ophthalmol* 113:791, 1995.

39. Zacksenhaus E, Bremner R, Jiang Z, Gill RM, Muncaster M, Sopta M, Phillips RA, Gallie BL. Unraveling the function of the retinoblastoma gene. *Adv Cancer Res* 61:115, 1993.

40. Gallie BL, Dunn JM, Chan HSL, Hamel PA, Phillips RA. The genetics of retinoblastoma: relevance to the patient. *Pediatr Clin N Am* 38:299, 1991.

41. Zhu X, Dunn JM, Phillips RA, Goddard AD, Paton KE, Becker A, Gallie BL. Preferential germline mutation of the paternal allele in retinoblastoma. *Nature* 340:312, 1989.

42. Zhu X, Dunn JM, Goddard AD, Squire JA, Becker A, Phillips RA, Gallie BL. Mechanisms of loss of heterozygosity in retinoblastoma. *Cytogenet Cell Genet* 59:248, 1992.

43. Parks MM, Zimmerman LE. Retinoblastoma. *Clin Proc Child Hosp DC* 16:77, 1960.

44. Eng C, Li FP, Abramson DH, Ellsworth RM, Wong FL, Goldman MB, Seddon J, Tarbell N, Boice JD. Mortality from second tumors among long-term survivors of retinoblastoma. *J Natl Cancer Inst* 85:1121, 1993.

45. Messmer EP, Heinrich T, Höpping W, De Sutter E, Havers W, Sauerwein W. Risk factors for metastases in patients with retinoblastoma. *Ophthalmology* 98:136, 1991.

46. Abramson DH, Ellsworth RM, Kitchin FD, Tung G. Second nonocular tumors in retinoblastoma survivors: are they radiation-induced? *Ophthalmology* 91:1351, 1984.

47. Hansen MF. Molecular genetic considerations in osteosarcoma. *Clin Orthop* 270:237, 1990.

48. Abramson DH, Frank CM. Second nonocular tumors in survivors of bilateral retinoblastoma: a possible age effect on radiation-related risk. *Ophthalmology* 105:579, 1998.

49. Becker LE, Hinton D. Primitive neuroectodermal tumors of the central nervous system. *Hum Pathol* 14:538, 1983.

50. Bindlish R, LaRoche GR. Successful treatment of neonatal trilateral retinoblastoma. *JAAPOS* 3:376, 1999.

51. Holladay DA, Holladay A, Montebello JF, Redmond KP. Clinical presentation, treatment, and outcome of trilateral retinoblastoma. *Cancer* 67:710, 1991.

52. Shields JA. Misconceptions and techniques in the management of retinoblastoma. *Retina* 12:320, 1992.

53. Ellsworth RM. The practical management of retinoblastoma. *Trans Am Ophthalmol Soc* 67:462, 1969.

54. White L. Chemotherapy in retinoblastoma: current status and future directions. *Am J Pediatr Hematol Oncol* 13:189, 1991.

55. Imhof SM, Mourits MP, Hofman P, Zonneveld FW, Schipper J, Moll AC, Tan KE. Quantification of orbital and mid-facial growth retardation after megavoltage external beam irradiation in children with retinoblastoma. *Ophthalmology* 103:263, 1996.

56. Bryne J, Fears TR, Whitney C, Parry DM. Survival after retinoblastoma: long-term consequences and family history of cancer. *Med Pediatr Oncol* 24:160, 1995.

57. Bech MN, Balmer A, Dessing C, Pica A, Munier F. First-line chemotherapy with local treatment can prevent external-beam irradiation and enucleation in low-stage intraocular retinoblastoma. *J Clin Oncol* 18:2881, 2000.

58. Murphree AL, Villablanca JG, Deegan WF, Sato JK, Malogolowkin M, Fisher A, Parker R, Reed E, Gomer CJ. Chemotherapy plus local treatment in the management of intraocular retinoblastoma. *Arch Ophthalmol* 114:1348, 1996.

59. Kingston JE, Hungerford JL, Madreperla SA, Plowman PN. Results of combined chemotherapy and radiotherapy for advanced intraocular retinoblastoma. *Arch Ophthalmol* 114:1339, 1996.

60. Shields CL, De Potter P, Himelstein BP, Shields JA, Meadows AT, Maris JM. Chemoreduction in the initial management of intraocular retinoblastoma. *Arch Ophthalmol* 114:1330, 1996.

61. Gallie BL, Budning A, DeBoer G, Thiessen JJ, Koren G, Verjee Z, Ling V, Chan HSL. Chemotherapy with focal therapy can cure intraocular retinoblastoma without radiotherapy. *Arch Ophthalmol* 114:1321, 1996.

62. Shields CL, Santos MC, Diniz W, Gunduz K, Mercado G, Cater JR, Shields JA. Thermotherapy for retinoblastoma. *Arch Ophthalmol* 117:885, 1999.

63. Hogan RN, Albert DM. Does retinoblastoma occur in animals? *Prog Vet Comp Ophthalmol* 1:73, 1991.

64. Donoso LA, Folberg R, Arbizo B. Retinal S antigen and retinoblastoma: a monoclonal antibody histopathologic study. *Arch Ophthalmol* 103:855, 1985.

65. Mirshahi M, Boucheix C, Dhermy P, Haye C, Faure JP. Expression of the photoreceptor specific S-antigen in human retinoblastoma. *Cancer* 57:1497, 1986.

66. Gavrieli Y, Sherman Y, Ben-Sasson SA. Identification of programmed cell death in situ via specific labeling of nuclear DNA fragmentation. *J Cell Biol* 119:493, 1992.

67. Bunt AH, Tso MO. Feulgen-positive deposits in retinoblastoma: incidence, composition, and ultrastructure. *Arch Ophthalmol* 99:144, 1981.

68. Hamel PA, Phillips RA, Muncaster M, Gallie BL. Speculations of the role of RB1 in tissue-specific differentiation, tumor initiation, and tumor progression. *FASEB J* 7:846, 1993.

69. Schlamp CL, Poulsen GL, Nork TM, Nickells RW. Nuclear exclusion of wild-type p53 in immortalized human retinoblastoma cells. *J Natl Cancer Inst* 89:1530, 1997.

70. Albert DM, Gonder JR, Papale J, Craft JL, Dohlman HG, Reid MC, Sunderman FW Jr. Induction of ocular neoplasms in Fischer rats by intraocular injection of nickel bisulfide. *Invest Ophthalmol Vis Sci* 22:768, 1982.

71. Brooks GF, Butel JS, Ornsteon LN, Jawetz E, Melnick JL, Adelberg EA. *Jawetz, Melnick and Adelberg's Medical Microbiology.* Norwalk, CT: Appleton and Lange, chap 45:1989.

72. Albert DM. The role of viruses in the development of ocular tumors. *Ophthalmology* 87:1219, 1980.

73. Livingston DM, Bradley MK. The Simian virus 40 large T antigen: a lot packed into a little. *Mol Biol Med* 4:63, 1987.

74. Albert DM, Rabson AS, Dalton AJ. In vitro neoplastic transformation of uveal and retinal tissue by oncogenic DNA viruses. *Invest Ophthalmol* 7:357, 1968.

75. Kobayashi M, Mukai N, Solish SP, Pomeroy ME. A highly predictable animal model of retinoblastoma. *Acta Neuropathol (Berl)* 57:203, 1982.

76. Mukai N, Kobayashi S, Oguri M. Ultrastructural studies of human adenovirus-produced retinoblastoma-like neoplasms in Sprague-Dawley rats. *Invest Ophthalmol* 13:593, 1974.

77. Mukai N, Nakajima T, Freddo T, Jacobson M, Dunn M. Retinoblastoma-like neoplasm induced in C3H/BifB/Ki strain mice by human adenovirus serotype 12. *Acta Neuropathol (Berl)* 39:147, 1977.

78. Mukai N, Nishida T, Nakajima T. A DNA virus-induced model of retinoblastoma. *Int Ophthalmol Clin* 20:223, 1980.

79. Kobayashi S, Mukai N. Retinoblastoma-like tumors induced in rats by human adenovirus. *Invest Ophthalmol* 12:853, 1973.

80. Nishida T, Mukai N, Solish SP, Pomeroy M. Effects of cyclic AMP on growth and differentiation of rat retinoblastoma-like tumor cells in vitro. *Invest Ophthalmol Vis Sci* 22:145, 1982.

81. Winther J. In vitro and in vivo growth of an intraocular retinoblastoma-like tumor in F-344 rats. *Acta Ophthalmol (Copenh)* 64:657, 1986.

82. Winther J, Jensen OA, Prause JU, Tommerup N. Characterization of an intraocular retinoblastoma-like tumour. *Acta Ophthalmol (Copenh)* 65:491, 1987.

83. Mukai N, Kalter SS, Cummins LB, Matthews VA, Nishida T, Nakajima T. Retinal tumor induced in the baboon by human adenovirus 12. *Science* 210:1023, 1980.

84. Albert DM, Papale JJ, Strumph P, Fournier GA. In vitro malignant transformation of hamster retina by herpes simplex virus. *Invest Ophthalmol Vis Sci* 24:1489, 1983.

85. Albert DM, Lahav M, Colby ED, Shadduck JA, Sang DN. Retinal neoplasia and dysplasia: I. Induction by feline leukemia virus. *Invest Ophthalmol Vis Sci* 16:325, 1977.

86. Reid TW, Albert DM, Rabson AS, Russell P, Craft J, Chu EW, Tralka TS, Wilcox JL. Characteristics of an established cell line of retinoblastoma. *J Natl Cancer Inst* 53:347, 1974.

87. Muncaster MM, Cohen BL, Phillips RA, Gallie BL. Failure of *RB1* to reverse the malignant phenotype of human tumor cell lines. *Cancer Res* 52:654, 1992.

88. Gallie BL, Albert DM, Wong JJY, Buyukmihci N, Puliafito CA. Heterotransplantation of retinoblastoma into the athymic "nude" mouse. *Invest Ophthalmol Vis Sci* 16:256, 1977.

89. Benedict WF, Dawson JA, Banerjee A, Murphree AL. The nude mouse model for human retinoblastoma: a system for evaluation of retinoblastoma therapy. *Med Pediatr Oncol* 8:391, 1980.

90. McFall RC, Sery TW, Makadon M. Characterization of a new continuous cell line derived from a human retinoblastoma. *Cancer Res* 37:1003, 1977.

91. Winther J, Overgaard J. Photodynamic therapy of experimental intraocular retinoblastomas: dose-response relationships to light energy and Photofrin II. *Acta Ophthalmol (Copenh)* 67:44, 1989.

92. Ohnishi Y, Murakami M, Wakeyama H. Effects of hematoporphyrin derivative and light on Y79 retinoblastoma cells in vitro. *Invest Ophthalmol Vis Sci* 31:792, 1990.

93. White L, Gomer CJ, Doiron DR, Szirth BC. Ineffective photodynamic therapy (PDT) in a poorly vascularized xenograft model. *Br J Cancer* 57:455, 1988.

94. Winther J, Overgaard J. Experimental studies of photodynamic therapy in a retinoblastoma-like tumor. *Acta Ophthalmol (Copenh)* 65:140, 1987.

95. Winther J, Ehlers N. Histopathological changes in an intraocular retinoblastoma-like tumor following photodynamic therapy. *Acta Ophthalmol (Copenh)* 66:69, 1988.

96. White L, Szirth BC, Benedict WF. Evaluation of response to chemotherapy in retinoblastoma heterotransplanted to the eyes of nude mice. *Cancer Chemother Pharmacol* 23:63, 1989.

97. White L. Responsiveness of retinoblastoma to local diaziquone: studies in a xenograft model. *Invest Ophthalmol Vis Sci* 31:787, 1990.

98. Hurwitz MY, Marcus KT, Chevez-Barrios P, Louie K, Aquilar-Cordova E, Hurwitz RL. Suicide gene therapy for treatment of retinoblastoma in a murine model. *Hum Gene Ther* 10:441, 1999.

99. Kyritsis AP, Tsokos M, Chader GJ. Control of retinoblastoma cell growth by differentiating agents: current work and future directions. *Anticancer Res* 6:465, 1986.

100. Sang DN, Anderson DJ. Retinoblastoma: HLA expression induced by retinoic acid. *Retina* 3:206, 1983.

101. Saulenas AM, Cohen SM, Key LL, Winter C, Albert DM. Vitamin D and retinoblastoma: the presence of receptors and inhibition of growth in vitro. *Arch Ophthalmol* 106:533, 1988.

102. Albert DM, Saulenas AM, Cohen S. Verhoeff's query: is vitamin D effective against retinoblastoma? *Arch Ophthalmol* 106:536, 1988.

103. Cohen SM, Saulenas AM, Sullivan CR, Albert DM. Further studies of the effect of vitamin D on retinoblastoma: inhibition with 1,25 dihydroxycholecalciferol. *Arch Ophthalmol* 106:541, 1988.

104. Howard MA, Wardwell S, Albert DM. Effect of butyrate and corticosteroid on retinoblastoma in vitro and in vivo. *Invest Ophthalmol Vis Sci* 32:1711, 1991

105. Del Cerro M, Notter MF, Seigel G, Lazar E, Chader G, Del Cerro C. Intraretinal xenografts of differentiated human retinoblastoma cells integrate with the host retina. *Brain Res* 583:12, 1992.

106. O'Brien JM, Marcus DM, Bernards R, Carpenter JL, Windle JJ, Mellon P, Albert DM. A transgenic mouse model for trilateral retinoblastoma. *Arch Ophthalmol* 108:1145, 1990.

107. Windle JJ, Albert DM, O'Brien JM, Marcus DM, Disteche CM, Bernards R, Mellon PL. Retinoblastoma in transgenic mice. *Nature* 343:665, 1990.

108. Kivelä T, Virtanen I, Marcus DM, O'Brien JM, Carpenter JL, Brauner E, Tarkkanen A, Albert DM. Neuronal and glial properties of a murine transgenic retinoblastoma model. *Am J Pathol* 138:1135, 1991.

109. Marcus DM, Carpenter JL, O'Brien JM, Kivela T, Brauner E, Tarkkanen A, Virtanen I, Albert DM. Primitive neuroectodermal tumor of the midbrain in a murine model of retinoblastoma. *Invest Ophthalmol Vis Sci* 32:293, 1991.

110. Harbour JW, Murray TG, Jamasaki D, Cicciarelli N, Hernandez E, Smith B, Windle J, O'Brien JM. Local carboplatin therapy in transgenic murine retinoblastoma. *Invest Ophthalmol Vis Sci* 37:1892, 1996.

111. Murray TG, Roth DB, O'Brien JM, Feuer W, Cicciarelli N, Markoe AM, Hernandez E, Smith BJ, Windle JJ. Local carboplatin and radiation therapy in the treatment of murine transgenic retinoblastoma. *Arch Ophthalmol* 114:1385, 1996.

112. Murray TG, Cicciarelli N, O'Brien JM, Hernandez E, Mueller RL, Smith BJ, Feuer W. Subconjunctival carboplatin therapy and cryotherapy in the treatment of transgenic murine retinoblastoma. *Arch Ophthalmol* 115:1286, 1997.

113. Albert DM, Marcus DM, Gallo JP, O'Brien JM. The antineoplastic effect of vitamin D in transgenic mice with retinoblastoma. *Invest Ophthalmol Vis Sci* 33:2354, 1992.

114. Vandewalle B, Hornez L, Wattez N, Revillion F, Lefebvre J. Vitamin-D_3 derivatives and breast-tumor cell growth: effect on intracellular calcium and apoptosis. *Int J Cancer* 61:806, 1995.

115. Skarosi S, Abraham C, Bissonnette M, Scaglione-Sewell B, Sitrin MD, Brastius TA. 1,25-Dihydroxyvitamin D_3 stimulates apoptosis in CaCoo-2 cells. *Gastroenterology* 112:A608, 1997.

116. Munker R, Kobayashi T, Elstner E, Norman AW, Uskokovic M, Zhang W, Andreeff M, Koeffler HP. A new series of vitamin D analogs is highly active for clonal inhibition differentiation, and induction of WAF1 in myeloid leukemia. *Blood* 88:2201, 1996.

117. Levin AJ. p53, the cellular gatekeeper for growth and division. *Cell* 88:323, 1997.

118. Brugarolas JJC, Gordon JI, Beach D, Jacks T, Hannon CJ. Radiation-induced cell cycle arrest compromised by p21 deficiency. *Nature* 377:552, 1995.

119. Sabet SJ, Darjatmoko SR, Lindstrom MJ, Albert DM. Antineoplastic effect and toxicity of 1,25-dihydroxy-16-ene-23-yne-vitamin D_3 in athymic mice with Y-79 human retinoblastoma tumors. *Arch Ophthalmol* 117:365, 1999.

120. Wilkerson CL, Darjatmoko SR, Lindstrom MJ, Albert DM. Toxicity and dose-response studies of 1,25-(OH)2-16-ene-23-yne vitamin D_3 in transgenic mice. *Clin Cancer Res* 4:2253, 1998.

121. Albert DM. Unpublished data.

122. Murray TG, O'Brien JM, Steeves RA, Smith BJ, Albert DM, Cicciarelli N, Markoe AM, Tompkins DT, Windle JJ. Radiation therapy and ferromagnetic hyperthermia in the treatment of murine transgenic retinoblastoma. *Arch Ophthalmol* 114:1376, 1996.

123. Al-Ubaidi MR, Font RL, Quiambao AB, Keener MJ, Liou GI, Overbeek PA, Baehr W. Bilateral retinal and brain tumors in transgenic mice expressing simian virus 40 large T antigen under control of the human interphotoreceptor retinoid-binding protein promotor. *J Cell Biol* 119:1681, 1992.

124. Howes KA, Lasudry JGH, Albert DM, Windle JJ. Photoreceptor cell tumors in transgenic mice. *Invest Ophthalmol Vis Sci* 35:342, 1994.

125. Dyson N, Howley PM, Munger K, Harlow E. The human papilloma virus-16 E7 oncoprotein is able to bind to the retinoblastoma gene product. *Science* 243:934, 1989.

126. Munger K, Werness BA, Dyson N, Phelps WC, Harlow E, Howley PM. Complex formation of human papillomavirus E7 proteins with the retinoblastoma tumor suppressor gene product. *EMBO J* 8:4099, 1989.

127. Howes KA, Ransom N, Papermaster DS, Lasudry JGH, Albert DM, Windle JJ. Apoptosis of retinoblastoma: alternative fates of photoreceptors expressing the HPV16-E7 gene in the presence or absence of p53. *Genes Dev* 8:1300, 1994.

128. Scheffner M, Werness BA, Huibregtse JM, Levine AJ, Howley PM. The E6 oncoprotein encoded by human papillomavirus types 16 and 18 promotes the degradation of p53. *Cell* 63:1129, 1990.

129. Mahon KA, Chepelinsky AB, Khillan JS, Overbeek PA, Piatigorsky J, Westphal H. Oncogenesis of the lens in transgenic mice. *Science* 235:1622, 1987.

130. Albert DM, Griep AE, Lambert PF, Howes KA, Windle JJ, Lasudry JGH. Transgenic models of retinoblastoma: what they tell us about its cause and treatment. *Trans Am Ophthalmol Soc* 92:385, 1994.

131. Griep AE, Kraweck J, Lee D, Liem A, Albert DM, Carabeo R, Drinkwater N, McCall M, Sattler C, Lasudry JGH, Lambert PF. Multiple genetic loci modify risk for retinoblastoma in transgenic mice. *Invest Ophthalmol Vis Sci* 39:2723, 1998.

132. Jacks T, Fazeli A, Schmitt EM, Bronson RT, Goodell MA, Weinberg RA. Effects of an Rb mutation in the mouse. *Nature* 352:295, 1992.

133. Lee EY, Chang CY, Hu N, Wang YC, Lai C-C, Herrup K, Lee W-H, Bradley A. Mice deficient for Rb are nonviable and show defects in neurogenesis and haematopoiesis. *Nature* 359:288, 1992.

134. Clarke AR, Maandag ER, Van Roon M, Van der Lugt NMT, Van der Valk M, Hooper ML, Berns A, Te Riele H. Requirement for a functional RB-1 gene in murine development. *Nature* 359:328, 1992.

135. Bernards R, Schackleford GM, Gerber MR, Horowitz JM, Friend SH, Schartl M, Bogenmann E, Rapaport JM, McGee T, Dryja TP, Weinberg RA. Structure and expression of the murine retinoblastoma gene and characterization of its encoded protein. *Proc Natl Acad Sci USA* 86:6474, 1989.

136. Zacksenhaus E, Gill RM, Phillips RA, Gallie BL. Molecular cloning and characterization of the mouse RB1 promoter. *Oncogene* 8:2343, 1993.

137. Howard E, Marcus DM, O'Brien JM, Albert DM, Bernards R. Five DNA tumor viruses undetectable in human retinoblastomas. *Invest Ophthalmol Vis Sci* 33:1567, 1992.

138. Bookstein R, Shew J-Y, Chen P-L, Scully P, Lee W-H. Suppression of tumorigenicity of human prostate carcinoma cells by replacing a mutated RB gene. *Science* 247:712, 1990.

139. Madreperla SA, Whittum-Hudson JA, Prendergast RA, Chen P-L, Lee W-H. Intraocular tumor suppression of retinoblastoma gene-reconstituted retinoblastoma cells. *Cancer Res* 51:6381, 1991.

140. Chen P-L, Chen Y, Shan B, Bookstein R, Lee W-H. Stability of retinoblastoma gene expression determines the tumorigenicity of reconstituted retinoblastoma cells. *Cell Growth Differ* 3:119, 1992.

141. Xu H-J, Sumegi J, Hu S-X, Banerjee A, Uzvolgyi E, Klein G, Benedict WF. Intraocular tumor formation of RB reconstituted retinoblastoma cells. *Cancer Res* 51:4481, 1991.

142. Uzvolgyi E, Classon M, Henriksson M, Huang H-JS, Szekely L, Lee W-H, Klein G, Sumegi J. Reintroduction of a normal retinoblastoma gene into retinoblastoma and osteosarcoma cells inhibits the replication associated function of SV40 large T antigen. *Cell Growth Differ* 2:297, 1991.

143. Sasabe T, Inana G. Mechanism of suppression of malignancy in hybrids between Y79 retinoblastoma and NIH3T3 cells. *Invest Ophthalmol Vis Sci* 32:2011, 1991.

11

METASTASES

Richard R. Dubielzig, Robin L. Grendahl, James C. Orcutt,
Nasreen A. Syed, and Kenneth B. Simons

ANIMALS

Historical Perspective. Lymphosarcoma, which is the most common secondary tumor in the globe of dogs and cats, is covered separately in the next chapter. Disease caused by metastasis to the globe is relatively rare in veterinary medicine. When they do occur, these tumors present unique challenges in both diagnosis and treatment. Veterinary ophthalmologists, oncologists, and general practitioners need to be aware of the consequences and significance of ocular metastasis from distant tumor sites. Not uncommonly, metastatic tumors to the eye will present as ocular disease prior to the detection of the primary tumor. In other cases, the primary tumor may already be known, and treatment may be in progress before ocular metastasis becomes a problem. The significance, prognosis, and treatment of the ocular disease will vary considerably depending on when in the sequence of events the ocular metastasis becomes apparent. Awareness of the likelihood of ocular metastasis may be important in the follow-up or staging of systemic cancer to oncologists.

In humans, clinical disease associated with ocular metastasis is rare. A survey of 8712 patients treated with radiation therapy in 1944 uncovered only six cases of ocular metastasis.[1] More recent studies using more sophisticated examination techniques have shown that a relatively high proportion of patients with metastatic cancer and particularly metastatic breast cancer have ocular metastases. In 1980, a study of 250 patients with a metastatic breast tumor showed that 27% had ocular metastases.[2] Postmortem studies of people with metastatic breast cancer have shown that a high proportion have metastatic lesions in the uveal tract, with the cases of choroidal metastasis far outnumbering anterior uveal metastases.[3,4] Histologic examination seems to uncover cases of micrometastases that may not have been apparent on clinical evaluation.

Although little is known about the epidemiology and the incidence of metastatic disease in dogs and cats, from the small number of cases seen by the author (R.R.D.) and reported in the literature, there does appear to be a higher risk of mammary carcinoma and hemangiosarcoma in dogs and pulmonary carcinoma in cats. Dogs tend to show a higher proportion of ciliary body and iridal metastases, whereas cats more commonly have choroidal metastases.

Epidemiology. In humans, approximately 50% of tumors metastatic to the globe are breast carcinomas.[5] Pulmonary carcinoma is the second most likely metastatic tumor,[3,4] and interestingly malignancies of the gastrointestinal (GI) tract are underrepresented in studies of ocular metastasis.[6] Case reports or small series have been described with ocular metastasis from a wide variety of different primary sites.

The author (R.R.D.) has examples of 23 cases in dogs and 14 cases in cats. An additional 16 cases have been reported in the literature in dogs[7–15] and six cases in cats.[15–21] Combining these numbers in dogs, there are a total of nine cases of mammary carcinoma with metastasis to the globe, and six cases of hemangiosarcoma as well as four cases of nasal carcinoma with metastasis by direct extension. There are three cases of oral melanoma and anaplastic carcinoma, and two each of osteosarcoma, anaplastic sarcoma, transitional cell carcinoma, and thyroid carcinoma. Solitary cases of endometrial carcinoma, pulmonary carcinoma, renal carcinoma, seminoma, and pancreatic carcinoma have been seen. In cats, there are six cases of pulmonary carcinoma and three of anaplastic carcinoma. There are three cases each of mammary carcinoma and squamous cell carcinoma, and two each of endometrial carcinoma and anaplastic sarcoma. Additionally, one case of sweat gland carcinoma has been reported. In dogs, 18 of 20 cases with localized tumor, metastatic disease was found in the ciliary body (Figure 11.1), whereas, in cats, 10 of 14 cases were choroidal (Figure 11.2).

It has been suggested that the choroidal metastases are more likely to be diagnosed in humans because features such as blurred vision and visual field deficits are more likely to be reported early in the disease process and less likely to be detected in animals. The disparity between the incidence of anterior uveal and posterior uveal metastasis between cats and dogs is less easy to explain. Experimental studies in rabbits suggest that local tissue factors account for the predilection for the anterior uveal tract in metastasis.[22]

Clinical Features. Metastatic ocular cancer may present a challenge to diagnosticians, especially when the ocular disease manifests prior to the discovery of the primary cancer. Some cases of metastatic cancer will present as primary mass lesions in the globe, in which case the treatment and prognosis may be greatly different for primary and secondary ocular tumors. With the exception of diffuse iris melanoma[23] and posttraumatic sarcoma in cats,[24] primary intraocular tumors in dogs and cats are unlikely to have life-threatening consequences. As a result, aggressive therapy for the ocular disease might present options that would salvage the function and appearance of the globe.[25] Enucleation may also be elected for primary tumors with the expectation that the animal will live a long and healthy life following surgery. Animals with solitary tumors metastatic to the globe, however, may have widespread systemic disease, and life-threatening consequences of neoplasia may be eminent. In these cases, dramatic therapy to restore vision or even to remove the globe may be contraindicated.

Ocular neoplasia, both primary and secondary, needs to be considered in all cases where there is unexplained glaucoma, intraocular hemorrhage, uveitis, or retinal detachment. The presence of a discernible mass may be obscured by opacification of the ocular media. Ultrasonography is useful in detecting mass lesions; however, the distinction

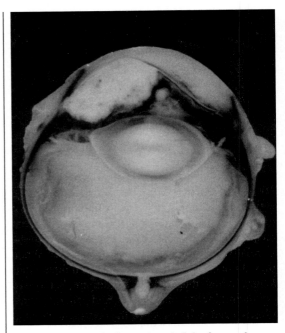

FIG. 11.1—A vertically sectioned globe from a dog with metastatic mammary carcinoma distorting the iris.

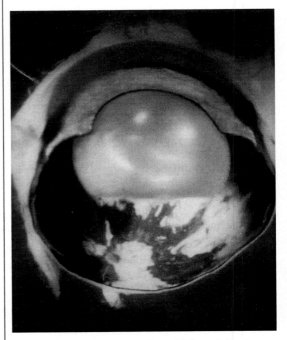

FIG. 11.2—A vertically sectioned feline globe shows angular regional retinal atrophy secondary to choroidal infarction caused by metastatic bronchial carcinoma.

among benign, malignant, inflammatory proliferative disease, or proliferative consequences of trauma, may be difficult. Because of the risk of malignant neoplasia, it is usually recommended that blind eyes with cloudy media be removed and submitted for histopathologic evaluation. If cosmetic scleral implants are to be used, then the ocular contents should be submitted for histopathologic evaluation. In all cases, prior to surgical treatment for suspected or known ocular neoplasia, appropriate radiography for detection of tumor at distant sites should be performed. The mammary glands, oral cavity, and lymph nodes should be examined carefully.

Morphology. Metastatic tumors to the globe may be solitary mass lesions in a relatively quiet eye; however, more often, these tumors are complicated mass lesions with hemorrhage, exudation, inflammation, or diffuse or multifocal involvement. Histologically, anaplastic mammary carcinomas offer little morphologic evidence of the origin of the primary tumor, and the body, with special consideration of the mammary gland and associated lymph nodes, needs to be evaluated carefully to verify the primary diagnosis. Cases of hemangiosarcoma involving the uveal tract appear only as intraocular hemorrhage on gross examination. Even histologically, identification of the neoplasm can be problematic. However, careful examination of the ciliary body stroma often demonstrates the typical histologic features of anaplastic mesenchymal cells tending to form fully developed vascular channels.

In cats with pulmonary carcinoma with metastasis of the choroid, the primary tumor can range from a large obvious neoplasm to small foci in the anterior lung lobes and thus can be difficult to detect radiographically. Pulmonary carcinomas have a strong tendency to infiltrate in blood vessels, and orbital and choroidal vascular invasion is the most common consequence. Choroidal infarction with angular areas of retinal atrophy are seen in otherwise quiet globes in some cases. Choroidal involvement and poor vascular profusion to the distal extremities are other consequences. Pain and scruffiness of the toes often coexist with ocular disease in affected cats. Histologically, the vasoinvasive tumors can be very well differentiated. Examples of stratified squamous epithelial or ciliated columnar epithelial with or without mucous secretion can be found. When tumors break out of the blood vessel, desmoplasia and invasive epithelial neoplasia are seen. Since the primary pulmonary tumor can easily be missed, some of the cases diagnosed as squamous cell carcinoma actually might be pulmonary carcinoma.[26]

Treatment and Prognosis. Treatment and prognosis of metastatic ocular cancer depend on the accurate diagnosis of the disease process. In all cases where ocular neoplasia is observed or suspected, the physical examination should include evaluation of organ systems known to be associated with intraocular metastasis. These include the mammary glands, oral cavity, systemic lymph nodes, and pulmonary radiography. The evaluation of the spleen, liver, and heart for hemangiosarcoma is useful in animals with a visible intraocular mass and no detectable primary. A clinician may choose to treat this as a primary ocular tumor and select an appropriate treatment modality to preserve the globe or its function or cosmetic appearance. Surgical or excisional laser ablation or cryosurgery may be elected to remove the mass. Wherever possible, tissue should be harvested for histopathologic evaluation. In cases where the mass is more extensive, evisceration with implantation of an intrascleral prosthesis is not recommended because of the likelihood of reoccurrence of even a benign neoplasm. Because most canine primary intraocular melanomas pose little danger of life-threatening disease, enucleation is usually considered to be curative. Practitioners must always keep the possibility of metastatic tumor in mind, and nucleated globes should always be submitted for histopathologic evaluation.

Cases in which a solitary mass is not observed present clinicians with a treatment dilemma. Globes that are visually impaired or painful with opaque media should be evaluated for intraocular or periocular neoplasia. Ultrasonography and radiography, and computed tomography (CT) or magnetic resonance imaging (MRI), might be variable. In cases where there is a blind eye with opaque media, enucleation with careful histopathologic evaluation is recommended to obtain a primary diagnosis. The risk of malignant neoplasia is important to exclude these cases. In some cases with retinal detachment or localized choroidal invasion, the primary disease may not be diagnosed on the initial evaluation. Frequent follow-up evaluations to monitor the course of disease may be necessary before the presence of malignant disease becomes manifest.

The therapy for systemic malignancy in animals is too broad a subject to be covered in this chapter. More is being learned all the time about effective therapy for systemic malignancies in dogs and cats. The appropriate systemic therapeutic regimen for malignant neoplasms is the domain of veterinary oncologists, and referral of affected animals is recommended where treatment to prolong life expectancy is sought.

HUMAN METASTATIC AND SECONDARY NEOPLASMS OF THE ORBIT

Tumors of the orbit may arise directly from orbital tissues (primary), invade from adjacent structures (secondary), or proliferate in the orbit after metastases from remote sites (metastatic). Secondary tumors may be either malignant or benign, but metastatic tumors by definition are malignant.

This chapter describes the more frequently encountered metastatic and secondary tumors of the orbit. Secondary lesions that originate from the lacrimal sac, globe, conjunctiva, and eyelid skin are described elsewhere. Primary orbital tumors are described in Chapter 1.

Human Metastatic Neoplasms of the Orbit. The orbit lacks normal lymphatic channels; therefore, metastatic tumors must reach the orbit via hematogenous routes. A distinction should be made between true hematogenously spread malignancies and lymphoid tumors that may be part of disseminated, systemic lymphoma or occur as a solitary lymphoid lesion in the orbit.[26]

Since Horner's original description of generalized carcinomatosis involving the orbit in 1864,[27] orbital metastases are increasing in reported frequency. The number of reports has grown substantially during the past 20 years.[28] This finding probably reflects extended survival among cancer patients due to modern treatment modalities, improved methods of diagnosis, and a greater index of suspicion for orbital metastases.

The relative prevalence of metastatic orbital tumors among patients with orbital disease varies. Shields and coworkers[29] biopsied 645 orbital masses; 16 (2.5%) were due to metastases from distant sites. Among 300 patients with proptosis, Silva[30] reported seven (2.3 %) with biopsy-proven metastatic orbital tumors. A retrospective pathologic review of 222 orbital tumors described 13 cases (5.9%) of metastases.[31] Rootman et al.[32] found that metastatic disease comprised 10.5% of all orbital tumors in a series of patients at the University of British Columbia.

The reported prevalence of orbital metastases among patients with known cancer elsewhere is approximately 2%.[33,34] In a series of 230 patients with known carcinoma, postmortem examination revealed five (2.3%) with metastatic orbital involvement and 23 (10%) with ocular involvement.[33]

Uveal metastases appear to be more common than those involving the orbit.[33,34] The relative frequency of intraocular to orbital metastases has been reported by several authors to range from 1:1 to 8:1.[28] Font and Ferry[35] reviewed 227 cases of metastatic carcinoma to the eye and orbit; only 28 cases of orbital metastases were reported. However, Albert et al.[36] found an equal number of ocular (five) and orbital (five) tumors in their series of 213 patients with known malignancies elsewhere.

Major surveys of orbital metastases have shown that, overall, breast, lung, prostate, GI, and renal cell carcinomas represent the largest groups of primary tumors from which orbital metastases arise. Cases in which the primary tumor is unknown also comprise a significant proportion of metastases. Furthermore, differences with regard to the site of primary neoplasm exist between children and adults. Among children, metastases typically arise from sarcomas and embryonal neural tumors.[26,36,37] Neuroblastoma, Ewing's sarcoma, and Wilms' tumor are the most common. By contrast, carcinomas predominate among adults. Table 11.1 summarizes findings of the major surveys of orbital metastases.

The site of primary neoplasm also varies depending on sex. The overall incidence of metastatic orbital involvement is greater among women because breast carcinoma is overwhelmingly the most common primary site for orbital metastases. Men exclusively experience

TABLE 11.1—Major surveys of orbital metastases

	Breast	Lung	Prostate	Gastrointestinal	Unknown	Other
Forrest[31]	3/13			1/13	3/13	6/13[b]
Hart[5,a]	5/14	5/14	0	0	4/14	0
Font and Ferry[35,a]	8/28	4/28	1/28	1/28	10/28	4/28[c]
Albert et al.[34,35,a]	3/5	1/5	1/5	0	0	0
Rootman et al.[32]	12/29	2/29	3/29	4/29	3/29	5/29[d]
Henderson[41]	19/41	6/41	0	2/41	1/41	13/41[e]
Shields et al.[38]	18/34	2/34	6/34	2/34	4/34	2/34[f]
Shields et al.[29]	12/16	1/16	2/16	1/16	1/16	0
Char (1986)	2/16	1/16	0	1/16	4/16	8/16[g]
Freedman and Folk[4,a]	26/54	3/54	4/54	2/54	4/54	14/54
Goldberg et al.[28]	13/38	2/38	4/38	3/38	3/38	13/38[h]

[a] Children not included.
[b] Six cases of neuroblastoma in children.
[c] Two renal cell carcinoma (Ca), 1 testicular Ca, and 1 pancreatic Ca.
[d] One cutaneous melanoma, 1 thyroid Ca, 1 liposarcoma, and 1 neuroblastoma.
[e] Seven neuroblastoma, 1 cutaneous melanoma, 1 hemangiopericytoma, 2 thyroid Ca, and 2 adrenal gland neoplasms.
[f] One cutaneous melanoma and 1 choroidal melanoma.
[g] One pheochromocytoma, 1 renal cell Ca, 3 neuroblastoma, 2 cutaneous melanoma, and 1 contralateal uveal melanoma.
[h] One Ca, 1 fibrosarcoma, 1 liposarcoma, 5 cutaneous melanoma, 1 neuroblastoma, 1 uterine Ca, 1 ovarian Ca, 1 pancreatic Ca, and 1 squamous cell Ca.

prostate cancer and also have a higher rate of GI, renal, and lung carcinoma.[26]

Orbital metastases may precede detection of a primary tumor elsewhere. Among 28 metastatic orbital tumors, Font and Ferry[35] noted 17 cases in which orbital involvement was detected before the primary neoplasm. Many patients fail to offer a prior history of cancer, especially when temporally remote. Careful documentation of the history is therefore essential in evaluating orbital tumors.

Clinical findings frequently observed include diplopia, proptosis, palpable mass, blepharoptosis, pain, conjunctival chemosis, visual loss, eyelid edema, strabismus, and epiphora.[38] Optic atrophy, choroidal folds, nasolacrimal duct obstruction and enophthalmos have been reported as well. Presentation at the time of diagnosis varies depending on the primary tumor and site of metastases. Enophthalmos caused by scirrhous breast carcinoma, and ecchymosis due to neuroblastoma, are specific findings helpful in diagnosis. Pain may be a prominent symptom in prostate carcinoma. Renal and thyroid carcinoma may present with orbital pulsations due to tumor vascularity or erosion through the orbital roof. Orbital metastases usually progress rapidly. Exceptions include breast and prostate carcinoma, which may demonstrate a more indolent course.

Diagnosis of metastatic orbital disease is facilitated through imaging studies, either CT or MRI.

Biopsy is usually necessary, but sometimes there is little histologic resemblance to the primary tumor. Histopathology, immunohistochemistry, and electron microscopy are helpful in determining the cells of origin. Tissue handling in anticipation of special tests must be considered and communicated to the pathologist before biopsy is undertaken.

The management of metastatic tumors is ideally approached through a multispecialty team of physicians that includes an ophthalmologist, an otolaryngologist, a head and neck surgeon, a neurosurgeon, a pathologist, a medical oncologist, and a radiation oncologist, often coordinated through a tumor board.

The following metastatic tumors will be discussed in detail: breast carcinoma, bronchogenic carcinoma, prostate carcinoma, neuroblastoma, GI carcinoma, and renal cell carcinoma.

BREAST CARCINOMA

EPIDEMIOLOGY. Breast carcinoma occurs in one of nine women in the United States,[37] accounting for 20% of cancer deaths among women, and 42% of all metastatic orbital disease originates from it. Among women, it is the most common primary malignancy that metastasizes to the eye and orbit.[4,28]

Orbital metastases from breast carcinoma most often occur in the fifth decade, and the majority of women have a history of breast cancer treatment.[32,39,40] Additionally, virtually all patients have other areas of dissemination by the time orbital disease is discovered. The interval from initial diagnosis of breast cancer to presentation with orbital metastases has been reported to be as long as 27 years,[4,40,41] with a mean interval of 4.5–7.6 years.[4,28,39,42]

Clinical Features. Clinical presentation varies depending on the cellular type of breast carcinoma and location of orbital involvement. The characteristic presentation consists of firm infiltration of the orbit, restricted extraocular movements, and ptosis. Proptosis may occur if the lesion is located posteriorly, whereas a palpable mass is apparent if the location is more anterior. Enophthalmos is frequently found with metastatic scirrhous breast carcinoma due to diffuse orbital infiltration, immobilization of the globe, and posterior retraction[26] (Figure 11.3A). Infiltration with restrictive ophthalmoplegia may progress until the globe becomes fixed or "frozen." Initially, the uninvolved eye may be incorrectly diagnosed with proptosis. Cline and Rootman[43] reviewed 26 cases of enophthalmos. Four were due to orbital metastases, three of which were metastatic scirrhous carcinoma. The fourth case was a desmoplastic carcinoma from an unknown primary site.

Diagnosis of metastatic breast carcinoma should be suspected in women who present with orbital symptoms and a history of breast cancer. Workup includes complete ophthalmologic evaluation with a dilated fundus examination to rule out more commonly encountered choroidal metastases. Orbital ultrasonography may confirm orbital involvement, but CT better depicts the size and extent of a lesion. The tumor usually appears diffuse with irregular borders on CT and may mold to adjacent orbital structures such as the sclera and bone (Figure 11.3B). In most cases, involvement is confined to soft tissues, with only occasional destruction of adjacent bone. Orbital biopsy is helpful and may be approached through a subciliary or lid-crease incision if located anterior to the equator. Tumors with a more posterior location may be biopsied either with fine-needle aspiration or orbitotomy.

MORPHOLOGY. Breast carcinoma can arise from either the ductal (90%) or lobular (10%) epithelium. Both infiltrating and noninfiltrating forms are found originating from the breast epithelial tissues. The most common form of breast cancer is the infiltrating ductal or "scirrhous" carcinoma, which accounts for roughly 75% of all breast carcinomas.[38]

Intraductal adenocarcinoma is the most common type of breast carcinoma that metastasizes to the orbit.[32] Some tumors resemble the primary neoplasm with differentiation into papillary-like growths that remain confined to intraductal structures and individual lobules. Orcutt et al.[44] described a case of ductal carcinoma that histopathologically revealed malignant cells forming linear single-file rows. The cells had eosinophilic cytoplasm and small hyperchromatic nuclei (Figure 11.3C).

Others tumors show little tendency to organize in such fashion and are highly invasive and anaplastic. Some are metaplastic with colloid- and mucus-secreting cells, squamous cells, and signet-ring cells.[45] Still other tumors may appear "histiocytoid" with large rounded cells resembling histiocytes. Unlike true histiocytes, these have a tendency to form a single-file arrangement and contain cytoplasmic mucinous vacuoles. This variant is often cicatricial with significant associated inflammation.[38]

Reifler and Davison[45] described a case of orbital metastatic lobular carcinoma that was histologically similar to a tumor concomitantly biopsied from the breast. Microscopically, there was diffuse infiltration of small carcinoma cells arranged concentrically around ducts. The cells had pale-staining cytoplasm and occasional fine vacuolization.

Due to histologic variation and poor differentiation frequently observed with metastatic breast carcinoma, it may be impossible to determine whether a tumor is of breast, lung, or GI origin. Immunocytochemistry greatly enhances diagnosis. GCDFP-15 is a mesenchymal specific antibody that defines a membrane-associated glycoprotein specific for breast, salivary, and sweat gland epithelium. It can be used to distinguish metastatic breast carcinoma from other poorly differentiated adenocarcinomas such as those

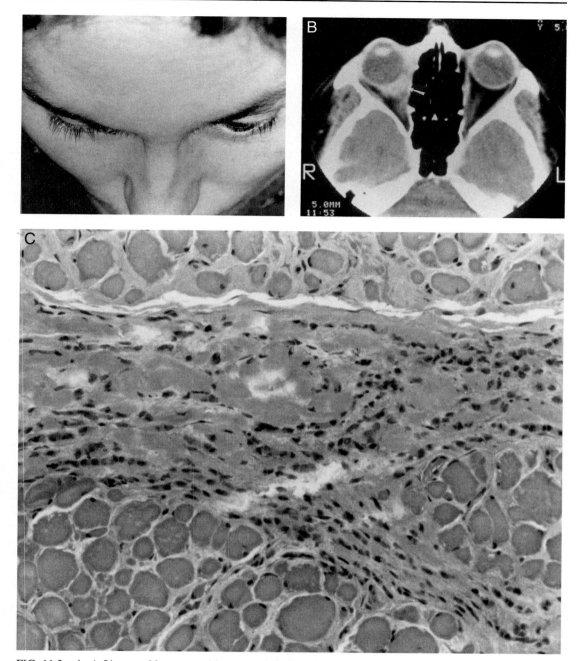

FIG. 11.3—**A:** A 51-year-old woman with metastatic infiltrating ductal breast carcinoma metastatic to the right orbit presented with a 6-month history of binocular diplopia and right enophthalmos. **B:** Orbital computed tomography shows an infiltrating mass (arrow) surrounding the right globe without bone involvement. **C:** The transseptal biopsy specimen shows fibroconnective tissue and muscle infiltrated by linear rows of malignant cells. (continued)

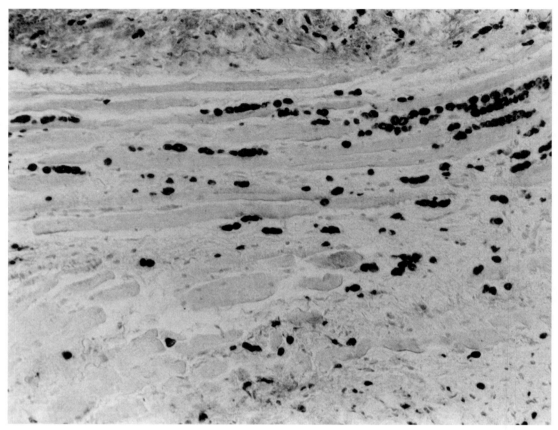

FIG. 11.3 (continued)—**D:** Immunocytochemical localization of low molecular weight cytokeratins within tumor cells. High molecular weight cytokeratins were also present.

originating from the lung or GI tract.[46] Additionally, cytokeratins (intermediate filament proteins) help to distinguish ductal breast carcinoma. Cytokeratins are a group of cytoplasmic intermediate filaments that can be divided into two general groups: "high" and "low" molecular weight cytokeratins. The pattern of reactivity to these two cytokeratin groups can define the cells of origin in a tumor as squamous (high molecular weight +; low molecular weight –), ductal (high molecular weight +; low molecular weight +), or simple (high molecular weight –; low molecular weight +)[46] (Figure 11.3D). Ductal breast carcinoma can, therefore, be differentiated from other carcinomas. Electron microscopy, although not specific, may show intracytoplasmic lumina and secretory granules.[32]

TREATMENT AND PROGNOSIS. Treatment possibilities for metastatic breast carcinoma include a combination of radiation, hormonal therapy, and chemotherapy. Prognosis for long-term survival is poor because orbital metastases are never the only metastatic site, and treatment is directed toward palliation of symptoms. In a study of 37 patients with metastatic disease to the orbit, 23 had metastatic breast carcinoma;[47] the median survival after completion of radiation treatment was 8.5 months.

Radiation therapy for metastatic disease is usually combined with hormonal manipulation or chemotherapy. The optimum amount of radiation is approximately 3000–4000 rad delivered in fractionated doses over a 3- to 4-week period.[47]

Hormonal manipulation is the first line of treatment for patients with receptor-positive tumors. The estrogen and progesterone receptor status in primary breast carcinoma is a useful prognostic indicator and serves to guide hormonal manipulation. Bullock and Yanes[42] were the first to demonstrate the presence of estrogen receptors in patients with breast carcinoma metastatic to the orbit. Later, Reifler and Davison[45] demonstrated the presence of both estradiol and progesterone receptors in infiltrating lobular carcinoma metastatic to the orbit. Approximately 50%–60% of women with breast tumors containing estrogen receptors respond favorably to endocrine therapy, whereas fewer than 15% of women with breast tumors lacking estrogen receptors have a favorable response.[48] In premenopausal patients, oophorectomy is the preferred method of endocrine manipulation, whereas tamoxifen is used to treat postmenopausal women. Medical adrenalectomy and treatment with androgens have also been advocated.

Serial measurements of serum carcinoembryonic antigen (CEA) have been followed in cases of metastatic breast carcinoma.[42] However, CEA levels may be normal and are less useful than steroid receptor status determination in the evaluation and treatment of women with breast carcinoma.[45]

Breast carcinoma is a chemosensitive tumor. Treatment of metastatic breast cancer with chemotherapeutic agents is indicated when patients experience rapidly progressive systemic dissemination. In most instances where chemotherapy is employed, estrogen receptor status is normal. A commonly employed regimen includes a combination of cyclophosphamide, methotrexate, fluorouracil, and prednisone.[32]

BRONCHOGENIC CARCINOMA

EPIDEMIOLOGY. Bronchogenic carcinoma is the number one deadly cancer in industrialized countries, and this is primarily due to the high prevalence of smoking.[49] Its peak incidence occurs between the ages of 40 and 70. The male-to-female ratio is 2:1, yet the incidence of lung cancer among women is rapidly increasing. Bronchogenic carcinoma is the most common primary neoplasm that metastasizes to the orbit in men.[4]

CLINICAL FEATURES. In contrast to breast carcinoma, lung cancer tends to metastasize early, reflecting the rapid growth and aggressive behavior of bronchogenic carcinoma.[4] Compared with most metastases, a shorter interval between diagnosis of the primary tumor and clinical evidence of metastatic disease is observed. Additionally, there are relatively more cases in which the primary malignancy is unknown at the time of metastatic presentation. Most patients present with a rapidly expanding orbital mass and globe displacement.[32] A pattern of infiltration is much less common with metastatic bronchogenic carcinoma, and enophthalmos is rarely seen.

Bronchogenic carcinoid is a neuroendocrine variant that carries a better long-term prognosis than bronchogenic carcinoma. With most cases of carcinoid metastases to the orbit, the primary tumor originates in the bronchus. Riddle et al.[50] reported 15 cases of carcinoid tumor metastatic to the eye or orbit, eight of which were of bronchial origin. Carcinoid syndrome, characterized by flushing, diarrhea, salivation, lacrimation, and respiratory wheezing, is due to elevated levels of serotonin and other bioactive amines liberated by a large tumor load. The syndrome rarely occurs in the setting of isolated orbital metastases; it more commonly occurs among patients with extensive hepatic metastatic disease.[51,52] Diagnosis of metastatic bronchogenic carcinoma is suggested when a middle-aged to elderly man with an extensive cigarette-smoking history presents with rapidly progressive proptosis or an orbital mass. If there is no history of lung cancer, a systemic workup for malignancy, including a chest radiograph, is indicated (Figure 11.4B).

Orbital imaging usually reveals a poorly marginated mass that is relatively dense compared with orbital fat and optic nerve, and isodense with the extraocular muscles (Figure 11.4A). CT may also demonstrate a relatively circumscribed mass with necrosis and calcifications.[32] Open biopsy and fine-needle aspiration biopsy (FNAB) facilitate diagnosis, but metastatic bronchogenic carcinoma is often poorly differentiated by the time it metastasizes to the orbit.

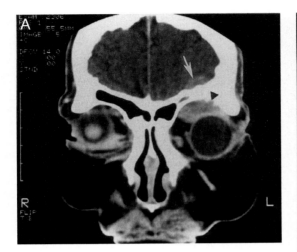

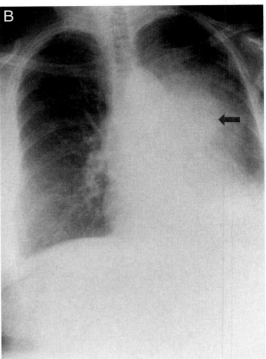

FIG. 11.4—Bronchogenic carcinoma. **A:** Orbital computed tomography of a 64-year-old woman shows an enhancing mass in the superior extraconal space of the left orbit indenting the globe. The scalloped appearance of bone indicates metaplastic bone reformation (arrowhead) with erosion through the orbital roof into the frontal sinus and epidural space (arrow). **B:** Chest radiograph shows a large, primary tumor involving the left upper lobe (arrow). (continued)

MORPHOLOGY. The most common cell type of bronchogenic neoplasm is adenocarcinoma, followed closely by squamous cell carcinoma, small cell carcinoma, and "mixed" forms.[49] Owing to its propensity for early metastasis and widespread dissemination at the time of diagnosis,[49] undifferentiated small cell carcinoma is the most common pathologic type of lung carcinoma metastasizing to the orbit.[32] Histologically, small cell carcinoma is composed of densely packed, small round or spindle-shaped cells that show poor differentiation and basophilic nuclei. Cells resemble lymphocytes, and this particular morphology is referred to as small blue cells (Figure 11.4C), the differential diagnosis of which includes lymphoma, neuroblastoma, idiopathic lymphoproliferative pseudotumor, rhabdomyosarcoma, and Ewing's sarcoma. Special techniques are often required to establish a precise diagnosis. Electron microscopy demonstrates neurosecretory dense-core granules.[28,32] Small cell carcinoma is also the variant most frequently associated with the elaboration of bioactive substances capable of inciting paraneoplastic syndromes.[49] Compared with small cell carcinoma, adenocarcinoma has a much lower incidence of orbital metastases. Neoplastic cells are generally cuboidal to columnar, frequently produce mucin,[49] and show cytoplasmic inclusions histologically and by electron microscopy.[28] Tumors often closely resemble breast or GI carcinoma. Immunohistochemical evaluation of high and low molecular weight cytokeratins may help to differentiate this tumor. Adenocarcinoma is typically positive for low molecular weight cytokeratins and negative for high molecular weight cytokeratins, whereas breast carcinoma is positive for both.[44]

Bronchial carcinoids, which arise from the Kulchitsky cells in the bronchial mucosa, rarely metastasize to the orbit. Although approximately 95% of carcinoid tumors arise in the GI tract,[52] the majority that metastasize to the orbit and eye are of bronchial origin.[50,53,54] Metastases typically retain recognizable

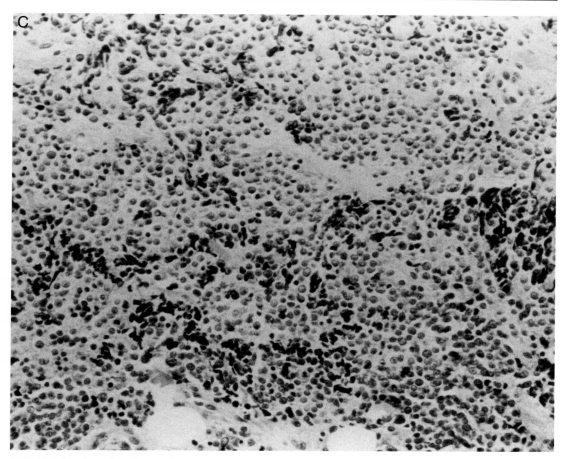

FIG. 11.4 (continued)—**C:** The biopsy specimen shows fibrous connective tissue infiltrated by sheets of poorly differentiated small cells, compatible with a metastatic small cell carcinoma from the lung.

histologic features resembling the primary tumor.[50] Carcinoid tumors have been called argentaffinomas because their cells contain neurosensory argyrophilic granules that are associated with the production of 5-hydroxyindoleacetic acid (5-HIAA). Silver stains and electron microscopy highlight the presence of the neurosensory granules. Additionally, 5-HIAA may be detected in the urine. Immunoperoxidase staining is reactive with antibodies against neuron-specific enolase, cytokeratin, synaptophysin, and chromogranin.[44,55]

TREATMENT AND PROGNOSIS. Treatment for metastatic lung carcinoma is primarily palliative, as only 1%–2% of patients with disseminated disease at diagnosis achieve lasting remissions. Correct diagnosis is essential for management because different treatment regimens are employed for small and non-small cell carcinomas.

Treatment with radiotherapy plus a combination chemotherapeutic regimen is recommended for small cell carcinoma metastatic to the orbit. Non-small cell carcinomas do not respond as well to chemotherapy, and patients with these tumors should be treated with palliative radiation. Treatment of carcinoid tumors metastatic to the orbit has not been well established. In general, lesions should be resected when possible. In cases where complete local resection cannot be achieved, radiation treatment has been advocated.[26]

PROSTATE CARCINOMA

EPIDEMIOLOGY. Prostatic carcinoma is the second leading cause of cancer-related death among men aged 50–75 years. The incidence, estimated to be 19% of all cancer in men, is second only to lung cancer.[56] Orbital metastases from prostate carcinoma are rare. In a series of 28 patients with tumors metastatic to the orbit, only one case of prostate carcinoma was observed.[35] Although rare, a review by Freedman and Folk[4] ranked prostatic carcinoma as the third most common known metastatic tumor involving the orbit.

Affected patients are usually men in their 70s. The peak age occurrence is older and the clinical progression is typically slower when compared with other types of orbital metastatic disease, reflecting the indolent nature of prostate carcinoma. Many patients have a history of prostate carcinoma, yet orbital involvement may be the initial presenting feature in some cases.

CLINICAL FEATURES. Patients frequently present with diplopia, exophthalmos, eyelid swelling, and decreased visual acuity.[57] Pain may be a more prominent feature of metastatic prostate carcinoma, owing to its propensity for bony metastases. Additionally, the ratio of orbital to ocular involvement is higher than other tumors and is probably due to metastatic involvement of orbital bone.

Bony lesions are characteristically osteoblastic. Although osteolytic lesions have been described, osteolysis usually occurs more commonly in the advanced stages.[57,58] Orbital spread can also involve soft tissue and may be seen as an expanding or cicatrizing lesion.[32] CT of osteoblastic lesions demonstrates new bone deposition and an increase in bone volume with irregular borders (Figure 11.5A).

Workup of suspected cases includes orbital CT, prostate examination, chest radiograph, bone scan, and determination of serum acid phosphatase and prostate–specific antigen levels. Acid phosphatase, which is normally released into the blood in small quantities by the prostate, can be markedly elevated in cases of advanced disease. In cases where primary prostate carcinoma is established, patients may not need orbital biopsy. However, if the diagnosis remains unclear after evaluation, orbital biopsy is helpful in establishing the diagnosis.

MORPHOLOGY. Adenocarcinoma is the most common histologic form of prostate carcinoma. Tumors may closely resemble the primary neoplasm, displaying small, closely spaced acini lined by a single layer of cuboidal epithelium. The neoplastic epithelium may be thrown into folds, imparting a cribriform pattern. The stroma between the glands is sometimes abundant and fibrous (Figure 11.5B). Individual cells display typical cytologic features of malignancy[56] and may contain mucin in intracytoplasmic vacuoles.[32] Occasionally, the orbital lesion is poorly differentiated and further analysis is necessary to establish diagnosis.

Histochemical markers and immunoperoxidase techniques are extremely helpful and can be readily employed with specimens from FNAB. Cell staining with the peroxidase-antiperoxidase method demonstrates yellowish brown intracytoplasmic precipitates,[59] indicating the presence of androgen receptors, thus confirming the diagnosis. Prostate-specific antigens (PSAs) are found normally in the cytoplasm of prostatic acinar ductal epithelium and can be demonstrated in benign hypertrophic as well as in malignant tissue. Staining for the presence of PSA by the immunoperoxidase technique may further aid in diagnosis (Figure 11.5C). Prostatic-specific acid phosphatase is an enzyme found in prostate tissue and can also be used to mark lesions originating from prostate origin.[60] However, it may not be as tissue specific as PSA. Prostatic-specific acid phosphatase has been found in other tissues, such as pancreatic islet cells, granulocytes,[61] and in seminal vesicular tissue.[62]

TREATMENT AND PROGNOSIS. Management of orbital metastases consists of hormonal manipulation and radiotherapy in an effort to produce palliation of symptoms. Treatment does not alter survival; the 5-year survival rate for patients with metastatic carcinoma is 25%, with only 10% surviving 10 years.[63]

The aim of endocrine manipulation is to deprive tumor cells of testosterone. This is readily achieved by orchiectomy or administration of estrogens (diethylstilbestrol) or synthetic agonists of luteinizing hormone-releasing hormone (LHRH).[56] Up to 40% of patients have complete or partial responses, with improvement of status in an additional 35%–40%.[32] Radiation therapy is also quite effective in palliation of symptoms, and doses are similar to those used in the treatment of other orbital metastases (i.e., 3000–4000 cGy in fractionated doses over a period of 3–4 weeks).

NEUROBLASTOMA

EPIDEMIOLOGY. Neuroblastoma is a highly malignant, solid tumor that arises from embryonic, sympathetic neuroblasts.[64] Approximately

60% of neuroblastomas originate from cells located in the abdominal sympathetic chain,[32,65] whereas the remainder arise from the adrenal medulla, ectopic adrenal tissue, or from the cervical or thoracic sympathetic chains.

Neuroblastoma represents 10%–15% of all childhood malignancies[66] and is the most common metastatic orbital lesion in children.[36] Neuroblastoma occurs most frequently in the young pediatric age group, with a median age of 2 years.[67]

In a retrospective review of 405 children with neuroblastoma, Musarella and colleagues[65] reported ophthalmologic involvement in nearly 20%. Ocular manifestations included Horner's syndrome, opsoclonus-myoclonus syndrome, and orbital metastases. These were the initial presenting signs in 33 children (8.1%) with neuroblastoma. Orbital metastases were present in 75% of those with ocular manifestations.

CLINICAL FEATURES. Orbital involvement with neuroblastoma is characterized by sudden onset of rapidly progressive proptosis, eyelid and periorbital swelling, ptosis, and ecchymosis[32] (Figure 11.6A). Ecchymosis results from hemorrhagic necrosis within a rapidly growing tumor that has surpassed its blood supply. The majority of orbital metastases originate from the abdomen[65], and bilateral involvement is observed in 20%–55% of cases.[64,65,68] Metastases directly invade the orbital bones and soft tissue. If the temporal orbit is involved, lytic bone lesions may be seen.[69]

Horner's syndrome occurs when a primary or metastatic tumor involves the cervical sympathetic ganglia. Opsoclonus-myoclonus may result from an antibody directed against a neuroblastoma antigen that cross-reacts with cerebellar tissue.[70] Other ophthalmic manifestations include retinal hemorrhages, dilated retinal veins, optic atrophy, papilledema, and strabismus.

Systemic findings include fever, malaise, and weakness. Catecholamines are liberated by the tumor and, if present in sufficient quantities, may produce flushing, systemic hypertension, and diarrhea.[71] The presence of urinary catecholamine metabolites may be helpful in the diagnosis.

Workup should be facilitated through prompt referral to a pediatric oncologist. CT of the abdomen or chest may demonstrate the primary tumor (Figure 11.6B). Orbital CT commonly shows a large, irregular, poorly circumscribed mass with associated bone destruction (Figure 11.6C). Lytic bone lesions are frequently observed, and lucent areas seen on CT reflect areas of tumor necrosis. Histologic diagnosis is usually required and facilitated through orbital biopsy. Bone scans, bone marrow biopsy, lymph node examination, and chest radiographs establish extent of disease.

MORPHOLOGY. Histologically, the tumor consists of undifferentiated, small round cells with well-defined hyperchromatic nuclei (Figure 11.6D). Cells are arranged into groups, and occasionally Homer Wright rosettes are observed. Mitotic figures and areas of necrosis are common. Electron microscopy may reveal the presence of neurosecretory dense-core vesicles, as well as prominent neurotubules and abortive axon formation.[69] Antibodies to neuron-specific enolase, synaptophysin, and chromogranin A may establish the diagnosis.[72]

TREATMENT AND PROGNOSIS. Treatment is approached through a multidisciplinary team directed by a pediatric oncologist. Chemotherapy is the mainstay of treatment for disseminated disease as well as palliative radiotherapy for periorbital lesions. The primary tumor may require surgical debulking.[69] Innovative approaches to management have included administration of high-dose combination chemotherapy plus supralethal doses of total body irradiation, followed by bone marrow rescue.[32] Outcome is influenced by age, stage, primary tumor site, and ophthalmic findings.[65] Favorable prognostic indicators include female gender, early diagnosis of the primary tumor, presentation before age 2 years, and primary cervical or thoracic location. The 2-year, relapse-free survival rate is 12% in children diagnosed after 2 years of age, and 75% before age 2.[67] Thoracic tumors are more favorable than those originating in the abdomen. Ophthalmic manifestations are closely related to the site and stage of tumor and outcome of the patient.[65] Horner's syndrome and the presence of opsoclonus-myoclonus are frequently associated with localized neuroblastoma. Patients with Horner's syndrome and myoclonus-opsoclonus had a 3-year survival rate of 78.6% and 100%, respectively. Orbital involvement almost always implies disseminated disease. Musarella and coworkers[65] reported an 11.3% 3-year survival rate in children with orbital metastases.

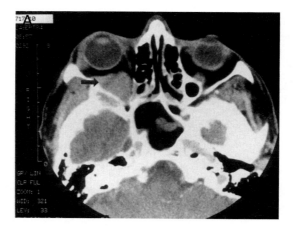

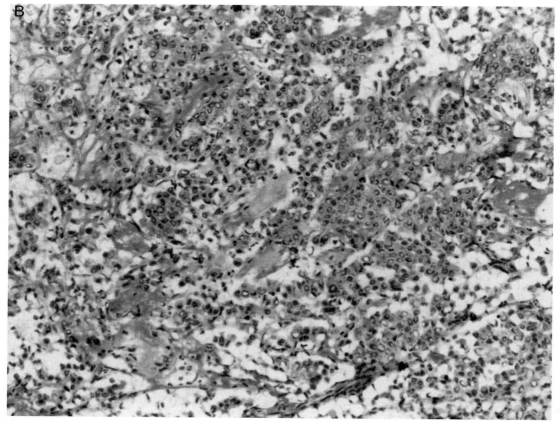

FIG. 11.5—A 76-year-old man with metastatic prostate carcinoma to the right orbit. The patient presented with 4 weeks of binocular diplopia, painless right periorbital swelling, proptosis, and right globe restriction. He had a history of prostate carcinoma that had been treated 4 years previously with radiotherapy. **A:** Computed tomography demonstrates metastatic prostate carcinoma in the posterior lateral orbit with extension into the middle cranial fossa (arrow). **B:** The biopsy specimen of the left orbit shows poorly differentiated prostate tumor with basophilic cells and nuclear pleomorphism. (continued)

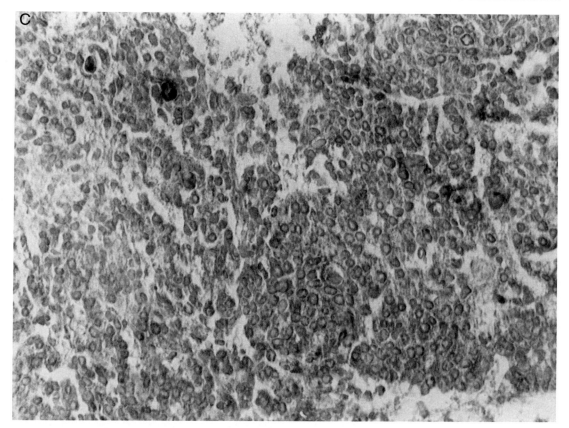

FIG. 11.5 (continued)—**C:** Immunocytochemical localization of prostate-specific antigen within tumor cell cytoplasm.

GASTROINTESTINAL CARCINOMA

EPIDEMIOLOGY. Carcinoma of the alimentary tract, colorectal carcinoma in particular, represents the second leading cause of cancer-associated deaths in the United States.[73] There is a slight male predominance, and presentation is rarely observed prior to age 40. In a combined series of 245 patients with metastatic orbital disease, Goldberg et al.[28] reported a 4.4% prevalence of orbital metastatic GI carcinoma. Overall, metastatic GI carcinoma to the orbit ranked sixth in this series. The majority of GI carcinomas that metastasize to the orbit originate from lower bowel adenocarcinoma and scirrhous carcinoma of the stomach.[32,40] Reports in the literature also describe metastases originating from the esophagus, small intestine, liver, and pancreas.[35,74]

CLINICAL FEATURES. Owing to the occult nature of GI carcinoma, orbital metastases may be the presenting sign of a latent primary neoplasm. Both orbital bone and soft tissue may be involved with metastases, and bony hyperostosis may be evident on CT. Orbital pain is not uncommon, especially if the tumor is mucin secreting.[32] Bilateral orbital involvement has been frequently observed among patients with GI metastases. Scirrhous gastric carcinoma may directly invade the extraocular muscles, causing acquired strabismus.[75]

Orbital imaging and biopsy help in establishing the diagnosis, while CT and imaging of the GI tract, liver, chest, and bones establish the extent of metastases elsewhere. Elevated blood levels of CEA are frequently measured when the tumor burden is significant. However, the CEA level is probably more important in following response to treatment, because a variety of other neoplasms may also produce an elevated CEA level.

MORPHOLOGY. GI neoplasms arise from the glandular structures lining the alimentary canal. Both colorectal adenocarcinoma and scirrhous carcinoma of the stomach may show varying degrees of differentiation into acinar structures and papillary patterns. Due to the undifferentiated nature of GI orbital metastases, diagnosis of the primary tumor may be difficult despite orbital biopsy. Some forms of metastatic gastric carcinoma to the orbit display an infiltrative pattern of neoplastic cells accompanied by a desmoplastic stroma. The presence of signet-ring cells is highly suggestive of gastric carcinoma. These cells contain abundant mucin that fills the cell cytoplasm and displaces the nucleus eccentrically against the cell membrane.[74] Large areas of extracellular mucin may be found as well. In metastatic colorectal adenocarcinoma, cells are arranged into a columnar, glandular pattern and display prominent cytoplasmic mucin formation. Abundant mucinous secretions may be also be observed. Electron microscopy shows tall, columnar cells with luminal brush borders as well as cytoplasmic filamentary webs in the apical regions of the cells.

TREATMENT AND PROGNOSIS. Management of orbital metastases originating from GI carcinoma primarily involves palliation of symptoms. Radiotherapy to the orbit has been the treatment of choice, but improved efficacy with systemic chemotherapy has been observed.[32]

Prognosis is generally poor with both gastric and colorectal carcinoma orbital metastases. Despite treatment, patients usually expire within a few months due to extensive metastatic disease.

RENAL CELL CARCINOMA

EPIDEMIOLOGY. Renal cell carcinoma represents 80%–90% of all malignant tumors of the kidney and 2% of all cancers in adults.[76] It usually presents during the fifth through the seventh decade and shows male predominance. The most common metastatic foci are lung and bone, yet renal cell carcinoma is capable of metastasizing to virtually every site in the body. The orbit and eye, however, are rarely involved. In a combined series of 245 patients with metastatic orbital disease, 17 tumors (3.2%) originated from the kidney.[28]

CLINICAL FEATURES. Renal cell carcinoma is often unpredictable. Wide variations in clinical

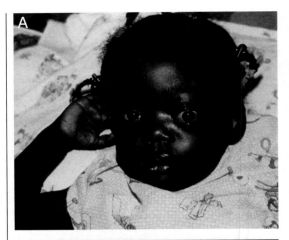

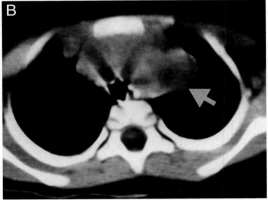

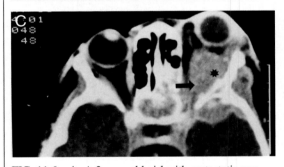

FIG. 11.6—**A:** A 3-year-old girl with metastatic neuroblastoma to the left orbit. **B:** Chest computed tomography shows a large primary neuroblastoma involving the thoracic sympathetic chain ganglion (arrow). **C:** Orbital computed tomography shows a mass (arrow) involving the left orbit, temporal fossa, and frontal lobe of brain. The scalloped appearance of bone indicates metaplastic bone (asterisk) reformation. (continued)

manifestations of orbital involvement are observed and have been confused with chalazion, orbital hemangioma, and melanoma.[77] Like breast carcinoma, a long latency period frequently exists

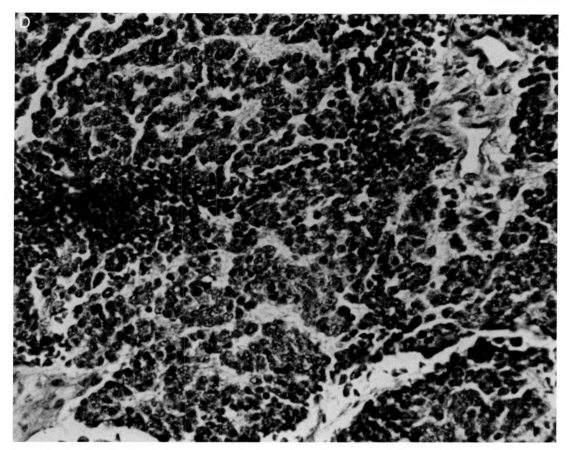

FIG. 11.6 (continued)—**D:** The bone marrow biopsy specimen shows poorly differentiated small cells.

between diagnosis of the primary tumor and manifestations of metastatic disease. Metastases have been noted as long as 25 years after nephrectomy for primary renal cell carcinoma.[78]

Patients usually present with the insidious onset of proptosis and globe displacement. Owing to the vascular nature of this tumor, pulsating exophthalmos may be a prominent feature. Furthermore, extensive orbital bone destruction with secondary central nervous system involvement may allow transmission of cerebral spinal fluid pulsations. Anteriorly located masses may be visible and are capable of severe external hemorrhage. Debulking of orbital metastases should be attempted with caution due to high tumor vascularity.

Diagnosis should be suspected in patients with a remote history of renal cell carcinoma and characteristic orbital findings. Additionally, patients with orbital symptoms alone should be ques-

tioned regarding the presence of hematuria, flank pain, and long-standing fever, as these may herald the presence of renal cell carcinoma. Orbital CT may reveal one or more discrete masses, which reflect this tumor's predilection for producing well-circumscribed, soft tissue lesions (Figure 11.7A and B). Biopsy of the orbital lesion may be necessary to establish the diagnosis. Systemic evaluation including imaging studies of the abdomen, chest, and long bones are important.

MORPHOLOGY. Gross pathologic examination typically shows a well-defined, discrete mass. Lesions are usually encapsulated, and hemorrhages are observed throughout the tumor.[76] Unlike other metastatic tumors to the orbit, renal cell carcinoma displays a highly characteristic histologic pattern. Tumors are composed of clear, round cells arranged into solid nests and

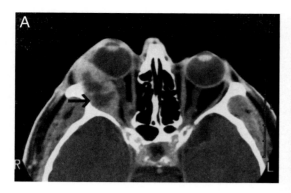
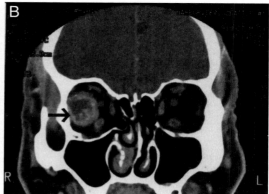
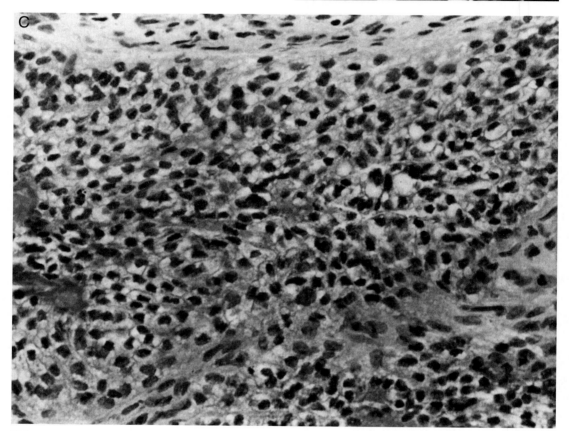

FIG. 11.7—**A:** Axial computed tomography of a 60-year-old man with widely metastatic renal cell carcinoma demonstrates a well-circumscribed mass in the lateral right orbit (arrow). **B:** Coronal computed tomography shows a well-circumscribed mass in the lateral right orbit (arrowhead). **C:** The biopsy specimen shows clear, round cells with abundant cytoplasm arranged into solid nests and surrounded by a fibrovascular stroma, similar to the primary tumor.

regularly compartmentalized by a fibrovascular stroma. Cells contain lipid-laden vacuoles, abundant cytoplasm, and irregularly shaped hyperchromatic nuclei with prominent nucleoli (Figure 11.7C). Glycogen may be a prominent cytoplasmic feature as well, and therefore cells stain positively with the periodic acid-Schiff (PAS) reaction.[79] Electron microscopy shows polyhedral cells with electron-lucent cytoplasm and darkly staining glycogen granules. Scattered mitochondria and sparse rough endoplasmic reticulum are observed.

TREATMENT AND PROGNOSIS. Management of orbital metastasis includes radiation therapy and tumor debulking. Renal cell carcinoma is highly vascular and prone to bleeding, and removal should be avoided in cases where the full extent of the lesion cannot be defined. Angiography to delineate the extent of tumor vascularity with subsequent embolization of feeding vessels has been advocated in severe cases. Decisions regarding surgical management should include consideration of the patient's overall systemic status. Radiotherapy is effective for the palliation of orbital symptoms. Renal cell carcinoma is not responsive to traditional chemotherapeutic modalities, but treatment with interferon and interleukin 2 is under investigation.[32]

The prognosis of metastatic orbital renal cell carcinoma is quite variable. Patients may survive years after presentation with orbital metastases or may succumb to their disease within months due to extensive systemic metastases.

Human Secondary Neoplasms of the Orbit. Secondary neoplasms of the orbit originate from contiguous anatomic areas, i.e., the paranasal sinuses, nasopharynx, conjunctiva, lacrimal sac, intracranial cavity, globe, and skin of the eyelids, nose, and forehead. The most common areas from which tumors invade are the eyelid skin,[29] the globe, and the maxillary and ethmoid sinuses.[40,80]

Malignant lesions directly invade through adjacent bone, whereas benign lesions displace volume into the orbit.[80] The nasolacrimal duct provides a direct route for invasion of nasal lesions, while foramina and fissures may serve as pathways for invasion of intracranial or sinus tumors.

Secondary orbital tumor involvement is more common than metastatic orbital disease. Among 645 orbital lesions biopsied at Wills Eye Hospital, 11% (70 cases) were secondary tumors of the orbit.[29] Tumor sources were intraocular (28 cases), eyelids (27), paranasal sinuses (8), and conjunctiva (7). Forrest[31] observed a similar relative incidence of secondary orbital tumors [20 cases (11%)] among 222 orbital tumors biopsied. Silva,[30] however, obtained orbital biopsies from 300 patients with proptosis and found 123 (41%) secondary orbital tumors. In the Mayo Clinic series (1948–1987), 607 secondary orbital neo-plasms among 1376 (44%) orbital tumors were reported.[81] The five most common secondary tumors in this series were mucocele, squamous cell carcinoma, meningioma, vascular malformation, and basal cell carcinoma.

Overall, secondary orbital tumors among children are infrequent. The Wills Eye Hospital series of childhood orbital neoplasms reported no secondary tumors other than invasion of the optic nerve by retinoblastoma.[82] At the University of Washington, however, we have observed esthesioneuroblastoma with secondary orbital involvement in three children. Secondary tumors such as orbital bone osteoma, fibrous dysplasia, ossifying fibroma, angiofibroma, and mucocele have also been described in children.[32,81,83,84]

Clinical signs and symptoms of secondary orbital tumors are similar to metastatic orbital lesions and reflect the site of primary involvement. Proptosis, visual loss, eyelid edema, diplopia, decreased motility, pain, globe displacement, chemosis, and palpable mass are frequently encountered.

Diagnosis is based on clinical suspicion and CT or MRI imaging of the orbits, paranasal sinuses, and intracranial cavity. Management should be approached through a multidisciplinary team of specialists, including an otolaryngologist, an oncologist, a radiation specialist, a neurosurgeon, and an ophthalmologist.

The following sections of this chapter discuss the more common malignant and benign tumors that secondarily invade the orbit. Specific epidemiology, clinical features, tumor morphology, treatment, and prognosis are addressed separately for each tumor. Tumors of the globe that secondarily involve the orbit are discussed in sections of this text that address primary globe tumors. Neoplasms originating from conjunctiva, lacrimal sac, and skin of the eyelids, face, and forehead are presented in Chapters 2–4.

NEOPLASMS OF THE SINUS AND NASOPHARYNX THAT INVADE THE ORBIT. Malignant tumors of the sinonasal tract constitute less than 1% of all systemic malignancies and about 3% of those arising in the upper respiratory tract.[85] Smith and Wheliss[86] observed eye and orbital involvement in 55% of 53 patients with histologically proven nasopharyngeal tumors. The reported incidence of orbital invasion from paranasal sinus malignancies varies between 55% and 81%.[86–89]

Sinonasal tract tumors invade the orbit by erosion of the bony walls, through preformed channels, or by perineural or perivascular invasion.[85] The presence and extent of orbital involvement depend on the primary tumor site, histopathology, and tumor aggressiveness. The majority of sinonasal tract malignancies that secondarily involve the orbit originate from the maxillary antrum, whereas the least common site of origin is the sphenoid sinus.[80,87] The interval between presentation of tumor and orbital involvement varies depending on type of neoplasm, but the majority (81%) invade the orbit within 1 year of initial presentation.[87]

Most secondary orbital tumors originating from the paranasal sinuses are carcinomas, with the majority being squamous cell. Johnson et al.[87] reviewed 47 cases of sinus tumors that had secondarily invaded the orbit. Their findings are outlined in Table 11.2.

EPITHELIAL MALIGNANCIES OF THE SINUS AND NASOPHARYNX. Epithelial malignancies of the sinus and nasopharynx commonly invade the orbit. In a combined series of patients with sinonasal tumors,[86] 60% were squamous cell carcinomas and 70% originated in the maxillary sinus.

In the Mayo Clinic series,[81] secondary epithelial neoplasms of the orbital were three times more common than primary epithelial tumors. Males outnumbered females by a ratio of nearly 3:1, and the peak incidence occurred during the fifth decade. Very few patients were younger than age 20.

Exposure to industrial fumes and wood dust has been associated with an increased incidence of sinonasal malignant tumors.[90] Furniture workers exposed to hardwood dust experience an increased incidence of adenocarcinoma of the ethmoid sinuses. Workers in the tanning process of shoe leather have an increased risk of developing epithelial malignancies of the sinonasal tract. Furthermore, nickel workers have an incidence of squamous cell and anaplastic carcinomas 250 times greater than the general population.[91,92]

Unlike metastatic lesions to the orbit, secondary epithelial lesions typically result in nonaxial displacement of the globe, away from the invading tumor. Lesions originating in the maxillary sinus displace the globe upward, and lesions arising from the ethmoid sinuses displace the globe inferiorly and temporally. Nasal symptoms such as airway obstruction, chronic sinusitis, and epistaxis are frequently encountered.

The clinical course demonstrates progressive destruction of the paranasal sinuses. A solid mass of tumor may invade the bony orbit, nasopharynx, sphenoid sinus, cribriform plate, pterygopalatine fossa, and base of the skull. Orbital involvement represents an advanced stage of disease, but in some cases may be the presenting sign. According to the American Joint Committee on Cancer (AJCC), secondary involvement of the orbit is by definition stage T3 or T4 (Table 11.3).[93] Patients

TABLE 11.2—Classification of 79 paranasal tumors that invaded the orbit

Squamous cell carcinoma (41)
Inverting papilloma (12)
Osteoma (7)
Adenocarcinoma (5)
Adenocystic carcinoma (4)
Chondrosarcoma (3)
Embryonal rhabdomyosarcoma (2)
Esthesioneuroblastoma (2)
Osteosarcoma (1)
Mucoepidermoid carcinoma (1)
Fibrosarcoma (1)

Number of cases are in parentheses.
From Johnson et al.[87]

TABLE 11.3—Maxillary sinus TNM staging for primary tumor (T)

TX	Primary tumor cannot be assessed.
TO	No evidence of primary tumor.
Tis	Carcinoma in situ.
T1	Tumor limited to the antral mucosa with no erosion or destruction of bone.
T2	Tumor with erosion or destruction of the infrastructure, including the hard palate and/or the middle nasal meatus.
T3	Tumor invades any of the following: skin of cheek, posterior wall of maxillary sinus, floor or medial wall of orbit, or anterior ethmoid sinus.
T4	Tumor invades orbital contents and/or any of the following: cribiform plate, posterior ethmoid or sphenoid sinuses, nasopharynx, soft palate, pterygomaxillary or temporal fossa, or base of skull.

From the American Joint Committee on Cancer.[93]

with tumors arising below an imaginary line drawn from the medial canthus to the angle of the mandible (Ohngren's line) have a better prognosis than do patients with tumors arising above this line.[85]

Patients presenting with chronic sinonasal complaints (longer than 6 weeks), nonaxial displacement of the globe, or other orbital manifestations should be evaluated for secondary orbital involvement of a sinonasal neoplasia. A complete ophthalmologic and otolaryngologic examination with attention to the cranial nerves is recommended. Axial and coronal thin-section CT of the sinuses, orbits, and intracranial cavity aids in the diagnosis and delineates extent of tumor involvement. It is important to establish extent of tumor involvement for appropriate therapy. CT findings include sinus opacification and a soft tissue mass eroding through the sinus wall. Most paranasal sinus tumors do not enhance with intravenous contrast,[94] but contrast is recommended for proper evaluation of surrounding structures. MRI provides more accurate imaging of soft tissues such as extraocular muscles, periorbital tissues, brain parenchyma, optic nerve, carotid artery, and cavernous sinus.[95] Bone, however, is better visualized through CT. Abnormal tissue should be biopsied either directly or endoscopically.

Despite the high frequency of secondary spread of these tumors, fewer than 10% of patients with malignant disease of the paranasal sinuses have lymph node metastases at presentation, and fewer yet exhibit distant metastases.[96] Patients should be evaluated for local and distant metastases and, if absent, local treatment may be curative.

Generally, radiotherapy of 4500–5000 cGy is administered, followed by a rest period of 2 weeks. The lesion is then resected. Sisson et al.[95] reported a 65% 5-year survival rate for patients treated with radiotherapy and surgery. Most of the patients in this study were made up of stage T3 and T4 maxillary antrum tumors and advanced ethmoid tumors.

The extent of local resection is dictated by the involvement of the surrounding structures. Forty years ago, orbital exenteration for tumors of the paranasal sinuses was routinely performed. However, studies have shown that preservation of the orbital contents in selected cases is safe.[97] Perry et al.[98] studied 41 patients with paranasal sinus tumors; 26 demonstrated orbital involvement and five required exenteration due to extensive periorbita invasion. The orbital contents were preserved in 21 cases where minimal or no involvement of the periorbita was observed grossly. These patients were treated with preoperative irradiation and removal of the tumor with sparing of the orbital contents. Only three of the 21 patients had recurrence about the orbital area. This study demonstrates that orbital exenteration does not improve prognosis if the periorbita is uninvolved.

Chemotherapy is reserved for patients with advanced or recurrent disease. Protocols described by Sisson et al.[95] include cisplatinum-based chemotherapy for squamous cell tumors and adriamycin-based chemotherapy for glandular malignancies. They reported an overall 5-year survival rate of less than 10% after chemotherapy, with local recurrence being the major cause of death.

Squamous Cell Carcinoma

EPIDEMIOLOGY. Although the majority of secondary squamous cell carcinomas are highly malignant, these tumors frequently have a long asymptomatic latency period prior to orbital invasion,[81] with most remaining clinically silent until they have extended beyond their sinus origin.[32]

CLINICAL FEATURES. Owing to their predilection for involvement of the maxillary antrum, oral manifestations such as trismus, tooth pain, and palatal erosion are common. Additionally, patients frequently complain of facial symptoms such as pain, paresthesias, cheek swelling, nasal obstruction, anosmia, and epistaxis. CT is the preferred method of imaging. Scanning typically shows a homogeneous soft tissue mass that enhances to some degree with contrast. Surrounding bone destruction is also very characteristic, but may be absent[81] (Figure 11.8A).

MORPHOLOGY. Squamous cell carcinomas typically extend locally, and death is usually a result of local invasion. Among 48 patients with squamous cell carcinoma of the maxillary antrum, Lavertu et al.[99] observed seven patients with nodal involvement and 25 with local recurrence of tumor after treatment with surgery and/or radiotherapy. The overall 5-year survival rates for patients with stage T3 and T4 disease were 31.8% and 6.7%, respectively.

Squamous cell carcinoma develops from the ciliated, columnar, respiratory epithelium lining

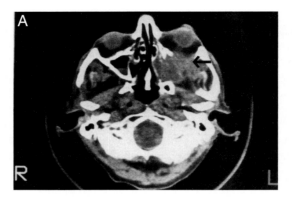

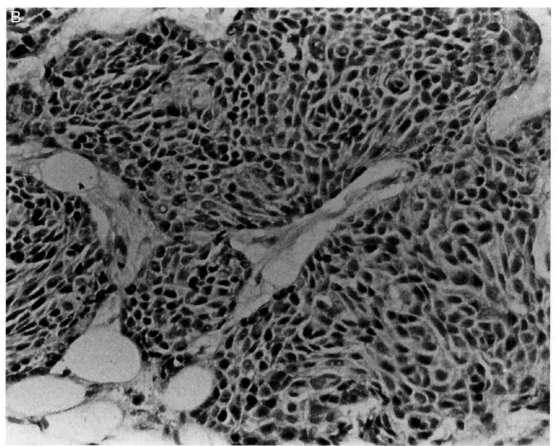

FIG. 11.8—**A:** A 61-year-old man presented with squamous cell carcinoma of the left maxillary sinus extending into the inferior orbit. Computed tomography discloses erosion of the orbital floor with extension into the orbit (arrow). **B:** The orbital biopsy specimen shows anaplastic squamous cells with little resemblance to normal epithelium. Treatment was by local excision, exenteration, and radiotherapy.

in the sinuses and anterior nasal cavity that has undergone malignant squamous metaplasia.[81,100] Tumors may be well-differentiated, keratinizing squamous carcinomas that resemble those found in other anatomic areas. According to Henderson,[81] the poorly differentiated and anaplastic types more commonly invade the orbit. As these become more anaplastic, the usual prickle-type cells become more polyhedral and may assume a spindle shape. Cellular boundaries may become indistinct, and foci of degeneration may appear and impart a pseudoglandular appearance (Figure 11.8B).

Immunohistochemical analysis typically shows cytoplasmic markers positive for high molecular weight cytokeratins, whereas low molecular weight cytokeratins are characteristically negative. This combination is highly suggestive of squamous cell carcinoma.[46]

On electron microscopy, cells typically show the formation of desmosomes. Variable amounts of scattered tonofilaments, polyribosomes, short segments of rough-surfaced endoplasmic reticulum, and mitochondria are observed in the cytoplasm.[69]

Adenoid Cystic Carcinoma

EPIDEMIOLOGY. Adenoid cystic carcinomas arise from a variety of anatomic structures, including the nasopharynx, paranasal sinuses, lacrimal, salivary, and mucous glands of the upper respiratory tract and skin.[101] A total of 19% of adenoid cystic carcinomas arise in the sinuses and nasopharynx, and their behavior and histopathology resemble those found elsewhere.[81]

In the Mayo Clinic series (1994), Henderson[81] reported a 4.2% relative incidence of adenoid cystic carcinomas among secondary epithelial malignancies. Tumors originated most commonly in the maxillary antrum, while the nasal cavity, ethmoid sinus, oral cavity, parotid gland, and lacrimal sac were other sites of origin. There were slightly more women than men reported, and the mean age was 50 years. These observations are similar to those for tumors arising in the lacrimal gland.

CLINICAL FEATURES. Adenoid cystic carcinoma is a locally aggressive tumor characterized by relentless progression and eventual death.[102] Spread is the hallmark of adenoid cystic carcinoma and is usually evident along the maxillary and mandibular divisions of the trigeminal nerve, resulting in pain

and hypesthesia. Spiro et al.[103] found that 14% of mucosal adenoid cystic carcinomas spread to the regional lymph nodes, whereas 40% metastasize hematogenously. Lung and bone are the most common sites of metastases, and systemic involvement is almost always associated with a failure of local control.[102] Interestingly, metastases may grow much slower than the primary tumor.

Diagnosis may be difficult because this tumor is sometimes clinically silent for long periods and imaging studies frequently fail to represent the full extent of local involvement accurately. With paranasal sinus involvement, the tumor diffusely infiltrates the subperiosteal spaces, resulting in bone involvement. Some degree of bony erosion and opacification of the paranasal sinuses is usually evident on CT.

MORPHOLOGY. Grossly, adenoid cystic carcinoma is an infiltrative, firm, grayish white mass. Microscopically, aggregates of closely packed, small cells with indistinct cell boundaries are seen. A hyalinized stroma surrounds the aggregates of cells, and a sharp demarcation line between cells and stroma is evident. The cellular islands contain circular, acellular spaces that vary in number and size. These spaces stain with mucicarmine, and their configuration may impart a Swiss-cheese appearance to the microscopic field.[81] In the past, adenoid cystic carcinomas were referred to as "cylindromas," owing to their appearance on light microscopy. Immunohistochemistry typically demonstrates cellular cytokeratins, and the stroma is vimentin positive.

Iwamoto and Jakobiec[104] compared the ultrastructure of the normal lacrimal gland and its epithelial tumors. Electron microscopy revealed that the cellular islands of adenoid cystic carcinoma were composed of three different types of cells. Type 1 cells contained either ductal-type granules or acinar-type granules, type 2 featured bundles of tonofilaments and resembled basal cells, and type 3 had features intermediate between those of basal cells and those of myoepithelial cells. The cystoid spaces within the cellular islands consisted of a peripheral zone of multilaminar basement membrane and a central zone containing thin fibrils.

MANAGEMENT AND PROGNOSIS. Adenoid cystic carcinoma located in the maxillary antrum (the most common paranasal sinus site of origin) has a very poor prognosis. Spiro et al.[101] reported a 15.6% survival rate at 5 years. Treatment of this tumor consists of pre- or postoperative irradiation and wide resection. Cure is rare, and recurrences may be found years to decades later.

Adenocarcinoma

EPIDEMIOLOGY. Adenocarcinoma accounts for only 4%–8% of all malignant neoplasms of the paranasal sinuses,[105-108] and secondary orbital involvement is uncommon. The reported incidence varies. Henderson[81] reported six cases among a total of 89 secondary epithelial orbital tumors, and Johnson et al.[87] reported five cases among 47 patients with secondary orbital neoplasms.

CLINICAL FEATURES. Clinical features and behavior are similar to those of adenoid cystic carcinoma. Adenocarcinomas typically grow rapidly in the ethmoid sinuses and nasal cavity.[109] There appears to be an increased incidence of the disease among employees of the woodworking industry.

MORPHOLOGY. Tumor pathology is variable, but tumors are frequently undifferentiated and highly dysplastic. Adenocarcinomas assume three basic growth forms: papillary, sessile, and alveolar-mucoid.[102] All three forms resemble adenocarcinomas found in the GI tract, especially those of the lower bowel. The papillary form may be mucinous and is usually the most localized of the three. It is also the form observed with increased frequency among woodworkers. Sessile adenocarcinomas have a broader base, retain little resemblance to their cells of origin, are more invasive, and carry a worse prognosis. Alveolar-mucoid carcinomas share this poorer prognosis and are characterized by an abundance of mucin in which individual and nests of cells reside. Immunohistochemical evaluation is positive for low molecular weight cytokeratins typical of adenocarcinomas found elsewhere.

Mucoepidermoid Carcinoma

EPIDEMIOLOGY. Mucoepidermoid carcinoma usually arises in the ductal epithelial cells of the salivary and lacrimal glands. Rarely, lesions originate from the paranasal sinuses to invade the orbit secondarily. A review of 47 sinus tumors secondarily invading the orbit reported a single case of a mucoepidermoid tumor that originated in the maxillary sinus.[87]

CLINICAL FEATURES. Rootman et al.[32] described a 47-year-old man who presented with decreased vision, an afferent pupillary defect, proptosis, pain, and limitation of adduction. CT showed opacification of the ethmoids, with multiple subtle focal areas of bony destruction and infiltration of the right orbit and bilateral medial canthi. FNAB displayed mucoepidermoid carcinoma.

MORPHOLOGY. Pathologically, the tumors are gritty lesions consisting of cords of poorly differentiated, neoplastic cells surrounded by a desmoplastic and inflammatory reaction.[32] Carcinomas are frequently divided into low-grade (well differentiated) and high-grade (poorly differentiated) tumors.[110] Grossly, low-grade tumors are well circumscribed, and about half contain large cystic spaces with mucin accumulation.[111] Histologically, they have large numbers of mucin-producing cells, with various numbers of epidermoid cells. Mucin may be extruded into the interstitium, where it accumulates into small lakes. The low-grade tumors stain positive for mucicarmine. High-grade tumors tend to be uniformly infiltrative, and cystic spaces are usually absent. If cystic spaces are found, they are typically secondary to tumor necrosis.[110] High-grade tumors have predominantly epidermoid cells and very rarely display mucous-bearing cells. Occasionally, squamous differentiation with the formation of epithelial pearls is seen.

MELANOMA. Melanomas that secondarily involve the orbit typically originate from the skin of the eyelids, forehead, cheek, or globe. Rarely, however, scattered melanocytes of the sinus epithelium give rise to melanomas.[100] Paranasal sinus melanomas represent only about 3.6% of all malignant sinonasal neoplasms[112] and are prone to spread locally with early metastasis.[109] Five-year survival ranges from 17% to 38%. Rootman et al.[32] described one patient with melanoma of the nasopharynx that secondarily invaded the orbit. Despite urgent radiotherapy, this patient died due to disseminated disease 6 months after the detection of orbital involvement.

Cutaneous melanoma and secondary orbital melanoma originating in the paranasal sinuses share similar histopathologic features. Cells may demonstrate spindle-shaped or epithelioid morphology, typically lack cohesiveness, and display numerous mitotic figures and prominent nucleoli. Cellular melanin pigment is frequently observed, yet may be absent in amelanotic varieties. Immunohistochemical analysis is a useful tool for diagnosis. HMB-45 is a monoclonal antibody to a cytoplasmic antigen found only in melanoma cells and junctional nevus cells. This marker is nearly 100% specific, with greater than 90% sensitivity.[46]

PAPILLOMA. Papillomas of the sinonasal tract are benign epithelial tumors that arise from squamous epithelium. The most common site of origin is the mucosa of the lateral nasal wall and the ethmoid air cells.[100] Despite their benign origins, lesions may destroy bone and recur when incompletely excised.[85] A small percentage are associated with malignant transformation, especially inverted papillomas, to squamous cell carcinoma.[87,100]

Pathologically, the tumor is an epithelial neoplasm that displays microscopic and macroscopic fingerlike projections similar to benign papillomas found elsewhere. The lesion is called *inverted* when it grows inward toward the stroma.

Biopsy is required to determine whether a papilloma is inverted. Local excision is the preferred treatment, with administration of radiotherapy in cases where malignant transformation has occurred.

OTHER SECONDARY ORBITAL EPITHELIAL NEOPLASMS. Odontogenic tumors such as ameloblastoma and ameloblastic fibrosarcoma may rarely involve the orbit. Ameloblastomas are benign, epithelial tumors that typically arise from the mandible. Occasionally, these arise in the maxilla, where they may extend to secondarily involve the orbit.[32] Treatment is palliative through radiotherapy and local resection.

ESTHESIONEUROBLASTOMA

Epidemiology. Esthesioneuroblastoma is a tumor of neural crest origin and arises from the olfactory sensory epithelium in the superior nasal cavity. Since its initial description by Berger and Luc in 1924,[113] this tumor has been referred to as neuroesthesioma, esthesioneuroblastoma, and olfactory neuroepithelioma.

Esthesioneuroblastoma occurs relatively infrequently, with a reported incidence of 1.5% among malignant tumors of the nasal fossae.[114] Despite its relative rarity, secondary orbital involvement is common.[115] A review of 38 cases of esthesioneuroblastoma at the Mayo Clinic revealed that ophthalmic signs or symptoms were present in 20 cases at the time of diagnosis.

Unlike with other orbital tumors of neural origin, such as retinoblastoma and neuroblastoma, the patients are typically older. The mean age in the Mayo Clinic series[81] was 37, but the tumors may occur any time from childhood to advanced age. The numbers of men and women affected are equal.

Clinical Findings. The most common ocular signs and symptoms are periorbital pain, epiphora, eyelid edema, proptosis, and globe injection.[115] Decreased vision, papilledema, diplopia, cranial nerve palsies, ptosis, a palpable mass, and enophthalmos have also been reported. Nonocular manifestations including nasal blockage, bloody nasal discharge, anosmia, cerebrospinal fluid rhinorrhea, and a pinkish red mass observed in the superior nasal cavity generally occur earlier in the disease than ophthalmic signs and symptoms.

Progression of this tumor is extremely variable. Some tumors demonstrate indolent behavior, with patients experiencing nonocular symptoms for years before diagnosis is established. Other lesions are quite aggressive, invading the orbit and other adjacent structures within a few months.

Esthesioneuroblastoma has a predilection for local tissue invasion, yet it has the capacity for metastasis to cervical lymph nodes and other distant sites.[116] Expansion into the base of the brain, paranasal sinuses, and orbit produces most of the associated complications. Lesions that erode through the ethmoid sinuses result in lateral displacement of the globe and limitation of abduction.[100] Papilledema, optic atrophy, ophthalmoplegia, and axial proptosis occur with more posterior involvement in the orbital apex.

Diagnosis may be difficult, and esthesioneuroblastoma has been mistaken for nasal carcinoma, nasal polyps, sinusitis, and cluster headache. However, with increased pathologic recognition, esthesioneuroblastoma is currently diagnosed more readily than in the past.[115] CT is helpful in delineating the extent of orbital involvement and typically illustrates a large, invasive, contrast-enhancing lesion with associated bone destruction[100] (Figure 11.9A). Suspicious orbital and sinus lesions should be biopsied for histologic and immunohistochemical evaluation.

Nasal or sinus biopsies usually are easier than obtaining orbital tissue.

Morphology. Gross pathologic examination shows a large, usually single, polypoid mass. It is frequently pedunculated and, when soft in consis-

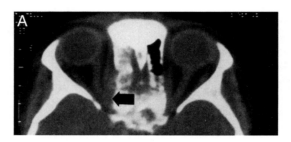

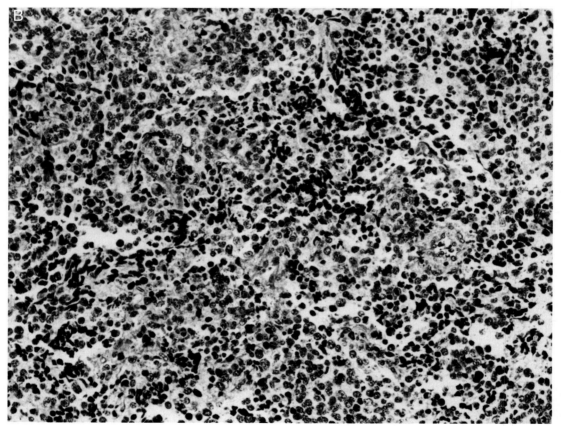

FIG. 11.9—**A:** A 12-year-old girl presented with lymphadenopathy and nasal stuffiness. Orbital computed tomography shows a mass in the right ethmoid sinus extending into the posterior medial right orbit. **B:** The tumor biopsy specimen shows small, round, poorly differentiated cells. Immunocytochemical analysis results were consistent with esthesioneuroblastoma. Left visual acuity deteriorated due to tumor expansion after diagnosis. Recovery of visual acuity was achieved after treatment with corticosteroids and radiation. The tumor was successfully treated with chemotherapy and radiation.

tency, is friable and bleeds easily. Pathologic evaluation with light microscopy reveals fairly uniform cells demonstrating a compact arrangement in nests and cords surrounded by a fibrovascular stroma.[117] Cell nucleoli are hyperchromatic, with scanty cytoplasm and frequent mitotic figures. Rosette and pseudorosette formations have been observed (Figure 11.9B).

Ultrastructural and immunohistochemical studies of esthesioneuroblastoma show a variable number of cells positive for neuron-specific enolase, cytokeratin, neurofilament intermediate filament, and S-100 protein.[44,117] Ultrastructural findings include round to oval cells arranged in a cell-to-cell pattern, with relatively sparse cell organelles. Many cell processes are present between the cell bodies and are joined by punctate adhesions and desmosomes.[117]

Management and Prognosis. Prognosis is related to extent of disease and subsequent therapy. Tumor staging and prognosis are presented in Table 11.4. Elkon et al.[118] found 5-year survival rates of 75% for Stage A, 60% for Stage B, and 41% for Stage C.

Treatment of Stage C disease includes wide local resection and radiotherapy, with pre- and postoperative chemotherapy. Esthesioneuroblastoma is particularly radiosensitive, and treatment with 3000–4000 cGy should be administered. Recommended antineoplastic drugs include vincristine and cyclophosphamide.

MENINGIOMA

EPIDEMIOLOGY. Meningiomas are benign neoplasms that arise from meningothelial cells of the arachnoid trabeculae. They are the second most common brain neoplasms after gliomas, representing 15%–20% of all intracranial tumors in adults[119] and 2% of intracranial tumors in children. Primary orbital involvement may occur when tumor arises from the arachnoid trabeculae of the optic nerve or arises from arachnoid nests within the orbit. Approximately 90% of meningiomas involving the orbit are secondarily derived from intracranial sites.[120,121] Furthermore, about one-third of intracranial meningiomas produce ophthalmic signs and symptoms.[122]

Most secondary meningiomas originate from the arachnoid near the sphenoid ridge and slowly encroach on the orbit. The olfactory groove, suprasellar, and basofrontal areas may cause vision loss but rarely encroach upon orbital tissues. Clinical manifestations of secondary orbital meningiomas typically begin during the fifth decade.[122] Meningiomas occur among females 2–3 times more frequently than among men.[120]

Patients with neurofibromatosis have a higher incidence of both intracranial and optic nerve sheath meningiomas.[122] Multicentric tumor occurrence is more common in this group as well. Additionally, Caucasians are probably more frequently affected than people of other races; however, no specific data support this observation.[122]

CLINICAL FEATURES. Clinical manifestations reflect the site of primary tumor involvement. Meningiomas may arise from the medial aspect of the sphenoid ridge and access the orbit through the superior orbital fissure or optic canal. Tumors originating from the lateral portion of the sphenoid wing grow forward into the lateral aspects of the orbit to produce proptosis combined with soft tissue swelling in the temporalis fossa[122] (Figure 11.10A). Hyperostosis of the bones at the orbital apex is characteristic of sphenoid-wing meningiomas and therefore should be suspected in patients with an orbital apex syndrome. Decreased vision may result but typically occurs much later in patients with secondary orbital involvement compared with patients with primary dural sheath meningiomas. Visual field defects, dyschromatopsia, proptosis, lid swelling,

TABLE 11.4—Staging and prognosis of esthesioneuroblastoma

Stage	Definition	% 5-Year survival rate
A	Confined to the nasal cavity	75
B	Confined to the nasal cavity and one or more paranasal sinuses	60
C	Extending beyond the nasal cavity or paranasal sinuses (includes orbit)	41

From Elkin et al. (page 96).[118]

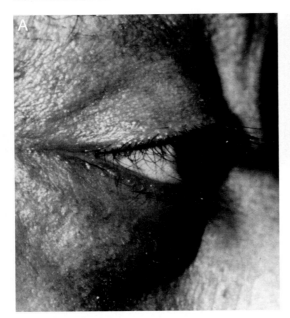

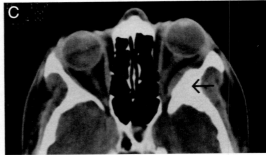

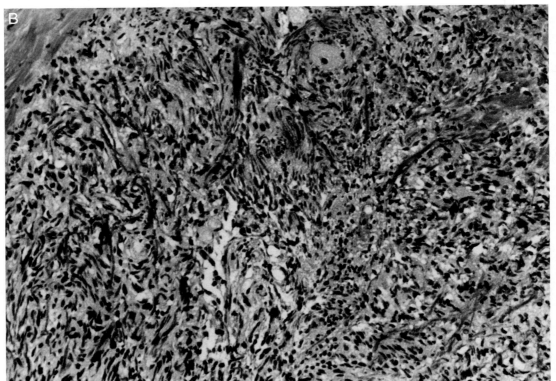

FIG. 11.10—**A:** A 45-year-old man presented with right, chronic, progressive proptosis. Fullness of the lower lid was present, but vision was normal and ductions were full. **B:** The sphenoid-wing meningioma was debulked at surgery. Tumor histology shows whorls and lobules of tightly packed, meningothelial cells. **C:** A 43-year-old woman with a left sphenoid wing meningioma. Computed tomography shows hyperostosis of the greater wing of the sphenoid bone secondary to tumor involvement (arrow).

an afferent pupillary defect, optic nerve swelling or atrophy, and decreased motility are also encountered. Opticociliary shunt vessels may be observed as well, but with much less frequency compared with primary optic nerve meningiomas.

Plain films demonstrate bony hyperostosis. Contrast-enhanced CT is the procedure of choice in evaluating sphenoid hyperostosis.[123] The CT typically shows an enhancing, soft tissue mass with calcifications expanding into the orbit from adjacent areas (Figure 11.10C). MRI with gadolinium enhancement provides excellent tumor delineation and is invaluable for evaluating intracranial tumor extension. Contrast angiography may demonstrate a tumor blush as well as delineate vascular supply.[41,124]

MORPHOLOGY. The histologic features of primary and intracranial meningiomas are similar.[125]

Grossly, the lesion is a firm, well-circumscribed mass. Several histologic variants have been described: meningotheliomatous, psammomatous, fibroblastic, transitional, and angioblastic.[125] The meningotheliomatous type is composed of neoplastic meningothelial cells resembling those normally present in the arachnoid. Cells with indistinct margins are arranged into lobules and whorls, resembling a syncytium of cells. Electron microscopy shows interdigitating cytoplasmic extension of adjacent cells. Psammomatous meningiomas are those tumors that display an abundance of concentrically laminated concretions. These *psammoma bodies* may be present in varying amounts. Lipid-laden xanthoma cells may also be present.

Fibroblastic meningiomas are composed of elongated, slender neoplastic meningothelial cells resembling fibroblasts. The cells are arranged into sheets and interwoven fascicles and are interspersed with various amounts of collagen (Figure 11.10D).[125] The transitional type shares features of both meningothelial and fibroblastic meningiomas. Angioblastic meningiomas resemble hemangiopericytomas or hemangioblastomas.

Electron microscopy frequently shows intercellular surface desmosomes with intracytoplasmic vimentin cytofilaments anchored to the desmosomes.[126] The combination of vimentin and desmosomal plaque protein is a diagnostic feature of meningioma. The coexpression of desmosomal and vimentin proteins by immunohistochemistry characterizes meningioma tumors.[126] Meningiomas are negative for glial fibrillary acidic protein,[127] whereas the S-100 protein shows a highly variable reaction.[126]

TREATMENT AND PROGNOSIS. Meningiomas typically demonstrate slow growth, and in fact may remain stable for long periods. Meningiomas rarely metastasize. Secondary tumors generally present with proptosis preceding vision loss, compared with optic nerve meningiomas where vision loss often occurs with minimal or no proptosis.

Management of secondary orbital meningiomas depends on their extent. Observation and primary surgical excision represent the mainstay of treatment. Invasion of vital structures, soft tissue, and bone may prevent complete excision, and therefore tumor debulkment may be the goal. Meningiomas are relatively insensitive to radiation;[128] however, some authors have advocated radiation therapy as adjuvant treatment for incompletely resected intracranial tumors. Chemotherapy is generally ineffective, but new modes of treatment may be helpful in the future.[32] Mifepristone or RU486 is an antiprogestational agent currently under investigation in the treatment of unresectable meningioma.

INTRAOCULAR METASTATIC DISEASE IN HUMANS

Neoplasms metastatic to intraocular structures, once thought to be extremely rare, are now widely thought to be more common than primary ocular tumors in adult humans. By definition, metastases are new foci of tumor that arise in locations remote from the primary site, in contrast to tumors that spread by direct extension to involve ocular structures.[129] This section discusses the clinical, gross pathologic and histopathologic features of metastatic tumors in humans, with the exception of the lymphomas and leukemias.

Historical Perspective. For nearly 100 years, intraocular metastasis was considered extremely rare. In 1872, Perl[130] contributed one of the first case reports of intraocular metastatic disease to medical literature, with a postmortem case of lung carcinoma metastatic to the choroid. Lemoine and McCleod[131] published a review of the literature in 1936, finding that 230 cases had been reported up to that time. Gotfredsen,[132] in 1944, in a large series, found only six intraocular metastases among 8712 patients with malignancies (incidence, 0.07%). By 1950, Greear[133] found that the number of cases totaled no more than about 300. In 1951, Spaeth[134] noted only four cases of intraocular metastases seen at the Wills Eye Hospital in a 10-year period. In 1966, Duke-Elder and Perkins[135] stated that metastatic cancer to the uvea is rare and that few surgeons have recorded more than one case.

In 1967, Albert et al.[22,34] published results of a clinical series and a review of the literature. They found five cases of choroidal metastases among 213 patients with known metastatic disease in their series (incidence, 2.3%) and estimated total cases of intraocular metastases to be approximately 463. This series by Albert et al. suggested a much higher incidence of intraocular metastasis than previously reported.[132] In 1971, Bloch and Gartner[136] published a series of 230 cases with autopsy-proven carcinomas and found 25 cases of intraocular metastasis (incidence, 11%) and were among the first to suggest metastasis as the most common intraocular tumor. In 1974, Ferry and Font[137,138] reviewed all of the cases of intraocular metastasis on record at the Armed Forces Institute of Pathology, which totaled 196. As part of their discussion, they used projections from the American Cancer Society and figures that had been previously reported in the literature to calculate and estimated 1150–25,300 new cases of intraocular metastasis, which far exceeded the estimates of new primary intraocular tumors for the same year.

More recently, Nelson et al.[139] estimated that the total incidence of intraocular metastasis from all sources is approximately 4%, although, in their own series of 52 intraocular metastases, only five of these tumors had been recognized clinically. Several authors postulate that the apparent increase in the incidence of intraocular metastases is due to several factors, including longer survival of many cancer patients, increased awareness, and improved methods of clinical detection of metastases by ophthalmologists and other specialists.[129,140,141] However, the incidence may be even higher than currently reported, due to patients who are too ill from their cancer to recognize or seek treatment for ocular disease or due to those in whom the metastasis remains asymptomatic.[129,137]

Primary Tumors. A wide variety of tumor types have been noted to metastasize to the eye. The vast majority of these tumors are carcinomas, as sarcomas rarely metastasize to intraocular structures.[137] Breast cancer is the most common primary tumor responsible for intraocular metastases in all reported series. It accounts for 40%–70% of all intraocular metastases.[41,129,137,142] The prevalence of intraocular metastases in the United States is estimated to be 10%–37%.[143] Almost all cases of intraocular metastases from breast carcinoma occur in females, but there have been several cases reported in men, of which at least two have been infiltrating ductal carcinoma.[144,145] The eye may be the first site of metastasis in up to 20%–30% of patients with metastatic breast carcinoma,[142] although intraocular metastasis is usually preceded by metastases to other organs, especially the lungs.[143] The average age of diagnosis is approximately 52 years,[143] and up to 92% of patients have a prior history of the primary malignancy. In general, intraocular metastases are discovered 2–5 years after diagnosis of the primary tumor, but metastases can occur months to many years following diagnosis of the primary.[41,143]

Lung carcinoma is the second most common primary tumor identified in cases of intraocular metastases and is the most common primary tumor identified in males. It comprises 10%–30% of all intraocular metastatic tumors.[129,142] Patients with intraocular metastases from the lung are less likely than patients with a primary arising in the breast to have a previous history of malignancy at the time the ocular metastasis is diagnosed. Lung carcinoma also tends to metastasize earlier than breast carcinoma.[138,146] In the future, metastases from lung carcinoma may increase as the number of advanced cases of lung carcinoma increases in women.[147]

Unknown primary tumor accounts for the third largest category of tumors with intraocular metastases. In 8%–16% of intraocular metastases, a primary source cannot be identified despite extensive workup.[129,137] A few malignancies, however uncommon, deserve special note. Cutaneous malignant melanoma has been reported to metastasize intraocularly and account for up to 4% of all intraocular metastases.[129] The intraocular metastases of cutaneous melanoma generally reflect widespread metastases and often coexist with central nervous system metastases.[148–151] One case of uveal melanoma metastatic to the opposite eye has been reported in the literature.[4] Another tumor of note is carcinoid, which has been reported to metastasize to intraocular structures and usually occurs as a solitary metastasis with an indolent growth pattern.[152] Carcinoid arising from the bronchial system is more likely to metastasize to the eye than is GI carcinoid.

Other tumors less commonly are responsible for metastases to the eye. Renal cell carcinoma may metastasize to the eye and often does so after several years of an apparently disease-free state.[77] Metastases from prostatic carcinoma has also been noted, although not at the rate that might be expected considering the increasing prevalence of the disease. Tumors metastatic from the GI tract are not uncommon and may arise from a primary tumor at any level along the alimentary canal, with a rate of about 7% in one series.[129] Other malignancies that more rarely metastasize to the eye include pancreatic carcinoma, thyroid carcinoma, testicular carcinoma, uterine carcinoma, cervical carcinoma, ovarian carcinoma, bladder carcinoma, hepatocellular carcinoma, osteogenic sarcoma, Ewing's sarcoma, and neuroblastoma.[129,153–158]

Other Epidemiologic Characteristics. Most clinical series do not address the issue of racial predilection. However, in the studies that do, whites are found to have a much higher incidence than blacks or Asians.[129,137,138] Of note, however, is that the rate of metastasis to the anterior segment is significantly higher than the rate of anterior segment primary malignant melanoma in blacks.[138] There is less agreement regarding sexual predilection when comparing different series. Ferry and Font[137] found a nearly equal distribution among the two genders: 52% female and 48% male. Hutchinson and Smith[146] describe a smaller series of patients in which they found a greater incidence of metastasis in males. In another series, Shields and Shields[129] found a greater incidence in females (70%) than in males (30%), likely due to the large number of cases of breast carcinoma in their series.

The age at diagnosis of intraocular metastasis tends to reflect the general age distribution of cancer. Most cases occur between the ages of 30 and 70, with an average age of approximately 52–60.[129,137,146] The incidence of intraocular metastasis in children is very low, although orbital metastasis is not uncommon.[142,146] Ewing's sarcoma and neuroblastoma have been reported to have intraocular metastases in children,[153] including one case report of a congenital metastasis of neuroblastoma in the anterior segment.[159]

Location. The vast majority of intraocular metastases involve the uveal tract, and, of these, the majority are located in the choroid (Figure 11.11). It is widely believed that since the uvea is so vascular, it is much more likely to have seeding of microemboli from a distant primary tumor. Since the eye itself has no lymphatic supply, metastatic disease may only reach ocular structures via hematogenous spread. Tumor emboli travel via the common and then internal carotid arteries and eventually enter the ophthalmic and posterior ciliary arteries to lodge most commonly in the choroidal bed.[129,137] Albert et al.[22] demonstrated this predilection for the uvea in an experimental rabbit model. They also postulated that local environmental factors may play a role in determining the growth of metastases. However, animals demonstrate a greater ability to support metastatic tumor growth in the anterior choroid versus the posterior choroid, whereas the opposite is true in humans.[146]

Early clinical series suggested a higher incidence of intraocular metastases in the left eye versus the right eye.[135] Authors theorized that the asymmetric branching of the carotid arteries from the aorta and the fact that the right common carotid arises from the innominate artery allow a more direct pathway for tumor emboli to the eye via the left common carotid. More recent series do not support this theory. Two large series have found no statistically significant difference between the incidence of metastatic disease on the right and left sides.[129,137] Up to 30% of cases

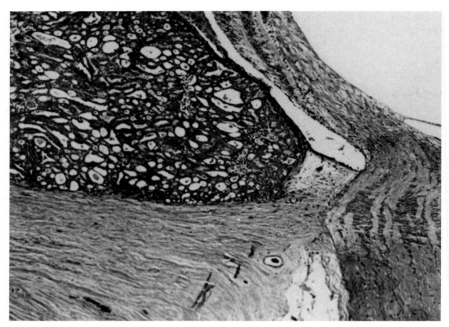

FIG. 11.11—Choroidal metastasis of an adenocarcinoma of unknown primary site. Hematoxylin-eosin, ×10.

with intraocular metastases may have bilateral ocular involvement.[129,150,154,156] Metastatic tumors tend to occur posterior to the equator and approximately 40% involve the macula.[134,142,146] Metastases may be single or multiple and may involve both the anterior and posterior segments of the eye.[4,137] Up to 32% of metastatic tumors may have multiple foci of involvement in an eye.[129]

Metastatic tumors with predominantly anterior segment involvement occur much less frequently than choroidal metastases. Anterior segment metastases primarily involve the iris and ciliary body, and account for approximately 5%–13% of all intraocular tumors.[4,129,138,141,146]

Metastases to the retina and/or vitreous are extremely rare. They probably account for less than 1% of all intraocular tumors. One clinical review of retinal metastases revealed an equal distribution of metastases from primary tumors of carcinomatous origin and from cutaneous malignant melanoma.[160]

Clinical Features. Choroidal metastases may remain asymptomatic or may present with blurry vision, metamorphopsia, or a scotoma that may be gradual or sudden in onset. In general, they tend to be painless.[129,161] Clinical appearance on ophthalmoscopy is that of one or more yellow, plaquelike lesions deep to the retina that tend to be relatively flat and may be fairly subtle. The overlying retinal pigment epithelium may show areas of golden-brown pigment clumping over the surface of the tumor. Ruptures of Bruch's membrane are less common with metastatic tumors versus primary choroidal melanoma; however, a metastatic tumor may occasionally appear as a significantly elevated, mushroom-shaped mass that can be difficult to distinguish from choroidal melanoma.[41,129] Multiple sites of involvement is highly suggestive of metastatic disease. Overlying serous retinal detachment is present in 75% of choroidal metastases.[4,129] The detachment may be shallow or bullous and may be associated with shifting subretinal fluid if extensive in nature.

The diagnosis of metastatic disease may not always be readily apparent from a patient's history or ophthalmic examination. The differential diagnosis of lesions with a clinical appearance similar to that of choroidal metastasis includes primary choroidal amelanotic melanoma or nevus, choroidal hemangioma, posterior scleritis,

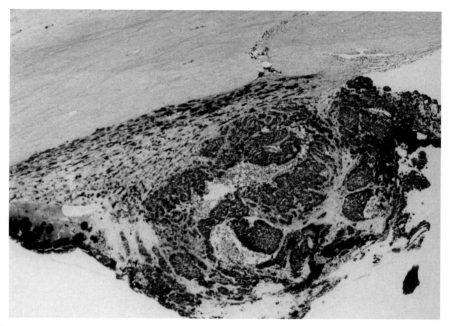

FIG. 11.12—Metastatic small cell carcinoma involving the ciliary body and iris root. Hematoxylin-eosin, ×13.

choroidal osteoma, inflammatory conditions of the retina and choroid, rhegmatogenous retinal detachment, Harada's disease, uveal effusion syndrome, and central serous chorioretinopathy.[162]

Iris and ciliary body metastases often share common symptoms, although the tumor may be asymptomatic in either location. They may cause decreased vision, pain, or redness, or the patient may note a spot on the iris. Ciliary body metastasis may remain undiagnosed for a long period, since a mass is often not readily apparent (Figure 11.12). The tumor may masquerade as a case of chronic uveitis or secondary glaucoma, may present as a peripheral mass behind the iris, with narrowing of the anterior chamber angle, or may cause a sector cataract or even subluxation of the lens. Sometimes the mass may be apparent after a patient's pupil has been dilated. A sentinel dilated episcleral vessel may be present in proximity to the tumor.[129,138,143] The ciliary body may become involved secondarily as a result of direct extension of a choroidal metastasis.

Metastases to the iris present with symptoms similar to those of ciliary body metastases. The clinical appearance is usually of a gray, white, yellowish, or pink mass on the iris. However, metastatic cutaneous melanoma may present as a dark mass.[148] The color of the tumor depends on its vascularity, and approximately one-third of iris metastases have prominent vascularity.[138] The tumor may appear gelatinous.[163] Angle involvement may be apparent on gonioscopy. The metastasis may release malignant cells into the anterior chamber and create a pseudohypopyon, confusing the clinical picture with that of endophthalmitis. Rubeosis iridis may be present with or without hyphema. Ferry and Font[138] comment that any case of uveitis with recurrent hyphema should be suggestive of intraocular metastasis.

Whereas primary iris melanomas tend to occur in the inferior 180° of the iris, metastatic tumors tend to occur in the superior 180°.[129] Seeding of the tumor along the iris surface is a prominent feature in approximately half of cases.[138] The differential diagnosis of iris metastases includes primary iris melanoma, melanotic and amelanotic types, iris nevus, leiomyoma, granulomatous uveitis,[164,165] and intraocular infections such as endophthalmitis.[129] Iris metastases tend to grow much more rapidly than primary iris melanoma.

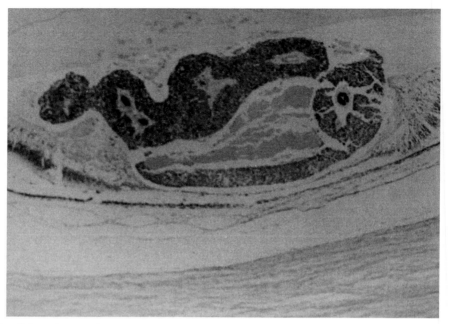

FIG. 11.13—Colon adenocarcinoma metastatic to the retina. Hematoxylin-eosin, ×13.

Retinal metastases, which are rare (Figure 11.13), may present with blurry vision or floaters, or as an inflammatory process. The lesion (or lesions) may appear as a white infiltrate with overlying vitreous cells. Metastatic cutaneous malignant melanoma may appear as a gray or black mass that can obscure underlying retinal detail.[129,151,160,166] Retinal lesions may be mistaken for retinal infarctions at an early stage. The diagnosis also may be confused with inflammatory or infectious retinitis such as *Candida* or cytomegalovirus.[160] Rarely, a metastatic process may present with only vitreous or aqueous cells, as is reported in one case of metastatic cutaneous malignant melanoma.[167]

Pathologic Features. Specimens of intraocular metastases usually are obtained at autopsy or in cases where enucleation was performed presuming the diagnosis of a primary tumor such as melanoma.[141] Biopsy specimens are not commonly encountered.

On gross examination of a sectioned globe with metastatic disease, one or more uveal masses may be evident. These may be diffuse, plaquelike lesions that are only mildly elevated but extend laterally to occupy a large area in the subretinal space, or, more rarely, the lesions may be dome shaped and indistinguishable from a choroidal melanoma. Choroidal lesions may extend anteriorly to involve the ciliary body. With ciliary body metastases, the tumor may appear as an amelanotic mass with lenticular opacity contiguous to the tumor. The lens may be subluxated by the mass. With either iris or ciliary body metastases, angle involvement may be evident and cellular debris may be evident in the anterior chamber.

In general, the histopathologic characteristics of a metastatic tumor depend on the nature of the primary tumor. However, many primary tumors are not of the well-differentiated variety, and metastases tend to be even less differentiated than the primary site. This lack of cellular differentiation may result in loss of the original characteristics of the tumor type.[41] In one series, in none of the cases in which intraocular metastatic disease was suspected could the primary tumor type be identified based on the histologic characteristics of the ophthalmic specimen.[146] Castro et al.[41] describe the general histologic characteristics of choroidal metastases. They observe that tumor emboli may lodge in small blood vessels, and the vessels subsequently rupture as the tumor contin-ues to enlarge. The tumor cells then continue to proliferate in the choroidal stroma and spread in a manner that follows the path of least resistance—hence the characteristic flat, plaquelike configu-ration. Retinal pigment epithelium in proximity to the tumor may show proliferation and accumula-tion of intracellular lipofuschin. This manifests as speckled pigmentation and yellow dots on fun-duscopic examination.

They note that Bruch's membrane is less fre-quently ruptured with metastases than with pri-mary choroidal melanoma. Polymorphonucleo-cytes may be seen around necrotic tumor cells, and degenerative changes may occur within the stroma. Stromal degenerative changes may involve disintegration of chromatophores and release of intracellular pigment. Eventually, the tumor may outstrip its blood supply, and tumor necrosis occurs. In addition, calcification of ves-sel walls may occur.[41] Metastases to the iris and ciliary body may exhibit an interesting growth pattern where the tumor spreads along the surface of intraocular structures in a layer that may only be one or two cell layers thick.[129,138]

When certain tumor types are suspected from a patient's history or histologic examination, addi-tional stains may be of use in establishing the diagnosis. Stains such as PAS, Alcian blue, and mucicarmine and use of hyaluronidase to demon-strate mucopolysaccharide, intracytoplasmic vac-uoles, or glycogen may be of use in certain tumors (e.g., those exhibiting abundant mucin) to help diagnose tissue of origin.[35,77,165] These stains may be of use in trying to differentiate primary mucin-secreting adenocarcinoma of the ciliary epithelium from metastatic disease, which may be difficult.[168] When trying to establish the diagnosis of carcinoid, stains such as the Grimelius stain (for agyrophil granules) and the Fontana-Masson stain (for argentaffin granules) may be extremely helpful.[53] With metastatic cutaneous malignant melanoma, the Fontana-Masson and the Perls' stain confirm the presence of melanin; however, the diagnosis of primary intraocular melanoma cannot be ruled out with these stains.[166] Electron microscopy may be of use in selected cases.

Immunohistochemical staining techniques may be of use for determining tissue origin.[169] Immunohistochemical staining for CEA may sug-gest a primary in the GI tract.[165] Similarly, immunohistochemical staining can be used for PSA.[53] If the amount of tissue in the specimen allows, analysis for estrogen and progesterone receptors in metastatic breast carcinoma may help to guide therapy for the metastasis.[45]

Diagnosis. In the case of suspected intraocular metastasis with a known primary tumor type, a workup for systemic metastases should be initi-ated, if it has not already been done. In patients without a known primary tumor, a complete sys-temic evaluation is in order. In females, a thor-ough workup for breast cancer should be done with a breast examination and mammograms.[42] Other areas of focus for both men and women include the lung, GI tract, kidney, thyroid gland, and pancreas.[129] Both men and women should have an evaluation of the reproductive organs, including ovaries, uterus, testicles, and prostate.

Laboratory evaluation, such as liver function tests (suggesting hepatic involvement), plasma CEA level,[141] and possibly PSA level, may also help make the diagnosis of metastatic disease.

In certain cases, fluorescein angiography may be of use in making the diagnosis of choroidal metastasis.[170] In general, most metastatic lesions are hypofluorescent in the arterial and early venous stages, in contrast to choroidal heman-gioma and melanoma, and show progressive hyperfluorescence in later frames.[129] The late phases of the angiogram also reveal a combina-tion of pinpoint and diffuse leaks as well as dis-crete large round leaks from the retinal pigment epithelium.[4] The angiogram is most useful for differentiating neoplastic from nonneoplastic conditions such as subretinal neovascular mem-branes, chorioretinal inflammation, and organ-ized hemorrhage.[129]

Standardized echography may help to distin-guish choroidal metastases from primary choroidal melanoma. It is less helpful for lesions of the anterior segment, although echography can help demonstrate the size and extent of intraocular involvement (Figure 11.14). On A scan, metastatic lesions display a sharp initial spike, medium to high internal reflectivity, irreg-ular internal structure, and usually poor vascu-larity.[4] B scan usually does not demonstrate orbital shadowing. Shifting subretinal fluid can

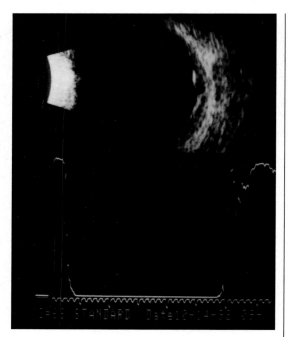

FIG. 11.14—Contact A scan and B scan demonstrate a diffusely thickened choroid with medium-high internal reflectivity characteristic of metastatic disease. (Courtesy of Michael F. Lewandowski, RDMS.)

diagnosis will influence the choice of treatment (i.e., surgical excision versus nonsurgical therapy). Ausburger[171] published a series of 19 cases of FNAB with details of the biopsy technique and specimen preparation. FNAB will not always yield enough tissue for a diagnosis, and all specimens should be reviewed by a pathologist experienced in the field of cytology.

Wedge biopsy of the ciliary body or choroid may be performed in selected cases where a tissue diagnosis is necessary. The procedure is usually performed via a scleral flap but does incur a certain amount of risk. The main concern with wedge biopsy is the risk of seeding of tumor cells from the biopsy site and the possibility of tumor microemboli via the episcleral vessels.

Treatment. Therapy of intraocular metastases is somewhat dependent on tumor type, tumor activity, and extent of intraocular involvement. Metastatic lesions may be discovered incidentally after systemic therapy for malignancy has already been initiated or completed. The intraocular lesions may have already responded to the therapy and not require any further treatment. In general, these inactive metastatic lesions are flat and do not have an overlying retinal detachment.[129]

In general, if the metastatic lesions appear active or are symptomatic, external beam irradiation is the mainstay of therapy. For choroidal metastases, the entire posterior segment is irradiated in a direct lateral field with a total dose of 3000–4000 cGy over a 1-month period.[45,141–143] In cases with iris involvement, a dose of 3000 cGy is used in a window that includes the anterior segment and lens. In select cases, brachytherapy with a radioactive episcleral plaque may be used effectively, usually in cases of solitary choroidal metastases. The radiation dose is generally about 3500 cGy.[129] Success of therapy is measured by a decrease in thickness of the tumor, resolution of secondary retinal detachment, decreased proliferation of the overlying retinal pigment epithelium, and, most importantly, resolution of the patient's symptoms.

Chemotherapy may be of use as an adjunctive therapy in some cases in which radiation has not been successful or as a primary therapy in cases where the primary tumor is exquisitely sensitive to the chemotherapeutic agents.[159] Chemotherapy

sometimes be demonstrated when an overlying retinal detachment is present.

The role of CT and MRI is not well defined with regard to intraocular tumors. Both may demonstrate the size and extent of the tumor but at present are not useful in differentiating metastatic from primary tumors. As MRI technique continues to be refined, this modality may become more useful in differentiating the two processes.

The radioactive phosphorus-uptake test [^{32}P] may also be employed in selected cases. This test is usually positive in cases of choroidal metastases, but it cannot differentiate between primary amelanotic melanoma and metastatic disease. It can help to differentiate malignant neoplasms from benign conditions such as choroidal hemangioma.[141]

FNAB is a well-established diagnostic technique for anterior segment lesions and has gained popularity for lesions of the posterior segment as well. In general, it should be reserved for those cases in which other diagnostic modalities have failed to yield a diagnosis and a specific tissue tends to be not as effective as radiation for most cases of intraocular metastases. In tumors that may be hormone sensitive (e.g., breast or prostate), hormonal therapy with agents such as tamoxifen may be of some benefit as an adjunctive treatment. With certain tumor types such as follicular carcinoma of the thyroid, other therapeutic modalities like radioactive iodine [^{131}I] may be effective.[161]

Enucleation should, in general, be reserved for those patients with a blind painful eye. Excisional biopsy is used in select cases of iris tumors but has to be weighed against the risks of surgery.

Prognosis. Overall, the prognosis for survival in patients with intraocular metastases is poor. The average survival with intraocular and orbital metastases of all tumor types in one series is 7.4 months.[4] The median survival with metastases to the anterior segment is somewhat shorter at 5.4 months.[138] Patients with breast cancer with intraocular metastases have a slightly longer survival time that depends on the stage of the tumor. Freedman and Folk[4] calculated a mean survival time following diagnosis of intraocular metastases of 873 days in Stage I and II breast carcinoma and of 139 days with Stages III and IV. They also calculated a mean survival time of 236 days with unidentified primary tumors. Other studies have found an average survival time of 6–17 months with breast carcinoma after the diagnosis of intraocular metastases.[41,141,143] Lung cancer has a more dismal survival time, with an average of 5.2 months.[141] These statistics reflect that intraocular metastases are often only a sign of more widespread systemic metastases and an advanced stage of the malignancy.

Summary. Intraocular metastases are now widely recognized to be the most common intraocular tumor in humans, although often they may go undiagnosed. Nearly any tumor type can metastasize to the eye, although most commonly breast and lung cancer are responsible. A variety of methods may be used to identify lesions as metastases and identify the primary tumor, but in a significant percentage a primary is never found. Most intraocular metastases can be treated palliatively, but the overall survival rate with metastatic disease remains rather poor.

ACKNOWLEDGMENT

This work was supported in part by an award from Research to Prevent Blindness, Inc.

REFERENCES

1. Godtfredsen E. On the frequency of secondary carcinoma of the choroid. *Acta Ophthalmol (Copenh)* 22:394, 1944.
2. Mewis L, Young SE. Breast carcinoma metastatic to the choroid: analysis of 67 patients. *Ophthalmology* 89:147, 1982.
3. Stephens RF, Shields JA. Diagnosis and management of cancer metastatic to the uvea: a study of 70 cases. *Ophthalmology* 86:1336, 1979.
4. Freedman MI, Folk JC. Metastatic tumors to the eye and orbit: patient survival and clinical characteristics. *Arch Ophthalmol* 105:1215, 1987.
5. Hart WM. Metastatic carcinoma to the eye and orbit. *Int Ophthalmol Clin* 2:465, 1962.
6. Siverberg E, Lubera JA. Cancer statistics. *CA* 39:3, 1989.
7. Barron CN, Saunders LZ, Jubb KV. Intraocular tumors in animals: III. Secondary intraocular tumors. *Am J Vet Res* 24:835, 1963.
8. Ladds PW, Gelatt KN, Strafuss AC, Mosier JE. Canine ocular adenocarcinoma of mammary origin. *J Am Vet Med Assoc* 156:63, 1970.
9. Szymanski CM. Bilateral metastatic intraocular hemangiosarcoma in a dog. *J Am Vet Med Assoc* 161:803, 1972.
10. Brodey RS, Pflugfelder C, Mikkilineni S, Twitchell MJ. Clinicopathologic conference. *J Am Vet Med Assoc* 172:837, 1978.
11. Whitley RD, Jensen HE, Andrews JJ, Simpson ST. Renal adenocarcinoma with ocular metastasis in a dog. *J Am Anim Hosp Assoc* 16:949, 1980.
12. Lavach JD. Disseminated neoplasia presenting with ocular signs: a report of two cases. *J Am Anim Hosp Assoc* 20:459, 1984.
13. Szymanski C, Boyce R, Wyman M. Transitional cell carcinoma of the urethra metastatic to the eyes in a dog. *J Am Vet Med Assoc* 185:1003, 1984.
14. Hogenesch H, Whiteley HE, Vicini DS, Helper LC. Seminoma with metastases in the eyes and the brain in a dog. *Vet Pathol* 24:278, 1987.
15. Bellhorn RW. Secondary ocular adenocarcinoma in three dogs and a cat. *J Am Vet Med Assoc* 160:302, 1972.
16. Hayden DW. Squamous cell carcinoma in a cat with intraocular and orbital metastases. *Vet Pathol* 13:332, 1976.
17. West CS, Wolf ED, Vainisi SJ. Intraocular metastasis of mammary adenocarcinoma in the cat. *J Am Anim Hosp Assoc* 15:725, 1979.
18. Miller WR, Merton DA. Ocular manifestations of metastatic sweat gland adenocarcinoma in a cat. *J Am Vet Med Assoc* 180:1100, 1982.
19. Cook CS, Peiffer RL, Stine PE. Metastatic ocular squamous cell carcinoma in a cat. *J Am Vet Med Assoc* 185:1547, 1984.

20. Murphy CJ, Canton DC, Bellhorn RW, Okihiro M, Cahoon B, Dufort R. Disseminated adenocarcinoma with ocular involvement in a cat. *J Am Vet Med Assoc* 195:488, 1989.

21. Hamilton HB, Severin GA, Nold J. Pulmonary squamous cell carcinoma with intraocular metastasis in a cat. *J Am Vet Med Assoc* 185:307, 1984.

22. Albert DM, Zimmerman AW Jr, Zeidman I. Tumor metastasis to the eye: Part III. The fate of circulating tumor cells to the eye. *Am J Ophthalmol* 63:733, 1967.

23. Duncan EE, Peiffer RL. Morphology and prognostic indicators of anterior uveal melanomas in cats. *Prog Vet Comp Ophthalmol* 1:25, 1991.

24. Dubielzig RR, Everitt J, Shadduck JA, et al. Clinical and morphologic features of post-traumatic ocular sarcomas in cats. *Vet Pathol* 27:62, 1990.

25. Nasisse MP, Davidson MG, Olivero DK, et al. Neodymium: YAG laser treatment of primary canine intraocular tumors. *Prog Vet Comp Ophthalmol* 3:152, 1993.

26. Shields JA. Metastatic cancer to the orbit. In: Shields JA, ed. *Diagnosis and Management of Orbital Tumors,* 1st ed. Philadelphia: WB Saunders, chap 18:1989.

27. Horner F. Carcinom der dura mater. *Klin Monatsbl Augenheilkd* 2:186, 1864.

28. Goldberg RA, Rootman J, Cline RA. Tumors metastatic to the orbit: a changing picture survey of ophthalmology. *Surv Ophthalmol* 35:1, 1990.

29. Shields JA, Bakewell B, Augsburger JJ, Flanagan JC. Classification and incidence of space-occupying lesions of the orbit: a survey of 645 biopsies. *Arch Ophthalmol* 102:1606, 1984.

30. Silva D. Orbital tumors. *Am J Ophthalmol* 65:318, 1968.

31. Forrest AW. Intraorbital tumors. *Arch Ophthalmol* 41:198, 1949.

32. Rootman J, Ragaz J, Cline R, Lapointe JS. Metastatic and secondary tumors of the orbit. In: Rootman J, ed. *Diseases of the Orbit.* Philadelphia: JB Lippincott, 405:1988.

33. Bloch RS, Gartner S. The incidence of ocular metastatic carcinoma. *Arch Ophthalmol* 85:673, 1971.

34. Albert DM, Rubenstein RA, Scheie HG. Tumor metastasis to the eye: I. Incidence in 213 adults with generalized malignancy. *Am J Ophthalmol* 63:723, 1967.

35. Font RL, Ferry AP. Carcinoma metastatic to the eye and orbit: III. A clinical pathologic study of 28 cases metastatic to the orbit. *Cancer* 38:1326, 1976.

36. Albert DM, Rubenstein RA, Scheie HG. Tumor metastasis to the eye: II. Clinical study in infants and children. *Am J Ophthalmol* 63:727, 1967.

37. Robbins SL, Kumar V. The female genital system and breast. In: Robbins LL, Kumar V, eds. *Basic Pathology,* 4th ed. Philadelphia: WB Saunders, chap 19:1987.

38. Shields CL, Shields JA, Peggs M. Metastatic tumors to the orbit. *Ophthalmic Plast Reconstr Surg* 4:73, 1988.

39. Burmeister BH, Benjamin CS, Childs WL. The management of metastases to eye and orbit from a carcinoma of the breast. *Aust NZ J Ophthalmol* 18:187, 1990.

40. Henderson JW. Metastatic carcinoma. In: Henderson JW, ed. *Orbital Tumors,* 1st ed. Philadelphia: WB Saunders, chap 16:1973.

41. Castro PA, Albert DM, Wang WJ, Ni C. Tumors metastatic to the eye and adnexa. *Int Ophthalmol Clin* 22:189, 1982.

42. Bullock JD, Yanes B. Ophthalmic manifestation of metastatic breast cancer. *Ophthalmology* 87:951, 1980.

43. Cline RA, Rootman J. Enophthalmos: a clinical review. *Ophthalmology* 91:229, 1984.

44. Orcutt JC, Reeh MJ, Gown AM, Lindquist TD. Diagnosis of orbital and periorbital tumors: use of monoclonal antibodies and cytoplasmic antigens (intermediate filaments). *Ophthalmic Plast Reconst Surg* 3:159, 1987.

45. Reifler DM, Davison P. Histochemical analysis of breast carcinoma metastatic to the orbit. *Ophthalmology* 93:254, 1986.

46. Dalley RW, Gown AM, Orcutt JC. Evaluation of orbital disease. In: Walsh TJ, ed. *Textbook of Neuro-ophthalmology: Clinical Signs and Symptoms,* 3d ed. Philadelphia: Lea and Febiger, chap 4:1992.

47. Glassburn JR, Klionsky M, Brady LW. Radiation therapy for metastatic disease involving the orbit. *Am J Clin Oncol* 7:145, 1984.

48. Winliff JL. Steroid hormone receptors in breast cancer. *Cancer* 53:630, 1984.

49. Robbins SL, Kumar V. The respiratory system. In: Robbins SL, Kumar V, eds. *Basic Pathology,* 4th ed. Philadelphia: WB Saunders, Chap 13:1987.

50. Riddle PJ, Font RL, Zimmerman LE. Carcinoid tumors of the eye and orbit: a clinicopathologic study of 15 cases, with histochemical and electron microscopic observations. *Hum Pathol* 13:459, 1982.

51. Honrubia FM, Davis WH, Moore MK. Carcinoid syndrome with bilateral orbital metastases. *Am J Ophthalmol* 72:1119, 1972.

52. Rush JA, Waller RR, Campbell RJ. Orbital carcinoid tumor metastatic from the colon. *Am J Ophthalmol* 89:636, 1980.

53. Shields CL, Shields JA, Eagle RC, Peyster RG, Conner BE, Green HA. Orbital metastasis from a carcinoid tumor: computed tomography, magnetic resonance imaging, and electron microscopic findings. *Arch Ophthalmol* 105:969, 1987.

54. Letter SW, *Surv Ophthalmol* 28:693, 1984.

55. Nida TY, Hall WA, Glantz MJ, Clark HB. Metastatic carcinoid tumor to the orbit and brain. *Neurosurgery* 31:949, 1992.

56. Robbins SL, Kumar V. The male genital system. In: Robbins SL, Kumar V, eds. *Basic Pathology,* 4th ed. Philadelphia: WB Saunders, chap 18:1987.

57. Boldt CH, Nerad JA. Orbital metastases from prostate carcinoma. *Arch Ophthalmol* 106:1403, 1988.

58. Plesnicar S. The course of metastatic disease originating from carcinoma of the prostate. *Clin Exp Metastasis* 3:103, 1985.

59. Taylor CR. Immunoperoxidase techniques: practical and theoretical aspects. *Arch Pathol Lab Med* 102:113, 1978.

60. Kopelman JE, Shorr N. A case of prostatic carcinoma metastatic to the orbit diagnosed by fine needle aspiration and immunoperoxidase staining for prostatic-specific antigen. *Ophthalmic Surg* 18:599, 1987.

61. Li CY, Lam KW. Immunohistochemical diagnosis of prostatic cancer with metastasis. *Cancer* 46:706, 1980.

62. Jobsis AC, DeVries GP. Demonstration of the prostatic origin of metastasis: an immunochemical method for formalin-fixed embedded tissue. *Cancer* 42:1788, 1978.

63. Chisholm CD. Treatment of advanced cancer of the prostate. *Semin Surg Oncol* 1:38, 1985. (Cited in Boldt CH, Nerad JA. Orbital metastases from prostate carcinoma. *Arch Ophthalmol* 106:1403, 1988.)

64. Alfano JE. Ophthalmological aspects of neuroblastomatosis: a study of 53 verified cases. *Trans Am Acad Ophthalmol Otolaryngol* 72:830, 1968.

65. Musarella MA, Chan HSL, Deboer G, Gallie BL. Ocular involvement in neuroblastoma: prognostic implications. *Ophthalmology* 91:936, 1984.

66. Brown GT, Walls RP, Murphee AL, Ortega J. Neonatal neuroblastoma metastatic to the iris. *Cancer* 52:929, 1983.

67. Maurer HM. Current concepts in cancer: solid tumors in children. *N Engl J Med* 299:1395, 1978.

68. Traboulsi EL, Shammuas LV, Massad M. Ophthalmologic aspects of metastatic neuroblastoma: report of 22 consecutive cases. *Orbit* 3:247, 1984.

69. Jacobiec FA, Font RL. Secondary tumors, muceceles, and metastatic tumors. In: Spencer WH, ed. *Ophthalmic Pathology*, vol 3, 3d ed. Philadelphia: WB Saunders, 2749:1986.

70. Altman AJ, Baehner RL. Favorable prognosis for survival in children with coincident opsoclonus-myoclonus and neuroblastoma. *Cancer* 37:846, 1976.

71. Harris GJ, Beattly RL. Acute proptosis in children. In: Lindberg JV, ed. *Oculoplastic and Orbital Emergencies*, 1st ed. East Norwalk, CT: Appleton and Lange, chap 8:1990.

72. Brodeur GM, Pritchard J, Berthold F, et al. Revisions of the international criteria for neuroblastoma diagnosis, staging, and response to treatment. *J Clin Oncol* 11:1466, 1993.

73. Robbins SL, Kumar V. The gastrointestinal tract. In: Robbins SL, Kumar V, eds. *Basic Pathology*, 4th ed. Philadelphia: WB Saunders, chap 16:1987.

74. Lubin JR, Grove AS, Zakov ZN, Albert DM. Hepatoma metastatic to the orbit. *Am J Ophthalmol* 89:268, 1980.

75. Arnold RW, Adams BA, Camoriano JK, Dyer JA. Acquired divergent strabismus: presumed metastatic gastric carcinoma to the medial rectus muscle. *J Pediatr Ophthalmol Strabismus* 26:50, 1988.

76. Cotran RS. The kidney and its collecting system. In: Robbins SL, Kumar V, eds. *Basic Pathology*, 4th ed. Philadelphia: WB Saunders, chap 14:1987.

77. Kindermann WR, Shields JA, Eiferman RA, Stephens RF, Stuart EH. Metastatic renal cell carcinoma to the eye and adnexae: a report of three cases and review of the literature. *Ophthalmology* 88:1347, 1981.

78. Bradham RR, Wannamaker CC, Prat-Thomas HR. Renal cell carcinoma metastases 25 years after nephrectomy. *JAMA* 223:921, 1973.

79. Henderson JW. Secondary epithelial neoplasms. In: Henderson JW, ed. *Orbital Tumors*, 1st ed. Philadelphia: WB Saunders, chap 15:1973.

80. Hesselink JR, Weber AL. Pathways of orbital extension of extraorbital neoplasms. *J Comp Assist Tomogr* 6:593, 1982.

81. Henderson JW. Secondary epithelial neoplasms. In: Henderson JW, ed. *Orbital Tumors*, 3d ed. New York: Raven, chap 17:1994.

82. Shields JA, Bakewell B, Augsberger JJ, Donoso LA, Bernardino V. Space occupying orbital masses in children: a review of 250 consecutive biopsies. *Ophthalmology* 93:379, 1986.

83. Margo CE, Weiss AW, Habal MB. Psammomatoid ossifying fibroma. *Arch Ophthalmol* 104:1347, 1986.

84. Moore AT, Buncic JR, Munro IR. Fibrous dysplasia of the orbit in childhood. *Ophthalmology* 92:12, 1985.

85. Myers EN, Carrau RL. Neoplasms of the nose and paranasal sinuses. In: Bailey BJ, ed. *Head and Neck Surgery: Otolaryngology*, 1st ed. Philadelphia: JB Lippincott, chap 86:1993.

86. Smith JL, Wheliss JA. Ocular manifestations of nasopharyngeal carcinoma. *Trans Am Acad Ophthalmol Otolaryngol* 65:659, 1961.

87. Johnson LN, Krohel GB, Yeon EB, Parnes SM. Sinus tumors invading the orbit. *Ophthalmology* 91:209, 1984.

88. Flores AD, Anderson DW, Doyle PJ, Jackson SM, Morrison MD. Paranasal sinus malignancy: a retrospective analysis of treatment methods. *J Otolaryngol* 13:141, 1984.

89. Gullane RJ, Conley J. Carcinoma of the maxillary sinus: a correlation of the clinical course with orbital involvement, pterygoid erosion, or pterygopalatine invasion and cervical metastases. *J Otolaryngol* 12:141, 1983.

90. Pedersen E, Hogetveit AC, Andersen A. Cancer of respiratory organs among workers at a nickel refinery in Norway. *Int J Cancer* 12:32, 1973.

91. Acheson ED, Pippard EC, Winter PD. Mortality of English furniture makers. *Scand J Work Environ Health* 10:211, 1984.

92. Acheson ED, Pippard EC, Winter RD. Nasal cancer in the Northamptonshire boot and shoe industry: is it declining? *Br J Cancer* 46:940, 1982.

93. American Joint Committee on Cancer. *Manual for Staging of Cancer,* 4th ed. Philadelphia: JB Lippincott, 45:1992.

94. Parsons C, Hodson N. Computed tomography of paranasal sinus tumors. *Radiology* 132:641, 1979.

95. Sisson GA, Toriumi DM, Atiyah RA. Paranasal sinus malignancy: a comprehensive update. *Laryngoscope* 99:143, 1989.

96. Harrison DFN. Critical look at the classification of maxillary sinus carcinomata. *Ann Otol Rhinol Laryngol* 87:3, 1978. (Cited in Parsons C, Hodson N. Computed tomography of paranasal sinus tumors. *Radiology* 132:641, 1979.)

97. Larson DL, Christ JE, Jesse RH. Preservation of the orbital contents in cancer of the maxillary sinus. *Arch Otolaryngol* 108:370, 1982.

98. Perry C, Levine PA, Williamson BR, Cantrell RW. Preservation of the eye in paranasal sinus cancer surgery. *Arch Otolaryngol Head Neck Surg* 114:632, 1988.

99. Lavertu P, Roberts JK, Kraus DH, Levine HL, Wood BG, Medendorp SV, Tucker HM. Squamous cell carcinoma of the paranasal sinuses: the Cleveland Clinic experience 1977–1986. *Laryngoscope* 99:1130, 1989.

100. Shields JA. Secondary orbital tumors. In: Shields JA, ed. *Diagnosis and Management of Orbital Tumors,* 1st ed. Philadelphia: WB Saunders, chap 20:1989.

101. Spiro RH, Huvos AG, Strong EW. Adenoid cystic carcinoma of salivary origin: a clinicopathologic study of 242 cases. *Am J Surg* 128:512, 1974.

102. Batsakis JG, Rice DH, Solomon AR. The pathology of head and neck tumors: squamous and mucous-gland carcinomas of the nasal cavity, paranasal sinuses, and larynx: Part 6. *Head Neck Surg* 2:497, 1980.

103. Spiro RH, Lewis JS, Hajdu SL, Strong EW. Mucous gland tumors of the larynx and laryngopharynx. *Ann Otol Rhinol Laryngol* 85:498, 1976.

104. Iwamoto T, Jakobiec FA. A comparative ultrastructural study of the normal lacrimal gland and its epithelial tumors. *Hum Pathol* 3:236, 1982.

105. Batsakis JG, Holtz F, Sueper RH. Adenocarcinoma of nasal and paranasal cavities. *Arch Otolaryngol* 77:625, 1963.

106. Jackson RT, Fits-Hugh GS, Constable WC. Malignant neoplasms of the nasal cavities and paranasal sinuses: a retrospective study. *Laryngoscope* 87:726, 1977.

107. Lederman M. Tumours of the upper jaw: natural history and treatment. *J Laryngol Otol* 84:364, 1970.

108. Mesar BW, Batsakis JG. Glandular tumors of the upper respiratory tract: a clinicopathologic assessment. *Arch Surg* 92:872, 1966.

109. Weber AL, Stanton AC. Malignant tumors of the paranasal sinuses: radiologic, clinical and histopathologic evaluation of 200 cases. *Head Neck Surg* 6:761, 1984.

110. Wagoner MD, Chuo N, Gonder R Jr, Grove AS, Albert DM. Mucoepidermoid carcinoma of the lacrimal gland. *Ann Ophthalmol* 14:383, 1982.

111. Evans RW, Cruickshank AH. Epithelial tumors of the salivary glands. Philadelphia: WB Saunders, 1970:120.

112. Holdcraft J, Gallagher J. Malignant melanomas of the nasal cavity and paranasal sinus mucosa. *Ann Otol Rhinol Laryngol* 78:5, 1960.

113. Berger L, Luc R. l'Esthesionepitheliome olfactif. *Bull Assoc Fr Pour Etude Cancer* 13:410, 1924.

114. Gerard-Marchant R, Micheau C. Microscopic diagnosis of olfactory esthesioneuromas: general review and report of five cases. *J Natl Cancer Inst* 35:75, 1965.

115. Rakes SM, Yeatts RP, Campbell RJ. Ophthalmic manifestation of esthesioneuroblastoma. *Ophthalmology* 92:1749, 1985.

116. Homzie MJ, Elkon D. Olfactory esthesioneuroblastoma: variables predictive of tumor control and recurrence. *Cancer* 46:2509, 1980.

117. Takahashi H, Ohar S, Yamada M, Ikuta F, Tanimura K, Honda Y. Esthesioneuroepithelioma: a tumor of true olfactory epithelium origin—an ultrastructural and immunohistochemical study. *Acta Neuropathol (Berl)* 75:147, 1987.

118. Elkin D, Hightower SL, Lim ML, Cantrell RW, Constable WC. Esthesioneuroblastoma. *Cancer* 44:1087, 1979.

119. Dutton JJ. Optic nerve sheath meningiomas. *Surv Ophthalmol* 37:167, 1992.

120. Graig WM, Gogel LF. Intraorbital meningiomas: a clinicopathologic study. *Am J Ophthalmol* 32:1663, 1949.

121. Wilson WB. Meningiomas of the anterior visual system. *Surv Ophthalmol* 26:109, 1992.

122. Shields JA. Optic nerve and meningeal tumors. In: Shields JA, ed. *Diagnosis and Management of Orbital Tumors,* 1st ed. Philadelphia: WB Saunders, chap 11:1989.

123. Zimmerman CF, Schatz N, Glaser JS. Magnetic resonance imaging of optic nerve meningiomas: enhancement with gadolinium-DTPA. *Ophthalmology* 97:585, 1990.

124. Jakobiec FA, Depot MJ, Kennerdell JS, et al. Combined clinical and computed tomographic diagnosis of orbital glioma and meningioma. *Ophthalmology* 91:137, 1983.

125. Marquardt MD, Zimmerman LE. Histopathology of meningiomas and gliomas of the optic nerve. *Hum Pathol* 13:226, 1982.

126. Henderson JW. Meningioma. In: Henderson JW, ed. *Orbital Tumors,* 3d ed. New York: Raven, chap 19:1994.

127. De Armond SJ, Eng LF, Rubinstein LF. The application of glial fibrillary acidic (GFA) protein immunohistochemistry in neurooncology: a progress report. *Pathol Res Pract* 168:374, 1980.

128. Kennerdell JS, Maroon JC, Malton M, Warren FA. The management of optic nerve sheath meningiomas. *Am J Ophthalmol* 106:450, 1988.

129. Shields JA, Shields CL. Metastatic tumors to the intraocular structures. In: Shields JA, Shields CL, eds. *Intraocular Tumors: A Text and Atlas.* Philadelphia: WB Saunders, 208:1992.

130. Perl M. Contributions to pathology of tumors. *Virchows Arch [A]* 56:437, 1872.

131. Lemoine AN, McLeod J. Bilateral metastatic carcinoma of the choroid: successful roentgen treatment of one eye. *Arch Ophthalmol* 16:804, 1936.

132. Godfredsen E. On the frequency of secondary carcinomas in the choroid. *Acta Ophthalmol (Copenh)* 22:394, 1944.

133. Greear JN Jr. Metastatic carcinoma of the eye. *Am J Ophthalmol* 33:1015, 1950.

134. Spaeth EB. Ocular tumors. *Arch Ophthalmol* 46:421, 1951.

135. Duke-Elder S, Perkins ES. Diseases of the uveal tract. In: Duke-Elder S, ed. *System of Ophthalmology,* vol 9: *Diseases of the Uveal Tract.* St Louis: CV Mosby, 919:1966.

136. Bloch RS, Gartner S. The incidence of ocular metastatic carcinoma. *Arch Ophthalmol* 85:673, 1971.

137. Ferry AP, Font RL. Carcinoma metastatic to the eye and orbit: II. A clinicopathologic study of 26 patients with carcinoma metastatic to the anterior segment of the eye. *Arch Ophthalmol* 29:472, 1975.

138. Ferry AP, Font RL. Carcinoma metastatic to the eye and orbit: I. A clinicopathologic study of 227 cases. *Arch Ophthalmol* 92:276, 1974.

139. Nelson CC, Hertzberg BS, Klintworth GK. A histopathologic study of 716 unselected eyes in patients with cancer at the time of death. *Am J Ophthalmol* 95:788, 1983.

140. Gillet RB. Metastatic carcinoma of the choroid. *Tex Med* 67:72, 1971.

141. Stephens RF, Shields JA. Diagnosis and management of cancer metastatic to the uvea: a study of 70 cases. *Ophthalmology* 86:1336, 1979.

142. Frank AR. Visual loss in the cancer patient. *Nebr Med J* 74:113, 1989.

143. Merrill CF, Kaufman DI, Dimitrov NV. Breast cancer metastatic to the eye is a common entity. *Cancer* 68:623, 1991.

144. Reynard M, Font RL. Two cases of uveal metastasis from breast carcinoma in men. *Am J Ophthalmol* 95:208, 1983.

145. Schlaen ND, Naves AE. Orbital and choroidal metastases from carcinoma of the male breast. *Arch Ophthalmol* 104:1344, 1986.

146. Hutchinson DS, Smith TR. Ocular and orbital metastatic carcinoma. *Ann Ophthalmol* 11:869, 1979.

147. Boring CC, Squires TS, Tong T. Cancer statistics, 1993. *CA* 43:7, 1993.

148. Oosterhuis JA, De Keizer RJ, De Wolff-Rouendaal D, et al. Ocular and orbital metastasis of cutaneous melanomas. *Int Ophthalmol* 10:175, 1987.

149. Shetlar DJ, Font RL, Ordonez N, et al. A clinicopathologic study of three carcinoid tumors metastatic to the orbit: immunohistochemical, ultrastructural, and DNA flow cytometric studies. *Ophthalmology* 97:257, 1990.

150. De Bustros S, Augsburger JJ, Shields JA, et al. Intraocular metastases from cutaneous malignant melanoma. *Arch Ophthalmol* 103:937, 1985.

151. Letson AD, Davidorf FH. Bilateral retinal metastases from cutaneous malignant melanoma. *Arch Ophthalmol* 100:605, 1982.

152. Bardenstein DS, Char DH, Jones C, et al. Metastatic ciliary body carcinoid tumor. *Arch Ophthalmol* 108:1590, 1990.

153. Green DM, Marinello MJ, Fisher J, et al. Ewing's sarcoma of the scapula with metastases to the lung and eye. *Am J Pediatr Hematol Oncol* 8:134, 1986.

154. Hauksson A, Bynke H, Trope C. A serious ovarian cystadenocarcinoma metastatic to both eyes. *Acta Obstet Gynecol Scand* 66:187, 1987.

155. Hertzanu Y, Vellet AD, Fain BA, et al. Eye metastases in carcinoma of the cervix: a case report. *S Afr Med J* 71:53, 1987.

156. Karnad A, Poskitt TR, Lines LG, Lefsky L. Simultaneous bilateral ocular metastases from a gastric carcinoma. *Ann Ophthalmol* 18:188, 1986.

157. Weisenthal R, Brucker A, Lanciano R. Follicular thyroid cancer metastatic to the iris: case report. *Arch Ophthalmol* 107:494, 1989.

158. Cole MD, Farah NB. The choroid: an unusual site for metastasis in patients with adenocarcinoma of the rectum—a case report. *Eur J Surg Oncol* 11:275, 1985.

159. Alio JL, Faci A, Garcia-Julian G, Martinez-Tello A. Anterior chamber metastasis from neuroblastoma. *J Pediatr Ophthalmol Strabismus* 19:299, 1982.

160. Leys AM, Van Eyck LM, Nuttin BJ, et al. Metastatic carcinoma to the retina: clinicopathologic findings in two cases. *Arch Ophthalmol* 108:1448, 1990.

161. Tang RA, Kellaway J, Young SE. Ophthalmic manifestations of systemic cancer. *Oncology* 5:59, 1991.

162. Michelson JB, Stephens RF, Shields JA. Clinical conditions mistaken for metastatic cancer to the choroid. *Ann Ophthalmol* 11:149, 1979.

163. Das BN, McLellan DR. Metastatic squamous carcinoma to the anterior uvea: clinicopathological report. *J R Coll Surg Edinb* 35:312, 1990.

164. Woog JJ, Albert DM, Dueker DK, et al. Metastatic carcinoma of the iris simulating iridocyclitis. *Br J Ophthalmol* 68:167, 1984.

165. Lieb WE, Shields JA, Shields CL, Spaeth GL. Mucinous adenocarcinoma metastatic to the iris, ciliary body, and choroid. *Br J Ophthalmol* 74:373, 1990.

166. Best SJ, Taylor W, Allen JP. Metastatic cutaneous malignant melanoma of the vitreous and retina. *Aust NZ J Ophthalmol* 18:397, 1990.
167. Cole EL, Zakov ZN, Meisler DM, Tuthill RJ. Cutaneous malignant melanoma metastatic to the vitreous. *Arch Ophthalmol* 104:98, 1986.
168. Jakobiec FA, Zimmerman LE, Spencer WH, et al. Metastatic colloid carcinoma versus primary carcinoma of the ciliary epithelium. *Ophthalmology* 94:1469, 1987.
169. Winkler CF, Goodman GK, Eiferman RA, Yam LT. Orbital metastases from prostatic carcinoma: identification by an immunoperoxidase technique. *Arch Ophthalmol* 99:1406, 1981.
170. Davis DL, Robertson DM. Fluorescein angiography of metastatic choroidal tumors. *Arch Ophthalmol* 89:97, 1973.
171. Augsburger JJ. Fine needle aspiration biopsy of suspected metastatic cancers to the posterior uvea. *Trans Am Ophthalmol Soc* 86:499, 1988.

12

OCULAR LYMPHOID PROLIFERATIONS

William C. Carlton, Amy K. Hutchinson, and Hans E. Grossniklaus

Lymphoproliferative diseases are common and interesting processes that can involve the globe, orbit, and/or the adnexa, usually as part of a systemic condition but occasionally as lesions confined to the ocular tissues.

ANIMALS

Ocular/adnexal lymphosarcoma is described in dogs, cattle, cats, and horses, but is common only in dogs, cats, and cattle. The principal location of the neoplasm differs in these species, as the neoplasm is principally intraocular in dogs and cats and orbital in cattle. Lymphosarcoma is described in the eyelids, but is rare in this location.

Bovine Ocular Lymphosarcoma

INCIDENCE AND CLINICAL FEATURES. Lymphosarcoma in cattle occurs in several anatomic locations, including the orbit.[1-3] Lymphosarcoma is the most common neoplasm of the orbit in cattle and its occurrence may be unilateral or bilateral. The retrobulbar region is generally one of multiple sites with lesions of lymphosarcoma, and many cattle have few to several enlarged lymph nodes.

Usually, the globe is not involved, but the periorbita, retrobulbar fat, and extraocular muscles are often infiltrated with neoplastic lymphocytes (Figure 12.1). The neoplasm may extend to the conjunctiva and sclera, but the cornea is rarely

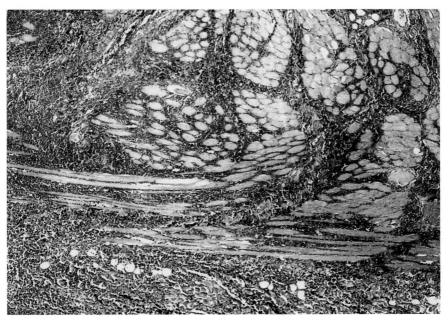

FIG. 12.1—Bovine; periorbita. Lymphosarcoma. Neoplastic cells infiltrate the periorbital tissues and separate the extraocular muscles. Hematoxylin-eosin, ×3.

involved.[3] Invasion of the eyeball was not observed in one series.[1]

The accumulation of the neoplastic tissue behind the globe produces a gradually progressive exophthalmos. In time, the eyelids will not close adequately, and the cornea will be affected by exposure keratitis and the conjunctiva by chemosis.

ETIOLOGY. Lymphosarcoma in cattle is caused by the bovine leukemia virus (BLV), a retrovirus.[4] The virus is spread horizontally and transmitted via infectious colostrum, milk, and saliva, and by mechanical means. Cattle with lymphosarcoma are positive for BLV by the BLV-agar gel immunodiffusion test.

PATHOLOGIC FEATURES. Ocular lymphosarcoma is generally one of several sites with neoplasm, and most cattle have neoplastic lymphoid tissues in such organs as the uterus, kidneys, abomasum, and visceral and peripheral lymph nodes.[2,3] The orbital neoplastic tissue may be composed of one of four principal cytologic forms. Thus, lymphosarcomas of ocular/adnexal sites have the cytologic type of the systemic neoplasm and may be placed in well-differentiated (Figure 12.2), intermediately differentiated, poorly differentiated, and immunoblastic categories.[5] The neoplastic lymphoid cells infiltrate the tissues of the orbit and may extend into the sclera. The neoplastic cells spread among the fibers of the extraocular muscles and surround the optic nerve but without invading the nerve.

BIOLOGIC FEATURES. Cattle with clinical signs indicative of ocular/orbital lymphosarcoma (exophthalmos) die within a few months from the diffuse involvement of such organs as the heart, kidneys, and liver.

TREATMENT. Treatment of orbital lymphosarcoma in cattle is seldom indicated because most cattle have disseminated disease and die within a few months of diagnosis. If a cow is pregnant and will deliver a calf in a few months, enucleation can be performed to relieve pain and suffering. Also, surgery might be used in a valuable cow with lymphosarcoma, which might be retained for superovulation and embryo transfer before her death.[2]

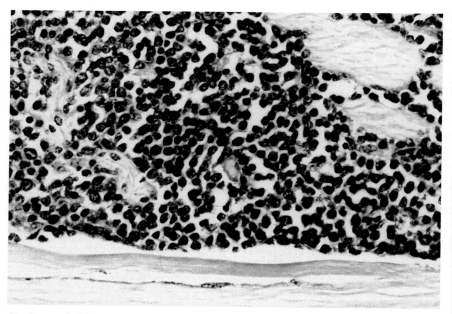

FIG. 12.2—Bovine; periorbita. Lymphosarcoma. Well-differentiated neoplastic lymphocytes infiltrate the periorbital tissue. Hematoxylin-eosin, ×350.

Canine Ocular Lymphosarcoma

INCIDENCE AND CLINICAL FEATURES. Lymphosarcoma is the most frequently diagnosed metastatic intraocular neoplasm,[6] but it also occurs in the orbit (Figure 12.3).[7,8] Most cases of intraocular lymphosarcoma are bilateral. Widespread systemic involvement either accompanies or precedes recognizable intraocular lymphosarcoma.

Clinical signs in dogs with intraocular lymphosarcoma include a variety of changes of the conjunctiva and cornea as well as iritis, uveitis, retinopathy, intraocular hemorrhage, and glaucoma.[6,9] The cornea is involved in globes with extensive infiltration at the limbus, episclera, and anterior uvea. The clinical appearance is that of an interstitial keratitis with dense corneal edema and deep vascularization. A dense white band may develop around the limbal margin of the cornea.

ETIOLOGY. The etiology of canine lymphosarcoma has not been determined, but an oncornaviral etiology has been suggested by the results of certain studies. Some lymphomas have been positive in the reverse transcriptive assay.[10]

PATHOLOGIC FEATURES. In intraocular lymphosarcoma, all segments of the globe may be invaded by neoplastic lymphoid cells, but the anterior uvea appears to be the primary site of metastasis. When only a few neoplastic lymphoid cells are present in the globe, they are generally found in the anterior ciliary body and root of the iris. When ocular involvement is more extensive, the anterior uvea is most severely infiltrated, with the choroid less so (Figures 12.4 and 12.5).

The extent of ocular involvement in metastatic ocular lymphosarcoma is highly variable, with some globes having scattered cells in the anterior uvea to globes containing large nodular masses that distort and replace the anterior uvea (Figures 12.6 and 12.7). When the involvement is nonnodular, the neoplastic lymphoid cells infiltrate the interstitial tissue and appear fairly evenly distributed. In some globes with less extensive infiltration, the neoplastic lymphoid cells are often perivascular and form collars or clumps of cells about small vessels (Figure 12.8). Neoplastic lymphoid cells often form a thin layer of cells on the anterior face of the iris (Figure 12.9) and may be free in the filtration angle and meshwork. When the anterior segment is extensively infiltrated, neoplastic lymphoid cells invade the cornea as orderly rows of cells between the collagen lamellae of the cornea stroma. Neoplastic lymphocytes may be well-differentiated (lymphocytic), intermediately differentiated (prolymphocytic) (Figure 12.10), poorly differentiated (lymphoblastic), and immunoblastic. Globes with lymphosarcoma may demonstrate a spectrum of secondary changes (Figure 12.11).

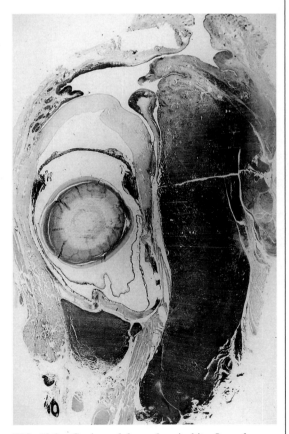

FIG. 12.3—Canine; globe and periorbita. Lymphosarcoma. The globe is distorted by large orbital lymphosarcoma that extends into the periorbital tissue. Hematoxylin-eosin, ×5.

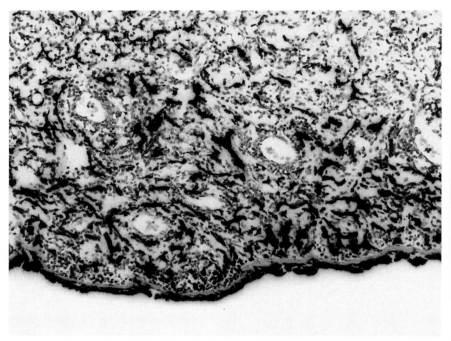

FIG. 12.4—Canine; globe, iris. Lymphosarcoma. Neoplastic lymphocytes are distributed throughout the iridic stroma. Hematoxylin-eosin, ×140.

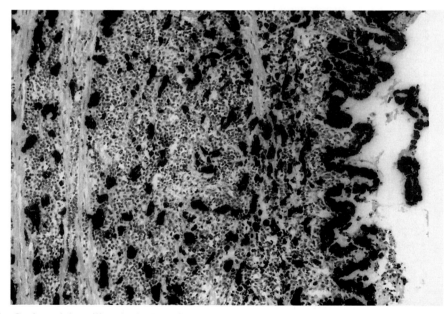

FIG. 12.5—Canine; globe, ciliary body. Lymphosarcoma. Neoplastic lymphocytic cells infiltrate the stroma and separate the ciliary muscle fibers. Hematoxylin-eosin, ×140.

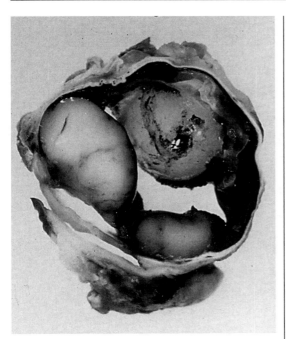

FIG. 12.6—Canine; globe. Lymphosarcoma. The sectioned globe contains two modular masses of lymphosarcoma.

BIOLOGIC FEATURES. Dogs with metastatic ocular lymphosarcoma have a very short life expectancy, as this lesion probably represents a late-stage occurrence in dogs with multicentric or alimentary lymphosarcoma.

TREATMENT. Because dogs with ocular lymphosarcoma have disseminated disease and a short life expectancy, excision is generally not indicated. However, palliative surgical procedures along with radiation therapy and chemotherapy may be used with some success to prolong a life with good quality.

Feline Ocular Lymphosarcoma

INCIDENCE AND CLINICAL FEATURES. The occurrence of intraocular metastatic lymphosarcoma is not uncommon, although few cases have been reported.[6,11–13] This is in contrast to the common occurrence of lymphosarcoma in cats. Lymphosarcoma also occurs as an orbital lesion.[8,14,15] Most of the described cases of ocular lymphosarcoma have been in cats with disseminated lymphosarcoma. Orbital lymphosarcoma is

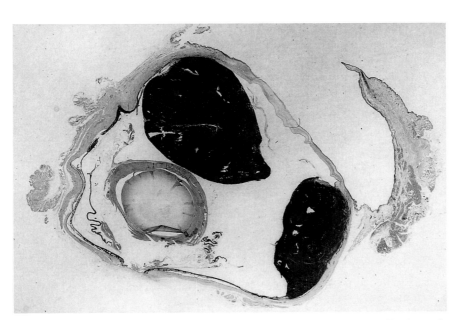

FIG. 12.7—Canine; globe. Lymphosarcoma. Darkly stained masses represent nodular collections of neoplastic lymphocytes. Hematoxylin-eosin, ×9.

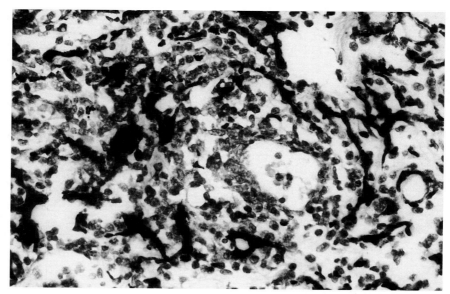

FIG. 12.8—Canine; globe, iris. Lymphosarcoma. Neoplastic lymphocytes are aggregated about the vessel in the iridic stroma. Hematoxylin-eosin, ×224.

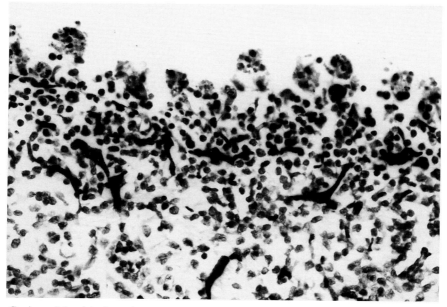

FIG. 12.9—Canine; globe, iris. Lymphosarcoma. Neoplastic lymphocytes are concentrated along the anterior face of an iris leaf. Hematoxylin-eosin, ×224.

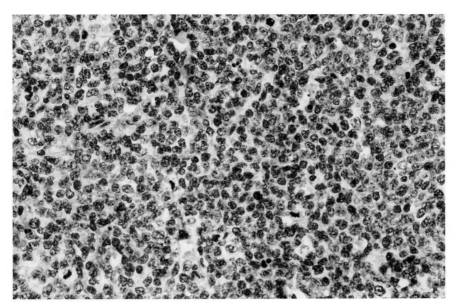

FIG. 12.10—Canine; globe. Lymphosarcoma. A sheet of lymphocytes of intermediate differentiation (prolymphocytic). Hematoxylin-eosin, ×350.

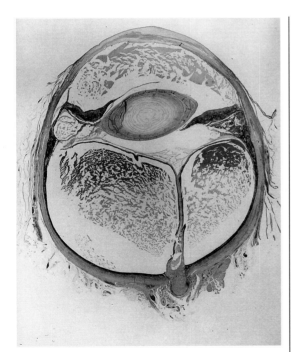

FIG. 12.11—Canine; globe. Lymphosarcoma. Neoplasm infiltrates the uvea and is accompanied by exudate in the anterior and posterior chambers, posterior synechia, retinal detachment, and presence of a subretinal exudate. Hematoxylin-eosin, ×6.

manifested by exophthalmos and intraocular lymphosarcoma by "uveitis" and by the presence of an intraocular mass (Figures 12.12 and 12.13). The lesion may present as a raised pink mass extending from the base of the iris to the papillary margin. In many cats with metastatic intraocular lymphosarcoma, the eyes have no clinical signs.

ETIOLOGY. A majority of cats with lymphosarcoma test positive for feline leukemia virus, a retrovirus that is horizontally transmitted and causes hematologic disease and immune suppression.[16,17] The incidence of positive reactions varies with age (more in younger cats) and distribution of lymphosarcoma (more in cats with multicentric lymphosarcoma).

PATHOLOGIC FEATURES. Lymphoid cells infiltrate various regions of the globe. The neoplasm apparently begins in the uvea from hematogenously deposited neoplastic lymphocytes. Mildly affected globes have infiltrates into the iris and ciliary body, with thickening of the iris and ciliary processes. When involvement is extensive, the lymphoid neoplasm replaces the anterior uvea, protrudes into the anterior chamber, and

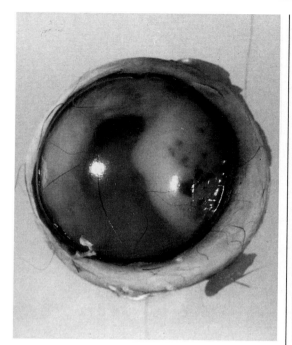

FIG. 12.12—Feline; globe. Lymphosarcoma. Neoplasm has markedly thickened the iris throughout most of its circumference.

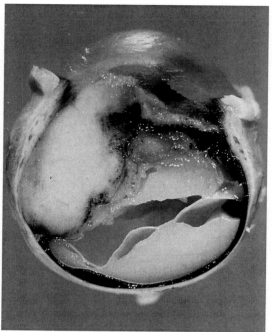

FIG. 12.13—Feline; globe. Lymphosarcoma. Neoplastic lymphocytes form a mass involving the iris, ciliary body, and choroid and protrude into the vitreal cavity.

infiltrates into the cornea and sclera (Figures 12.14 and 12.15). Larger masses have areas of necrosis with viable neoplastic cells forming cuffs about some blood vessels. The neoplasm extends into the choroid with resultant exudative retinal detachment and may break out of the globe into the periocular tissues and infiltrate extraocular muscles (Figure 12.16). Neoplastic lymphoid cells occur as dense solid masses or as infiltrating columns within such tissues as the cornea and sclera. The lymphoid cells vary somewhat in cytologic features, but are generally of moderate size, round cells with round to oval-shaped, often vesicular nuclei, some of which have prominent nucleoli (Figure 12.17).

Biologic Features. Lymphosarcoma has a rather short clinical course in cats, with about 75% dead within 8 weeks of detection.[18]

Treatment. Treatment of cats with ocular/orbital lymphosarcoma includes surgery, radiation therapy, and chemotherapy. The nature of the neoplasm lends to its diagnosis by fine-needle aspirational

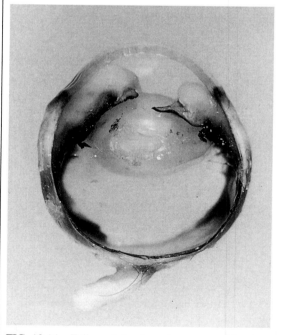

FIG. 12.14—Feline; globe. Lymphosarcoma. Neoplastic lymphocytes enlarge and replace the anterior uvea.

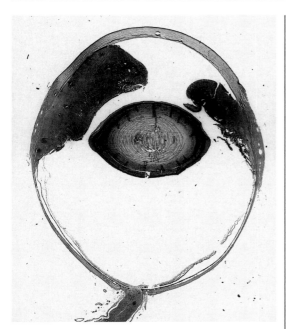

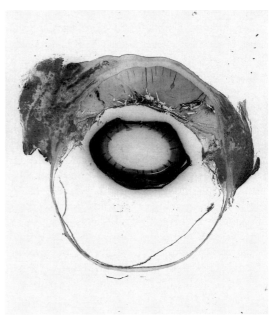

FIG. 12.15—Feline; globe. Lymphosarcoma. Neoplastic lymphocytes thicken and replace the anterior uvea, and neoplasm is especially extensive on the left side of the anterior uvea. Hematoxylin-eosin, ×9.

FIG. 12.16—Feline; globe. Lymphosarcoma. Neoplastic lymphocytes have penetrated the sclera and invaded the periocular tissues and cornea. Hematoxylin-eosin, ×10.

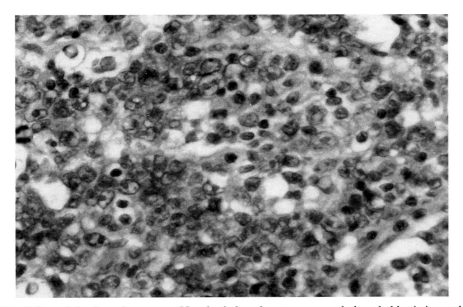

FIG. 12.17—Feline; globe. Lymphosarcoma. Neoplastic lymphocytes are mostly lymphoblastic in cytologic features with vesicular nuclei and prominent nucleoli. Hematoxylin-eosin, ×560.

biopsy. Frequently, the diagnosis is made upon the examination of an enucleated globe that has been removed due to complications of the lymphoma. Radiation and chemotherapy have been attempted with equivocal results.

Equine Ocular Lymphosarcoma

INCIDENCE AND CLINICAL FEATURES. Lymphosarcoma is an uncommon disease in horses, which are affected less frequently than are cattle, dogs, and cats. Ocular involvement is probably rare and has included involvement of the globe,[19] third eyelid,[19,20] eyelids,[21] and orbit.[19] Intraocular involvement results in bilateral "uveitis," and the neoplasm causes enlargement of the third eyelid and swelling of the eyelids. Lymphosarcoma of the eyelids thickens the eyelids and causes narrowing of the palpebral fissure.[21] Systemically, peripheral lymphadenopathy and/or abdominal masses (stomach, intestines, and mesentery) are present in most affected horses.

ETIOLOGY. No information is available on a cause of lymphosarcoma in horses.

PATHOLOGIC FEATURES. Intraocular metastatic lymphosarcoma is manifested in the few cases described as a bilateral "uveitis" with variable uveal infiltrates (Figure 12.18). Neoplastic cells infiltrate the interstitial tissues of the anterior uvea (Figure 12.19), and some cells are free in the anterior and posterior chambers (Figure 12.20). In such organs as the third eyelid and eyelids, the lymphosarcoma is characterized as a solid sheet of uniform lymphoid cells subdivided by fibrous septae. The neoplastic cells are round, have prominent round nuclei with prominent nucleoli in some, and have scant cytoplasm.

BIOLOGIC FEATURES. The course of the clinical disease in equine lymphosarcoma is variable depending on the principal organs affected with the neoplasm. Lymphosarcoma in horses may present as primary marrow involvement and thrombocytopenia, as an alimentary form, or as a peripheral lymphadenopathy. Four of the six horses with ocular lesions also had peripheral lymphadenopathy.[19]

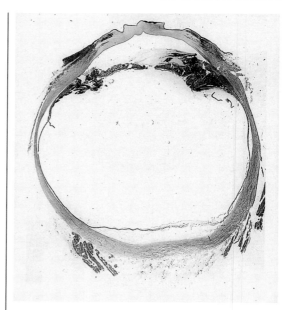

FIG. 12.18—Equine; globe. Lymphosarcoma. Neoplasm involves the anterior uvea with involvement more severe in the uvea of the right side of the globe. Hematoxylin-eosin, ×5. (Slide provided by Dr. M. McCracken.)

TREATMENT. Horses with ocular lesions have systemic lymphosarcoma as well and are not often treated. Successful surgical removal has been achieved with a case of lymphosarcoma of the third eyelid.[20]

HUMANS

Historical Perspective. Historically, the subject of ocular lymphoid tumors has been "mired in confusion and controversy."[22] The distinction between ophthalmic "benign" lymphoid proliferation and "malignant" lymphoma has yet to be clearly defined. Modern immunologic and molecular biologic techniques utilized to distinguish between benign and malignant lymphoid proliferations have reinforced the concept that "lymphoproliferative disorders may represent a continuous spectrum of disease that is not separable in a conceptual sense."[23] Nonetheless, ocular lymphoproliferative lesions fall into several definable categories that occur with varying frequencies in different locations in the orbit, eye, and ocular adnexa (Table 12.1). We consider *lymphoma* a subset of

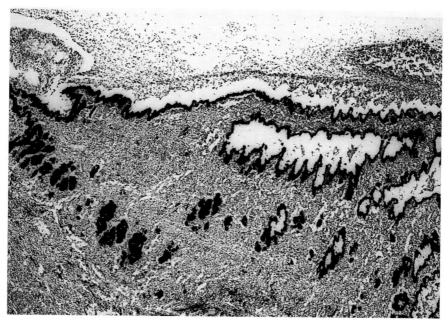

FIG. 12.19—Equine; globe, ciliary body. Lymphosarcoma. Neoplastic lymphocytes diffusely infiltrate the ciliary body and occur in the vitreal space interior to ciliary processes. Hematoxylin-eosin, ×35.

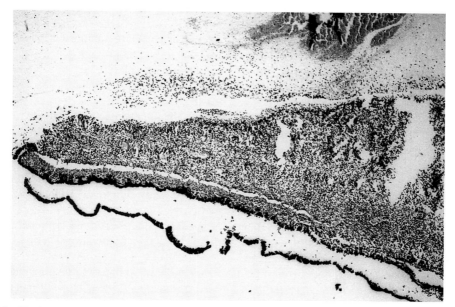

FIG. 12.20—Equine; globe, iris. Lymphosarcoma. Neoplastic lymphocytes diffusely infiltrate the iris, and some are present in the exudate in the anterior chamber. Hematoxylin-eosin, ×35.

TABLE 12.1—Characteristics of some lymphoproliferations of the orbit, ocular adnexa, and globe

Neoplasm	Ophthalmic site	Associated disease	Patients
Small lymphocytic proliferations	Orbit Conjunctiva	Systemic lymphoma	Female>male Adults
Large cell lymphoma	Uvea Retina Vitreous	Systemic lymphoma CNS lymphoma	Female>male Adults
Burkitt lymphoma			
African	Orbit	Visceral lymphoma	Children
Non-African	Orbit	Nodal lymphoma	Children
AIDS-related	Orbit	Nodal lymphoma	HIV positive
Hodgkin's disease	Orbit Eye	Systemic Hodgkin's disease	Adults
Lymphoplasma cytoid proliferations	Orbit	Multiple myeloma Waldenstrom's	Male>female Adults

CNS, central nervous system.

"lymphoproliferative (lymphoid) lesions." In this chapter, we discuss and classify the types of lymphoid proliferations that occur in and around the eye, describe what is known about the epidemiology of these lesions, present the clinical features and morphology of each type of lesion, and review treatment and prognosis.

Terminology. Ocular lymphocytic proliferations have been classified as extranodal because of their origin in tissue other than lymph nodes or traditionally recognized lymphoid organs. Additionally, conjunctival and orbital lymphomas have been considered to be part of the mucosal associated lymphoid tissue (MALT)-derived lymphomas.[24] Within the orbit, eye, and ocular adnexa, various lymphoid proliferations have been described, including benign (reactive) lymphoid hyperplasia (BLH), atypical lymphoid hyperplasia (ALH), malignant lymphoma, large cell lymphoma, Hodgkin's disease, Burkitt's lymphoma, cutaneous T-cell lymphoma (mycosis fungoides), and various lymphoplasmacytoid tumors.[25,26] A brief overview of the terminology associated with each of these types of lymphoid proliferations is presented in the next paragraph.

Although lymphocytes are normally present between the acini of the lacrimal gland and lymphocytes and plasma cells are located in the substantia propria of the conjunctiva,[27] the orbit, eye, and ocular adnexa are devoid of lymph nodes.[28] Any lymphoproliferative lesion of the ocular region is considered abnormal, even though the cells composing the lesion may have normal morphologic and cytologic features. In fact, any type of

ophthalmic lymphoid proliferation may be associated with extraophthalmic (systemic) involvement.[29] BLH describes a lymphocytic proliferation composed of a mixture of lymphocytes, histiocytes, plasma cells, and other inflammatory cells in a reactive pattern.[25,26] The older term *pseudolymphoma* has also been applied to BLH.[24] ALH is used to describe intermediate lesions. Malignant lymphoma is reserved for those lesions that are composed of monoclonal proliferations of lymphocytes. BLH, ALH, and malignant lymphoma can be considered to comprise a spectrum of non-Hodgkin's lymphoid tumors.[26] Malignant lymphoma of large cell type, previously known by the now obsolete terms "reticulum cell sarcoma" and "histiocytic lymphoma," is considered separately because of its distinct clinicopathologic presentation in the eye.[25] Currently, the Working Formulation and the Rappaport Classification (Table 12.2) are most commonly used to classify malignant lymphoma. Other lymphoid proliferations of the orbit, eye, and ocular adnexa that are discussed in this chapter include Hodgkin's disease, Burkitt's lymphoma, cutaneous T-cell lymphoma (mycosis fungoides), and lymphoplasmacytoid tumors.

Epidemiology. Lymphoid tumors (masses) have been documented in almost every part of the eye and ocular adnexa, although they are most commonly found in the orbit and conjunctiva.[25] Primary extraocular lymphomas appear to be found in decreasing order of frequency in the orbit, conjunctiva, and eyelid.[29] Based on series most representative of ophthalmic practice, malignant lymphoma, ALH, and BLH account for approximately

TABLE 12.2—Working Formulation and Rappaport Classification of malignant lymphoma

Working Formulation	Rappaport Classification
Low grade	
Small lymphocytic	Lymphocytic, well differentiated
Follicular, predominantly small cleaved cell	Nodular, poorly differentiated lymphocytic
Follicular, mixed small small and large cell	Nodular, mixed lymphocytic and histiocytic
Intermediate grade	
Follicular, large cell	Nodular, histiocytic
Diffuse, small cleaved cell	Diffuse, poorly differentiated lymphocytic
Diffuse, mixed small and large cell	Diffuse, mixed lymphocytic and histiocytic
Diffuse, large cell	Diffuse, histiocytic
High grade	
Large cell, immunoblastic	Diffuse, histiocytic
Lymphoblastic	Lymphoblastic lymphoma
Small noncleaved cell	Undifferentiated, Burkitt's and non-Burkitt's

Modified from Robbins et al. (page 711).[42]

8%–13% of all orbital space-occupying lesions.[30–33] In a series of 2455 surgically excised conjunctival lesions in adults, malignant lymphoma and lymphoid hyperplasia accounted for 3% of the lesions.[34] Primary intraocular lymphoid proliferations are less common than ocular adnexal lymphoma. The largest series to date of primary intraocular lymphomas includes 32 patients.[35] The incidence of intraocular BLH is unknown.[25] Patients with systemic malignant lymphoma occasionally have ocular involvement. In an autopsy series of 1269 patients with systemic lymphoma, 1.3% had orbital involvement[36] and, in another series of 60 patients who died with systemic lymphoma, four (6.6%) had intraocular involvement.[37]

The majority of ocular and ocular adnexal lymphoid proliferations occur in patients in decades 5–7 of life and are thus rarely seen in children,[33,38] except for Burkitt's lymphoma, which primarily involves children. Burkitt's lymphoma can be divided into three forms, all of which may involve the orbit.[39] The African form of Burkitt's lymphoma, which is the most common tumor found in children in tropical Africa,[40,41] typically invades the maxilla and, by extension, the orbit. Orbital involvement is seen in up to 50% of cases.[39] The age of maximum susceptibility is 5–6 years.[33] Orbital involvement in non-African (American) Burkitt's lymphoma is less common than in the African form. American Burkitt's lymphoma most often arises in the terminal ileum and spreads to regional lymph nodes and bone marrow, with a median age of onset at 10–11 years.[33]

The acquired immune deficiency syndrome (AIDS) or HIV-related form of Burkitt's lymphoma is similar to the American form, although it tends to arise in lymph nodes and a variety of other sites and has a higher incidence of central nervous system (CNS) involvement.[39]

Epstein-Barr virus (EBV) has been implicated as a possible etiologic factor in the pathogenesis of Burkitt's lymphoma, most strongly in the African form. Immunocompetent patients can mount a T-cell response to the virus, whereas patients with AIDS and other disorders have impaired immunocompetence, resulting in uncontrolled B-cell proliferation.[39,42]

Patients with HIV infection have an increased incidence of malignant lymphoma when compared with age-matched counterparts, including a higher incidence of extranodal lymphoma.[43] Orbital[44–46] and intraocular[43,47] large cell lymphoma have been reported in patients with AIDS. One series of autopsies of 25 patients with AIDS reported that one patient had an orbital lymphoma,[46] but the true incidence of orbital lymphoma in patients with AIDS is unknown.[4]

Clinical Features. The clinical features of lymphoid proliferations of the orbit, eye, and ocular adnexa vary according to the nature of the lymphocytic proliferation and the site at which it occurs.

LYMPHOID TUMORS OF SMALL LYMPHOCYTIC TYPE. This category includes BLH, ALH, and malignant lymphoma, all of which have similar

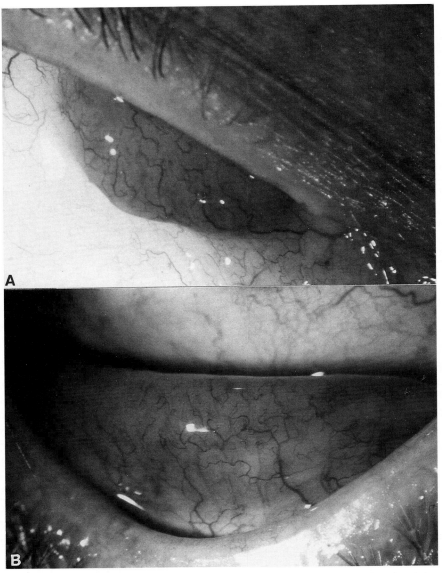

FIG. 12.21—This 43-year-old man developed bilateral conjunctival "salmon patch" lesions involving the right bulbar (**A**) and left tarsal (**B**) conjunctiva.

clinical presentations. Malignant lymphoma of large cell type is discussed separately because of its unique clinical features.

Lymphoid tumors may occur in the conjunctiva, uvea, ocular adnexa, or orbit. In a study of 117 lymphoid tumors occurring in the orbit, conjunctiva, and the eyelid, the majority occurred in the orbit (68%), followed by the conjunctiva (28%) and eyelid (8%).[29] The median age of

patients at the time of presentation is 61 years, with a range of 17–93 years.[29] The male-to-female ratio is approximately 1:1.4.[29] Presenting complaints include insidious proptosis, displacement of one or both eyes, and a mass or swelling.[26,29] Common physical findings include a palpable mass, proptosis, and ptosis. Conjunctival lymphoid tumors have a characteristic "salmon patch" appearance (Figures 12.21 and 12.22).

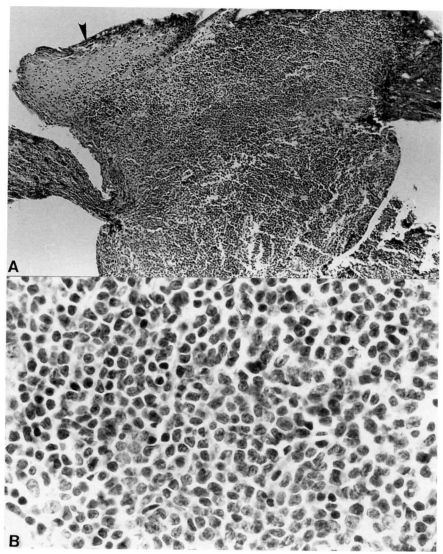

FIG. 12.22—**A:** Biopsy of the bulbar conjunctival lesion from the patient in Figure 12.21 shows conjunctival epithelium (arrowhead) overlying substantia propria that is infiltrated with mononuclear cells. Hematoxylin-eosin, ×25. **B:** Higher magnification shows the infiltrate to be composed of monotonous cells with condensed chromatin and cleaved or irregular nuclei. A diagnosis of malignant lymphoma was made. Hematoxylin-eosin, ×160.

Visual and motility disturbances are relatively uncommon.[26,29] Both benign and malignant orbital lymphoid tumors are usually unilateral. Previous reports have noted that bilateral tumors are more likely to be malignant lymphoma rather than benign or reactive lesions,[26,48] although currently it is unclear whether that is the case.

Extraocular lymphoid tumors tend to involve the lacrimal gland in the anterior, superior orbit and may be difficult to distinguish from other lacrimal gland tumors, although computed tomography (CT) may assist in making the distinction. Orbital lymphoid tumors have a characteristic CT appearance, tending to mold or conform to orbital bones and the globe like putty (Figure 12.23), whereas epithelial malignancies of the lacrimal gland tend to compress or destroy adjacent bone.[26] Additionally, orbital lymphomas

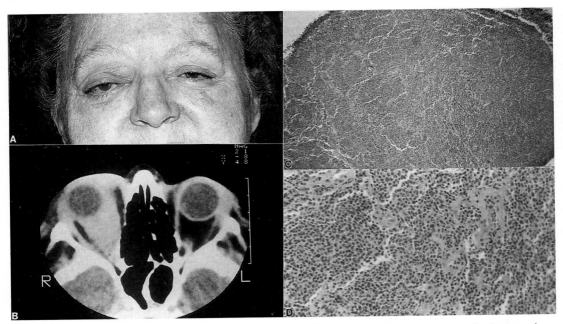

FIG. 12.23—**A:** This 67-year-old woman was evaluated for fullness of the right superior orbit. **B:** Computed tomography demonstrated a superomedial orbital mass that conformed to bone and the globe like putty. **C:** A biopsy of the mass showed sheets of small round cells. Hematoxylin-eosin, ×25. **D:** Higher magnification showed a monotonous proliferation of small lymphocytes consistent with a malignant lymphoma of small lymphocytic ("well differentiated" lymphocytic lymphoma). Hematoxylin-eosin, ×100.

tend to be ovoid or oblong masses, whereas epithelial malignancies are more rounded.[26] Despite these observations, CT is not considered useful in distinguishing malignant lymphoma from BLH. One study found that malignant lymphomas are more likely to have a homogeneous appearance than are reactive lesions, and that bone destruction, although rare, was confined to malignant lymphoma.[49] Another report noted that bone destruction occurred in a reactive inflammatory process.[50]

Intraocular lymphoid tumors are less common than extraocular or adnexal lesions. BLH of the uvea typically occurs as a unilateral condition. The mean age of patients at the time of onset is 5 years (range, 30–94 years). The disease is slightly more common in females than males and in whites than nonwhites.[51] The most common presenting complaint is decreased vision. Physical findings are based on the location of the uveal BLH and include iris thickening, proptosis secondary to extrascleral involvement, glaucoma, choroidal thickening with or without retinal detachment, and iridocyclitis.[51] Primary intraocular malignant lymphoma is most commonly of large cell type.

MALIGNANT LYMPHOMA, LARGE CELL TYPE. Extraocular or orbital involvement by large cell lymphoma is less common than presentation in the eye itself. The clinical features of orbital large cell lymphoma are similar to those of other orbital lymphoid tumors, although patients with large cell lymphoma are more likely to have systemic involvement than those with small lymphocytic lymphoma. CNS involvement may result in visual field defects, muscle palsies, or papilledema.[25] Orbital CT of patients with large cell lymphoma reveals destruction of bone more often than in patients with other types of lymphoma.

Intraocular large cell lymphoma is often associated with extraocular disease. The mean age of onset of symptoms is 60 years, although the disease has been reported in a 27-year-old patient.[35,52] In a series of 32 patients reported by Freeman and coworkers, the disease was found to be more common in women than in men.[35] Other series have found equal gender distributions.[53]

The two clinically recognized patterns of intraocular involvement by large cell lymphoma are vitreoretinal and uveal, with the former being more common than the latter.[35] Vitreoretinal large cell lymphoma is thought to be part of multicentric CNS lymphoma, whereas uveal large cell lymphoma probably occurs secondary to involvement outside the CNS.[35] The majority of patients with uveal large cell lymphoma have bilateral ocular disease and associated visceral involvement. Overlapping of the vitreoretinal and uveal types occurs.[25]

Presenting complaints in both types of large cell lymphoma include painless decrease in vision and floaters.[35] Patients are often initially diagnosed with chronic uveitis that is poorly responsive to corticosteroids.[53] Physical findings in patients with vitreoretinal large cell lymphoma include keratic precipitates, aqueous cells, pseudohypopyon, vitreous cells, and haze (Figure 12.24), and retinal infiltrates sometimes simulating a perivasculitis.[25] These patients may have small tumor detachments of the retinal pigment epithelium, giving a leopard-spot appearance that may be appreciated on fluorescein angiography (Figures 12.24 and 12.25). Occasionally, intraocular large cell lymphoma may mimic an infectious necrotizing retinitis with gray-to-white opacification of the retina and associated hemorrhage. Retinal artery obstruction has been reported in association with large cell lymphoma.[54] Ophthalmoscopic findings in patients with uveal large cell lymphoma include distinctive yellow-white fundus lesions and clear vitreous. The lesions may be multiple and discrete or may coalesce to form large masses. Uveal lymphoma may occasionally include predominantly retinal lesions.[55] Large cell lymphoma should be considered in older patients with uveitis of unknown etiology; delays in the diagnosis of intraocular large cell lymphoma are common.[25,35]

MISCELLANEOUS LYMPHOID TUMORS. Other lymphoid tumors occurring in and around the eye include Burkitt's lymphoma, cutaneous T-cell lymphoma (mycosis fungoides), Hodgkin's disease, and lymphoplasmacytoid tumors, including multiple myeloma (discussed below). Rare lesions including angiocentric lymphoma (malignant angioendotheliomatosis), angiolymphoid hyperplasia with eosinophilia (Kimura's disease), and sinus histiocytosis with massive lymphadenopathy (Rosai-Dorfman disease) may occur, but are not discussed here.

BURKITT'S LYMPHOMA. The three types of clinical profiles of affected patients have been described above. This section focuses on the presenting symptoms and physical findings associated with the disease.

The African variety of Burkitt's lymphoma typically arises in the maxilla and may enlarge to involve the orbit, resulting in rapidly progressive proptosis, upward displacement of the globe, and sometimes visual loss. The tumor may invade the globe or cause such severe displacement as to result in exposure keratopathy.[26,39]

The American form of Burkitt's lymphoma classically arises in the terminal ileum, most likely in Peyer's patches. Orbital involvement with rapidly progressive unilateral proptosis may occur from enlargement of a primary tumor arising in the ethmoid sinus.[26,56] Other less common presentations are fulminant bilateral proptosis[26,57] and meningeal carcinomatosis.[26,58]

The HIV-related form of Burkitt's lymphoma most often arises in lymph nodes and sometimes may primarily involve the bone marrow.[39]

CUTANEOUS T-CELL LYMPHOMA (MYCOSIS FUNGOIDES). The term *cutaneous T-cell lymphoma* is used to encompass a spectrum of diseases that are characterized by clonal proliferations of T lymphocytes arising in or predominantly involving the skin.[59] A classification of cutaneous T-cell lymphoma has been discussed by Meekins and coworkers.[59] According to this classification, cutaneous T-cell lymphoma may be the most common type of lymphoma affecting adults in the United States.[60] The disease is more common in men than women and typically occurs in patients over age 45.[59] Mycosis fungoides and the Sézary syndrome are variants that account for approximately one-third of patients with cutaneous T-cell lymphoma.

Ophthalmic involvement in patients with cutaneous T-cell lymphoma may be more common

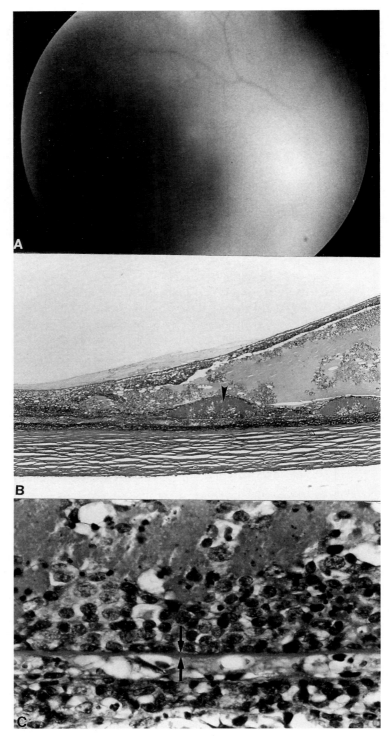

FIG. 12.24—**A:** An 87-year-old woman was evaluated for retinal infiltrates and a hazy vitreous. **B:** Examination of her enucleated blind right eye showed a necrotic retina infiltrated with atypical mononuclear cells. The same cells were present underlying retinal pigment epithelial detachments (arrowhead). Hematoxylin-eosin, ×10. **C:** Close inspection showed large cell lymphoma present internally and externally to Bruch's membrane (between the arrows). Hematoxylin-eosin, ×160. (Case presented by Curtis E. Margo, MD, at the 1988 Theobald Society Meeting.)

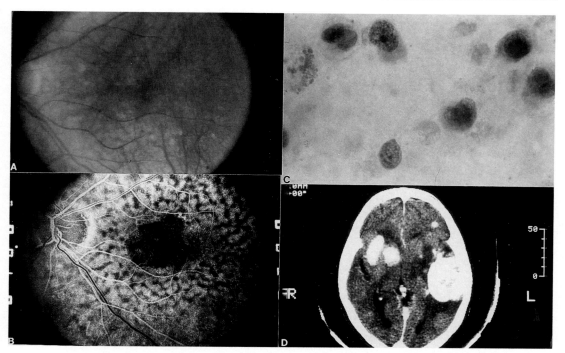

FIG. 12.25—**A:** The left eye of this 68-year-old woman with a history of "chronic uveitis" demonstrates vitreous haze and a "leopard spot" appearance at the level of the retinal pigment epithelium. **B:** Fluorescein angiography highlights the "leopard spot" appearance that is due to small tumor detachments of the retinal pigment epithelium. **C:** Cells obtained from a vitreous biopsy specimen show increased nuclear-to-cytoplasmic ratios, heterochromatin, nuclear membrane infoldings, and prominent nucleoli. The diagnosis is large cell lymphoma. Papanicolaou, ×400. **D:** The patient subsequently developed cerebral infiltrates of large cell lymphoma demonstrated by computed tomography.

than previously recognized and may provide an early clue to the sometimes elusive diagnosis. In a recent study, 17 patients with cutaneous T-cell lymphoma underwent ophthalmic examination.[60] The most frequent ophthalmic finding, seborrheic blepharoconjunctivitis, was noted in 13 (76%) of the patients. Other common findings included cicatricial ectropion (59%), diffuse conjunctivitis (41%), meibomianitis (29%), chalazia (18%), maderosis (18%), punctate epithelial defects of the cornea (59%), and keratitis sicca (24%). Although patients in that study were not compared with age-matched controls, the authors suggested that nonspecific ocular signs such as those listed above may be clues to the diagnosis of T-cell lymphoma in its early epidermotrophic stage, and ophthalmologists evaluating patients with persistent seborrheic blepharoconjunctivitis should inquire regarding cutaneous lesions elsewhere.[60]

The traditionally recognized ocular findings of cutaneous T-cell lymphoma are uncommon and generally occur in the more advanced stages of the disease. These findings include conjunctival and caruncle infiltrates, necrotizing or ulcerative keratitis, anterior and posterior uveitis, retinal and vitreous infiltrates, optic atrophy, papilledema, orbital involvement, and eyelid tumors (Figure 12.26), which may be single or multiple and rapidly enlarge, simulating orbital cellulitis.[59–67]

HODGKIN'S DISEASE. Hodgkin's disease rarely affects ocular structures. When it does occur, it is generally seen in patients with long-standing histories of the disease.[26,68,69] Visual pathway involvement has been reported as the initial manifestation of the disease in at least one instance.[70] Hodgkin's disease has a bimodal age distribution, with the early peak at 15–24 years and the second peak after age 45.[42] Orbital involvement

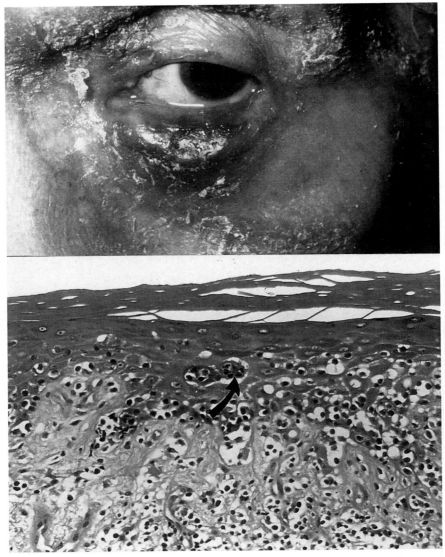

FIG. 12.26—**A:** This 77-year-old woman was evaluated for a left lower eyelid ectropion and a cutaneous lesion that involved the eyelid and cheek. **B:** Biopsy of the eyelid showed a dermal and epidermal infiltrate of irregular lymphocytes, some of which formed Pautrier microabscesses (arrow). The diagnosis is cutaneous T-cell lymphoma. Hematoxylin-eosin, ×63. (Case presented by Godfrey Heathcote, MD, at the 1992 Eastern Ophthalmic Pathology Society Meeting.)

is characterized by a unilateral or bilateral progressively enlarging mass.[26]

Intraocular findings that have been reported in patients with Hodgkin's disease include anterior granulomatous uveitis with keratic precipitates, Koeppe nodules, and diffuse vitreous reaction.[25] Soft exudates may be found in the retinas.[25,71,72]

LYMPHOPLASMACYTOID TUMORS. This category of tumors includes multiple myeloma, Waldenström's macroglobulinemia, extramedullary plasmacytoma, small lymphocytic lymphoma with plasmacytoid features, and other neoplasms composed of B cells with hybrid cellular characteristics representing a cross between plasma cells and

TABLE 12.3—Ocular involvement in multiple myeloma

Orbit
  Invasion of bone by tumor
  Compression of optic nerve
  Proptosis
  Ptosis
  Motility disturbance

Conjunctiva
  Crystal deposition
  Tumor infiltrate
  Hemostasis

Cornea
  Crystal deposition
  Copper deposition in Descemet's membrane

Anterior chamber
  Angle closure glaucoma
  Secondary glaucoma

Lens
  Subluxation
  Copper deposition

Uvea
  Iritis
  Pars plana/plicata cysts
  Choroidal tumors
  Choroidal infiltrates

Vitreous
  Hemorrhage

Retina
  Subretinal deposits
  Retinal vein occlusion
  Dysproteinemic fundus with hemorrhages, soft
    exudates venous beading, vascular tortuosity, and
    occlusion
  Microaneurysms
  Exudative retinal detachment
  Detachment of retinal pigment epithelium

Optic nerve
  Disc edema
  Neoplastic infiltration

Sclera
  Neoplastic infiltration

Extraocular muscles
  Amyloid infiltration

lymphocytes. Multiple myeloma, which is the prototype of these disorders,[26] is a neoplasm of plasma cells characterized by the production of a monoclonal immunoglobulin; "punched-out" lesions of the skull, vertebrae, and ribs; anemia; hypercalcemia; and increased susceptibility to infections.[73] The disease generally occurs in patients between the ages 40 and 70, and is twice as common in men as in women.[26,73] The ocular manifestations of multiple myeloma may be due to direct invasion by tumor cells or indirectly via production of the abnormal immunoglobulin (Table 12.3).[74,75]

Orbital involvement by plasma cell tumors is rare[76] and may be seen as part of multiple myeloma, as a solitary plasmacytoma (Figure 12.27), as an extension of plasmacytoma arising in a paranasal sinus, or as a primary orbital solitary plasmacytoma.[77,78] Solitary plasmacytoma of the orbital bone presents as a single osteolytic lesion and is associated with eventual development of multiple myeloma in some cases (Figure 12.27).

Waldenström's macroglobulinemia is a clinical term designating a malignant proliferation of lymphocytes secreting monoclonal immunoglobulin M (IgM) (or rarely IgA), causing increased serum viscosity, and most commonly affecting older men.[73] The most common pathologic diagnosis in patients with the disease is small lymphocytic lymphoma with plasmacytoid features, but the clinical syndrome occasionally occurs with other lymphomas if they secrete enough IgM. The disease rarely affects the orbit. The most common ocular manifestation of Waldenström's macroglobulinemia is congestive retinopathy caused by high levels of circulating IgM.[76]

Morphology. In this section, the gross and histologic appearances of ophthalmic lymphoproliferative lesions are discussed. Additionally, the use of immunohistochemical and molecular biologic techniques are reviewed as aids in distinguishing benign from malignant lesions.

SMALL LYMPHOCYTIC LYMPHOID TUMORS

GROSS APPEARANCE. The gross appearance of all lymphoid proliferations (BLH, ALH, and malignant lymphoma) is similar. The tumors have a "fish flesh" creamy-to-yellow appearance.

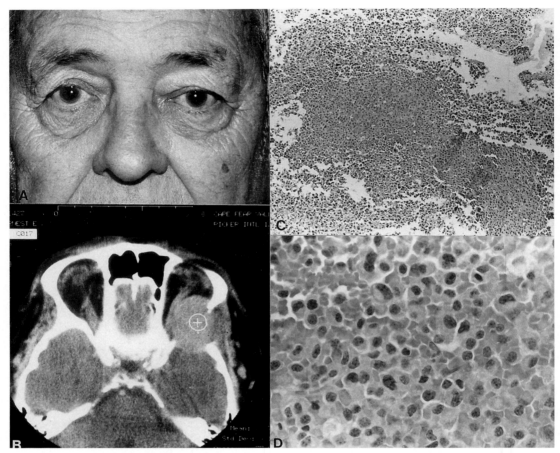

FIG. 12.27—**A:** This 69-year-old man was evaluated for proptosis of the left eye. **B:** Computed tomography showed a left posterolateral orbital mass with bone destruction. **C:** A biopsy of the mass showed sheets of round cells with abundant eosinophilic cytoplasm. Hematoxylin-eosin, ×25. **D:** The tumor cells displayed atypical, eccentric nuclei with coarsely clumped chromatin and abundant cytoplasm with a prominent Golgi zone. The diagnosis is solitary plasmacytoma. Hematoxylin-eosin, ×160. (Case presented by Mark W. Scroggs, MD, at the 1989 Eastern Ophthalmic Pathology Society Meeting.)

Highly vascularized lesions may be reddish. Because of a paucity of fibrous stroma, lymphoid lesions are typically friable.

HISTOLOGIC AND CYTOLOGIC APPEARANCE. Several distinctive histologic features are useful in making the diagnosis of BLH[22] (Figure 12.28). Scant fibrous stroma may help distinguish lymphoid tumors from inflammatory pseudotumors in which fibrosis may be a significant feature. The cells making up BLH are small lymphocytes with dark, round, bland nuclei and few mitotic figures. A polymorphic population of cells is present. Plasma cells, histiocytes, and eosinophils are often found. Germinal centers containing mitotically active large lymphocytes and tingible-body macrophages (macrophages that contain intracytoplasmic basophilic inclusions indicative of a rapid mitotic turnover) surrounded by a mantle of small lymphocytes suggest a reactive process. Similarly, plump, reactive endothelial cells are more common in BLH than in malignant lymphoma. Generally, BLH lesions have fewer than five mitotic figures per high-power field outside the reactive follicles, whereas follicular lymphoma may have increased mitotic activity in interfollicular zones.[22]

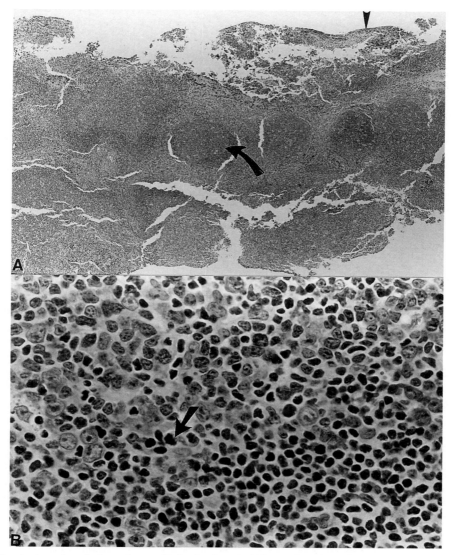

FIG. 12.28—**A:** A conjunctival specimen with benign lymphoid hyperplasia is surfaced by squamous mucosa (arrowhead) and contains lymphoid follicles (curved arrow) of lymphocytes surrounded by mantle zones. Hematoxylin-eosin, ×10. **B:** Mitotic figures (arrow) are confined to the follicular center in the top left of the field. Small lymphocytes are present in the mantle zone in the lower right of the field. Hematoxylin-eosin, ×160.

ALH represents a somewhat controversial group of borderline or indeterminate lymphoid lesions[22] that appear as monotonous and monomorphic sheets of cells (Figure 12.29). Remnants of follicles known as *abortive* or *pseudo*follicles (also called *naked* germinal centers) may be present. Within these follicles, mitotic activity is sparse or absent. Similar follicle-like structures may be present in mantle cell (centrocytic) lymphoma, and ALH might represent an evolving lymphoma. Individual cell nuclei in ALH are somewhat larger than in BLH. Chromatin is more open, and small nucleoli may be seen. The lymphocyte cytoplasm may be more abundant in ALH than in BLH. Multinucleated giant cells may be identified in ALH. ALH may also appear as a mixed population of cells in which a predominantly small

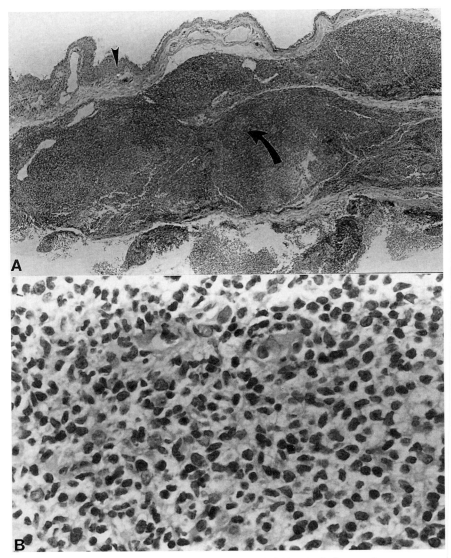

FIG. 12.29—**A:** This conjunctival specimen with atypical lymphoid hyperplasia contains squamous mucosa (arrowhead) on the surface and a diffuse infiltrate with abortive follicles (curved arrow). Hematoxylin-eosin, ×10. **B:** The infiltrate is composed of small mature lymphocytes and larger lymphocytes with moderately open chromatin patterns and punctate nucleoli. Hematoxylin-eosin, ×160.

lymphocytic line coexists with a subpopulation of larger lymphoid and histiocytic cells. In these lesions, mitotic activity is more prevalent.

There are several histologic classification schemes for malignant lymphoma, including the Working Formulation and Rappaport Classification (Table 12.2). These classifications are based on the general concepts that follicular (nodular) architecture portends a better prognosis than does a diffuse pattern and that small cell type generally implies more indolent disease than does large cell type. The prognostic significance of the follicular or diffuse nature of the lesion is unknown for ophthalmic lymphomas. The majority of ophthalmic lymphomas are classified as diffuse, with only about 10%–15% clas-

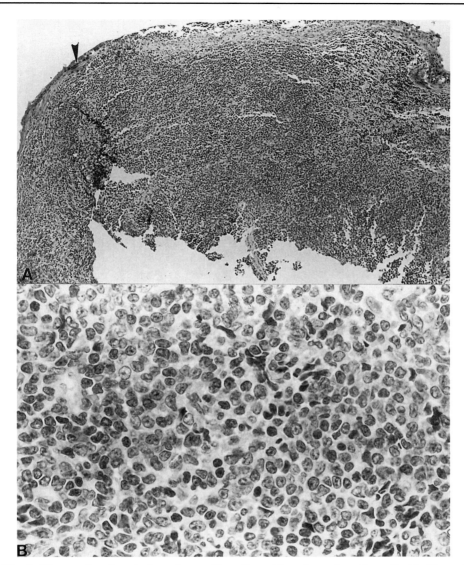

FIG. 12.30—**A:** The tarsal conjunctival specimen with malignant lymphoma from the patient in Figure 12.21 shows squamous mucosa (arrowhead) overlying a monotonous sheet of lymphocytes. Hematoxylin-eosin, ×25. **B:** Close inspection shows the tumor cells to have nuclei with slightly open chromatin, nuclear membrane infoldings, and small nucleoli. This is a predominantly small cleaved cell lymphoma (poorly differentiated lymphoma in the Rappaport Classification). Hematoxylin-eosin, ×160.

sified as follicular. Features that help distinguish follicular lymphoma from BLH are a decrease in mitotic figures in the center of the neoplastic follicles, endothelial cells not as reactive, inconspicuous tingible-body macrophages, and eosinophils and plasma cells are scarce in the former. Of the diffuse lymphomas, about half contain a mixture of small and large lymphocytes (mixed lymphocytic and histiocytic in the Rappaport Classification) and the other half are small lymphocytic or predominantly small cleaved cell (well-differentiated lymphocytic or poorly differentiated lymphocytic in the Rappport Classification) (Figure 12.30). The concept that many ocular adnexal lymphomas represent mantle cell (centrocytic, intermediate cell type) lymphomas is now emerging.[78] Extraocular lymphoma may represent an example of lymphoma arising in *m*ucosal *a*ssociated *l*ymphoid *t*issue (MALToma).

The size of the lymphocytes may be gauged by comparing the size of the nucleus with an adjacent endothelial cell or histiocyte nucleus. If the lymphocyte nucleus is the same size or smaller than the nonlymphoid nucleus, it is termed *small*. If the lymphocyte nucleus is consistently larger than the nonlymphoid nucleus, it is termed *large* (Figure 12.31). Nuclear membranes with infoldings are designated as *cleaved* nuclei. Optimal fixation and preservation of tissue is necessary for appropriate histologic evaluation and classification of lymphoproliferative disorders. Our laboratory uses B5, a mercury-based fixative. An alternative fixative is Zenker's solution. For comparison, the specimen shown in Figure 12.23 was fixed in formalin and those in Figures 12.22 and 12.30 were fixed in B5.

IMMUNOHISTOLOGIC AND MOLECULAR BIO-LOGIC FEATURES. It is difficult to determine the "benign" versus "malignant" nature of lymphoproliferative lesions of the ocular adnexa, since histologically "benign" lesions may be associated with extraocular (systemic) disease.[29] Pathologists have attempted to clarify the malignant potential (tendency of a given lesion to be associated with systemic disease) of lymphoproliferative tumors by studying immunophenotypic and genotypic features.

Immunohistochemical techniques have been used to identify the antigenicity of cells composing lymphoid infiltrates. Antigenic determinants such as CD antigens and immunoglobulin heavy and light chains may be used to identify the cell that displays the marker (i.e., B versus T lymphocytes versus macrophages), and thus the composition of the lymphoid tumor can be determined (Table 12.4). Studies that have correlated the histologic features of lymphoid proliferations of the orbit and adnexa with immunophenotypic features have revealed that the majority of lesions histologically classified as BLH have polyclonal features (a mixture of histiocytes, B and T lymphocytes, plasma cells,

etc.), whereas lesions classified as malignant lymphoma tend to have monoclonal immuno-histologic features.[27,29,51,79–81] Fresh-frozen tissue for surface marker immunophenotypic study is recommended, and fresh tissue is needed if suspension studies (flow cytometry) are to be done. Specific guidelines for differentiating polyclonal lymphoid proliferations from monoclonal B-cell lymphoma have been established (Table 12.5).[29]

Despite the usefulness of immunophenotyping in assessing clonality and thereby distinguishing benign lymphoid hyperplasia from B-cell lymphoma, this determination has little prognostic significance since similar percentages of patients with ocular adnexal lymphoid hyperplasia and B-cell lymphoma (29% and 35%, respectively) demonstrate prior, concurrent, or subsequent extraophthalmic lymphoma.[29] Further study of the genotypic features of extranodal lymphoid proliferations has provided some insight into the relationship between histologically benign and immunophenotypically polyclonal ocular lesions (BLH) and extraocular malignant lymphoma. Jakobiec, Knowles, and others have used molecular genetic (genotypic) analysis to identify gene rearrangements preceding immunoglobulin production in B lymphocytes and the expression of cell-surface antigen recognition receptors in T lymphocytes. Small clones of lymphocytes comprising as few as 2%–5% of cells in an infiltrate can be found to possess the same rearranged DNA sequences with genetic probes. Thus, studies of immunophenotypically polyclonal BLH lesions have revealed that the majority of these lesions harbor monoclonal or oligoclonal B-cell proliferations that theoretically may give rise to monoclonal B-cell lymphoma.[80–82] Jakobiec, Knowles, and coworkers proposed a scheme for lymphoid tumor progression analogous to that for melanocytic and squamous lesions. Even though they frequently contain occult clonal B-cell populations, lesions classified as BLH are only occasionally associated with extraocular lymphoma.[81] Therefore, classifying and treating BLH as malignant lymphoma based on the presence of gene rearrangement is not warranted at this time, and further investigation for more reliable markers of malignant transformation is needed.

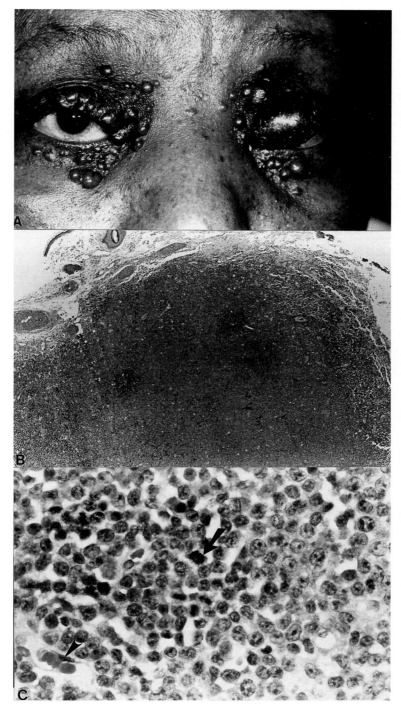

FIG. 12.31—**A:** This 58-year-old woman was evaluated for bilateral eyelid masses. **B:** A biopsy showed a diffuse monotonous infiltrate of mononuclear cells in the dermis. Hematoxylin-eosin, ×10. **C:** The tumor cells are large in comparison with an adjacent endothelial cell (arrowhead) and contain vesiculated nuclei with prominent nucleoli and scattered mitoses (arrow). The lesion was classified as a large cell lymphoma, immunoblastic. Hematoxylin-eosin, ×160.

TABLE 12.4—Monoclonal antibodies and cell markers for lymphocytes, natural killer cells, and monocytes-histiocytes

Cell type	Monoclonal/marker	Cell type	Monoclonal/marker
T lymphocytes	OKT 1 OKT 3 OKT 11 Leu 1	B lymphocytes	Leu 14 B 1 OKB 2 BA-1
T suppressor/Ig cytotoxic cells	OKT 5 OKT 8 Leu 3a	Plasma cells	surface OKT 10
Cytoplasmic Ig T-helper/inducer cells	OKT 4 Leu 3a	Histiocytes	OKM 1 OKM 5 OKT 6
Natural killer cells	OKM 1 OKT 10 Leu 7		M221

Modified from Jacobiec and Font.[22]

TABLE 12.5—Guidelines to determine polyclonal lymphoid proliferations from monoclonal B-cell lymphoma

1. Determine proportion of T and B cells
    A. If > 40% T cells, polyclonal
    B. If > 60% B cells, possible B-cell lymphoma
2. Determine kappa to lambda light-chain ratio by flow cytometry
    A. If between 0.3 and 6.3, probable polyclonal lesion
    B. If <0.1 or >6.9, probable monoclonal B-cell lymphoma
3. Identify anomalous immunophenotypic profile (lack of surface Ig on B cells, expression of CD 5 on B cells)—these are characteristic of malignant lymphoma

Malignant Lymphoma, Large Cell Type

GROSS APPEARANCE. Ophthalmic large cell lymphoma occurs in the uvea, retina, and vitreous. Specimens submitted for pathologic examination are either vitreous aspirates or enucleated eyes.[35] In enucleation specimens, the lymphoma commonly infiltrates the uvea, sensory retina, or both (Figure 12.24). Tumor cells may be located between the sensory retina and choroid, producing a neoplastic detachment of the retinal pigment epithelium (RPE) (Figures 12.24 and 12.25). The tumor may also infiltrate the iris and occlude the anterior chamber angle.[25]

HISTOLOGIC AND CYTOLOGIC APPEARANCE. The histologic appearance of large cell lymphoma in enucleated eyes includes lymphoma infiltration of the uvea, primarily the choroid. The tumor cells percolate through Bruch's membrane and are present as small mounds underlying the RPE (Figure 12.24). These small detachments of the RPE account for the funduscopic and fluorescein angiographic "leopard spot" appearance. There may be atrophy of the RPE overlying tumor infiltrates. Occasionally, tumor cells may be present in the retina particularly in a perivascular configuration. The involved eye may exhibit changes secondary to tumor infiltration, including ischemic and hemorrhagic changes. The optic nerve and vitreous may be infiltrated with lymphoma cells, depending on the severity of the involvement.

The cytologic evaluation of intraocular large cell lymphoma is of practical importance, since vitreous biopsy specimens are not infrequently evaluated to rule out large cell lymphoma in older adults with chronic uveitis of undetermined origin. It should be noted that considerable experience is required to evaluate these specimens. We recommend that the surgeon obtain approximately 0.5–1.0 ml of undiluted specimen via a pars plana vitrectomy approach. Our laboratory immediately dilutes the specimen with an equal volume of 95% ethyl alcohol. We process the specimen by the Millipore filter technique and modified Papanicolaou stain, although the cytospin technique and Wright-Giemsa stain are alternatives. The overall cellularity and cellular constituency of the specimen should be evaluated. For a diagnosis of large cell lymphoma, the specimen should be reasonably cellular and there should be a paucity of inflammatory cells, particularly polymorphonuclear leukocytes. Granulomatous inflammation should be excluded. Individual cells and clumps of cells with malignant cytologic features, including large size, chromatin margination, nuclear membrane infoldings, and prominent nucleoli, should be noted (Figure 12.25). Mitotic figures may occasionally be present. Wilson and coworkers have reported that immunohistochemical analysis may assist in the evaluation of these specimens.[83] Techniques such as genotyping cells in the vitreous biopsy specimen by using polymerase chain reaction may prove beneficial in the evaluation of intraocular lymphoma.

MISCELLANEOUS LYMPHOID TUMORS. The gross appearance of the entities in this category is similar to other lymphoid proliferations. The histologic appearance of the entities in this category is described as follows.

BURKITT'S LYMPHOMA. The three clinical types of Burkitt's lymphoma have a similar histopathologic appearance. The tumor is composed of tightly packed, small lymphocytes with interspersed tingible-body macrophages giving a "starry sky" appearance (Figure 12.32). Tumor cells have coarse chromatin and 2–5 nucleoli, and display striking mitotic activity.

CUTANEOUS T-CELL LYMPHOMA. This disease is characterized by cutaneous infiltration by neoplastic T lymphocytes that accumulate in the epidermis and superficial dermis. The lymphocytes may cluster around epidermal Langerhans cells to form Pautrier microabscesses (Figure 12.26), and individual cells are characterized by prominent nuclear infoldings.

HODGKIN'S DISEASE. Hodgkin's disease is composed of infiltrates of mononuclear malignant Hodgkin's cells and binucleate malignant Reed-Sternberg cells whose nuclei have a "fried egg" appearance. Variants of neoplastic cells, including lacunar cells, may be present. Variable numbers of lymphocytes, eosinophils, plasma cells, histiocytes, and sometimes polymorphonuclear leukocytes are present in Hodgkin's disease. The four histologic types of Hodgkin's disease are lymphocyte predominance, nodular sclerosis, mixed cellularity, and lymphocyte depletion. Reed-Sternberg cells are absent and lymphocytes are abundant in lymphocyte-predominant Hodgkin's disease. The nodular sclerosis type features nodules of tumor divided by lamellar bands of fibrous tissue, lacunar cells, and Reed-Sternberg cells. The mixed-cellularity type is intermediate in histologic appearance between lymphocyte-predominance and lymphocyte-depletion Hodgkin's disease. Lymphocyte-depletion Hodgkin's disease contains pleomorphic malignant cells with rare classic Reed-Sternberg cells, fibrosis, and few lymphocytes.

LYMPHOPLASMACYTOID PROLIFERATIONS. These lesions are characterized by plasma cells and plasmacytoid lymphocytes. Plasma cells contain eccentric nuclei, and the nucleus has a clockface or cartwheel chromatin pattern. A paranuclear pale halo or Hof zone (Golgi zone) is present. Plasmacytomas contain plasma cells with increased nuclear-to-cytoplasmic ratios, atypical nuclear characteristics, and multinucleate cells. Waldenström's macroglobulinemia, a clinical diagnosis, is usually caused by a neoplastic proliferation of small lymphocytes with plasmacytoid features. Intranuclear periodic acid-Schiff (PAS)-positive inclusions (Dutcher bodies) may be present.

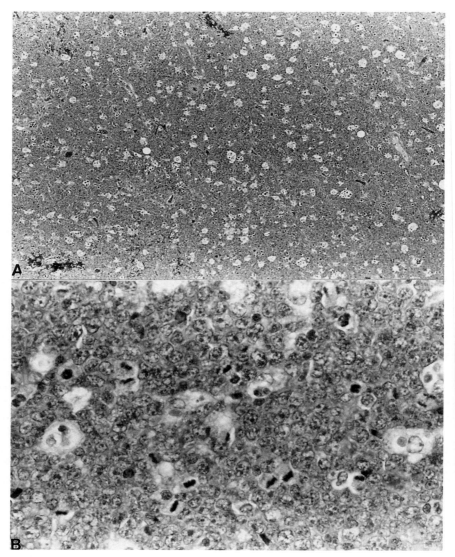

FIG. 12.32—**A:** This case of orbital African Burkitt's lymphoma exhibits a "starry sky" appearance due to tingible-body macrophages. Hematoxylin-eosin, ×25. **B:** The tumor is composed of small, monomorphous round cells with vesicular nuclei. Tingible-body macrophages and numerous mitotic figures are scattered throughout. Hematoxylin-eosin, ×160.

Diagnosis and Treatment

ORBITAL LYMPHOPROLIFERATIVE LESIONS. If an orbital lymphoma is suspected on the basis of clinical findings, a thorough evaluation for systemic disease should be performed. The evaluation should include a physical examination including palpation of the liver, spleen, and lymph nodes; complete blood count with differ-

ential; chest x-ray; CT scan of the chest, abdomen, and orbits; and serum electrophoresis.

If the findings on systemic workup are normal, an orbital biopsy should be performed. In general, an incisional biopsy is recommended so that adequate tissue may be removed for light-microscopic examination and immunohistochemical studies. This implies a minimum of 1 g of tissue. The lesion should be completely excised, if possible, without damaging surrounding structures. If the biopsy reveals lymphoma, bone marrow aspirations and biopsy should be performed for staging. In patients with previously documented malignant lymphoma presenting with an orbital mass, fine-needle aspiration biopsy may be considered and treatment instituted if the cells are compatible with the previous pathology.

Treatment varies depending on the histopathology of the lesion. In a diagnosis of BLH, the appropriate treatment is local radiotherapy with shielding of the globe. Some authors recommend 1500–2000 cGy,[26] whereas others recommend 2500–3000 cGy.[84] If the diagnosis is ALH and the findings on systemic workup are normal, local orbital radiotherapy using 2500–3000 cGy is advocated.[26] For a diagnosis of malignant lymphoma with normal findings on systemic workup, local radiotherapy using 2000–4000 cGy should be used.[84] If the findings on systemic workup are abnormal, the patient should be treated with appropriate therapy in conjunction with an oncologist. Often concurrent radiotherapy to the orbit and CNS is required. Burkitt's lymphoma is sensitive to chemotherapeutic agents, including cyclophosphamide, vincristine, and methotrexate. Cases of Burkitt's lymphoma refractory to chemotherapy may be treated with 3000 cGy of external radiation. The treatment of cutaneous T-cell lymphoma includes low-dose superficial irradiation, psoralen longwave ultraviolet-light therapy, and topical nitrogen mustard. Palliative chemotherapy is recommended for patients with disseminated disease (Sézary syndrome). Leukophoresis and antithymocyte globulin are under investigation as potentially useful treatments.[59] Multiple myeloma is treated with appropriate systemic chemotherapy. Additionally, orbital radiotherapy using 3000–4000 cGy may be recommended. For localized lymphoplasmacytoid lesions, treatment is less aggressive and may consist of simple excision.

INTRAOCULAR LYMPHOPROLIFERATIVE LESIONS. Primary lymphoproliferative lesions of the uvea are often misdiagnosed, with an average 13-month delay in diagnosis unless the index of suspicion is high. Freeman and coworkers recommend physical examination, CT of the head, and cerebrospinal fluid examination in all patients with ocular and/or systemic large cell lymphoma. Enlarged or suspicious lymph nodes should be biopsied. Iris lesions from intraocular large cell lymphoma appear as homogeneous diffuse solid masses on ultrasound. Fluorescein angiography may be nonspecific, showing early hyperfluorescence and late staining; the "leopard spot" appearance may be suggestive. CT may reveal an associated orbital or conjunctival mass, which may aid in the diagnosis. Biopsy may be performed on accessible involved anterior orbital or conjunctival tissue. Iridectomy or fine-needle aspiration biopsy may be used if the iris is involved. Cytologic and immunohistochemical analysis of a vitreous biopsy specimen may be useful in establishing the diagnosis of the vitreoretinal form of the disease (see above).[35,83] A trial of systemic corticosteroids or low-dose irradiation may be useful if the diagnosis is uncertain, as BLH often responds well to both treatments. A diagnostic enucleation may be required if malignant melanoma cannot be excluded.

Treatment is based on the nature of the lymphoproliferative lesion. If BLH is highly suspected or diagnosed by pathologic examination of tissue, systemic corticosteroids are used. If the lesion does not resolve with corticosteroid treatment, then low-dose irradiation (100–200 cGy) is recommended.

Suspected cases of intraocular large cell lymphoma are often diagnosed by vitreous biopsy for posteriorly located lesions and by fine-needle aspiration biopsy or iridectomy for anteriorly located lesions. Radiation is the mainstay of therapy for intraocular large cell lymphoma. Chemotherapy may be useful for large cell lymphoma that involves the viscera, but is relatively ineffective in large cell lymphoma of the eye. Treatment also depends whether the lymphoma involves the CNS.[35]

Prognosis

SMALL LYMPHOCYTIC LYMPHOID TUMORS. The most important prognostic factor in patients with an ocular adnexal infiltrate is the extent of disease discovered after thorough staging at the time of presentation (Table 12.6).[29,84] The vast majority of patients presenting with a clinical stage-IE lesion have a benign, indolent course regardless of histopathology or immunophenotype.[29] In a series

TABLE 12.6—Clinical stages of Hodgkin's disease and malignant lymphoma (Ann Arbor Classification)

Stage	Distribution of disease
I	Single lymph node region (I) or single extralymphatic site (IE)
II	Two or more lymph node regions on same side of diaphragm alone (II) or with contiguous extralymphatic organ/tissue (IIE)
III	Lymph node regions on both sides of diaphragm (III) may include speen (IIIS) and/or limited contiguous extralymphatic organ (IIIE) or site (IIIES)
IV	Multiple/disseminated foci of involvement of one or more extralymphatic organ/tissue with or without lymphatic involvement

Modified from Robbins et al. (page 715).[42]

of 117 ocular adnexal proliferations, 86% of all patients presenting with a clinical stage-IE unilateral or bilateral ocular adnexal lymphoid infiltrate, regardless of histopathology or immunophenotype, were alive, well, and free of lymphoma during a median follow-up of 51 months.[29]

Anatomic site was also helpful in predicting prognosis in the aforementioned series. Lymphoid infiltrates of the conjunctiva were associated with a lower incidence of extraocular lymphoma (20%) than were those of the orbit and eyelid (35% and 67%, respectively).[29] Other studies have not found the presenting site to be a significant prognostic factor.[84] Similarly, bilaterality is not a consistently reliable prognostic factor.[84] Adnexal lymphomas of small lymphocytic (well-differentiated lymphocytic lymphoma, Rappaport Classification) and intermediate cell types were associated with a lower incidence of extraocular involvement than has been found with ocular adnexal lymphomas of all other histologic types (27% and 46%, respectively).[28] Other studies have found that patients with low-grade lymphoma have increased 5-year survivals when compared with patients with intermediate-grade lymphomas (70% and 25%, respectively).[84] These grades were derived from the Working Formulation and *intermediate grade* is not the *intermediate cell type*. Intraocular BLH rarely progresses with systemic disease.[25]

LARGE CELL LYMPHOMA. The prognosis of patients with intraocular large cell lymphoma is generally poor. The median survival time from onset of symptoms was 35 months, and the mean time from diagnosis to death was 26 months (range, 0–124 months).[35] Longer survivals have been reported in patients with simultaneous CNS and ocular irradiation.[25]

MISCELLANEOUS LYMPHOID TUMORS

BURKITT'S LYMPHOMA. These tumors respond well to aggressive chemotherapy. Although relapses may occur, treatment at present results in 50% long-term survival rates in patients without underlying disease, such as HIV infection.[42,85]

CUTANEOUS T-CELL LYMPHOMA. The prognosis of this disorder depends most heavily on the extent of the disease at the time of diagnosis. Other prognostic factors include age, associated symptoms, and whether the disease is epidermotrophic or nonepidermotrophic. The median survival is 3–5 years after histologic diagnosis.[59]

HODGKIN'S DISEASE. The most important prognostic factor in patients with Hodgkin's disease is tumor burden.[58,86] Patients with Stage-I and Stage-IIA disease have nearly 100% 5-year survival after treatment. Even patients with Stage-IVA and Stage-IVB disease may be expected to have a 50% 5-year disease-free survival with aggressive treatment. Nevertheless, long-term survivors after chemotherapy and radiotherapy have increased risks of developing second malignancies such as acute leukemia, malignant lymphoma, and carcinoma.[42,87,88]

LYMPHOPLASMACYTOID TUMORS. Prognosis varies depending on the underlying diagnosis. Patients with multiple myeloma usually survive less than 2 years, although changing treatment protocols may increase survival. Patients with other lymphoplasmacytoid tumors tend to have a much better prognosis, and solitary orbital plasmacytoma requires only excision.

REFERENCES

1. Smith HA. The pathology of malignant lymphoma in cattle: a study of 113 cases. *Pathol Vet* 2:68, 1965.
2. Rebhun WC. Orbital lymphosarcoma in cattle. *J Am Vet Med Assoc* 180:149, 1982.
3. Rebhun WC. Diseases of the bovine orbit and globe. *J Am Vet Med Assoc* 175:171, 1979.
4. Burny A, Bruek C, Chantrenne H, Cleuter Y, Dekegel D, Ghysdael J, Kettman R, Leckereq M, Leunen J, Mammericky M, Portelette D. Bovine leukemia virus: molecular biology and epidemiology. In: Klein G, ed. *Viral Oncology.* New York: Raven, 231:1980.
5. Jarrett WFH, Mackey CJ. Neoplastic diseases of the hematopoietic and lymphoid tissues. *Bull WHO* 50:21, 1974.
6. Saunders LZ, Barron CN. Intraocular tumors in animals: IV. Lymphosarcoma. *Br Vet J* 120:25, 1964.
7. Bloom F, Meyer LM. Malignant lymphoma (so-called leukemia) in dogs. *Am J Pathol* 21:683, 1945.
8. Morgan RV. Ultrasonography of retrobulbar diseases of the dog and cat. *J Am Anim Hosp Assoc* 25:393, 1989.
9. Cello RM, Hutcherson B. Ocular changes in malignant lymphoma of dogs. *Cornell Vet* 52:492, 1962.
10. Amstrong SJ, Souja PN, De Wreghitt TG, Nagington J, Mohy BWJ, Owen LN. Studies on a possible viral etiology of canine lymphosarcoma and mammary tumors. *Br J Cancer* 38:175, 1978.
11. Carlton WW. Intraocular lymphosarcoma: two cases in Siamese cats. *J Am Anim Hosp Assoc* 12:83, 1976.
12. Meincke JE. Reticuloendothelial malignancies with intraocular involvement in the cat. *J Am Vet Med Assoc* 148:157, 1966.
13. Corcoran K, Peiffer RL, Koch S. Histopathology of feline ocular lymphosarcoma: 49 cases. *Vet Comp Ophthalmol* 5:35, 1995.
14. Bloom F. Unilateral exophthalmus associated with leukemia in a cat. *Vet Med* 32:29, 1937.
15. Gilger BC, McLaughlin SA, Whitley RD, Wright JC. Orbital neoplasms in cats: 21 cases (1974–1990). *J Am Vet Med Assoc* 201:1083, 1992.
16. Jarrett WFH, Martin WB, Crighton GW, Dalton RG. Leukemia in the cat: transmission experiments with leukemia (lymphosarcoma). *Nature* 202:566, 1964.
17. Hardy WDJ, McLelland AJ, MacEwen EG, Hess PW, Hayes AA, Zuckerman EE. The epidemiology of the feline leukemia virus. *Cancer* 39(suppl):1850, 1977.
18. Jarrett WFH, Crighton GW, Dalton RG. Leukemia and lymphosarcoma in animals and man: I. Lymphosarcoma or leukemia in domestic animals. *Vet Rec* 79:693, 1966.
19. Rebhum WC, Bertone A. Equine lymphosarcoma. *J Am Vet Med Assoc* 184:720, 1984.
20. Glaze MB, Gossett KA, McCoy DJ, Kreeger JM. A case of equine adnexal lymphosarcoma. *Equine Vet J* 10(suppl):83, 1990.
21. Murphy C, Lavoie JP, Groff J, Hacker D, Pryor P, Bellhorn RW. Bilateral eyelid swelling attributable to lymphosarcoma in a horse. *J Am Vet Med Assoc* 194:939, 1989.
22. Jakobiec FA, Font RL. Orbit. In: Spencer WH, ed. *Ophthalmic Pathology: An Atlas and Textbook.* Philadelphia: WB Saunders, 2663:1986.
23. Garner A. Orbital lymphoproliferative disorders. *Br J Ophthalmol* 76:47, 1992.
24. Isaacson PG, Wright DH. Extranodal lymphoma. In: Anthony PP, MacSween RNM, eds. *Recent Advances in Histopathology.* Edinburgh: Churchill Livingstone, 159:1987.
25. Shields JA, Shields CL. Intraocular lymphoid tumors and leukemias. In: Shields JA, Shields CL, eds. *Intraocular Tumors: A Text and Atlas.* Philadelphia: WB Saunders, 489:1992.
26. Shields JA. Lymphoid tumors and leukemias. In: Shields JA, ed. *Diagnosis and Management of Orbital Tumors.* Philadelphia: WB Saunders, 316:1989.
27. Jakobiec FA, Lefkowitch J, Knowles DM. B and T lymphocytes in ocular disease. *Ophthalmology* 91:635, 1984.
28. Jakobiec FA, Knowles DM. An overview of ocular adnexal lymphoid tumors. *Trans Am Ophthalmol Soc* 137:420, 1989.
29. Knowles DM, Jakobiec FA, McNally LA, Burke JS. Lymphoid hyperplasia and malignant lymphoma occurring in the ocular adnexa (orbit, conjunctiva, and eyelids): a prospective multiparametric analysis of 108 cases during 1977 to 1987. *Hum Pathol* 21:959, 1990.
30. Shields JA. Incidence of orbital tumors and pseudotumors: lymphoid proliferations. In: Shields JA, ed. *Diagnosis and Management of Orbital Tumors.* Philadelphia: WB Saunders, 316:1989.
31. Shields JA, Bakewell B, Augsberger JJ, Flanagan JC. Classification and incidence of space-occupying lesions of the orbit: a survey of 645 biopsies. *Arch Ophthalmol* 102:1606, 1984.
32. Kennedy RE. An evaluation of 820 orbital cases. *Trans Am Ophthalmol Soc* 131:134, 1984.
33. Henderson JW, Farrow GM. *Orbital Tumors,* 2d ed. New York: Brian and Decker, 1980.
34. Grossniklaus HE, Green WR, Luckenbach M, Chan CC. Conjunctival lesions in adults: a clinical and histopathologic review. *Cornea* 6:78, 1987.
35. Freeman LN, Schachat AP, Knox DL, Michels RG, Green WR. Clinical features, laboratory investigations, and survival in ocular reticulum cell sarcoma. *Ophthalmology* 94:1631, 1987.

36. Rosenberg SA, Diamond HD, Jaslowitz B, Craven LF. Lymphosarcoma: a review of 1269 cases. *Medicine (Baltimore)* 40:31, 1961.

37. Nelson CC, Hertzberg BS, Klintworth GK. A histopathologic study of 716 unselected eyes in patients with cancer at the time of death. *Am J Ophthalmol* 95:788, 1983.

38. Shields JA, Bakewell B, Augsberger JA, Donoso LA, Bernadino V. Space-occupying orbital masses in children: a review of 250 consecutive biopsies. *Ophthalmology* 93:379, 1986.

39. Brooks LH, Downing JD, McClure JA, Engel HM. Orbital Burkitt's lymphoma in a homosexual man with acquired immune deficiency. *Arch Ophthalmol* 102:1533, 1984.

40. Templeton AC. Orbital tumors in African children. *Br J Ophthalmol* 55:254, 1971.

41. Karp LA, Zimmerman LE, Payne T. Intraocular involvement in Burkitt's lymphoma. *Arch Ophthalmol* 85:295, 1971.

42. Robbins SL, Cotran RS, Kumar V. *Pathologic Basis of Disease*, 3d ed. Philadelphia: WB Saunders, chap 15:1984.

43. Stanton CA, Sloan DB, Slusher MM, Greven CM. Acquired immunodeficiency syndrome-related primary intraocular lymphoma. *Arch Ophthalmol* 110:1614, 1992.

44. Antle CM, White VA, Horseman DE, Rootman J. Large cell orbital lymphoma in a patient with acquired immune deficiency syndrome: case report and review. *Ophthalmology* 97:1494, 1990.

45. Tien DR. Large cell lymphoma in AIDS. *Ophthalmology* 98:412, 1991.

46. Jabs DA, Green WR, Fox R, Polk BF, Bartlett JG. Ocular manifestations of acquired immune deficiency syndrome. *Ophthalmology* 96:1092, 1989.

47. Schanzer MC, Font RL, O'Mallet RF. Primary ocular lymphoma associated with the acquired immune deficiency syndrome. *Ophthalmology* 98:88, 1991.

48. McNally L, Jakobiec FA, Knowles DM. Clinical, morphologic, immunophenotypic, and molecular genetic analysis of bilateral ocular adnexal neoplasms in 17 patients. *Am J Ophthalmol* 103:555, 1987.

49. Westcott S, Carner A, Moseley IF, Wright JE. Orbital lymphoma versus reactive lymphoid hyperplasia: an analysis of the use of computed tomography in differential diagnosis. *Br J Ophthalmol* 75:722, 1991.

50. Frohman LP, Kupersmith MJ, Lang J, et al. Intracranial extension and bone destruction in orbital pseudotumor. *Arch Ophthalmol* 104:380, 1986.

51. Ryan SJ, Zimmerman LE, King FM. Reactive lymphoid hyperplasia: an unusual form of intraocular pseudotumor. *Trans Am Acad Ophthalmol Otolaryngol* 76:652, 1972.

52. Cooper EL, Riker JL. Malignant lymphoma of the uveal tract. *Am J Ophthalmol* 34:1153, 1951.

53. Sloas HA, Starling J, Harper DG, Cupples HP. Update of ocular reticulum cell sarcoma. *Am J Ophthalmol* 91:480, 1981.

54. Gass JD, Trattler HL. Retinal artery obstruction and atheromas associated with non-Hodgkin's large cell lymphoma (reticulum cell sarcoma). *Arch Ophthalmol* 109:1134, 1991.

55. Ridley ME, McDonald R, Sternberg P, et al. Retinal lymphoid proliferation manifestations of ocular lymphoma (reticulum cell sarcoma). *Ophthalmology* 99:1153, 1992.

56. Blakemore WS, Ehrenberg M, Fritz KJ, et al. Rapidly progressive proptosis secondary to Burkitt's lymphoma: origin in the ethmoid sinuses. *Arch Ophthalmol* 101:1741, 1983.

57. Zak TA, Tisher JE, Afshani E. Infantile non-African Burkitt's lymphoma presenting as bilateral fulminant exophthalmos. *J Pediatr Ophthalmol Strabismus* 19:294, 1982.

58. Donoso LA, Magargal LE, Eiferman RA. Meningeal carcinomatosis secondary to malignant lymphoma (Burkitt's pattern). *J Pediatr Ophthalmol Strabismus* 18:48, 1981.

59. Meekins B, Proia AD, Klintworth GK. Cutaneous T-cell lymphoma presenting as a rapidly enlarging ocular adnexal tumor. *Ophthalmology* 92:1288, 1985.

60. Leib ML, Lester H, Braunstein RE, Edelson RL. Ocular findings in cutaneous T-cell lymphoma. *Ann Ophthalmol* 23:182, 1991.

61. Saga T, Ohno S, Matsuda H, Ogasawara M, Kokichi K. Ocular involvement by a peripheral T-cell lymphoma. *Arch Ophthalmol* 102:399, 1984.

62. Sherman MD, Van Dalen JTW, Conrad K. Bilateral orbital infiltration as the initial sign of a peripheral T-cell lymphoma presenting in a leukemic phase. *Ann Ophthalmol* 22:93, 1990.

63. Keltner JL, Fritsch E, Cykiert RC, Albert DM. Mycosis fungoides: intraocular and central nervous system involvement. *Arch Ophthalmol* 95:645, 1977.

64. Foerester HC. Mycosis fungoides with intraocular involvement. *Trans Am Acad Ophthalmol Otolaryngol* 64:308, 1960.

65. Whitbeck EG, Spiers ASD, Hussain M. Mycosis fungoides: subcutaneous and visceral tumors, orbital involvement and ophthalmoplegia. *J Clin Oncol* 1:270, 1983.

66. Stenson S, Ramsay DL. Ocular findings in mycosis fungoides. *Arch Ophthalmol* 99:272, 1981.

67. Leitch RJ, Rennie IG, Parsens MA. Ocular involvement in mycosis fungoides. *Br J Ophthalmol* 77:126, 1993.

68. Fratkin JD, Shammas HF, Miller SD. Disseminated Hodgkin's disease with bilateral orbital involvement. *Arch Ophthalmol* 96:102, 1978.

69. Patel S, Rootman J. Nodular sclerosing Hodgkin's disease of the orbit. *Ophthalmology* 90:1433, 1983.

70. Sweeny PJ, Hardy RW, Steinberg MC. An unusual case of progressive visual loss. Presented at the ninth annual Neuro-ophthalmic Pathology Symposium, St Louis, February, 1977.

71. Primbs GB, Mousees WE, Irvine AR. Intraocular Hodgkin's disease. *Arch Ophthalmol* 66:477, 1961.

72. Brinane-van Geertruyden M. Retinal lesions in Hodgkin's disease. *Arch Ophthalmol* 56:94, 1955.

73. Orellana J, Friedman AH. Ocular manifestations of lymphoid proliferations, multiple myeloma, Waldenstrom's macroglobulinemia, and benign monoclonal gammopathy. *Surv Ophthalmol* 26:157, 1981.

74. Shakin EP, Augsburger JJ, Eagle RD, et al. Multiple myeloma involving the iris. *Arch Ophthalmol* 106:524, 1988.

75. Maisel JM, Miller F, Sibony PA, Maisel LM. Multiple myeloma presenting with ocular inflammation. *Ann Ophthalmol* 19:170, 1987.

76. DeSmet MD, Rootman J. Orbital manifestations of plasmacytic lymphoproliferations. *Ophthalmology* 94:995, 1987.

77. Gonnering RS. Bilateral primary extramedullary orbital plasmacytomas. *Ophthalmology* 94:267, 1987.

78. McCormick SA, Datta B, McNally LM. Mantle cell lymphoma of the orbit: criteria for classification, incidence and prognostic implicators. *Invest Ophthalmol Vis Sci* 34(suppl):827, 1993.

79. Medeiros LJ, Harris NL. Lymphoid infiltrates of the orbit and conjunctiva: a morphologic and immunophenotypic study of 99 cases. *Am J Surg Pathol* 13:459, 1989.

80. Medeiros LJ, Harris NL. Immunohistologic analysis of small lymphocytic infiltrates of the orbit and conjunctiva. *Hum Pathol* 21:1126, 1990.

81. Jakobiec FA, Neri A, Knowles DM. Genotypic monoclonality in immunophenotypically polyclonal orbital lymphoid tumors: a model of tumor progression in the lymphoid system. *Ophthalmology* 94:980, 1987.

82. Knowles DM, Athen EA, Ubriaco A, McNally L, et al. Extranodal noncutaneous lymphoid hyperplasias represent a continuous spectrum of B-cell neoplasia: demonstration by molecular genetic analysis. *Blood* 73:1635, 1989.

83. Wilson DJ, Braziel R, Rosenbaum JT. Intraocular lymphoma: immunopathogenic analysis of vitreous biopsy specimens. *Arch Ophthalmol* 110:1455, 1992.

84. Erickeson BA, Harris GJ, Enk CA, et al. Periocular lymphoproliferative diseases: natural history, prognostic factors and treatment. *Radiology* 185:63, 1992.

85. Magrath IT. Malignant non-Hodgkin's lymphoma in children. *Hematol Oncol Clin North Am* 1:477, 1987.

86. Spect L, Nordentof AM, Cold S, et al. Tumor burden as the most important prognostic factor in early stage Hodgkin's disease. *Cancer* 61:1719, 1988.

87. Tucker MA, Coleman CN, Cox RS, et al. Risk of second cancer after treatment of Hodgkin's disease. *N Engl J Med* 318:76, 1988.

88. Grossniklaus HE, Farhi DC, Jacobson BR, Abbuhl NF. Malignant lymphoma of the conjunctiva following Hodgkin's disease. *Br J Ophthalmol* 72:212, 1988.

13

THE PHAKOMATOSES

Guy G. Massry and Marilyn C. Kincaid

The phakomatoses (phakoma, mother spot) are a group of neuro-oculo-viscero-cutaneous disorders unique to humans and are characterized by hamartomatous lesions throughout the body. Although each clinical entity is a unique disease process, there can be significant overlap among the manifestations of each.[1] In his original evaluation of three of these clinical entities—neurofibromatosis (von Recklinghausen's disease), tuberous sclerosis (Bourneville's syndrome), and cerebroretinal angiomatosis (von Hippel's disease)—van der Hoeve coined the term *phakomatoses*.[2,3] Since van der Hoeve's description, a number of other entities have been included among the phakomatoses. These include encephalotrigeminal angiomatosis (Sturge-Weber syndrome), ataxia telangiectasia (Louis-Bar syndrome), and racemose hemangiomatosis (Wyburn-Mason syndrome). At present, various other disorders have been suggested as belonging to the family of phakomatoses. Recent textbooks have included such entities as the linear nevus sebaceus syndrome, Klippel-Trenaunay-Weber syndrome, Rendu-Osler-Weber syndrome, and the basal cell nevus syndrome in this group.[4–6]

Clearly, there is confusion regarding inclusion into this unique group of disorders. However, the classification notwithstanding, the importance of the phakomatoses lies in identifying their varied clinical presentations, understanding the salient features of each disorder, identifying those patients at risk of illness and death, and offering appropriate treatment modalities and genetic and family counseling when appropriate.

In this chapter, the historical background, and the ocular and nonocular features of the six classic phakomatoses, are briefly described. Examples of the ocular histopathologic presentation of each entity is also reviewed. This is not meant to be an exhaustive review of the literature on the phakomatoses, but instead a useful reference for ophthalmologists who may encounter any or all of these diseases.

NEUROFIBROMATOSIS

Neurofibromatosis (NF) was first described by Friedrich Daniel von Recklinghausen in 1882.[7] It is an autosomally dominant inherited disorder with an extremely high penetrance and variable expressivity.[1,8] The clinical manifestations of NF may develop congenitally, in infancy, adolescence, or adulthood.[9] The neural crest cell line is primarily affected, especially the Schwann cells and melanocytes. There are two distinct variants of the disorder, NF-1 and NF-2, each with a distinct presentation and its own diagnostic criteria.

NF-1 (von Recklinghausen's disease) is the more common form of NF, occurring in 0.05% of the population,[10] with an incidence of approximately 1/3000,[11] making it one of the most common dominantly transmitted diseases in humans. The NF-1 gene has been localized to chromosome 17,[12] and the gene product identified.[13]

To establish the diagnosis of NF-1, two or more of the following characteristics must be evident: six or more café au lait spots 15 mm or larger in adults, or 5 mm or larger in children; two or more neurofibromas of any type, or one plexiform neurofibroma; freckling in axillary or inguinal regions; a visual pathway glioma; two or more Lisch's nodules; characteristic osseous lesions; or a first-degree relative who has NF-1 by these criteria.[13]

NF-2 (bilateral acoustic NF) is less common than NF-1, occurring in 1/50,000 live births.[14] It is also inherited in an autosomal dominant fashion with high penetrance, but rather than chromosome 17, the NF-2 gene is found on chromosome 22.[15,16] The gene product, which has been named *schwannomin* or *merlin,* also appears to be a tumor suppressor.[17] The diagnostic criteria for NF-2 include bilateral acoustic neuromas, or a first-degree relative with NF-2 and either unilateral acoustic neuroma or two of the following: meningioma, glioma, schwannoma, neurofibroma, or premature posterior subcapsular cataract.[13]

Cutaneous Involvement. Cutaneous involvement may be varied, but the main triad of lesions include café au lait spots, fibroma molluscum, and plexiform neurofibromas,[9] with the latter two being different types of neurofibromas.

Café au lait spots are pigmented macular lesions with irregular edges that vary from large to small and tend to involve the trunk, but may be found anywhere on the body (Figure 13.1). Histopathologically, they demonstrate an increased number of giant pigment granules in melanocytes in the basal layer of the epidermis.[9] The number and size of the lesions tend to increase with age.[4]

The fibroma molluscum, which is the most common type of neurofibroma, typically pre-

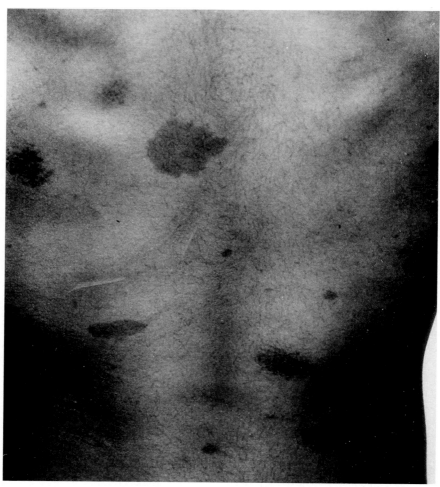

FIG. 13.1—Café au lait lesions of the skin of the back in von Recklinghausen's neurofibromatosis. (Courtesy of S.M. Chung, MD.)

sents as an isolated small pedunculated nodule (Figure 13.2). Histopathologically, it consists of enlarged cutaneous nerves with hyperplastic Schwann cells and connective tissue elements.[9] The plexiform neurofibroma represents a diffuse proliferation of perineural tissue surrounding irregularly arranged nerves. It has classically been described as having a "bag of worms" consistency upon palpation.[4] A less common form of neurofibroma, elephantiasis neuromatosa, results from diffuse Schwann cell proliferation within the dermis, resulting in marked thickening and folding of the skin (Figure 13.2). Finally, axillary and inguinal freckling (in areas devoid of sun exposure) is also a common skin manifestation of NF-1.

In contrast to NF-1, NF-2 typically is devoid of cutaneous manifestations. Rarely, a few café au lait spots or minimally elevated papules may be present.[4]

Central Nervous System Involvement. Nervous system findings in NF are common. Neurofibromas of the peripheral nerves in NF-1 and central nervous system (CNS) meningiomas and gliomas in NF-1 and NF-2 can lead to significant morbidity and mortality. There is an established association of optic nerve gliomas with NF-1. Of patients with optic nerve gliomas, 10%–50% have NF-1.[18,19] Conversely, of all patients with NF-1, 15% have optic nerve gliomas.[20,21] Intracranial gliomas in NF-1 may involve not only the optic nerve, but also any part of the central visual pathway, including the chiasm. Chiasmal involvement may lead to disease of the hypothalamic-pituitary axis.

Patients with NF-1 also exhibit a tendency toward learning difficulty and mental deficiency.[4] The intellectual impairment typically presents by school age, is nonprogressive, and is not related to other manifestations of the disease.[8]

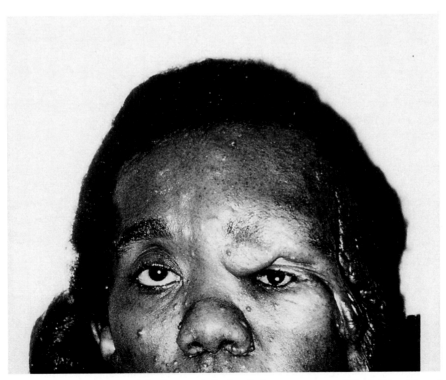

FIG. 13.2—Small fibroma mollusca of the face, and elephantiasis neuromatosa of the left temple and ear area, in a patient with von Recklinghausen's neurofibromatosis. (Courtesy of S.M. Chung, MD.)

The primary neurologic manifestation of NF-2 is bilateral acoustic neuromas, although neurofibromas, meningiomas, and gliomas also occur. Acoustic neuromas are schwannomas arising from the vestibular nerve. Patients present in the second and third decades of life with decreased hearing, tinnitus, and dysequilibrium.[4] The tumors can be removed surgically, usually with associated deficits in seventh nerve function and hearing. Neurologic examination, brainstem auditory evoked responses, and magnetic resonance imaging aid in making the diagnosis.

Skeletal and Visceral Involvement. Osseous manifestations of NF-1 include progressive kyphoscoliosis, pseudoarthroses (nonhealing fractures), defects in the orbital wall, and enlarge-

ment of the sella turcica.[4] Visceral involvement includes hamartomatous lesions of the gastrointestinal tract[22] that may lead to intestinal obstruction and pheochromocytomas,[23,24] in addition to a variety of malignant tumors.[4]

Ophthalmic Involvement. The hallmark of eyelid involvement in NF-1 is the plexiform neurofibroma of the upper lid. This lesion characteristically causes ptosis and an S-shaped contour deformity of the upper lid, and, as previously mentioned, has a bag-of-worms consistency when palpated (Figure 13.3). Café au lait spots and neurilemomas can also manifest on the eyelids.[4]

Hamartomas of the iris, Lisch's nodules, are the most common ocular finding in NF-1[4] and are a reliable marker for the disorder[25] (Figure 13.4). They are present in 92% of children with NF-1

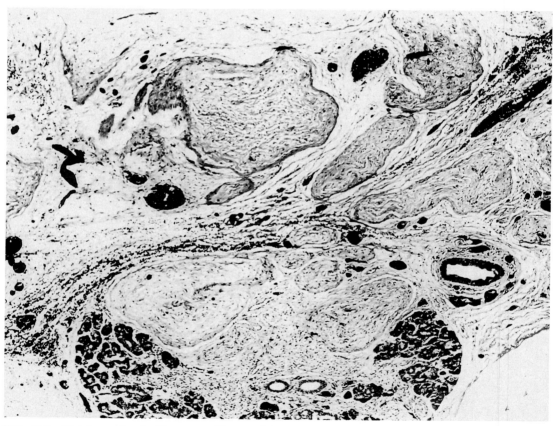

FIG. 13.3—Histology of a plexiform neurofibroma of the upper lid and orbit. Numerous nerve fibers are intermixed with normal lacrimal glands and ducts, which appear dark in this figure. Hematoxylin-eosin, original magnification ×12.5.

over the age of 5, and they increase in number with age.[26] Clinically, Lisch's nodules are gelatinous, dome-shaped lesions located on the iris surface or deep within the stroma. They are tan to brown in color, primarily bilateral, yet asymmetric, and can be barely visible by slit-lamp biomicroscopy to 2 mm in diameter. They can appear hypopigmented on a dark iris. Histopathologically, they resemble iris nevi. Light and electron microscopy demonstrate them to be melanocytic hamartomas.[27,28]

Congenital glaucoma is associated with NF-1, and is typically ipsilateral to the upper eyelid involved with a plexiform neurofibroma. The underlying mechanism of the glaucoma has been postulated to be a goniodysgenesis[29] or angle obstruction by hamartomatous tissue.[28,30]

Hamartomas may also involve the entire uveal tract[22,28] or only the choroid.[31,32] Clinically, choroidal hamartomas appear as ill-defined yellow-white to light brown lesions, which may be single, multiple, diffuse, or localized to the posterior pole.[22,26,31] Lewis and Riccardi demonstrated choroidal hamartomas to be present in 51% of white patients with NF-1, with none being present in black patients.[26] Histopathologically, they are composed of both neuronal and melanocytic elements. Ovoid bodies, onionlike formations that contain fine neuronal fibers and resemble tactile nerve endings, have been demonstrated in choroidal hamartomas by light and electron microscopy.[33,34] Ovoid bodies are composed of lamellae of Schwann cell processes arranged around axons.

Proptosis may be another finding in patients with NF-1. It may result from an optic nerve glioma, orbital neurofibroma, or a defect in the bony structure of the orbit.[4] The latter finding usually leads to pulsating exophthalmos or, less frequently, enophthalmos. Other ocular associations in NF-1 include hamartomas of the conjunctiva,[22,35] prominent corneal nerves,[4] astrocytic hamartomas of the retina,[36,37] and combined retinal-retinal pigment epithelial hamartomas.[37]

As previously mentioned, gliomas of the visual pathway occur in NF-1 and rarely in NF-2, and can be a significant cause of visual morbidity. Gliomas are slow-growing and locally invasive tumors. When involving the optic nerve, they can present with a unilateral decrease in visual acuity, strabismus, proptosis, and optic atrophy.[4] Patients may also be asymptomatic, and computed tomography (CT) and magnetic resonance imaging (MRI) can help in confirming the diagnosis (Figure 13.5). Since optic nerve gliomas can also arise in the setting of previously normal CT or MRI scans, continued surveillance is necessary.[38] Chiasmal tumors have a worse prognosis than prechiasmal lesions, as they may involve the hypothalamus or obstruct the third ventricle, with resultant hydrocephalus.[39]

Histopathologically, gliomas are pilocytic astrocytomas composed of astrocytes, oligodendrocytes, and a mucopolysaccharide ground substance (Figure 13.6). No mitotic figures occur, and degenerative changes referred to as Rosenthal fibers may be identified. These appear as eosinophilic, cigar-shaped, irregular swellings of cell processes and are not specific for pilocytic astrocytoma. Treatment options for optic gliomas are controversial and include observation, radiation, and surgery.[4]

NF-2 is associated with few ocular findings compared with NF-1. Unilateral or bilateral posterior subcapsular cataracts occur in approximately 40% of cases.[40,41] Optic nerve meningiomas[14] and gliomas[42] have also been reported, as has papilledema from increased intracranial pressure[43] and morning glory optic disc anomaly,[44] all of which can cause visual loss.[45]

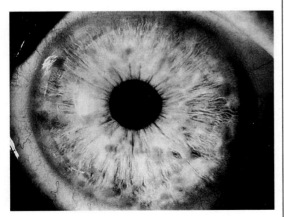

FIG. 13.4—Lisch's nodules are seen as irregular rounded lesions on the surface of the iris. (Courtesy of S.M. Chung, MD.)

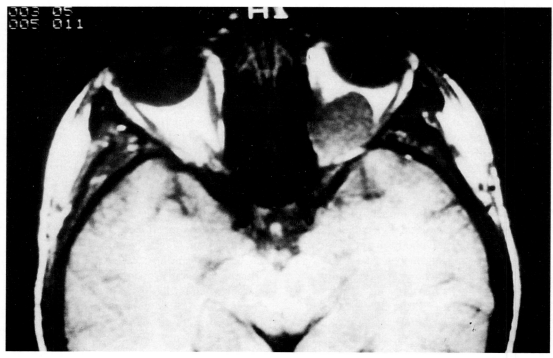

FIG. 13.5—Magnetic resonance image of an optic nerve glioma on the right. The orbital fat appears white in this T-1 weighted image. (Courtesy of S.M. Chung, MD.)

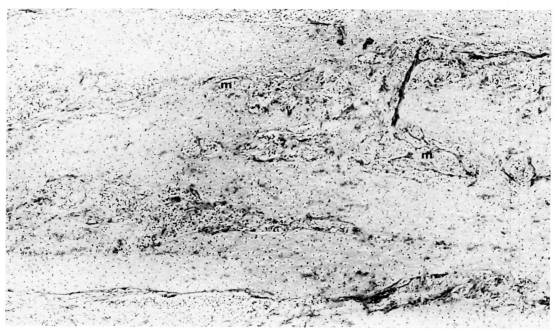

FIG. 13.6—Histopathology of an optic nerve glioma. The optic nerve is diffusely hypercellular and thickened by the neoplastic astrocytes. There is some reactive meningeal hyperplasia also (m). Hematoxylin-eosin, original magnification ×31.

TUBEROUS SCLEROSIS

In 1880, Bourneville described a 15-year-old girl with epilepsy, mental retardation, and a vesiculopapular rash on the nose, cheek, and forehead.[4] Postmortem examination demonstrated tumors of the brain and kidney. Although previous reference had been made to solitary manifestations of tuberous sclerosis (TS) (Bourneville's disease),[46] Bourneville was the first to describe the syndrome. In 1908, Vogt suggested a triad of findings that define the disease: adenoma sebaceum, epilepsy, and mental retardation.[47] The astrocytic hamartoma (phakoma) of the retina, now considered characteristic of TS, was not described until 1920 by van der Hoeve,[48] who was also the first to characterize the histopathology of the phakoma a few years later.[2] Finally, in 1979, primary and secondary diagnostic criteria were established for the disease.[4]

TS occurs equally in both sexes and is diagnosed earlier (average age, 8) if mental retardation is present; if not, the average age at diagnosis is 17.[46] It is transmitted in an autosomal dominant fashion with a high degree of penetrance and variable expressivity, leading to varied and potentially subtle presentations of the disorder. This, in turn, may lead to missed diagnosis, thus affecting appropriate genetic counseling unless there is a high index of suspicion for the disorder. In addition, the spontaneous mutation rate of the gene for TS, localized to the long arm of chromosome 9,[49] has been documented as high. Because of the subtle presentations of the disorder, many patients previously believed to have new mutations were probably descendants of patients with undiagnosed TS, with a consequent overestimation of the rate of spontaneous mutation.[1]

Cutaneous Manifestations. A consistent cutaneous manifestation of TS is the adenoma sebaceum, a reddish brown papular "butterfly" rash found on the malar region of the face and chin (Figure 13.7). The papules are usually 1–2 mm in diameter, but can be as large as 7 mm.[46] Adenoma sebaceum occurs in 80%–90% of patients, typically manifesting after age 2 and becoming more

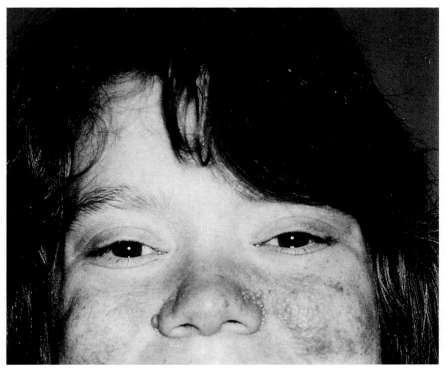

FIG. 13.7—A patient with tuberous sclerosis, showing the typical malar facial rash. (Courtesy of S.M. Chung, MD.)

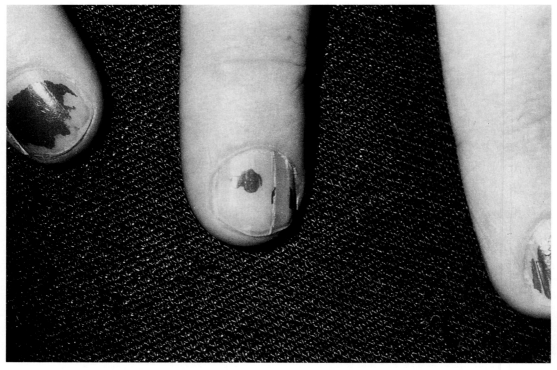

FIG. 13.8—Fingernails of the same patient as in the preceding figure, showing the characteristic longitudinal grooves. (Courtesy of S.M. Chung, MD.)

prominent with age. Adenoma sebaceum is a misnomer; the lesion was originally described as a benign tumor of sebaceous gland origin. We now recognize it to be an angiofibroma.[49] Angiofibromas are composed of hyperplastic connective and vascular tissue that secondarily displaces surrounding sebaceous glands.

Hypopigmented cutaneous macules are referred to as ash leaf spots because of their resemblance to ash leaves in size and shape. They are seen in 80% of affected patients[4] and may be present on any part of the body. The lesion is best seen with a Woods ultraviolet light. Skin biopsy is specific, disclosing lesions composed of melanocytes with small melanosomes containing reduced amounts of melanin. Ash leaf spots may be present congenitally and are typically the earliest cutaneous manifestation of TS. Consequently, they may be of diagnostic help in determining the etiology of infantile spasms, developmental delay, or mental retardation in early childhood.[4]

Shagreen patches (fibrous plaques) are localized areas of fibrous infiltration of the skin and are seen in 20% of patients with TS.[50,51] These cutaneous masses are yellowish brown with a waxy appearance, and are usually discovered on the eyelids, lumbosacral region, or legs. Subungual fibromas of the fingernails and toenails, identical histopathologically to adenoma sebaceum, may also be present and cause characteristic longitudinal grooves clinically (Figure 13.8). Finally, café au lait spots indistinguishable from those seen in patients with NF can be observed.[9]

Central Nervous System Involvement. Infantile spasms (salaam spasms) are often the presenting feature of TS in children.[51] These seizures are repetitive, myoclonic, muscular spasms that involve the neck, trunk, and limbs for seconds, and occur in bouts of 10–50.[46] The name *salaam spasms* was coined because affected children appear to be giving the traditional Arabic "salaam" greeting. The seizures in TS change

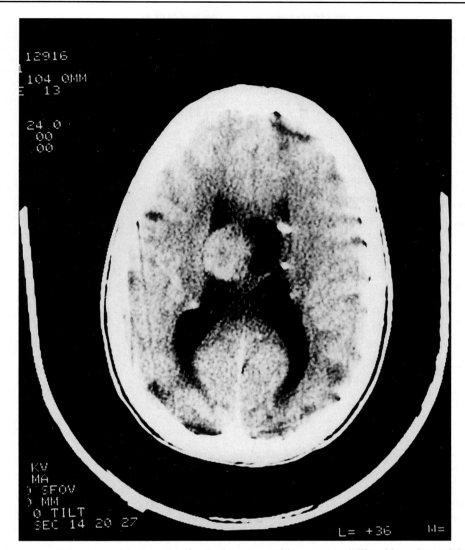

FIG. 13.9—Computed tomographic scan showing brain stones (white areas) and dilated lateral ventricles. This is the same patient as in Figure 13.7. (Courtesy of S.M. Chung, MD.)

with age, becoming grand mal in 93% of children.[50] Although the etiology of infantile spasms is quite varied, their association with TS is frequent enough that 25% develop other evidence of TS within 4 years,[52,53] making it essential to seek out ocular and other common characteristics of TS in these children.

Mental retardation was considered to be part of the original triad of TS. We now know that only 50%–60% of affected patients are mentally deficient.[1,46,50] The mental deficiency and seizure disorder that accompany TS result from benign periventricular tumors (astrocytic hamartomas) and sclerotic "tuber"-like lesions in the gray matter. Microscopically, these tumors are composed of an increased number of fibrillary astrocytes associated with abnormally large and bizarre cells with multiple nuclei and prominent nucleoli.[46] There are also areas of vacuolization and calcification with a paucity of neurons.[46] Malignant astrocytomas have also been described.[51]

Neuroimaging is helpful in identifying areas of involved brain. CT may pick up benign calcified tumor nodules (brain stones) (Figure 13.9) and may be helpful in identifying asymptomatic carriers of the disease. No correlation between CT findings and extent of neurologic disease has been found.[54] MRI typically reveals a high signal intensity in the cerebral cortex, presumably correlating with CNS hamartoma.[55] Finally, cranial ultrasonography has detected ependymal nodules in children with TS before CT could define the lesion.[56]

Visceral Involvement. The principal visceral tissues affected in TS include the heart and kidney. Echocardiograms reveal that cardiac rhabdomyomas occur in approximately 43% of patients with TS.[57] Most are asymptomatic and primarily affect the interventricular septum or ventricular wall.[57] There is an occasional association with arrhythmia, or pulmonary or aortic valve stenosis.

Kidney lesions include cysts and angiomyolipomas. The two may be found alone or in combination and, like the heart tumors, are primarily asymptomatic. Symptomatic patients may develop hematuria, pain, and frank renal failure, with uremia and hypertension.[58]

Ocular Involvement. The primary ocular manifestation of TS is the retinal astrocytic hamartoma (phakoma), which is present in more than 50% of patients. The lesion can be present in any location within the fundus, but has a predilection for the juxtapapillary area (Figure 13.10). There may be single or multiple lesions present and up to 33% are bilateral.[4]

Retinal astrocytic hamartomas may present in three distinct forms[47] that may represent different stages of evolution of the same lesion. The first type is a flat, translucent, noncalcified lesion located in the most superficial layers of the retina. At the other end of the spectrum is the classic "mulberry"-like, nodular, large tumor, which is highly calcified. There is also an intermediate type, whose clinical appearance lies somewhere between the other two forms.

Histopathologically, the phakoma consists of elongated astrocytes with long processes and long oval nuclei.[46] They are supplied by large-bore vessels and may contain calcium and hyalin.

The natural history of phakoma is generally benign, and thus it does not require medical or

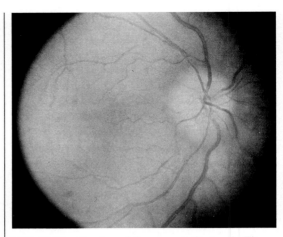

FIG. 13.10—Fundus of the same patient as in Figure 13.7, showing a "buried" astrocytic hamartoma. The optic nerve appears elevated, but there are none of the other signs of true papilledema. The opposite eye was normal. (Courtesy of S.M. Chung, MD.)

surgical treatment. Rarely, exudative retinal detachment or vitreous hemorrhage occur. Because astrocytic hamartoma is a benign lesion, it is important not to confuse it with other potentially serious conditions that may mimic its appearance. Such lesions may include retinoblastoma, *Toxocara* granulomas, and toxoplasmosis retinitis.

WYBURN-MASON SYNDROME

Arteriovenous malformations (AVMs) of the retina were first described by Magnus.[59] In 1943, Wyburn-Mason established the association of retinal AVMs with similar intracranial vascular anomalies.[60] The association of retinal and intracranial AVMs has since been referred to as Wyburn-Mason syndrome or sometimes Bonnet-Dechaume-Blanc syndrome.

In his original article, Wyburn-Mason found that 81% of patients with retinal AVMs had concomitant intracranial AVMs, predominantly in the midbrain. Conversely, of those patients with evidence of midbrain AVMs, 70% had retinal AVMs.[60] These percentages were based solely on clinical data, as cerebral angiography was still in its early stages. As such, the percentages have proven to be overestimated. More recent work reviewing reports of retinal AVMs in the literature has documented an association with intracranial AVMs to be 23%, and intracranial AVMs to be associated with retinal AVMs 8% of the time.[61] Diagnosis of AVMs in these cases was made by autopsy, angiogram, or at surgery.

Wyburn-Mason syndrome typically presents before age 30, affects men and woman equally, and with few exceptions presents unilaterally.[62] Although two cases of hereditary retinal AVMs have been reported,[60,63] no distinct pattern exists. In addition to the retina and CNS, the orbit (8%), eyelids (2%), oronasopharynx (7%), skin, lung, and spine (all 1%) can be involved.[64] AVMs of the orbit and eyelids may cause ptosis, proptosis, dilated conjunctival vessels, and an enlarged optic foramen radiologically.[4] Involvement of the mandible may lead to severe oral hemorrhage during or after dental procedures.[65]

Central Nervous System and Systemic Involvement. AVMs are the most common form of intracranial hamartoma.[62] As previously mentioned, the primary site of CNS involvement is the midbrain, typically ipsilateral to the retinal lesion. Symptoms attributable to intracranial involvement can be widespread, but commonly include headache and vomiting.[4] Recurrent cerebral and subarachnoid hemorrhage may lead to lapses in consciousness, while hemiparesis (plegia), Parinaud's syndrome, and other evidence of midbrain disease may be evident. Interestingly, seizures are uncommon.[65] Treatment of intracranial AVMs is difficult because they often lie deep within brain tissue and are surgically inaccessible.

Retinal Involvement. The retinal lesion (AVM) consists of a direct communication of a dilated and tortuous artery and vein. Retinal AVMs are congenital lesions that are generally stable and have a preponderance for the posterior pole and superotemporal retina.[64] The lesion is typically found on routine ophthalmic examination. Occasionally, it may be discovered in patients with acute or progressive painless decrease in vision. This may be attributed to vitreous hemorrhage,[66] compression of anterior visual pathway nerve fibers,[4] or microvascular leakage into the macula from incompetent vessels.[66] Central retinal vein occlusions, branch retinal artery occlusions, and neovascular glaucoma have also been described.[67]

To clarify the varied presentation of retinal AVMs, Archer has subdivided them into three groups.[63] Group 1 AVMs consist of an abnormal capillary plexus interposed between an artery and vein. These tend to be stationary, well demarcated to a sector of the retina, asymptomatic, and not associated with systemic vascular malformations. Group 2 lesions involve a direct communication between a branch artery and vein. Because of the lack of an intervening capillary network, the venous end of this group is exposed to high flow with secondary *arterialization.* This may occasionally lead to localized vascular decompensation with subsequent retinal edema and exudate. However, most patients are asymptomatic, discovered on routine examination, with lesions localized to one quadrant of the retina, and do not have associated systemic AVMs. Group 3 AVMs consist of widespread dilation and tortuosity of major retinal vessels involving large segments of the retinal vasculature. This is the subgroup of patients who have various degrees of vascular decompensation, loss of vision, and intracranial and systemic involvement.

Histopathologically,[68,69] because of the arterialization of the veins, it may be difficult to distinguish arteries from veins. The vessels may be so large as to occupy the full thickness of the retina. The vessel walls are exceedingly thickened due to variable but extensive fibromuscular coats and fibrohyalin adventitial layers. The associated retina may undergo secondary cystic and pigmentary degeneration, and ganglion cells and nerve fibers may be lost as a result of optic nerve compression. Grossly, the vessels may extend full thickness through the retina into the intracranial compartment.

Therapy for affected patients is limited. Retinal lesions with vascular incompetency may be amenable to laser therapy if they are not overly extensive.[4] An attempt is made to occlude the afferent feeder artery if it is not of the large-bore type. Similar treatment of large-caliber vessels is associated with a significant risk of severe hemorrhage.

Morbidity and mortality in Wyburn-Mason syndrome are directly linked to hemorrhagic events in the CNS and retina. Most of the Group 1 and 2 retinal AVM patients are asymptomatic and do not need further workup or treatment.

Conversely, those patients with Group 3 lesions have an increased risk of intracranial and retinal complications, severe neurologic deficits, visual loss, and even death. Ophthalmologists play an important role in diagnosing this condition and initiating appropriate treatment and referral when appropriate.

ATAXIA TELANGIECTASIA

Progressive cerebellar ataxia, oculocutaneous telangiectasia, and recurrent sinopulmonary infections constitute the syndrome we know today as ataxia telangiectasia (AT) or Louis-Bar syndrome.[70] It was first described, in part, by Madame Louis-Bar, when she reported a young man with cerebellar ataxia and telangiectasia of the skin and conjunctiva.[71] In the ensuing years, Boder and Sedgwick further elucidated the syndrome in their description of eight patients with the disorder and coined the name *ataxia telangiectasia.* They noted the autosomal recessive inheritance pattern, frequent association with sinopulmonary infections, and peculiarity of eye movements.[72]

The first clinical manifestation of the disorder is cerebellar ataxia, which presents soon after the child begins to walk. Telangiectasias involving the bulbar conjunctiva usually become evident between ages 3 and 7,[4] and eventually involve the ears, face, hard and soft palate, and extensor surfaces of the extremities.[73] Other features of the syndrome include thymic hypoplasia, with a range of cellular and humoral deficiencies,[74] frequent sinopulmonary infections,[75] and an increased incidence of malignancy.[76,77] The disorder is the only one of the phakomatoses that is inherited in an autosomal recessive manner. One of the genes responsible for the disorder has been localized to chromosome 11.[78]

Ophthalmic Involvement. The primary ophthalmic manifestation of AT is bilateral bulbar conjunctival telangiectasia, which is eventually present in all cases.

The characteristic oculomotor abnormality is an inability to initiate voluntary saccades (both horizontal and vertical) or to mobilize the eyes for the fast phase of vestibular nystagmus. Soon afterward, pursuit movements are lost, followed by total ophthalmoplegia of the supranuclear type.[79–81] As the eye-movement disorder progresses, head thrusts, such as those observed in oculomotor apraxia, develop. In the latter condition, however, only horizontal saccades are involved, and there are normal random saccades. Inability to maintain fixation and nystagmus are also observed.

Cutaneous Involvement. Cutaneous telangiectasia manifests itself between the ages of 3 and 7.[4] The face and palate are usually the first to become involved. As the child becomes older, the antecubital and popliteal areas and the dorsum of the hands and feet follow.[82] Other skin manifestations include café au lait spots, vitiligo, premature graying of the hair, seborrheic and atopic dermatitis, early loss of subcutaneous fat, generalized atrophy of skin, and cutaneous infections.[4,70]

Central Nervous System and Visceral Involvement. The hallmark of this disorder is progressive cerebellar ataxia that eventually leaves patients wheelchair bound. Concomitantly with the ataxia, patients develop choreoathetosis and myoclonic jerks.[70] Mental retardation occurs, but typically not until adolescence. Neuropathologically, there is marked atrophy of the cerebellar cortex, primarily affecting the Purkinje and granular cells.[83–85] There is associated reduction in various neurotransmitters,[86] with eventual degeneration of cerebellar nuclei, spinal cord and, potentially, the entire CNS.[86,87]

Thymic hypoplasia is a consistent abnormality seen in AT. Associated with this is an increased risk of immunologic abnormalities and sinopulmonary infections. Infections occur in over 80% of patients according to some reports and may dominate the clinical picture, leading to bronchiectasis and, ultimately, respiratory failure and death.[70] Also, patients are prone to develop leukemia, malignant lymphoma, and other systemic malignancies.

Over 50% of patients have glucose intolerance associated with hyperinsulinism, insulin resistance, and hyperglycemia.[88] Female patients have poorly developed secondary sexual characteristics, males display hypogonadism, and 75% of patients demonstrate growth retardation.[70]

Ophthalmologists play a secondary role in treating AT, helping neurologists make the diagnosis in children presenting with characteristic neurologic manifestations. Unfortunately, the prognosis is poor, as most patients succumb to respiratory infection, lymphoma, leukemia, or other malignancies.

VON HIPPEL-LINDAU DISEASE

Von Hippel-Lindau (VHL) disease is characterized by retinal and cerebellar hemangioblastomas, and tumors and cystic lesions of visceral tissue. Von Hippel characterized the clinical appearance of the retinal angioma[89] and then described the histopathologic features of the lesion.[90] Lindau later established the association of the retinal tumors with cerebellar hemangiomatous cysts.[91] Since that time, the eponym *von Hippel-Lindau disease* has been used to describe the disorder. Conversely, if only retinal angiomas are present, the disorder is simply referred to as *von Hippel's disease.*

VHL disease is unique as compared with the other phakomatoses in that cutaneous manifestations are rarely present. It is transmitted in an autosomal dominant fashion in 25% of cases,[9] with irregular penetrance, variable expressivity, and no sexual predilection. The gene for the disorder has been localized to chromosome 3,[92] and has been described as a tumor-suppressor gene.[93] It is uncommon for individuals to manifest all clinical characteristics of the syndrome, and there is a familial tendency toward clustering of certain features.[93]

Central Nervous System Involvement. The most common CNS lesion present in VHL disease is cerebellar hemangioblastoma, occurring in 35%–75% of patients.[94,95] The tumor is usually cystic, but a solid presentation occurs in approximately 20% of patients.[4] Patients usually present in the third decade with symptoms attributable to increased intracranial pressure, such as headache; or cerebellar dysfunction, such as vertigo, problems with gait, or nystagmus. However, symptomatic presentation has occurred as late as the seventh decade. Fortunately, the tumors are usually well circumscribed from surrounding tissue and can be resected completely, although recurrences are not uncommon.[4] This tumor is the most common cause of death in VHL disease.

Medullary and spinal cord hemangioblastomas also occur in VHL disease. In the medulla, they can lead to death secondary to compression of cardiorespiratory centers. Spinal cord lesions typically occur in the upper cervical region and are usually clinically silent.

Visceral Involvement. Renal cell carcinoma occurs in approximately 25% of patients[94,96] and can lead to death from metastatic disease or uremia.[94,96,97] The tumor typically presents with findings of hematuria, obstructive nephropathy, or an abdominal mass.[98] Tumor diagnosis is usually made in the fifth decade and, as such, is the latest of the life-threatening manifestations to present in VHL disease. It is thought that the association between renal cell carcinoma and VHL disease is probably greater, and, as more patients survive the cerebellar disease, the numbers will prove this true.[95,98]

Pheochromocytomas have been reported in 3%–10% of patients with VHL disease,[4] often bilaterally. Most cases, however, are clustered in specific families, so the percentages may be misleading. Other visceral manifestations of VHL are nonlethal and include adenomas of the epididymis and kidney, and cystic lesions of the liver, epididymis, lung, adrenals, bone, ovary, and omentum.[9]

Ocular Manifestations. The first observed manifestation of VHL disease is usually the retinal angioma.[94,97] The lesion is frequently asymptomatically diagnosed in the second or third decade, but can be present at birth. The angioma begins as a localized microvascular abnormality similar to the microaneurysm seen in diabetes.[99] As the tumor progresses, it becomes a globular, reddish, slightly elevated vascular lesion fed by a dilated retinal artery and drained by a dilated retinal vein. It has a predilection for the midperiphery, but may occur in a juxtapapillary location, often being confused for a swollen disc or other tumor. Rarely, the angioma may manifest adjacent to the intraorbital portion of the optic nerve. Approximately 50% of tumors are bilateral, and 33% are multifocal in one eye.[98]

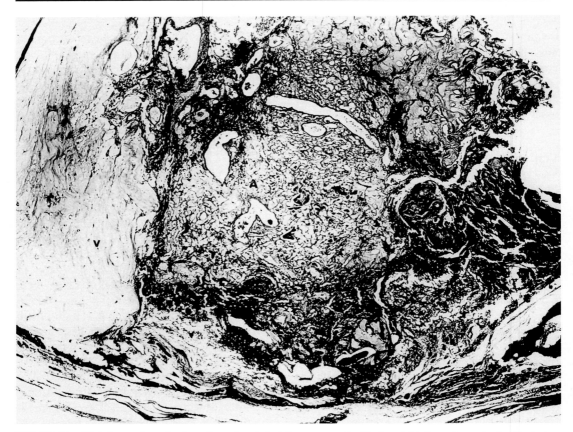

FIG. 13.11—Histology of a retinal angioma located at the ora serrata. To the *right,* there is marked retinal pigment epithelial hyperplasia. The retina is replaced by a large angioma (A) with variable-sized vascular channels. No normal retina is recognizable. To the *left,* is collapsed vitreous (v) with neovascularization. This lesion had been treated with cryopexy, but this had failed and the eye was blind. Hematoxylin-eosin, original magnification ×7.8.

Although the natural history of retinal angiomas in VHL disease in variable, untreated tumors may eventually decrease vision as a result of retinal exudation and hemorrhage. The vascular leakage may present locally or distant from the lesion, and may be so severe that extensive exudative retinal detachment may occur. In these cases, untreated eyes may develop neovascularization, rubeotic glaucoma, and phthisis bulbi.[9]

Fluorescein angiography demonstrates early rapid filling of the retinal angioma from its arterial feeder vessel, with subsequent intense hyperfluorescence. The draining retinal vein can be distinguished from its arterial counterpart by its later filling and early laminar flow. As the stages of the angiogram progress, there is diffuse leakage of dye from incompetent vascular endothelium in the tumor.[100]

By light microscopy, retinal angiomas are of the capillary variety and are composed of aberrant capillary channels with associated intervening lipid-laden stromal cells (foam cells) (Figure 13.11). The origin of the stromal foam cell is obscure, having been linked to microglia, neuroepithelium, macrophages, pericytes, and endothelial cells.[101] Mottow-Lippa and coworkers have suggested an origin from pluripotent vasoformative stem cells that can differentiate into either stromal or endothelial cells.[102] Recent work suggests that foam cells are the true neoplastic component of hemangioblastoma. These cells undergo a second mutation, and are thus homozygous for the abnormal gene, in a manner similar to retinoblastoma. They express vascular endothelial growth factor, thereby inducing the vascular tumor.[103]

Normal retinal capillaries do not have fenestrations. However, endothelial cells of retinal angioma in VHL disease have been shown by electron microscopy to be fenestrated.[102,104] This fenestrated architecture accounts for the clinical and angiographic finding of vascular insufficiency to the tumor. Additionally, focal thickening of basement membrane and pericyte loss are observed.

Retinal angiomas have been treated in a number of ways depending on their size, location, and the clarity of the optical media. Photocoagulation, diathermy, and cryotherapy have been successful in directly ablating angiomas that are 1–2 disc diameter or smaller.[105] Special attention must be given to the judicious application of therapy, as potential complications include vitreous and subretinal hemorrhage, and retinal hole formation. Whereas smaller lesions can be treated in a single session, larger lesions have required multiple sessions of therapy, and there have still been tumor recurrences.

Feeder-vessel laser ablation has been used to treat small vessels with some success;[99] however, similar treatment with larger vessels has been less successful, with a higher rate of complications.[106] Cryotherapy, used in repeated sessions, has been successful in treating larger tumors that have failed photocoagulation, are anteriorly located, or are in eyes with poor optical media.[107] Finally, other techniques, such as perforating diathermy[108] and eye-wall resection,[109] have been described.

Many patients with retinal lesions will eventually develop some loss of vision. The size of the lesion, and if and when treatment was initiated, play an important role in determining final visual outcome. However, it is clear that untreated eyes may become blind and require enucleation. Consequently, ophthalmologists must monitor patients and family members closely, and begin appropriate therapy when warranted. Additionally, since ophthalmologists are often the first to identify patients with potentially fatal VHL disease, it is important to have a thorough understanding of the genetic and systemic implications. Once identified, patients must be appropriately referred for workup, including a careful family history, imaging of the brain, spinal cord, and abdomen, and necessary laboratory tests.

STURGE-WEBER SYNDROME

In 1860, Schirmer established the association of the facial port-wine stain (angioma) with glaucoma,[4] and, 19 years later, Sturge reported a child with an extensive hemifacial angioma who concomitantly had buphthalmos and seizures.[110] The seizures began as partial and contralateral to the facial angioma and then became generalized. Sturge also noted a discrepancy between the color of the choroid in the two eyes, with the eye ipsilateral to the facial angioma being darker and redder. Sturge postulated that the seizure disorder and glaucoma were due to vascular lesions similar to the port-wine stain involving the ipsilateral brain and choroid.

Weber established a clinical correlate to Sturge's hypothesis of angiomatous involvement of the brain when he reported the roentgenographic appearance of the brain in a patient with this yet-unnamed syndrome. He demonstrated parallel dark streaks on skull films ipsilateral to the patient's facial lesion and concluded that they were due to calcium deposits secondary to the presence of an intracranial angioma.[111] The eponym *Sturge-Weber syndrome* (SWS) was then coined.

Today, we know the complete form of the disorder to consist of a facial hemangioma with ipsilateral intracranial and choroidal hemangiomas, glaucoma, and seizure disorder. It is felt that this constellation of findings results from abnormalities in the primitive vasculature in the developing cephalic neuroectoderm.[112] There is no racial or sexual predilection for the syndrome,[113] and no distinct hereditary pattern has been established.[4]

Cutaneous Involvement. The facial angioma (nevus flammeus, port-wine stain) is the most apparent manifestation of the disorder. It typically involves half of the face in the distribution of the first and second branches of the trigeminal nerve; hence the name *encephalotrigeminal angiomatosis*. On rare occasion, the angioma crosses the midline, presents bilaterally, or involves the lower face and neck. The lesion is usually congenital, but becomes more obvious as it becomes darker and more nodular with age.[113] Intracranial involvement leading to seizures is usually not present if there is no supraorbital angiomatous involvement,[114] while glaucoma is typically present only when the facial angioma involves the upper lid.[9] Microscopically, cutaneous angioma consists of dilated and telangiectatic dermal capillaries lined by a single layer of endothelial cells.[4]

Historically, treatment has consisted of cosmetics, but laser therapy has been applied. Laser treatment is most successful in the darker and more nodular lesions, and is fraught with the complications of pigmentary changes and scarring.[115]

Central Nervous System Involvement. Neurologic manifestations of SWS include seizures in 80% of patients, hemiplegia (paresis) in 31% of patients, and mental deficiencies in 54% of patients.[116] These are primarily related to the intracranial angioma and the maldevelopment or atrophy of the cerebral cortex associated with the lesion. The seizures typically begin as focal and contralateral to the facial lesion, but may become generalized with age.

The angioma may involve the leptomeninges, characteristically in the subarachnoid space. Its pathology was first described by Kalischer in 1901, who noted that there were numerous delicate entwined blood vessels enmeshed in the pia mater, with an underlying small cerebral hemisphere on the side of the brain ipsilateral to the facial lesion.[4] Grossly, the angioma consists of numerous small venules of uniform caliber.

Calcification of the intracranial angioma is progressive and can be noted as early as 1 year of age on skull x-ray. The double-contoured lines on skull films that Weber referred to have been labeled *railroad tracks*[4] and tend to become more pronounced in adolescence and in the teens, becoming stable after the second decade of life.[9]

Ophthalmic Involvement. The most common ocular finding in SWS is the choroidal hemangioma occurring in 40% of cases.[116,117] This lesion typically presents as a relatively flat yellow-orange lesion in the posterior pole.[4] Alternatively, especially in the young, it may be diffuse and difficult to identify, presenting with only choroidal darken-

ing ("tomato catsup" fundus).[118] In this situation, its presence is best established by comparing the color of the fundus to the color of the opposite eye. This is in contrast to isolated choroidal hemangiomas seen in patients without SWS, which usually manifest as well-circumscribed, elevated choroidal masses.[4]

Symptoms from choroidal tumors, if present, develop in young adulthood.[9] These include progressive hyperopia, visual loss from retinal and choroidal degeneration, focal ossification overlying the lesions, and partial to total exudative retinal detachment.[116] Fluorescein angiography characteristically demonstrates early hyperfluorescence as the tumor fills, with later staining and dye leakage from the tumor. Ultrasonography reveals high internal reflectivity. In most cases, neither of these diagnostic modalities is necessary.

Although many authors have referred to these hamartomas as cavernous hemangiomas of the choroid, most, in fact, are of the mixed cavernous and capillary variety.[119] They are composed of delicate vascular channels lined by flat endothelial cells, separated by fine intervascular septa.

Treatment for these lesions consists of hyperopic correction when appropriate, and on rare occasion photocoagulation, cryotherapy, diathermy, or local irradiation if exudation decreases vision and is amenable to therapy.[4]

The other major ocular feature of SWS is glaucoma, which occurs in approximately 30% of patients;[120] is commonly congenital, unilateral, and ipsilateral to the facial angioma; and present if the upper lid is involved.[9] Exceptions to all of these typical presentations have been described. Additionally, there is an increased risk of chronic open-angle glaucoma in adult patients who did not develop glaucoma as children.[4]

Many theories as to the pathogenesis of the glaucoma in SWS have been postulated. The two most accepted postulates include a trabeculodysgenesis similar to that seen in congenital glaucoma without SWS,[121] and increased episcleral venous pressure secondary to multiple arteriovenous shunts present in an episcleral hemangioma.[122] Both of these theories have been supported on clinical and histopathologic grounds, and Weiss has proposed a dual theory including components of both.[123] Other hypotheses include an abnormality of the sympathetic nerve supply to the eye, transudation of fluid from the choroidal lesion, and outflow obstruction similar to that seen in adults with chronic open-angle glaucoma.[116]

Treatment of glaucoma associated with SWS may be difficult. Medical therapy rarely is successful, and the results of surgical procedures, including goniotomy and trabeculotomy, are worse than that in children with primary congenital glaucoma.[4] A combined trabeculectomy-trabeculotomy procedure has also been attempted in a small group of patients without sustained control of intraocular pressure.[124] In addition to attaining only moderate success, surgery on glaucoma patients with SWS also carries an increased risk of potential complications, including expulsive choroidal hemorrhage and intraoperative choroidal effusion.[117,124,125]

REFERENCES

1. Beck RW, Hanno R. The phakomatoses. *Int Ophthalmol Clin* 25:97, 1985.
2. Van der Hoeve J. Eye diseases in tuberose sclerosis of the brain and in Recklinghausen's disease. *Trans Ophthalmol Soc UK* 43:534, 1923.
3. Van der Hoeve J. The Doyne memorial lecture: eye symptoms in phakomatoses. *Trans Ophthalmol Soc UK* 52:380, 1932.
4. Ebert EM, Boger III WP, Albert DM. Phakomatoses. In: Albert DM, Jakobiec, FA, eds. *Principles and Practice of Ophthalmology,* vol 6, 2d ed. Philadelphia: WB Saunders, 1999:5117.
5. Gold DH, Weingeist TA. *The Eye in Systemic Disease.* Philadelphia: JB Lippincott, 1990:439 and 617.
6. Taylor D. *Pediatric Ophthalmology.* Boston: Blackwell Scientific, 1990:583.
7. Crump T. Translation of case reports in: Ueber die multiplen Fibrome der Haut und ihre Beziehung zu den multiplen Neuromen, by F. v. Recklinghausen. *Adv Neurol* 29:259, 1981.
8. Riccardi VM. Von Recklinghausen neurofibromatosis. *N Engl J Med* 305:1617, 1981.
9. Font RL, Ferry AP. The phakomatoses. *Int Ophthalmol Clin* 12:1, 1972.
10. Ariel IM. Tumors of the peripheral nervous system. *Cancer J Clin* 33:282, 1983.
11. Brownstein S. Neurofibromatosis. In: Gold DH, Weingeist TA, eds. *The Eye in Systemic Disease.* Philadelphia: JB Lippincott, 1990:447.
12. Barker D, Wright E, Nguyen K, et al. Gene for von Recklinghausen neurofibromatosis is in the pericentromeric region of chromosome 17. *Science* 236:1100, 1987.
13. Gutmann DH, Aylsworth A, Carey JC, Korf B, Marks J, Pyentz RE, Rubenstein A, Viskochil D. The diagnostic evaluation and multidisciplinary

14. Richards SC, Bachynski BN. Ophthalmic manifestations of neurofibromatosis type 2. *Int Pediatr* 5:270, 1990.
15. Rouleau GA, Wertelecki W, Haines JL, et al. Genetic linkage of bilateral acoustic neurofibromatosis to a DNA marker on chromosome 22. *Nature* 329:246, 1987.
16. Wertelecki W, Rouleau GA, Superneau DW, Forehand LW, Williams JP, Haines JL, Gusella JF. Neurofibromatosis 2: clinical and DNA linkage studies of a large kindred. *N Engl J Med* 319:278, 1988.
17. Rettele GA, Brodsky MC, Merin LM, Teo C, Glasier CM. Blindness, deafness, quadriparesis, and a retinal malformation: the ravages of neurofibromatosis 2. *Surv Ophthalmol* 41:135, 1996.
18. Ladekarl S. Von Recklinghausen's glioma of the optic nerve and chiasm. *Acta Ophthalmol (Copenh)* 42:127, 1964.
19. Lloyd LA. Gliomas of the optic nerve and chiasm in childhood. *Trans Am Ophthalmol Soc* 71:488, 1973.
20. Lewis RA, Gerson LP, Axelson KA, Riccardi VW, Whitford RP. Von Recklinghausen neurofibromatosis: II. Incidence of optic gliomata. *Ophthalmology* 91:929, 1984.
21. Listernick R, Charrow J, Greenwald MJ, Esterly NB. Optic gliomas in children with neurofibromatosis type 1. *J Pediatrics* 114:788, 1989.
22. Kobrin JL, Blodi FC, Weingeist TA. Ocular and orbital manifestations of neurofibromatosis. *Surv Ophthalmol* 24:45, 1979.
23. DeAngelis LM, Kelleher MB, Post KD, Fetell MR. Multiple paragangliomas in neurofibromatosis: a new neuroendocrine neoplasia. *Neurology* 37:129, 1987.
24. Modlin IM, Farndon JR, Shepherd A, Johnston IDA, Kennedy TL, Montgomery DAD, Welbourn RB. Phaeochromocytomas in 72 patients: clinical and diagnostic features, treatment and long-term results. *Br J Surg* 66:456, 1979.
25. Lubs MLE, Bauer M, Formas ME, Djokic B. Iris hamartomas in the diagnosis of neurofibromatosis 1. *Int Pediatr* 5:261, 1990.
26. Lewis RA, Riccardi VM. Von Recklinghausen neurofibromatosis: incidence of iris hamartomata. *Ophthalmology* 88:348, 1981.
27. Perry HD, Font RL. Iris nodules in von Recklinghausen's neurofibromatosis: electron microscopic confirmation of their melanocytic origin. *Arch Ophthalmol* 100:1635, 1982.
28. Brownstein S, Little JM. Ocular neurofibromatosis. *Ophthalmology* 90:1595, 1983.
29. Politi F, Sachs R, Barishak R. Neurofibromatosis and congenital glaucoma: a case report. *Ophthalmologica* 176:155, 1978.
30. Grant WM, Walton DS. Distinctive gonioscopic findings in glaucoma due to neurofibromatosis. *Arch Ophthalmol* 79:127, 1968.
31. Klein RM, Glassman L. Neurofibromatosis of the choroid. *Am J Ophthalmol* 99:367, 1985.

32. Savino PJ, Glaser JS, Luxenberg MN. Pulsating enophthalmos and choroidal hamartomas: two rare stigmata of neurofibromatosis. *Br J Ophthalmol* 61:483, 1977.

33. Wolter JR. Nerve fibrils in ovoid bodies with neurofibromatosis of the choroid. *Arch Ophthalmol* 73:696, 1965.

34. Kurosawa A, Kurosawa H. Ovoid bodies in choroidal neurofibromatosis. *Arch Ophthalmol* 100:1939, 1982.

35. Insler MS, Helm C, Napoli S. Conjunctival hamartoma in neurofibromatosis. *Am J Ophthalmol* 99:731, 1985.

36. Bloch FJ. Retinal tumor associated with neurofibromatosis (von Recklinghausen's disease): report of a case. *Arch Ophthalmol* 40:433, 1948.

37. Destro M, D'Amico DJ, Gragoudas ES, Brockhurst RJ, Pinnolis MK, Albert DM, Topping TM, Puliafito CA. Retinal manifestations of neurofibromatosis: diagnosis and management. *Arch Ophthalmol* 109:662, 1991.

38. Massry GG, Morgan CF, Chung SM. Evidence of optic pathway gliomas after previously negative neuroimaging. *Ophthalmology* 104:930, 1997.

39. Seiff SR, Brodsky MC, MacDonald G, Berg BO, Howes EL Jr, Hoyt WF. Orbital optic glioma in neurofibromatosis: magnetic resonance diagnosis of perineural arachnoid gliomatosis. *Arch Ophthalmol* 105:1689, 1987.

40. Kaiser-Kupfer MI, Freidlin V, Datiles MB, Edwards PA, Sherman JL, Parry D, McCain LM, Eldridge R. The association of posterior subcapsular lens opacities with bilateral acoustic neuromas in patients with neurofibromatosis type 2. *Arch Ophthalmol* 107:541, 1989.

41. Pearson-Webb MA, Kaiser-Kupfer MI, Eldridge R. Eye findings in bilateral acoustic (central) neurofibromatosis: association with presenile lens opacities and cataracts but absence of Lisch nodules [letter to the editor]. *N Engl J Med* 315:1553, 1986.

42. Dossetor FM, Landau K, Hoyt WF. Optic disk glioma in neurofibromatosis type 2. *Am J Ophthalmol* 108:602, 1989.

43. Thomas DA, Trobe JD, Cornblath WT. Visual loss secondary to increased intracranial pressure in neurofibromatosis type 2. *Arch Ophthalmol* 117:1650, 1999.

44. Brodsky MC, Landau K, Wilson RS, Botshauser E. Morning glory disc anomaly in neurofibromatosis type 2. *Arch Ophthalmol* 117:839, 1999.

45. Ragge NK, Baser ME, Klein J, Nechiporuk A, Sainz J, Pulst S-M, Riccardi VM. Ocular abnormalities in neurofibromatosis 2. *Am J Ophthalmol* 120:634, 1995.

46. Williams R, Taylor D. Tuberous sclerosis. *Surv Ophthalmol* 30:143, 1985.

47. Nyboer JH, Robertson DM, Gomez MR. Retinal lesions in tuberous sclerosis. *Arch Ophthalmol* 94:1277, 1976.

48. Van der Hoeve J. Eye symptoms in tuberous sclerosis of the brain. *Trans Ophthalmol Soc UK* 40:329, 1920.

49. Fryer AE, Chalmers A, Connor JM, et al. Evidence that the gene for tuberous sclerosis is on chromosome 9. *Lancet* 1:659, 1987.

50. Lagos JC, Gomez MR. Tuberous sclerosis: reappraisal of a clinical entity. *Mayo Clin Proc* 42:26, 1967.

51. Monaghan HP, Krafchik BR, MacGregor DL, Fitz CR. Tuberous sclerosis complex in children. *Am J Dis Child* 135:912, 1981.

52. Pampiglione G, Pugh E. Infantile spasms and subsequent appearance of tuberous sclerosis syndrome. *Lancet* 2:1046, 1975.

53. Pampiglione G, Moynahan EJ. The tuberous sclerosis syndrome, and clinical and EEG studies in 100 children. *J Neurol Neurosurg Psychiatry* 39:666, 1976.

54. Kingsley DPE, Kendall BE, Fitz CR. Tuberous sclerosis: a clinico-radiological evaluation of 110 cases with particular reference to atypical presentation. *Neuroradiology* 28:38, 1986.

55. Roach ES, Williams DP, Laster DW. Magnetic resonance imaging in tuberous sclerosis. *Arch Neurol* 44:301, 1987.

56. Frank LM, Chaves-Carballo E, Earley LM. Early diagnosis of tuberous sclerosis by cranial ultrasonography. *Arch Neurol* 41:1302, 1984.

57. Waziri M. Tuberous sclerosis. In: Gold DH, Weingeist TA, eds. *The Eye in Systemic Disease*. Philadelphia: JB Lippincott, 1990:450.

58. Hendren WG, Monfort GJ. Symptomatic bilateral renal angiomyolipomas in children. *J Urol* 137:256, 1987.

59. Magnus H. Aneurysma arteriosa-venosum retinale. *Virchows Arch Pathol Anat Physiol* 60:38, 1874.

60. Wyburn-Mason R. Arteriovenous aneurysm of the mid-brain and retina, facial naevi, and mental changes. *Brain* 66:163, 1943.

61. Bech K, Jensen OA. On the frequency of coexisting racemose haemangiomata of the retina and brain. *Acta Psychiatr Neurol Scand* 36:47, 1961.

62. Mansour AM, Schwartz TL. Wyburn-Mason syndrome. In: Gold DH, Weingeist TA, eds. *The Eye in Systemic Disease*. Philadelphia: JB Lippincott, 1990:455.

63. Archer DB, Deutman A, Ernest JT, Krill AE. Arteriovenous communications of the retina. *Am J Ophthalmol* 75:224, 1973.

64. Mansour AM, Walsh JB, Henkind P. Arteriovenous anastomoses of the retina. *Ophthalmology* 94:35, 1987.

65. Theron J, Newton TH, Hoyt WF. Unilateral retinocephalic vascular malformations. *Neuroradiology* 7:185, 1974.

66. Bernth-Petersen P. Racemose haemangioma of the retina: report of three cases with long term follow-up. *Acta Ophthalmol (Copenh)* 57:669, 1979.

67. Mansour AM, Wells CG, Jampol LM, Kalina RE. Ocular complications of arteriovenous communications of the retina. *Arch Ophthalmol* 107:232, 1989.

68. Cameron ME, Greer CH. Congenital arteriovenous aneurysm of the retina: a postmortem report. *Br J Ophthalmol* 52:768, 1968.

69. Krug EF, Samuels B. Venous angioma of the retina, optic nerve, chiasm and brain: a case report with postmortem observations. *Arch Ophthalmol* 8:871, 1932.

70. Waldmann TA, Misiti J, Nelson DL, Kraemer KH. Ataxia telangiectasia: a multisystem hereditary disease with immunodeficiency, impaired organ maturation, x-ray hypersensitivity, and a high incidence of neoplasia. *Ann Intern Med* 99:367, 1983.

71. Louis-Bar D. Sur un syndrome progressif comprenant des telangiectasies capillaires cutanees et conjunctivales symmetriques: a disposition naevoide et des troubles cerebelleux. *Confin Neurol* 4:32, 1941.

72. Boder E, Sedgwick RP. Ataxia telangiectasia: a familial syndrome of progressive cerebellar ataxia, oculo-cutaneous telangiectasia and frequent pulmonary infections. *Pediatrics* 21:526, 1970.

73. Miller NR. Ataxia telangiectasia. In: Gold DH, Weingeist TA, eds. *The Eye in Systemic Disease.* Philadelphia: JB Lippincott, 1990:439.

74. Eisen AH, Karpati G, Laszlo T, Andermann F, Robb JP, Bacal HL. Immunologic deficiency in ataxia telangiectasia. *N Engl J Med* 272:18, 1965.

75. Karpati G, Eisen AH, Andermann F, Bacal H, Robb JP. Ataxia telangiectasia: further observations and report of eight cases. *Am J Dis Child* 110:51, 1965.

76. Becker Y. Cancer in ataxia-telangiectasia patients: analysis of factors leading to radiation-induced and spontaneous tumors. *Anticancer Research* 6:1021, 1986.

77. Morrell D, Cromartie E, Swift M. Mortality and cancer incidence in 263 patients with ataxia-telangiectasia. *J Natl Cancer Inst* 77:89, 1986.

78. Savitsky K, Bar-Shira A, Gilad S, et al. A single ataxia telangiectasia gene with a product similar to PI-3 kinase. *Science* 268:1749, 1995.

79. Cogan DG, Chu FC, Reingold D, Barranger J. Ocular motor signs in some metabolic diseases. *Arch Ophthalmol* 99:1802, 1981.

80. Smith JL, Cogan DG. Ataxia-telangiectasia. *Arch Ophthalmol* 62:364, 1959.

81. Baloh RW, Yee RD, Boder E. Eye movements in ataxia-telangiectasia. *Neurology* 28:1099, 1978.

82. Reed WB, Epstein WL, Boder E, Sedgwick R. Cutaneous manifestations of ataxia-telangiectasia. *JAMA* 195:746, 1966.

83. Aguilar MJ, Kamashita S, Landing BH, et al. Pathologic observations in ataxia telangiectasia: a report of 5 cases. *J Neuropathol Exp Neurol* 27:659, 1968.

84. Terplan KL, Krauss RF. Histopathological brain changes in association with ataxia-telangiectasia. *Neurology* 19:446, 1969.

85. Paula-Barbosa MM, Ruela C, Tavares MA, Pontes C, Saraiva A, Cruz C. Cerebellar cortex ultrastructure in ataxia-telangiectasia. *Ann Neurol* 13:297, 1983.

86. Perry TL, Kish SJ, Hinton D, Hansen BA, Becker LE, Gelfand EW. Neurochemical abnormalities in a patient with ataxia-telangiectasia. *Neurology* 34:187, 1984.

87. De Leon GA, Grover WD, Huff DS. Neuropathologic changes in ataxia telangiectasia. *Neurology* 26:947, 1976.

88. McFarlin DD, Straber W, Waldmann JA. Ataxia-telangiectasia. *Medicine (Baltimore)* 51:281, 1972.

89. Von Hippel E. Uber eine sehr seltene Erkrakung der Netzhaut: klinische Beobachtungen. *Graefes Arch Ophthalmol* 59:83, 1904.

90. Von Hippel E. Die anatomische Grundlage der von mir beschrienbenen "Òsher sheltenen Erkrakung der Netzhaut." *Graefes Arch Ophthalmol* 79:350, 1911.

91. Lindau A. Studien ueber Kleinhirn/cysten: Bau, Pathogenese, und Beziehungen zur Angiomatosis Retinae. *Acta Pathol Microbiol Scand Suppl* 1:1, 1926.

92. Seizinger BR, Rouleau GA, Ozelius LJ, et al. Von Hippel-Lindau disease maps to the region of chromosome 3 associated with renal cell carcinoma. *Nature* 332:268, 1968.

93. Neumann HPH, Wiestler OD. Clustering of features of von Hippel-Lindau syndrome: evidence for a complex gene locus. *Lancet* 337:1052, 1991.

94. Hardwig PW, Robertson DM. Von Hippel-Lindau disease: a familial, often lethal, multisystem phakomatosis. *Ophthalmology* 91:263, 1984.

95. Horton WA, Wong V, Eldridge R. Von Hippel-Lindau disease: clinical and pathological manifestations in nine families with 50 affected members. *Arch Intern Med* 136:769, 1976.

96. Maher ER, Yates JRW, Harries R, et al. Clinical features and natural history of von Hippel-Lindau disease. *Q J Med* 77:1151, 1990.

97. Melmon KL, Rosen SW. Lindau's disease: review of the literature and study of a large kindred. *Am J Med* 36:595, 1964.

98. Hardwig PW. Von Hippel-Lindau disease. In: Gold DH, Weingeist TA, eds. *The Eye in Systemic Disease.* Philadelphia: JB Lippincott, 1990:453.

99. Welch RB. Von Hippel-Lindau disease: the recognition and treatment of early angiomatosis retinae and the use of cryosurgery as an adjunct to therapy. *Trans Am Ophthalmol Soc* 68:367, 1970.

100. Haining WM, Zweifach PH. Fluorescein angiography in von Hippel-Lindau disease. *Arch Ophthalmol* 78:475, 1967.

101. Kawamura J, Garcia JH, Kamijyo Y. Cerebellar hemangioblastoma: histogenesis of stroma cells. *Cancer* 31:1528, 1973.

102. Mottow-Lippa L, Tso MOM, Peyman GA, Chejfec G. Von Hippel angiomatosis: a light, electron microscopic, and immunoperoxidase characterization. *Ophthalmology* 90:848, 1983.

103. Chan C-C, Vortmeyer AO, Chew EY, et al. *VHL* gene deletion and *VEGF* gene expression detected in the stromal cells of retinal angioma. *Arch Ophthalmol* 117:625, 1999.

104. Jakobiec FA, Font RL, Johnson FB. Angiomatosis retinae: an ultrastructural study and lipid analysis. *Cancer* 38:2042, 1976.

105. Gass JDM. Treatment of retinal vascular anomalies. *Trans Am Acad Ophthalmol Otolaryngol* 83:432, 1977.

106. Goldberg MF, Koenig S. Argon laser treatment of von Hippel-Lindau retinal angiomas: I. Clinical and angiographic findings. *Arch Ophthalmol* 92:126, 1974.

107. Annesley WH, Leonard BC, Shields JA, Tasman WS. Fifteen year review of treated cases of retinal angiomatosis. *Trans Am Acad Ophthalmol Otolaryngol* 83:446, 1977.

108. Cardoso RD, Brockhurst RJ. Perforating diathermy coagulation for retinal angiomas. *Arch Ophthalmol* 94:1702, 1976.

109. Peyman GA, Rednam KRV, Mottow-Lippa L, Flood T. Treatment of large von Hippel tumors by eye wall resection. *Ophthalmology* 90:840, 1983.

110. Sturge WA. A case of partial epilepsy apparently due to a lesion of one of the vasomotor centers of the brain. *Trans Clin Soc Lond* 12:162, 1879.

111. Weber FP. Right-sided hemi-hypertrophy resulting from right-sided congenital spastic hemiplegia, with a morbid condition of the left side of the brain, revealed by radiograms. *J Neurol Psychopathol* 3:134, 1922.

112. Enjolras O, Riche MC, Merland JJ. Facial port-wine stains and Sturge-Weber syndrome. *Pediatrics* 76:48, 1985.

113. Person JR, Perry HO. Recent advances in the phakomatoses. *Int J Dermatol* 17:1, 1978.

114. Alexander GL, Norman RM. *The Sturge-Weber Syndrome.* Bristol, England: John Wright and Sons, 1960.

115. Tan OT, Gilchrest BA. Laser therapy for selected cutaneous vascular lesions in the pediatric population: a review. *Pediatrics* 82:652, 1988.

116. Tripathi BJ, Tripathi RC, Cibis GW. Sturge-Weber syndrome. In: Gold DH, Weingeist TA, eds. *The Eye in Systemic Disease.* Philadelphia: JB Lippincott, 1990:443.

117. Christensen GR, Records RE. Glaucoma and expulsive hemorrhage mechanisms in the Sturge-Weber syndrome. *Ophthalmology* 86:1360, 1979.

118. Susac JO, Smith JL, Scelfo RJ. The "tomato-catsup" fundus in Sturge-Weber syndrome. *Arch Ophthalmol* 92:69, 1974.

119. Witschel H, Font RL. Hemangioma of the choroid: a clinicopathologic study of 71 cases and a review of the literature. *Surv Ophthalmol* 20:415, 1976.

120. Cibis GW, Tripathi RC, Tripathi BJ. Glaucoma in Sturge-Weber syndrome. *Ophthalmology* 91:1061, 1984.

121. Hoskins HD Jr, Shaffer RN, Hetherington J. Anatomical classification of the developmental glaucomas. *Arch Ophthalmol* 102:1331, 1984.

122. Phelps CD. The pathogenesis of glaucoma in Sturge-Weber syndrome. *Ophthalmology* 85:276, 1978.

123. Weiss DI. Dual origin of glaucoma in encephalotrigeminal haemangiomatosis: a pathogenetic concept based upon histopathologic and haemodynamic considerations. *Trans Ophthalmol Soc UK* 93:477, 1973.

124. Board RJ, Shields MB. Combined trabeculotomy-trabeculectomy for the management of glaucoma associated with Sturge-Weber syndrome. *Ophthalmic Surg* 12:813, 1981.

125. Bellows AR, Chylack LT, Epstein DL, Hutchinson BT. Choroidal effusion during glaucoma surgery in patients with prominent episcleral vessels. *Arch Ophthalmol* 97:493, 1979.

EXPERIMENTAL OCULAR ONCOLOGY: ANIMAL MODELS

Jeffrey I. Everitt, John A. Shadduck, and Herbert E. Whiteley

A variety of spontaneous, induced, and transplantation ocular oncology models have been developed in animals. These laboratory animal models serve as an important tool for studies of ocular tumor pathobiology and immunology, and provide useful information for the clinical management of human ocular neoplasia. Recently, the development of transgenic animal technology has provided tumor biologists with an extremely powerful means by which to dissect the molecular mechanisms that control the oncogenic process. The ability now exists to design and construct animal models of human neoplastic disorders by a stable integration of exogenous genetic information into the animal genome. This exciting new technology greatly expands the role of animal models in all areas of oncology, including experimental studies of tumors of the globe and adnexal structures.

Experimental studies of ocular tumors are important because there are many uncertainties and controversies concerning the natural history and clinical management of the most common human ocular neoplasms: the melanocytic tumors. The clinical management of ocular neoplasms presents special challenges, due to the need to consider both preservation of vision as well as life. There is an important need to develop and characterize animal models that will aid in the evaluation of new therapeutic modalities for the management of eye cancer. Unfortunately, despite recent advances in the generation of new laboratory rodent models of ocular cancer, and the availability of several well-characterized and well-studied transplantation models, there is still a paucity of relevant intraocular tumor systems in large laboratory animal species. Induced and spontaneous tumor models in these species are needed to provide ophthalmologists with globes that can be subjected to funduscopic studies and manipulated in the clinical setting.

In addition to adding to our understanding of the pathobiology of ocular neoplastic disease, experimental studies of ocular neoplasms have added greatly to our understanding of general tumor biology. Molecular studies of human hereditary retinoblastoma resulted in an understanding of the role of the retinoblastoma gene and contributed to our present understanding of the genetic predisposition to familial cancer. This finding in turn led to the discovery of an entire class of cancer susceptibility genes, the tumor-suppressor genes.[1] The experimental study of ocular melanocytic tumors may provide special insights into pigment cell pathobiology and the control of metastases.[2] The development and characterization of novel animal model systems to study the biology of ocular neoplasia will undoubtedly play a major role in future studies of these difficult and important disease processes.

TRANSPLANTABLE INTRAOCULAR NEOPLASMS

The anterior chamber of the eye has been used as a site for experimental transplantation of numerous cells and tissues for many years. The hospitality of this site has been recognized for more than 100 years, when tumor cells were placed in the anterior chamber of a rabbit's eye and were found to survive.[3,4] This chapter deals with several areas, including the immunologic response and use of the anterior chamber as a site for study of intraocular melanoma, and mentions the various types of neoplasms introduced into the anterior chamber for the study of tumor biology and treatment regimens.

The immune response to antigens exposed by the intraocular route has produced a variable but unique set of immunologic responses.[3] This response, termed *anterior chamber associated immune deviation* (ACAID), was first identified and characterized by Kaplan and Streilein[5] and further developed by Niederkorn and colleagues.[6,7] The phenomenon of immunologic privilege associated with the anterior chamber has been known for many years. This deviant immune response is characterized by impaired cell-mediated or delayed-type immunity, normal humoral antibody production, impaired in vivo lymphocyte proliferation to antigens, presence of cytotoxic T cells in the spleen and cervical lymph nodes, and induction of T-suppressor cells.[3]

The degree and type of immunologic response to tumors transplanted into the anterior chamber of the eye depend on the antigenicity of the neoplastic cells in relation to the host. Neoplasms that demonstrate large differences in histocompatibility at major histocompatibility loci induce a transient immune suppression but then are rejected by the host. This type of reaction causes destruction of the tumor but also significant "bystander" reaction, with subsequent damage to other portions of the globe. When P-91 mastocytoma cells (a mutagenic line of P-815 mastocytoma cell) are injected into syngeneic hosts such as the DBA/2 strain of mouse, the neoplasm is rejected by delayed-type hypersensitivity. This T-cell-mediated process causes significant destruction of associated ocular structures.[8] Conversely, if these neoplastic cells are injected into allogeneic C57BL/6 mice, the cells are rejected without concomitant destruction of surrounding tissue.[8,9] This second type of response was determined using the UV5C25 fibrosarcoma cell line injected into syngeneic BALB/c hosts. These neoplasms were infiltrated by mononuclear cells and were completely rejected without damage to normal ocular structures (Figure 14.1).[9] Further studies using these tumors showed that the neoplasms were infiltrated by mononuclear cells (tumor-infiltrating lymphocytes) that were directly cytolytic to tumor cells and had functional characteristics of cytotoxic T cells; this was produced in conjunction with normal systemic delayed-type hypersensitivity without nonspecific tissue destruction.[10]

When P815 mastocytoma cells are injected intracamerally into syngeneic BALB/c mice, the cells grow uninhibited in the anterior chamber, with subsequent destruction of the globe and local invasion into surrounding structures such as the brain.[6,7] These P815 mastocytoma cells originated from DBA/2 mice and are not different in major histocompatibility loci from the host BALB/c mice, differing only at minor loci. These neoplasms continue to proliferate in the eye without distinct immunologic reaction to the neoplasm; however, when P815 cells are introduced at other sites, such as subcutaneously, they will be rejected. Similarly, when P815 cells are injected into the contralateral eye, they will grow transiently and then be rejected.[3,6,7]

In general, it appears that when injected intracamerally (in the anterior chamber), neoplastic cells that demonstrate differences in a single class of histocompatibility loci induce rejection by a delayed-type hypersensitivity with associated destruction of ocular tissue. Tumors that have multiple differences in major histocompatibility loci are rejected with precision and without bystander ocular damage. Transplanted tissue that differs from the host only by minor histocompatibility antigens, and thus is weakly immunogenic, suppresses the immune response and the tumor continues to grow.

Experimental Melanomas. Cutaneous melanoma cells, when injected into the globe, have been used as a model for uveal melanoma to study growth, metastasis, and treatment regimens. The Greene hamster melanoma has been the basic model used for many years.[11] Cutaneous hamster melanoma cells are injected into the choroid of weanling Syrian golden hamsters. The neoplastic cells grow and invade the choroidal region, eventually filling the entire globe with subsequent perforation through the sclera.

Generally, 1 week after injection, neoplastic cells remained within the choroid; by 2 weeks after injection, they had penetrated Bruch's membrane and expanded to fill mostly the vitreal cavity. This proliferative and infiltrative nature continued to the point where the entire globe and orbit were involved by 4–6 weeks.[11] The large neoplastic masses often contained areas of necrosis and hemorrhage, with little recognizable choroidal or retinal tissue left.[11] Because of the small size of the hamster eye, Greene melanoma cells were transplanted into the iris of rabbits. Neoplastic cells showed rapid growth with

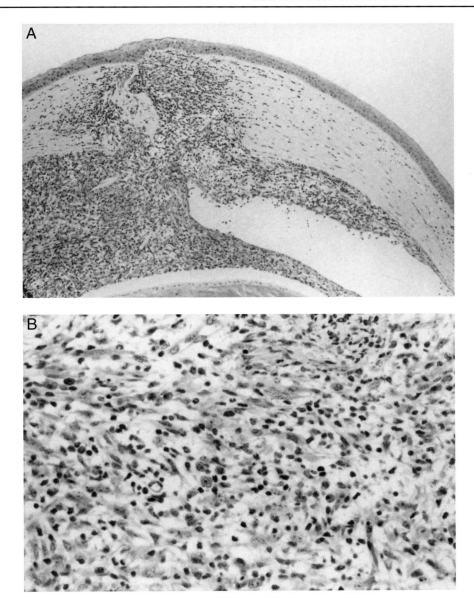

FIG. 14.1A and B—Cutaneous fibrosarcoma (UV5C25) in a BALB/c mouse. This neoplasm expresses tumor-specific antigens, is infiltrated by mononuclear cells, and is being rejected without destruction of surrounding ocular structures. **A,** ×82; **B,** ×330. (Courtesy of J. Niederkorn and M. Kripke.)

expansion of the tumor with vascularization; about 10 days after injection, however, necrosis occurred.[12] Use of this model for the examination of treatment regimens may be complicated by host immune responses similar to the ACAID phenomenon.

The B16 murine melanoma cells have been administered via intracameral injections to study metastatic potential and treatment regimens with novel chemotherapeutic agents.[5] The advantage of this model is that the origin, tumor-specific antigens, and genetic background of B16 melanoma have been characterized.[13,14] Investigators have used the highly metastatic subline Queens melanoma (Figure 14.2) and nonmetastatic B16F10 subline. The

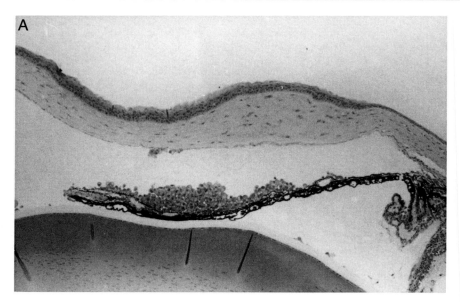

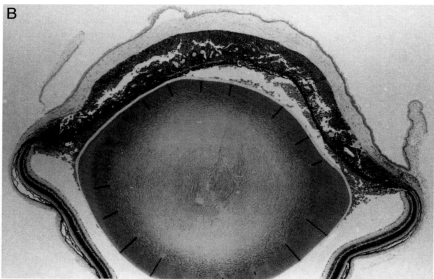

FIG. 14.2—**A:** Queens murine melanoma 6 days after injection. **B and C:** Queens murine melanoma 12 days after injection. (continued)

B16F10 subline does not metastasize unless the host has been immunosuppressed and subjected to traumatic enucleation.[14,15]

Metastatic potential and effect of treatment have also been studied using human uveal melanoma cells (OCM1) injected intracamerally and intravenously into nude mice (Figure 14.3).[16] These cells have a propensity to metastasize to the liver.[16] These studies also showed evidence that cell surface gangliosides may be important in metastatic cell adhesion.[16]

Attempts to develop a model of intraocular murine melanoma by using melanomas of the Sinclair miniswine have been made, but the ability to consistently reproduce intraocular melanomas using this model has been poor.[17,18]

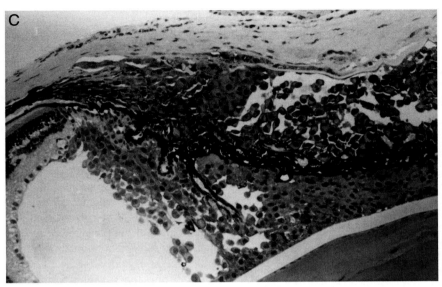

FIG. 14.2 (continued)—The neoplasm is proliferating in the anterior chamber and in and along the iris. It has infiltrated into the ciliary cleft. **A,** ×82; **B,** ×33; **C,** ×165. (Courtesy of J. Niederkorn.)

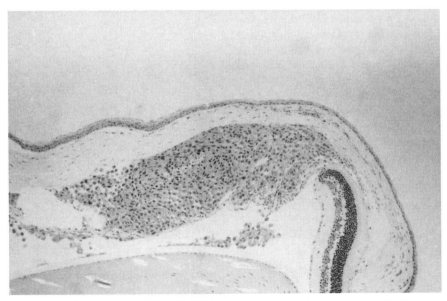

FIG. 14.3—Human uveal melanoma cell line (OCM1) injected into a nude mouse eye. ×82. (Courtesy of J. Niederkorn and J. Kan-Mitchell.)

Other Intraocular Neoplastic Models. The anterior chamber of both the rabbit eye and the rat eye has been used as a site for growth of neoplastic tissue, including studies of tumor pathophysiology and response to treatment regimens. Investigations with this model have included studies of the intraocular growth of endometrium in rabbits as a model for endometriosis,[19] intraocular carcinoid tumors,[20] and intraocular retinoblastoma-like neoplasms in rats.[21]

VIRALLY INDUCED INTRAOCULAR NEOPLASMS

Rodent Models of Virally Induced Retinoblastoma. Intraocular neoplasms diagnosed as retinoblastomas have been induced in CD rats given high intraocular doses of human adenovirus type 12 (Huie strain).[22,23] These experimental tumors are composed primarily of small, uniform hyperchromatic, undifferentiated cells arrayed in uniform tubular alignment or in columnar patterns suggestive of neuroepithelium. Microscopic features of retinoblastoma present in these experimentally induced tumors include incomplete Homer-Wright rosettes and cilia with a 9 + 0 doublet microtubular pattern. These tumors did not have Flexner-Wintersteiner rosettes, fleurettes, or photoreceptor differentiation, although ganglioneuronic differentiation was present.[24] Ultrastructural features of the adenoviral-induced tumors include intercellular junctions, triple-membrane structures, annulate lamellae, coated vesicles, microtubules, and neurofilaments.[24] Adenovirus-12-induced intraocular tumors occur with variable incidence, depending on the age at which the animals are inoculated and whether methylnitrosourea is used as a chemical cocarcinogen. Tumors are most easily produced if the rats are inoculated intravitreously within a few hours after birth, and the latent period is shortened if methylnitrosourea is used as a pretreatment. The incidence ranges from 5% to 45%, with a latency period of between 40 and 360 days.[23]

Experimental intraocular neoplasms with features identical to those already described are consistently and rapidly induced when a rat-origin, human adenovirus-12-transformed cell line is transplanted to the vitreous of newborn inbred CDF rats.[25] In this model, all of 39 CDF rats developed clinical evidence of tumors within 30 days of implantation. The lesions appear identical to those induced by adenovirus 12 in situ. These tumors grow relatively slowly, although they can eventually distort the globe and perforate the eye.[26]

Ohashi and colleagues reported that 11 of 54 hamsters given intraocular inoculations of the human JC papovavirus as newborns subsequently developed intraocular neoplasms.[27] Eight of these tumors were diagnosed as retinoblastomas, based on the presence of high mitotic index, Homer-Wright rosettes, ciliary structure, and neuronal processes with microtubules and microfilaments. These hamsters also developed neoplasms of the central and peripheral nervous system. Similar ocular tumors were produced in mice following intraocular inoculation of adenovirus 12.[28]

Feline Sarcoma Virus-Induced Uveal Melanomas. Uveal melanomas were produced by injection of Gardner strain feline sarcoma virus intraocularly in 10- to 15-day-old kittens.[29] Approximately 90% of injected eyes develop anterior uveal neoplasms that resemble spontaneous anterior uveal melanomas of people. Clinically, these tumors arise as flat hyperpigmented iridal plaques at the site of viral inoculation. The tumors are generally detectable by 40 days after viral injection and are always recognizable by 60 days. A variable clinical course is noted, with some lesions showing rapid and destructive progression after an initial period of relatively slow growth.

The tumors arise in the iris and enlarge as a discrete mass or diffuse thickening within the iris and/or ciliary body.[30] Microscopically, injected eyes have hypertrophy and hyperplasia of uveal melanocytes as early as 14 days after injection. These spindle-shaped melanocytes often demonstrate atypias. Progressive tumors demonstrate pigmented epithelioid, pigmented spindle-shaped, and nonpigmented spindle-shaped cells that invade the iris stroma (Figure 14.4). These neoplastic lesions invade the ciliary body from the iris and can grow quite large. In the larger tumors, epithelioid cells become increasingly common and can predominate. Secondary tumors arise at extraocular sites, but these do not resemble the metastatic spread of human intraocular melanoma and are believed to represent transformation of local fibroblasts by the fibrosarcoma virus.[29]

CHEMICALLY INDUCED OCULAR NEOPLASMS

Intraocular Tumor Models. Intraocular neoplasms have been induced in laboratory animals

A

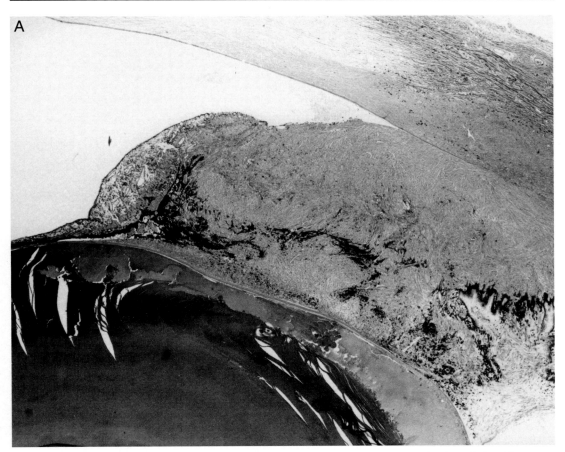

FIG. 14.4—**A:** Feline sarcoma virus-induced intraocular melanoma in a cat 47 days after inoculation. Tumor has arisen at the virus injection site at the base of the iris, infiltrating the iris and ciliary body, and resulting in adhesions to lens and cornea. ×25. (continued)

by a variety of chemical agents. Intraocular instillation of carcinogenic nickel subsulfide in rats led to the induction of multiple intraocular tumors, which histologically were diagnosed as melanomas, retinoblastomas, gliomas, and unclassified malignant neoplasms (Figure 14.5).[31] This tumor induction system resulted in intraocular neoplasms characterized by short latency period, high tumor incidence, and ease of tumor detection. Extraocular orbital tumors have also been induced by the local deposition of carcinogenic nickel compounds (Figure 14.6).[32]

Most efforts to create chemically induced intraocular tumors have been aimed at the creation of models of melanocytic tumors. Uveal melanomas have been induced in rats by the

intraocular instillation of nickel subsulfide[31] and nickel sulfide,[33] subcutaneous injection of urethan,[34] and intraocular implantation of platinum foil and cellophane film.[35] Intraocular instillation of nickel compounds is carcinogenic in nonrodent species, as evidenced by studies resulting in intraocular melanoma-like neoplasms in nickel subsulfide-treated Japanese common newts (*Cynops purrhogaster*).[36]

The small size of the globe and uncertain natural history and metastatic potential of induced intraocular melanocytic lesions in rodents limits the utility of small animal models for relevant studies of human intraocular tumor biology. Until recently, with the exception of retrovirus-induced uveal melanoma in cats, there were no animal

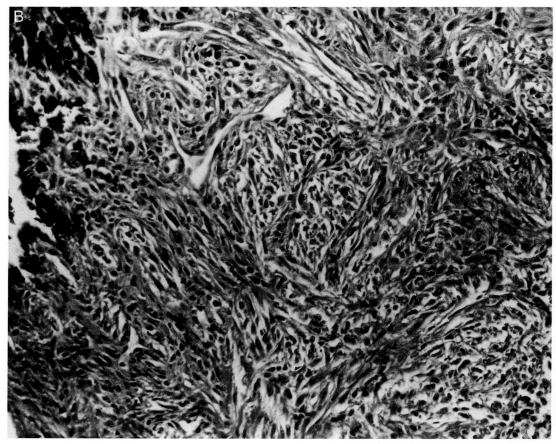

FIG. 14.4 (continued)—**B:** High magnification of the neoplasm demonstrating interwoven fascicles of spindle-shaped melanocytes. ×500.

models of primary uveal melanoma described in eyes large enough to document the clinical evolution of ocular proliferative lesions. Most experimental studies that required ocular manipulation used the Greene cutaneous hamster melanoma model implanted into the eye of the rabbit.[12] Although the rabbit eye permits serial funduscopic photography, the transplant aspect of the model makes it irrelevant to the study of in situ tumor development and progression.

Recently, a rabbit model was described in which primary uveal melanocytic lesions were induced in the choroid of rabbits following the chronic topical application of 7,12-dimethyl-benz(*a*)anthracene (DMBA).[37,38] Four weekly topical doses of DMBA to the choroid of Dutch (pigmented) rabbits, followed by 12 weekly doses of croton oil as a promoter, resulted in a spectrum of melanocytic proliferations, including hyperplasia and benign nevi with varying grades of cytologic atypia.[38] DMBA had been previously used to create animal models of cutaneous melanocytic lesions[39] as well as an animal model of conjunctival primary acquired melanosis.[40] To date, no experimental regimens have been described that result in chemically induced melanoma in a rabbit or other large animal model.

Other Chemically Induced Eye Tumors. Chronic exposure of the Grey short-tailed opossum (*Monodelphis domestica*) to ultraviolet radiation (UVR) leads to the formation of cutaneous and corneal neoplasms.[41] The tumors that

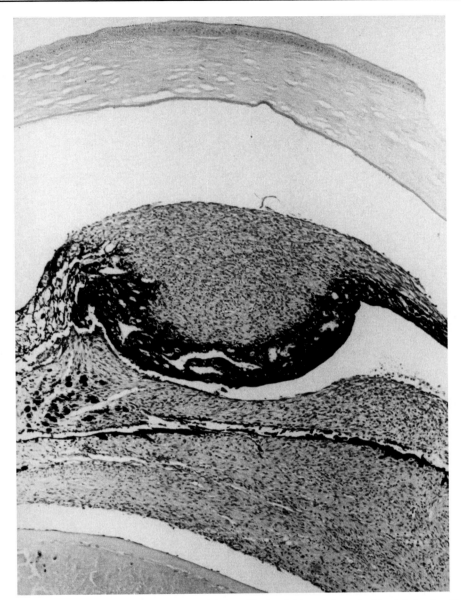

FIG. 14.5—Tumor (spindle cell melanoma) of the iris in a Fischer 344 rat injected with nickel subsulfide 8 months previously. ×270.

arise appear to be fibroblastic neoplasms of the corneal stroma. The ability of this animal to photoreactivate pyrimidine dimers in cutaneous and corneal DNA, in conjunction with its susceptibility to UVR-induced tumors, makes it a valuable model with which to determine whether pyrimidine dimers are involved in UVR tumorigenesis.

Although chemically induced ocular tumors are not common in carcinogenesis bioassays using laboratory rodents,[42] the eye is a site of tumor formation in a fish carcinogenesis model. Medaka (*Oryzias latipes*) given a single brief exposure to methylazoxymethanol acetate develop a spectrum of neoplastic retinal lesions with histologic features of medulloepitheliomas and retinoblastomas.

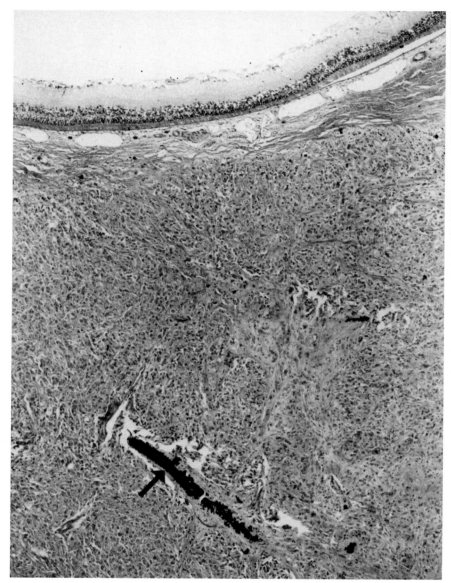

FIG. 14.6—Optic nerve meningioma induced by extraocular deposition of nickel subsulfide (arrow). ×86.

This animal model is being examined for its suitability for molecular studies of the retinoblastoma tumor suppressor gene.[43]

TRANSGENIC ANIMAL MODELS

Transgenic animals are constructed using molecular genetic techniques to produce animals that have functional genes added to the genome or have alterations of specific genes believed to be important in disease processes. Using these new experimental animal systems, many complex issues in the pathobiology of ocular neoplasia can be studied in vivo, including tissue-specific expression of oncogenes in tumor growth, and the role of oncogenes and tumor-suppressor genes in specific cell types. Transgenic animals are produced by three different methods of introduction of genes into the germline: (1) direct microinjection of DNA into the male pronucleus of the one-cell embryo, (2) retroviral infection of preimplantation or postimplantation embryos, and (3) injection of embryonic stem cells into the blastocyst. Following transgene introduction, multiple factors affect the expression of the transgene, such as DNA methylation, integration site in the genome, and the regulatory elements employed. Among the many transgenic species, the mouse has been the laboratory animal of choice due to short gestation period, large litter size, easy maintenance, and well-characterized genetics. One of the major challenges facing future studies in ocular carcinogenesis is the need to develop transgenic animal models of ocular neoplasia in species suitable for experiments that require larger-size globes.

Retinoblastoma Model. An intraocular model has been established in transgenic mice in which retinal and midbrain tumors develop that are reminiscent of human retinoblastoma.[44] This transgenic model was created by the introduction of a gene containing the protein coding region of the simian virus 40 (SV40) T antigen (*Tag*) driven by the promoter of the luteinizing hormone β-subunit gene. These mice develop heritable ocular tumors with complete penetrance. Retinal tumors are first observed at about 2 months of age and fill the vitreous cavity by 5–6 months of age. These tumors share histologic, ultrastructural, and immunohistochemical similarity with human retinoblastomas.[45] A specific association has been shown between the *Rb* encoded protein p105 and *Tag* antigen in mouse retinoblastoma cells. This finding, along with the occurrence of tumors in these transgenic mice, provides in vivo evidence that oncogenesis is due to the ocular-specific expression of an *Rb*-binding oncoprotein that can functionally inactivate the *Rb* protein. This transgenic model should offer significant advantages to previous adenoviral models and transplantation models for the study of the pathogenesis and treatment of this malignant disorder.

Lens Oncogenesis Model. The study of oncogenesis in the epithelial tissue of the lens provides a model system for the examination of the events that occur after an oncogene product is produced in a differentiating mammalian tissue. The regulatory region of the mouse α-crystallin gene is used to target SV40 tumor antigen expression in the eye lens in transgenic mice. SV40 oncogene products begin to accumulate at midgestation, and the animals develop lens tumors that invade neighboring ocular tissues.[46] This experimental murine tumor system enables investigators to examine the qualitative and quantitative aspects of the processes that mediate the role of differentiation and proliferation in oncogenesis.[47] Studies using these mice should help elucidate important factors in the ocular microenvironment that might explain the paucity of naturally occurring lens tumors in animals and humans.[48]

Retinal Pigment Epithelium Melanoma Model. Spontaneous ocular melanomas arose in a transgenic mouse line Tg(Tyr-SV40E)Mi1-13 that carried an integrated fusion gene containing the SV40 early region under the control of a tyrosinase promoter expressed in pigment cells.[49] The ocular melanomas in this model rapidly enlarged the globe, starting as early as 4 weeks of age. All mice examined had histologic evidence of neoplastic or preneoplastic lesions. Histologically, the melanomas were pleomorphic, with both epithelioid and spindle cells. The majority of tumors were predominately epithelioid and were positive for S-100 and HMB-45 reactivity. Premelanosomes or melanosomes were found frequently in the epithelioid cells and occasionally in the spindle variants, even in those without obvious pigmentation.

The majority of the melanomas in this model appear to originate in the retinal pigment epithelium (RPE), with a few arising in the choroid or at the interface of the RPE and choroid. Histogenetic origin from the RPE was shown by genetic ablation of choroidal melanocytes in this model.[50] Early preneoplastic hyperplasias with atypia were noted in the RPE associated with hypomelanotic or amelanotic areas. There is clear histopathologic evidence for a progression of RPE lesions in these transgenic mice. Local invasion and distal metastasis are common, with spread to lymph nodes, lung, bone, muscle, and brain. Notably, there were no liver metastases. These mice will prove useful for experimental studies of the etiology, progression, metastasis, and treatment of RPE melanomas.

Tumors of the Ciliary Body and Retinal Pigment Epithelium. A line of transgenic mice has been developed in which the c-Ha-rasT24 oncogene was placed behind the promoter I region of the murine γ-glutamyl transferase gene gGT.[51] Bilateral ocular neoplasms and proliferations arose in these mice, originating from the pigmented ciliary epithelium and RPE. The proliferative lesions showed a progression from hyperplasia through adenoma to adenocarcinoma. The lesions arise prenatally, with many mice having adenomas at birth. By day 27 postnatally, most mice had adenocarcinomas arising in the region of the ciliary body.

CONCLUSIONS

Expanding our understanding of the etiology, natural history, and progression of human ocular neoplastic disorders will require experimental studies in laboratory animal models. Although there are relatively few spontaneous or induced ocular tumor models in animals that provide a suitable eye for clinical documentation and manipulation, the future is bright for a whole new era in comparative oncology. Transgenic technology, with the specific targeting of genes by powerful molecular approaches, will enable the transfer of existing murine technology to large animal species. In this manner, new animal models will be created that specifically recapitulate relevant aspects of human neoplastic disorders.

REFERENCES

1. Knudson AG. Hereditary cancers: clues to mechanisms of carcinogenesis. *Br J Cancer* 59:661, 1989.
2. Folberg R. Tumor progression in ocular melanomas. *J Invest Dermatol* 100:326S, 1993.
3. Steinlein JW. Immune regulation and the eye: a dangerous compromise. *FASEB J* 1:199, 1987.
4. Barke CF, Billingham RE. Immunologically privileged sites. *Adv Immunol* 25:1, 1977.
5. Kaplan HJ, Streinlein JW. Immunologically privileged sites require a functioning spleen? *Nature* 251:553, 1974.
6. Niederkorn JY, Streilein JW, Shadduck JA. Deviant immune responses to allogeneic tumors injected intracamerally and subcutaneously in mice. *Invest Ophthalmol Vis Sci* 20:355, 1981.
7. Niederkorn JY, Streilein JW. Immunogenetic basis for immunologic privilege in the anterior chamber of the eye. *Immunogenetics* 13:227, 1981.
8. Niederkorn JY, Knisely TL. Immunologic analysis of a destructive pattern of intraocular tumor resolution. *Curr Eye Res* 7:515, 1988.
9. Knisely TL, Luckenbach MW, Fischer BJ, Niederkorn JY. Destructive and nondestructive patterns of immune rejection of syngeneic intraocular tumors. *J Immunol* 138:4515, 1987.
10. Knisely TL, Niederkorn JY. Emergence of a dominant, cytotoxic T lymphocyte antitumor effector from tumor-infiltrating cells in the anterior chamber of the eye. *Cancer Immunol Immunother* 30:323, 1990.
11. Albert DM, Shadduck JA, Liu H, Sunderman FW, Wagoner MD, Dohlman HG, Papale J. Animal models for the study of uveal melanoma. *Int Ophthalmol Clin* 20:143, 1980.
12. Romer TJ, Van Delft JL, De Wolff-Rouendaal D, Jager MJ. Hamster Greene melanoma implanted in the anterior chamber of the rabbit eye: a reliable tumor model? *Ophthalmic Res* 24:119, 1992.
13. Sanborn G, Niederkorn JY, Kan-Mitchell J, Albert D. Prevention of metastasis of intraocular melanomas in mice treated with difluoromethylornithine. *Graefes Arch Clin Exp Ophthalmol* 230:72, 1992.
14. Poste G, Fidler IJ. The pathogenesis of cancer metastasis. *Nature* 283:139, 1980.
15. Niederkorn JY, Mellon J, Pidherney M, Mayhew E, Anand R. Effect of antibodies on the metastatic spread of intraocular melanomas in a nude mouse model of human uveal melanoma. *Curr Eye Res* 12:47, 1993.
16. Niederkorn JY. Enucleation and consort with immunologic impairment promotes metastasis of intraocular melanomas in mice. *Invest Ophthalmol Vis Sci* 25:1080, 1984.
17. Burns RP, Tidwell N. Experimental ocular malignant melanoma in Sinclair swine. *Curr Eye Res* 5:257, 1986.
18. Feeney-Burns L, Burns RP, Gao CL. Ocular pathology in melanomatous Sinclair miniature swine. *Am J Pathol* 131:62, 1988.
19. Rock JA, Prendergast RA, Bobbie D, Green WR, Parmley TH, Dubin NH. Intraocular endometrium in the rabbit as a model for endometriosis. *Fertil Steril* 59:232, 1993.
20. Nilsson O, Bilchik AJ, Adrian TE, Modlin IM. Intraocular transplantation of carcinoid tumors from mastomys and humans. *J Pathol* 160:347, 1990.
21. White L, Zirth BC, Benedict WF. Evaluation of response to chemotherapy in retinoblastoma heterotransplanted to eyes of nude mice. *Cancer Chemother Pharmacol* 23:63, 1989.
22. Kobayashi S, Mukai N. Retinoblastoma-like tumors induced in rats by human adenovirus. *Invest Ophthalmol Vis Sci* 12:853, 1973.
23. Kobayashi S, Mukai N. Retinoblastoma-like tumors induced by human adenovirus type 12 in rats. *Cancer Res* 34:1646, 1974.
24. Mukai N, Kobayashi S, Oguri M. Ultrastructural studies of human adenovirus-produced retinoblastoma-like neoplasms in Sprague-Dawley rats. *Invest Ophthalmol Vis Sci* 13:593, 1974.

25. Kobayashi S, Mukai N, Solish SP, Pomeroy ME. A highly predictable animal model of retinoblastoma. *Acta Neuropathol (Berl)* 57:203, 1982.

26. Winther J. In vitro and in vivo growth of an intraocular retinoblastoma-like tumor in F-344 rats. *Acta Ophthalmol (Copenh)* 64:657, 1986.

27. Ohashi T, ZuRhein GM, Varakis JN, Padgett BL, Walker DL. Experimental (JC virus-induced) intraocular and extraocular orbital tumors in the Syrian hamster. *J Neuropathol Exp Neurol* 37:667, 1978.

28. Mukai N, Nakajima T, Freddo T, Jacobson M, Dunn M. Retinoblastoma-like neoplasm induced in C3H/BifB/Ki strain mice by human adenovirus serotype 12. *Acta Neuropathol (Berl)* 39:147, 1977.

29. Albert DM, Shadduck JA, Craft JL, Niederkorn JY. Feline uveal melanoma model induced with feline sarcoma virus. *Invest Ophthalmol Vis Sci* 20:606, 1981.

30. Shadduck JA, Albert DM, Niederkorn JY. Feline uveal melanomas induced with feline sarcoma virus: potential model of the human counterpart. *J Natl Cancer Inst* 67:619, 1981.

31. Albert DM, Gonder JR, Papale J, Craft JL, Dohlman HG, Reid MC, Sunderman FW. Induction of ocular neoplasms in Fischer rats by intraocular injection of nickel subsulfide. *Invest Ophthalmol Vis Sci* 22:768, 1982.

32. Yoshitomi K, Everitt JI, Boorman GA. Primary optic nerve meningiomas in F344 rats. *Vet Pathol* 28:79, 1991.

33. Everitt JI, Shadduck JA. Retinoblastoma, experimental rat and hamster. In: Jones TC, Mohr U, Hunt RD, eds. *ILSI Monogr Lab Anim Pathol Spec Senses.* Berlin: Springer-Verlag, 1991:114–115.

34. Kendry G, Roe FJC. Melanotic lesions of the eye in August hooded rats induced by urethan or *N*-hydroxyurethan given during the neonatal period: a histopathological study. *J Natl Cancer Inst* 43:749, 1969.

35. Evgen'eva TP. Pigmented tumors in rats induced by introduction of platinum and cellophane films into the chamber of the eye. *Bull Exp Biol Med* 14:1296, 1972.

36. Okamoto M. Induction of ocular tumor by nickel subsulfide in the Japanese common newt, *Cynops pyrrrhogaster. Cancer Res* 47:5213, 1987.

37. Folberg R, Baron J, Reeves RD, Stevens RH, Tse DT. Primary melanocytic lesions of the rabbit choroid following topical application of 7,12-dimethylbenz(*a*)-anthracene: preliminary observations. *J Toxicol Cutan Ocul Toxicol* 9:313, 1990.

38. Pe'er J, Folberg R, Massicotte SJ, Baron J, Ginderdeuren RP, Zimmerman B, Meyer ML, Worsey H. Clinicopathologic spectrum of primary uveal melanocytic lesions in an animal model. *Ophthalmology* 99:977, 1992.

39. Pawloski A, Lea PJ. Nevi and melanoma induced by chemical carcinogens in laboratory animals: similarities and differences with human lesions. *J Cutan Pathol* 10:81, 1983.

40. Folberg R, Baron J, Reeves RD, Stevens RH, Bogh LD. Animal model of conjunctival primary acquired melanosis. *Ophthalmology* 96:1006, 1989.

41. Ley RD, Applegate LA, Fry RJM, Sanchez AB. Photoreactivation of ultraviolet radiation-induced skin and eye tumors of *Monodelphis domestica. Cancer Res* 51:6539, 1991.

42. Yoshitomi K, Boorman GA. The eye and associated glands. In: Boorman G, Eustis S, Elwell M, MacKenzie W, eds. *Pathology of the Fischer Rat.* New York: Academic, 1990:259.

43. Ostrander GK, Shim JK, Hawkins WE, Walker WW. A vertebrate model for investigation of retinoblastoma. *Proc Am Assoc Cancer Res* 33:109, 1992.

44. Windle JJ, Albert DM, O'Brien JM, Marcus DM, Disteche CM, Bernards R, Mellon PM. Retinoblastoma in transgenic mice. *Nature* 243:665, 1990.

45. Kivela T, Virtanen I, Marcus DM, O'Brien JM, Carpenter JL, Brauner E, Tarkkanene A, Albert DM. Neuronal and glial properties of a murine transgenic retinoblastoma model. *Am J Pathol* 138:1135, 1991.

46. Mahon KA, Chepelinsky AB, Khillian JS, Overbeck PA, Piatigorsky J, Westphal H. Oncogenesis of the lens in transgenic mice. *Science* 235:1622, 1984.

47. Nakamura T, Mahon KA, Miskin R, Dey A, Kuwabara T, Westphal H. Differentiation and oncogenesis: phenotypically distinct lens tumors in transgenic mice. *New Biol* 1:193, 1989.

48. Griep AE, Westphal H. Differentiation versus proliferation of transgenic mouse lens cells expressing polyoma large T antigen: evidence for regulation by an endogenous growth factor. *New Biol* 2:727, 1990.

49. Bradl M, Klein-Szanto A, Porter S, Mintz B. Malignant melanoma in transgenic mice. *Proc Natl Acad Sci USA* 88:164, 1991.

50. Mintz B, Klein-Szanto AJP. Malignancy of eye melanomas originating in the retinal pigment epithelium of transgenic mice after genetic ablation of choroidal melanocytes. *Proc Natl Acad Sci USA* 89:11, 421, 1992.

51. Chevaz-Barrios P, Schaffner DL, Barrios R, Overbeek PA, Lebovitz RM, Lieberman MW. Expression of the rasT24 oncogene in the ciliary pigment epithelium and retinal pigment epithelium results in hyperplasia, adenoma, and adenocarcinoma. *Am J Pathol* 143:20, 1993.

I N D E X

ISBN 0-8138-2388-9

90000